Silver, Kempe, Bruyn & Fulginiti's
Handbook of
Pediatrics

Silver, Kempe, Bruyn & Fulginiti's

Handbook of Pediatrics

SIXTEENTH EDITION

GERALD B. MERENSTEIN, MD, FAAP

Professor
Department of Pediatrics
University of Colorado Health Sciences Center:
   The Children's Hospital
Denver, Colorado

DAVID W. KAPLAN, MD, MPH

Associate Professor
Head, Adolescent Medicine
Department of Pediatrics
University of Colorado Health Sciences Center:
   The Children's Hospital
Denver, Colorado

ADAM A. ROSENBERG, MD

Associate Professor
Department of Pediatrics
University of Colorado Health Sciences Center:
   The Children's Hospital
Denver, Colorado

APPLETON & LANGE
Norwalk, Connecticut/San Mateo, California

0-8385-3639-5

Copyright © 1991 by Appleton & Lange
A Publishing Division of Prentice Hall
Copyright © 1987 by Appleton & Lange

91 92 93 94 95 / 10 9 8 7 6 5 4 3 2 1

Prentice Hall International (UK) Limited, *London*
Prentice Hall of Australia Pty. Limited, *Sydney*
Prentice Hall Canada, Inc., *Toronto*
Prentice Hall Hispanoamericana, S.A., *Mexico*
Prentice Hall of India Private Limited, *New Delhi*
Prentice Hall of Japan, Inc., *Tokyo*
Simon & Schuster Asia Pte. Ltd., *Singapore*
Editora Prentice Hall do Brasil Ltda., *Rio de Janeiro*
Prentice Hall, *Englewood Cliffs, New Jersey*

ISBN 0-8385-3639-5
ISSN 0440-1921

PRINTED IN THE UNITED STATES OF AMERICA

Table of Contents

The Authors

Steven H. Abman, MD
Assistant Professor, Department of Pediatrics, University of Colorado
Health Sciences Center: The Children's Hospital, Denver.

Mark J. Abzug, MD
Assistant Professor, Department of Pediatrics, University of Colorado
Health Sciences Center: The Children's Hospital, Denver.

Roger M. Barkin, MD
Chairman, Department of Pediatrics, Rose Medical Center; Professor
of Surgery, University of Colorado Health Sciences Center, Denver.

Stephen Berman, MD
Associate Professor, Department of Pediatrics, University of Colorado
Health Sciences Center: The Children's Hospital, Denver.

David W. Boyle, MD
Assistant Professor, Department of Pediatrics, University of Indiana
School of Medicine, Indianapolis.

David Burgess, MD
Assisant Professor, Department of Pediatrics, University of
Colorado Health Sciences Center: The Children's Hospital, Denver.

Nancy Cohen Carlson, MD
Assistant Professor, Department of Pediatrics, University of Colorado
Health Sciences Center: The Children's Hospital, Denver.

Michael R. Clemmons, MD
Assistant Professor, Department of Pediatrics, University of Colorado
Health Sciences Center: The Children's Hospital, Denver.

Mark A. Colloton, MS, PA-C
Assistant Professor, Department of Pediatrics, University of Colorado
Health Sciences Center: The Children's Hospital, Denver.

Robert E. Eilert, MD
Chairman, Department of Orthopedic Surgery, The Children's Hospital; Assistant Clinical Professor, Department of Orthopedics, University of Colorado Health Sciences Center, Denver.

Philip P. Ellis, MD
Professor and Chairman, Department of Ophthalmology, University of
Colorado Health Sciences Center, Denver.

Benjamin A. Gitterman, MD
Associate Professor, Department of Pediatrics, University of Colorado Health Sciences Center; Director, Pediatric Clinic, Denver General Hospital.

Ronald W. Gotlin, MD
Associate Professor, Department of Pediatrics, and Head, Section of Endocrinology, University of Colorado Health Sciences Center: The Children's Hospital, Denver

K. Michael Hambidge, MD, ScD
Professor, Department of Pediatrics, University of Colorado Health Sciences Center: The Children's Hospital, Denver.

Taru Hays, MD
Associate Professor, Department of Pediatrics, University of Colorado Health Sciences Center: The Children's Hospital, Denver.

Brenda L. Huffman, MD
Formerly Chief Resident and Instructor in Pediatrics, Department of Pediatrics, University of Colorado Health Sciences Center: The Children's Hospital, Denver.

David W. Kaplan, MD, MPH
Associate Professor, Department of Pediatrics, and Head, Adolescent Medicine, University of Colorado Health Sciences Center: The Children's Hospital, Denver.

Ruth S. Kempe, MD
Associate Professor of Psychiatry and Pediatrics, University of Colorado Health Sciences Center, Denver.

Jay Kincannon, MD
Dermatology Resident, Department of Dermatology, University of Colorado Health Sciences Center, Denver.

Gary M. Lum, MD
Associate Professor, Department of Pediatrics, and Head, Section of Nephrology, University of Colorado Health Sciences Center: The Children's Hospital, Denver.

Kathleen A. Mammel, MD
Assistant Professor, Department of Pediatrics, University of Colorado Health Sciences Center: The Children's Hospital, Denver.

Gerald B. Merenstein, MD, FAAP
Professor, Department of Pediatrics, University of Colorado Health Sciences Center: The Children's Hospital, Denver.

Paul G. Moe, MD
Professor of Pediatrics and Neurology, Department of Pediatrics, University of Colorado Health Sciences Center: The Children's Hospital, Denver.

John W. Ogle, MD
Assistant Professor and Director, Child Health Associate Program, Department of Pediatrics, University of Colorado Health Sciences Center: The Children's Hospital, Denver.

W. Davis Parker, Jr., MD
Associate Professor, Department of Pediatrics, University of Colorado Health Sciences Center: The Children's Hospital, Denver.

David S. Pearlman, MD
Clinical Professor, Department of Pediatrics, University of Colorado Health Sciences Center; Senior Staff Physician, Pediatrics, National Jewish Center for Immunology and Respiratory Medicine, Denver.

Lee Ann Pearse, MD
Assistant Professor of Clinical Pediatrics, Department of Pediatrics, University of Miami School of Medicine, Miami, Florida.

Adam A. Rosenberg, MD
Associate Preofessor, Department of Pediatrics, University of Colorado Health Sciences Center: The Children's Hospital, Denver.

Barry H. Rumack, MD
Professor, Department of Pediatrics, and Head, Section of Clinical Pharmacology and Toxicology, University of Colorado Health Sciences Center; Director, Rocky Mountain Poison & Drug Center, Denver.

Robert F. St. Peter, MD
Robert Wood Johnson Clinical Scholar, University of California at San Francisco/ Stanford University, San Francisco.

Michael S. Schaffer, MD
Associate Professor, Department of Pediatrics, University of Colorado Health Sciences Center: The Children's Hospital, Denver.

Barton D. Schmitt, MD
Professor, Department of Pediatrics, University of Colorado Health Sciences Center: The Children's Hospital, Denver.

Alan R. Seay, MD
Associate Professor of Pediatrics and Neurology and Head, Section of Child Neurology, Department of Pediatrics, University of Colorado Health Sciences Center: The Children's Hospital, Denver.

Judith M. Sondheimer, MD
Associate Professor and Head, Section of Gastroenterology and Nutrition, Department of Pediatrics, University of Colorado Health Sciences Center: the Children's Hospital, Denver.

Steven B. Spedale, MD
Instructor in Pediatrics and Fellow in Neonatology, Department of Pediatrics, University of Colorado Health Sciences Center: The Children's Hospital, Denver.

David G. Spoerke, MS, RPh

Dale William Steele, BA, MD
Formerly Instructor and Chief Resident, Department of Pediatrics, University of Colorado Health Sciences Center: The Children's Hospital, Denver.

Linda C. Stork, MD
Assistant Professor, Department of Pediatrics, University of Colorado Health Sciences Center: The Children's Hospital, Denver.

Elaine Van Gundy, MD
Department of Pediatrics, National Jewish Hospital, Denver.

William L. Weston, MD
Professor of Dermatology and Pediatrics and Chairman, Department of Dermatology, University of Colorado Health Sciences Center: The Children's Hospital, Denver.

Mary Zavadel, MD
Formerly Chief Resident and Instructor, Department of Pediatrics, University of Colorado Health Sciences Center: The Children's Hospital, Denver.

Preface

Handbook of Pediatrics offers a convenient, up-to-date source of practical information on the care of children from infancy through adolescence. Focusing on the clinical aspects of pediatric care, the sixteenth edition covers a wide range of topics, including development and growth of the healthy child, ambulatory care, preventive medicine, and diagnosis and treatment of common pediatric disorders. Pertinent physiologic and pharmacologic principles support the wealth of clinical information.

Audience

Handbook of Pediatrics serves the needs of all health professionals involved in the day-to-day care of pediatric patients. **Medical students and house officers** working in hospitals or ambulatory care facilities will appreciate the concise descriptions of diseases and the accessibility of information. **Nurses and practicing physicians,** particularly those in primary care, will find the Handbook a ready reference for a broad spectrum of information; chapters are included on dermatology, cardiology, otolaryngology, and other relevant pediatric subspecialties.

New to This Edition

The sixteenth edition of *Handbook of Pediatrics* represents a major revision and reorganization of this classic. Reflecting the original intent of Drs. Silver, Kempe, Bruyn and Fulginiti, the book provides an up-to-date digest of pediatric information. The new team of editors and contributors has revised, reorganized, and updated the book to enhance its usefulness in today's practice. The latest medical advances and therapeutic recommendations are included, with increased emphasis on ambulatory care, cost effectiveness, and sensitivity and specificity of diagnostic tests.

More than half of the 32 chapters are totally new; many others have major revisions. Many new tables and illustrations have been added to increase the accessibility of information.

New chapters included the following:
- Ambulatory Pediatrics
- Fluid & Electrolyte Disorders
- Drug Therapy
- The Newborn Infant: Assessment & General Care
- The Newborn Infant: Diseases & Disorders

- Adolescence
- Poisons & Toxins
- Immunization Procedures, Vaccines, Antisera, & Skin Tests
- Heart
- Respiratory Tract
- Allergic Diseases

Continuing Features

- Normal values of blood chemistry, urine, bone marrow, peripheral blood, feces, sweat, and cerebrospinal fluid.
- Descriptions of the most commonly used laboratory tests.
- Index to Pediatric Emergencies on the inside front cover.

Acknowledgements

We wish to thank the authors who contributed to this edition and all those whose work on previous editions has carried over to this one, particularly Drs. Silver, Kempe, Bruyn and Fulginiti.

We wish to express our gratitude to our readers throughout the world who have provided us with helpful suggestions. Comments and suggestions for future editions can be sent to us in care of Appleton & Lange, 2755 Campus Drive, Suite 205, San Mateo, CA 94403.

Gerald B. Merenstein
David W. Kaplan
Adam A. Rosenberg

Denver, Colorado
January, 1991

NOTICE

Not all of the drugs mentioned in this book have been approved by FDA for use in infants or in children under age 6 or age 12. Such drugs should not be used if effective alternatives are available; they may be used if no effective alternatives are available or if the known risk of toxicity of alternative drugs or the risk of nontreatment is outweighed by the probable advantages of treatment.

Because of the possibility of an error in the article or book from which a particular drug dosage is obtained, or an error appearing in the text of this book, our readers are urged to consult appropriate references, including the manufacturer's package insert, especially when prescribing new drugs or those with which they are not adequately familiar.

—The Authors

Pediatric History & Physical Examination | 1

Benjamin A. Gitterman, MD

HISTORY

For many pediatric problems, the history is the single most important factor in arriving at a correct diagnosis. The physician's interaction with the patient and the parents during the history-taking process is also the first stage in the psychotherapeutic management of the patient. Socioeconomic, cultural, and educational factors may influence the caregiver–patient communication process. Assurance of confidentiality should be part of the process.

The outline in Figure 1–1 should be modified and adapted as appropriate for the age of the child and the reason for the consultation.

Source of History and Reason for Referral

The history and reason for the consultation should be obtained from the parent or whoever is responsible for the care of the child. Much valuable information can also be obtained from the child. Adolescents should be interviewed alone when possible; they may be uncomfortable discussing sensitive information in the presence of their parents.

Identifying Information

Name, address, and telephone number; sex; date and place of birth; race, religion and nationality; referred by whom; father's and mother's names, occupations, and business telephone numbers.

Chief Complaint (CC)

Patient's or informant's own brief account of the complaint and its duration.

Source of history and reason for referral	Operations
Identifying information	Accidents and injuries
Chief complaint	Medications
History of present illness	Family history
Birth history	Personal history
Development	Social history
Nutrition	Habits
Illnesses	Review of systems
Immunizations and tests	

Figure 1–1. Taking a pediatric history.

History of Present Illness (HPI)

(1) When was the patient last entirely well?

(2) How and when did the condition begin?

(3) Progress of disease; order and date of onset of new symptoms.

(4) Specific symptoms and physical signs that may have developed.

(5) Pertinent negative data obtained by direct questioning.

(6) Aggravating and alleviating factors.

(7) Significant medical attention and medications given, and over what period of time.

(8) In acute infections, statement of type and degree of exposure, and interval since exposure.

(9) For the well child, factors of significance and general condition since last visit.

(10) Examiner's opinion about the reliability of the informant.

Birth History

A. Antenatal: Health of mother during pregnancy, prenatal care, diet, infections (eg, rubella) and other illnesses, vomiting, bleeding, preeclampsia-eclampsia and other complications, Rh typing and serologic tests, pelvimetry, medications, x-ray procedures, amniocentesis.

B. Natal: Duration of pregnancy, kind and duration of labor, type of delivery, sedation and anesthesia (if known), birth weight, state of infant at birth, resuscitation required, onset of respiration, first cry, special procedures.

C. Neonatal: Apgar score, color (cyanosis, pallor, jaundice), cry, twitching, excessive mucus, paralysis, convulsions, fever, hemorrhage, congenital abnormalities, birth injury. Difficulty in sucking, rashes, feeding difficulties. Length of hospital stay, discharge weight.

Development

(1) Milestones: age when first raised head, rolled over, sat alone, pulled up, walked with help, walked alone, talked (meaningful words, sentences). (See Chapter 2.)

(2) Urinary continence during night; during day.

(3) Control of defecation.

(4) Comparison of development with that of siblings and parents.

(5) Any period of failure to grow or unusual growth.

(6) School grade, quality of work.

Nutrition

A. Breast or Formula Feeding: Type, duration, major formula changes, time of weaning, difficulties.

B. Supplements: Vitamins (type, amount, duration), iron, fluoride.

C. Solid Foods: When introduced, how taken, types, unusual family dietary habits (vegetarian, etc), balancing of food groups.

D. Appetite: Food likes and dislikes, idiosyncrasies, allergies, attitude of child to eating.

Illnesses

A. Hospitalizations.

B. Infections: Age, types, number, severity.

C. Contagious Diseases: Age, measles, rubella, chickenpox, mumps, pertussis, diphtheria, scarlet fever. Complications of any of above.

D. Other Serious Noninfectious Illnesses.

Immunizations & Tests

Indicate type, number, reactions, age of child.

A. Inoculations: Diphtheria, tetanus, pertussis, measles, rubella, mumps, *Haemophilus influenzae,* others.

B. Oral Immunizations: Poliomyelitis.

C. Serum Injections: Passive immunizations.

D. Tests: Tuberculin, serology, others.

Operations

Type, age, complications; reasons for operations; apparent response of child.

Accidents & Injuries

Nature, severity, sequelae.

Medications

Chronic use of medications; allergies to medications.

Family History

(1) Father and mother (age and condition of health).

(2) Siblings (age, condition of health, significant previous illnesses and problems).

(3) Stillbirths, miscarriages, abortions; age at death and cause of death of members of immediate family.

(4) Tuberculosis, allergy, blood dyscrasias, mental or nervous diseases, diabetes, cardiovascular diseases, kidney diseases, hypertension, rheumatic fever, neoplastic diseases, congenital abnormalities, convulsive disorders, others.

(5) Health of contacts.

Personal History

A. Relations with Other Children: Independent or clinging to mother; negativistic, shy, submissive; separation from parents; hobbies; easy or difficult to get along with. How is child similar to or different from siblings? How does child relate to others?

B. School Progress: Preschool activity (child care, Head Start, preschool, etc), academic performance, special aptitudes or problems, reaction to school.

Social History

A. Family Structure: Adults in the home and their relationship to child; stability of family situation; sources of income; home (size, number of rooms, living conditions, sleeping facilities), type of neighborhood, access to play facilities. Who cares for child if both parents work outside of home?

B. Family Support Systems: Relatives nearby or close friends to provide support and give parents "time off."

C. Child care arrangements and satisfaction.

D. School: Public or private, students per classroom, satisfaction with school.

E. Insurance: Type of medical coverage, if any.

Habits

A. Sleeping: Hours, disturbances, snoring, restlessness, dreaming, nightmares.

B. Recreation: Exercise and play.

C. Elimination: Urinary, bowel.

D. Behavioral Concerns: Excessive bed-wetting, masturbation, thumb-sucking, nail-biting, breath-holding, temper tantrums, tics, nervousness, undue thirst, others. Similar disturbances among members of family, School problems (learning, perceptual).

E. Adolescent Habits: Smoking, alcohol or substance abuse, sexual activity, use of birth control, knowledge regarding STDs. These questions need not be asked immediately but should be routine if appropriate to the patient's age.

F. Dental Hygiene: Self-care habits (brushing, flossing), most recent preventive check.

G. Safety: Use of infant or child restraining devices in automobiles, careful storage of medicines and toxic substances, covering of electrical outlets, other (age-appropriate) safety measures.

H. Family Health Habits as Models: Smoking, alcohol, exercise, safety, diet.

Review of Systems

A. General Review: Unusual weight gain or loss, fatigue, fevers, pattern of growth, recent behavioral changes.

B. Skin: Rashes, lumps, itching, dryness, color changes, changes in hair or nails, easy bruising.

C. Eyes: Vision, last eye examination, glasses or contact lenses, pain, redness, excessive tearing, double vision.

D. Ears, Nose, and Throat: Frequent colds, sore throat, sneezing, stuffy nose, nasal discharge or postnasal drip, mouth breathing, snoring, otitis, hearing, adenitis, allergies.

E. Dental: Age at eruption of deciduous and permanent teeth; bleeding gums, condition of teeth, other concerns.

F. Cardiorespiratory System: Frequency and nature of disturbances. Dyspnea, chest pain, cough, sputum, wheezing, history of pneumonia, cyanosis, syncope, tachycardia.

G. Gastrointestinal System: Swallowing problems, spitting, vomiting, diarrhea, constipation, type of stools, abdominal pain or discomfort, jaundice, changes in bowel movements, blood in stools.

H. Genitourinary System: Enuresis, dysuria, frequency, polyuria, pyuria, hematuria, character of stream, vaginal discharge, menstrual history, bladder control, abnormalities of genitalia.

I. Neuromuscular System: Headache, nervousness, dizziness, tingling, convulsions, habit spasms, ataxia, muscle or joint pains, postural deformities, exercise tolerance, gait. Screening for scoliosis.

J. Endocrine System: Disturbances of growth, excessive fluid intake, polyphagia, goiter, thyroid disease, age of onset of pubertal changes.

PHYSICAL EXAMINATION

Every child should have a complete systematic examination at regular intervals (Fig 1–2). The examination should not be restricted to those portions of the body considered to be involved on the basis of the presenting complaint.

Vital signs	Neck
General appearance	Thorax
Skin	Lungs
Lymph nodes	Heart
Head	Abdomen
Face	Male and female genitalia
Eyes	Rectum and Anus
Nose	Extremities
Mouth	Spine and Back
Throat	Neurologic examination
Ears	Developmental assessment

Figure 1–2. The physical examination.

Approaching the Child

Adequate time should be allowed for the child and the examiner to become acquainted. The child should be treated as an individual whose feelings and sensibilities are well developed, and the examiner's conduct should be appropriate to the age of the child. A friendly manner, quiet voice, and slow and easy approach will help to facilitate the examination. If the examiner is not able to establish a friendly relationship but feels that it is important to proceed with the examination, this should be done in an orderly, systematic manner in the hope that the child will then accept the inevitable.

The examiner's hands should be washed in warm water before the examination begins and should be warm.

Observing the Child

Although the very young child may not be able to speak, much information can be obtained by an observant and receptive examiner. The total evaluation of the child should include impressions obtained from the time the child first enters the room; it should not be based solely on the period during which the patient is on the examining table. This is also the best time to assess the interaction between parent and child; the examiner's impressions should be recorded.

In general, more information is obtained by careful inspection than by any other method of examination.

Holding the Child for Examination

Much of the examination can be performed while the child is held in the parent's lap or over the parent's shoulder. Certain parts of the examination can sometimes be done more easily with the child prone or held against the parent so that the examiner cannot be seen.

Removal of Clothing

Clothes should removed gradually to prevent chilling and to avoid resistance from a shy child. To save time and to avoid creating unpleasant associations with the caregiver in the child's mind, undressing the child and taking the temperature are best performed by the parent. The marked degree of modesty that some children exhibit should be respected.

Sequence of Examination

In most cases, it is best to begin the examination of the young child with an area that is least likely to be associated with pain or discomfort. The ears and throat should usually be exam ined last. The examiner should develop a regular sequence of examination that can be adapted to each child as required by special circumstances.

Painful Procedures

Before performing a disagreeable, painful, or upsetting examination, the examiner should tell the child (1) what is likely to happen and how the child can assist, (2) that the examination is necessary, and (3) that it will be performed as rapidly and as painlessly as possible.

Vital Signs

Record temperature, pulse rate, and respiratory rate (TPR); blood pressure (see Chapter 19); weight; and height. The weight should be recorded at each visit; the height should be determined at monthly intervals during the first year, at 3-month intervals during the second year, and twice a year thereafter. The height, weight, and head circumference of the child should be compared with standard charts and the approximate percentiles recorded. Multiple measurements at intervals are of more value than single ones, since they give information regarding the pattern of growth. The blood pressure should also be compared with standard percentiles. During the first years of life, the temperature should be taken by rectum (except for routine temperatures of the premature infant and infants under age 1 month, when axillary temperatures are sufficiently accurate).

General Appearance

Does the child appear well or ill? Degree of prostration; degree of cooperation; state of comfort, nutrition, and consciousness; abnormalities; gait, posture, and coordination; estimate of intelligence; reaction to parents, physician, and examination; nature of cry and degree of activity; facies and facial expression.

Skin

Color (cyanosis, jaundice, pallor, erythema), texture, eruptions, hydration, edema, hemorrhagic manifestations, scars, dilated vessels and direction of blood flow, hemangiomas, café au lait areas and nevi, mongolian spots, pigmentation, turgor, elasticity, subcutaneous nodules, sensitivity, hair distribution, character, desquamation, capillary refill.

Practical notes:

(1) Loss of turgor, especially of the calf muscles and skin over the abdomen, is evidence of dehydration.

(2) The soles and palms are often bluish and cold in early infancy; this finding is of no significance.

(3) The degree of anemia cannot be determined reliably by inspection, since pallor (even in the newborn) may be normal and not due to anemia.

(4) To demonstrate pitting edema in a child, it may be necessary to exert prolonged pressure.

(5) A few small pigmented nevi are commonly found, particularly in older children.

(6) Spider nevi occur in about one-sixth of children under age 5 years and almost half of older children.

(7) "Mongolian spots" (large, flat, black or blue-black areas) are frequently present over the lower back and buttocks; they have no pathologic significance.

(8) Cyanosis will not be evident unless at least 5 g of reduced hemoglobin is present; therefore, it develops less easily in an anemic child.

(9) Carotenemia is usually most prominent over the palms and soles and around the nose and spares the conjunctiva.

(10) Striae and wrinkling may indicate rapid weight gain or loss.

Lymph Nodes

Location, size, sensitivity, mobility, consistency. One should routinely attempt to palpate suboccipital, preauricular, anterior cervical, posterior cervical, submaxillary, sublingual, axillary, epitrochlear, and inguinal lymph nodes.

Practical notes:

(1) Enlargement of the lymph nodes occurs much more readily in children than in adults.

(2) Small inguinal lymph nodes are palpable in almost all healthy young children. Small, mobile, nontender shotty nodes are commonly found as residua of previous infection.

Head

Size, shape, circumference, asymmetry, cephalhematoma, bossae, craniotabes, control, molding, bruits, fontanelles (size, tension, number, abnormally late or early closure), sutures, dilated veins, scalp, hair (texture, distribution, parasites), face, transillumination.

Practical notes:

(1) The head is measured at its greatest circumference; this is usually at the mid forehead anteriorly and around to the most prominent portion of the occiput posteriorly. The ratio of he

circumference to circumference of the chest or abdomen is usually of little value.

(2) Fontanelle tension is best determined with the child quiet and in the sitting position.

(3) Slight pulsations over the anterior fontanelle may occur in normal infants.

(4) Although bruits may be heard over the temporal areas in normal children, the possibility of an existing abnormality should be ruled out.

(5) Craniotabes may be found in normal newborn infants (especially premature infants) and for the first 2–4 months of life.

(6) A positive Macewen sign ("cracked pot" sound when skull is percussed with one finger) may be present normally as long as the fontanelle is open.

(7) Transillumination of the skull can be performed by means of a flashlight with a sponge rubber collar so that it fits tightly when held against the head.

Face

Symmetry, paralysis, distance between nose and mouth, depth of nasolabial folds, bridge of nose, distribution of hair, size of mandible, swellings, hypertelorism, Chvostek's sign, tenderness over sinuses.

Eyes

Photophobia; visual acuity; muscular control and conjugate gaze; nystagmus; mongolian slant; Brushfield's spots; epicanthic folds; lacrimation; discharge; lids; exophthalmos or enophthalmos; conjunctiva; pupillary size, shape, and reaction to light and accommodation; color of iris; media (corneal opacities, cataracts); fundi; visual fields (in older children).

Practical notes:

(1) Newborn infants usually will open their eyes if placed prone, supported with one hand on the abdomen, and lifted over the examiner's head.

(2) Not infrequently, one pupil is normally larger than the other. This sometimes occurs only in bright or subdued light.

(3) Examination of the fundi should be part of every complete physical examination.

(4) Dilation of the pupils may be necessary for adequate visualization of the eyes.

(5) A mild degree of strabismus may be present during the first 6 months of life but should be considered abnormal after that time.

(6) To test for strabismus in a very young or uncooperative

child, note where a distant source of light is reflected from the surface of the eyes; the reflection should be present on corresponding portions of the 2 eyes.

(7) Small areas of capillary dilatation are commonly seen on the eyelids of normal newborn infants.

(8) Most infants produce visible tears during the first few days of life.

Nose

Exterior, shape, mucosa, patency, discharge, bleeding, pressure over sinuses, flaring of nostrils, septum.

Mouth

Lips (thinness, downturning, fissures, color, cleft), teeth (number, position, caries, mottling, discoloration, notching, malocclusion or malalignment), mucosa (color, redness of Stensen's duct, enanthems, Bohn's nodules, Epstein's pearls), gums, palate, tongue, uvula, mouth breathing, geographic tongue (usually normal).

Practical note: If the tongue can be extended as far as the alveolar ridge, there will be no interference with nursing or speaking. Frenectomy is not a preventive measure for being "tongue-tied."

Throat

Tonsils (size, inflammation, exudate, crypts, inflammation of the anterior pillars), epiglottis, mucosa, hypertrophic lymphoid tissue, postnasal drip, voice (hoarseness, stridor, grunting, type of cry), speech).

Practical notes:

(1) Before examining a child's throat, it is advisable to examine the mouth. Permit the child to handle the tongue blade, nasal speculum, and flashlight in order to overcome fear of the instruments. Then ask the child to stick out the tongue and say "Ah," louder and louder. In some cases, this may allow an adequate examination. In others, a child who is cooperative enough may be asked to "pant like a puppy"; while this is being done, the tongue blade is applied firmly to the rear of the tongue. Gagging need not be elicited in order to obtain a satisfactory examination. In still other cases, it may be expedient to examine one side of the tongue at a time, pushing the base of the tongue first to one side and then to the other. This may be less unpleasant and is less apt to cause gagging.

(2) Young children may have to be restrained to obtain a

adequate examination of the throat. Eliciting a gag reflex may be necessary if the oropharynx is to be adequately seen.

(3) The small child's head may be restrained satisfactorily by the parent's hands placed at the level of the child's elbows while the arms are held firmly against the sides of the child's head.

(4) A child who can sit up can be held on the parent's lap, back against the parent's chest. The child's left hand is held in the parent's left, the right hand in the right, and the hands are placed against the child's groin or lower thighs to prevent slipping. If the throat is to be examined in natural light, the parent faces the light. If artificial light and a head mirror are used, the light should be behind the parent. In either case, the physician uses one hand to hold the head in position and the other to manipulate the tongue blade.

(5) Young children seldom complain of sore throat even in the presence of significant infection of the pharynx and tonsils.

Ears

Pinnas (position, size), canals, tympanic membranes (landmarks, mobility, perforation, inflammation, discharge), mastoid tenderness and swelling, hearing.

Practical notes:

(1) A test for hearing is an important part of the physical examination of every infant and child. If a parent says that the child does not hear well, this must be investigated until disproved.

(2) The ears of all sick children should be examined.

(3) When actually examining the ears, it is often helpful to place the speculum just within the canal, remove it and place it lightly in the other ear, remove it again, and proceed in this way from one ear to the other, gradually going farther and farther, until a satisfactory examination is completed.

(4) In examining the ears, use as large a speculum as possible and insert it no farther than necessary, both to avoid discomfort and to avoid pushing wax in front of the speculum so that it obscures the field. The otoscope should be held balanced in the hand by holding the handle at the end nearest the speculum. One finger should rest against the child's head to prevent injury resulting from sudden movement.

(5) Pneumatic insufflation to test mobility of the tympanic membrane should always be part of the examination.

(6) The child may be restrained most easily if lying prone.

(7) Low-set ears are present in a number of congenital syndromes, including several associated with mental retardation. The ears may be considered low-set if they are below a line

drawn from the lateral angle of the eye to the external occipital protuberance.

(8) Congenital anomalies of the urinary tract are frequently associated with abnormalities of the pinnas.

(9) To examine the ears of an infant, it is usually necessary to pull the auricle backward and downward; in the older child, the external ear is pulled backward and upward.

Neck

Position (torticollis, opisthotonos, inability to support head, mobility), swelling, thyroid (size, contour, bruit, isthmus, nodules, tenderness), lymph nodes, veins, position of trachea, sternocleidomastoid (swelling, shortening), webbing, edema, auscultation, movement, tonic neck reflex.

Practical note: In the older child, the size and shape of the thyroid gland may be more clearly defined if the gland is palpated from behind.

Thorax

Shape and symmetry, veins, retractions and pulsations, beading, Harrison's groove, flaring of ribs, pigeon breast, funnel shape, size and position of nipples, breasts, length of sternum, intercostal and substernal retraction, asymmetry, scapulas, clavicles, scoliosis.

Practical note: At puberty, in normal children, one breast usually begins to develop before the other. Tenderness of the breasts is relatively common in both sexes. Gynecomastia is not uncommon in boys.

Lungs

Type of breathing, dyspnea, prolongation of expiration, cough, expansion, fremitus, flatness or dullness to percussion, resonance, breath and voice sounds, rales, wheezing.

Practical notes:

(1) Breath sounds in infants and children normally are more intense and more bronchial, and expiration is more prolonged, than in adults.

(2) Most of the young child's respiratory movement is produced by abdominal movement; there is very little intercostal motion.

(3) If the stethoscope is placed over the child's mouth and the sounds heard by this route are subtracted from the sounds heard through the chest wall, the difference usually represents the amount produced intrathoracically.

Heart

Location and intensity of apex beat, precordial bulging, pulsation of vessels, thrills, size, shape, auscultation (rate, rhythm, force, quality of sounds—compare with pulse with respect to rate and rhythm; friction rub—variation with pressure), murmurs (location, position in cycle, intensity, pitch, effect of change of position, transmission, effect of exercise) (see Chapter 19).

Practical notes:

(1) Many children normally have sinus dysrhythmia. The child should be asked to take a deep breath to determine its effect on the rhythm.

(2) Extrasystoles are not uncommon in childhood.

(3) The heart should be examined with the child erect, recumbent, and turned to the left.

Abdomen

Size and contour, visible peristalsis, respiratory movements, veins (distention, direction of flow), umbilicus, hernia, musculature, tenderness and rigidity, rebound tenderness, tympany, shifting dullness, pulsation, palpable organs or masses (size, shape, position, mobility), fluid wave, reflexes, femoral pulsations, bowel sounds.

Practical notes:

(1) The abdomen may be examined with the child prone in the parent's lap, held over the shoulder, or seated or the examining table facing away from the doctor. These positions may be particularly helpful where tenderness, rigidity, or a mass must be palpated. In the infant, the examination may be aided by having the child suck at a "sugar tip" or nurse at a bottle.

(2) Light palpation, especially for the spleen, often will give more information than deep palpation.

(3) Umbilical hernias are common during the first 2 years of life. They usually disappear spontaneously.

Male Genitalia

Circumcision, meatal opening, hypospadias, phimosis, adherent foreskin, size of testes, cryptorchidism, scrotum, hydrocele, hernia, pubertal changes. Tanner stage should be noted.

Practical notes:

(1) In examining a suspected case of cryptorchidism, palpation for the testicles should be done before the child has fully undressed or become chilled or had the cremasteric reflex stimulated. In some cases, examination while the child is in a warm bath may be helpful. The boy should also be examined while

sitting in a chair holding his knees with his heels on the seat; the increased intra-abdominal pressure may push the testes into the scrotum.

(2) To examine for cryptorchidism, one should start above the inguinal canal and work downward to prevent pushing the testes up into the canal or abdomen.

(3) The penis of an obese boy may be so obscured by fat as to appear abnormally small. If this fat is pushed back, a penis of normal size is usually found.

Female Genitalia

Vagina (imperforate, discharge, adhesions), hypertrophy of clitoris, pubertal changes. Tanner stage should be noted.

Practical note: Digital or speculum examination is rarely indicated before puberty.

Rectum & Anus

Irritation, fissures, prolapse, imperforate anus. Note muscle tone, character of stool, masses, tenderness, sensation.

Practical note: The rectal examination should be performed with the little finger (inserted slowly). Examine the stool on glove finger (gross, microscopic, culture, guaiac) as indicated.

Extremities

A. General: Deformity, hemiatrophy, bowleg (common in infancy), knock-knee (common at age 2–3 years), paralysis, edema, temperature, posture, gait, stance, asymmetry.

B. Joints: Swelling, redness, pain, limitation, tenderness, motion, rheumatic nodules, carrying angle of elbows, tibial torsion.

C. Hands and Feet: Extra digits, clubbing, simian lines, curvature of little finger, deformity of nails, splinter hemorrhages, flatfeet (feet commonly appear flat during first 2 years of life), abnormalities of feet, dermatoglyphics, width of thumbs and big toes, syndactyly, length of various segments, dimpling of dorsa, temperature.

D. Peripheral Vessels: Presence, absence, or diminution of arterial pulses.

Practical note: Normal femoral arterial pulsations during the newborn period do not definitely exclude coarctation.

Spine & Back

Posture; curvatures; rigidity; webbed neck; spina bifida; pilonidal dimple or cyst; tufts of hair; mobility; mongolian spots; tenderness over spine, pelvis, and kidneys.

Neurologic Examination (after Vazuka)

A. Cerebral Function: General behavior, level of consciousness, intelligence, emotional status, memory, orientation, illusions, hallucinations, cortical sensory interpretation, cortical motor integration, ability to understand and communicate, auditory-verbal and visual-verbal comprehension, visual recognition of object, speech, ability to write, performance of skilled motor acts.

B. Cranial Nerves:

1. I (olfactory)–Identification of odors; disorders of smell.

2. II (optic)–Visual acuity, visual fields, ophthalmoscopic examination.

3. III (oculomotor), IV (trochlear), and VI (abducens)–Ocular movements, strabismus, ptosis, dilatation of pupil, nystagmus, pupillary accommodation, pupillary light reflexes.

4. V (trigeminal)–Sensation of face, corneal reflex, masseter and temporal muscle reflexes, maxillary reflex (jaw jerk).

5. VII (facial)–Wrinkling forehead, frowning, smiling, raising eyebrows, asymmetry of face, strength of eyelid muscles, taste on anterior portion of tongue.

6. VIII (vestibulocochlear)–

a. Cochlear–Hearing, lateralization, air and bone conduction, tinnitus.

b. Vestibular–Caloric tests.

7. IX (glossopharyngeal) and X (vagus)–Pharyngeal gag reflex; ability to swallow and speak clearly; sensation of mucosa of pharynx, soft palate, and tonsils; movement of pharynx, larynx, and soft palate; autonomic functions.

8. XI (accessory)–Strength of trapezius and sternocleidomastoid muscles.

9. XII (hypoglossal)–Protrusion of tongue, tremor, strength of tongue.

Practical note: Cranial nerve function is usually observed in young children. Formal testing is not realistic in most cases.

C. Cerebellar Function: Finger to nose; finger to examiner's finger; rapidly alternating pronation and supination of hands; ability to run heel down other shin and to make a requested motion with foot; ability to stand with eyes closed, walk normally, walk heel to toe; tremor; ataxia; posture; arm swing when walking; nystagmus; abnormalities of muscle tone and speech.

D. Motor System: Muscle size, consistency, and tone; muscle contours and outlines; muscle strength; myotonic contraction; slow relaxation; symmetry of posture; fasciculations; tremor; resistance to passive movement; involuntary movement.

E. Reflexes:

1. Deep–Bicep, brachioradialís, tricep, patellar, and Achilles reflexes; rapidity and strength of contraction and relaxation.

2. Superficial–Abdominal, cremasteric, plantar, and gluteal reflexes.

3. Neonatal–Babinski, Landau, Moro, rooting, suck, grasp, and tonic neck reflexes.

Developmental Assessment

Both a history for "milestones" and developmental screening tests are part of the routine physical evaluation.

Practical note: Screening devices are not diagnostic of particular problems but merely indicate a need for further developmental evaluation.

2 | Development & Growth

David Burgess, MD

Development and growth are continuous dynamic processes occurring from conception to maturity and taking place in an orderly sequence that is approximately the same for all individuals. At any particular age, however, wide variations can be found among normal children; these variations reflect the active response of the growing individual to numberless hereditary and environmental factors.

Development signifies maturation of organs and systems, acquisition of skills, ability to adapt more readily to stress, and ability to assume maximum responsibility and to achieve freedom in creative expression. Growth signifies increase in size.

DEVELOPMENT

To give comprehensive pediatric care, the physician and other health care providers should know something about normal development at all ages and should be particularly familiar with development during the earliest years, since they occupy a unique position as family adviser during this period.

Screening Tests

In accordance with the Guidelines for Health Supervision put forth by the American Academy of Pediatrics, a two-stage developmental screening program was developed for use in the primary health care setting to detect developmental delays in infancy and the preschool years. The first stage consists of the Revised Prescreening Developmental Questionnaire (R-PDQ) (Fig 2–1) or the Key Denver Developmental Screening Test items (DDST) (or both), followed by the complete DDST (Fig 2–2) as a second-stage screening test for children identified as suspect.

R-PDQ Age: (____ yr _//_ mo _2_ completed wks)

	For Office Use
39. Gets To Sitting Can your baby get to a sitting position without help? <div align="right">(Yes) No</div>	(11) GM
40. Imitates Speech Sounds Write down 2 or 3 words that your baby tries to imitate with a recognizable sound (not necessarily complete words). In your judgment does (s)he try to imitate words? <div align="right">Yes (No)</div>	((11)) L *DELAY*
41. Bangs 2 Cubes Held in Hands Without your moving his/her hands can your baby bang together 2 small blocks? Rattles and pan lids do not count. <div align="right">Yes (No)</div>	*No DELAY* (12-1) FMA

Figure 2–1. Revised Prescreening Developmental Questionnaire.

A. First-Stage Screening: The R-PDQ is a parent-answered questionnaire designed to achieve 3 goals:

(1) To make parents more aware of the development of their children.

(2) To document systematically the developmental progress of individual children.

(3) To facilitate early identification of children whose development may be delayed.

Administration of the R-PDQ consists of the following steps (the appropriate R-PDQ form must be used depending on the age of the child):

(1) The child's R-PDQ age is calculated.

(2) The R-PDQ is given to the child's caregiver, who completes it based on available instructions. All appropriate questions must be answered.

(3) Delays are identified. A delay is an item passed by 90% of children (in the original DDST norming studies) at a younger age than the child being screened.

Children who have no delays on the R-PDQ are considered developmentally normal. If a child has one or more delays, second-stage screening with the DDST should be administered as soon as possible.

The Key Denver Items (KDI) were identified to save time and cost in screening with the DDST. The KDI are a subset of 39

Figure 2-2. Denver Developmental Screening Test.

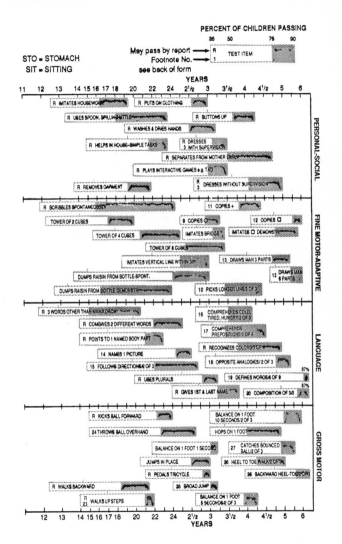

Figure 2-2 (cont'd). Denver Developmental Screening Test.

DDST items (rather than the entire set of 105 items) that require administration of only 3 or 4 key items per screen. Key DDST items are identified by a black outline of the age bars.

Administration of the KDI (Fig 2–3) consists of the following steps:

(1) The child's age is calculated and an age line drawn.

(2) The key DDST items immediately to the left but not touching the age line are identified, administered, and interpreted as detailed in the DDST manual.

(3) Delays are identified. Delays are key DDST items that are failed or refused and are located completely to the left of the child's age line.

(4) If the child fails or refuses one or more of the key DDST items, second-stage screening should be completed with the DDST.

B. Second-Stage Screening: The use of the R-PDQ and the KDI will identify between 10 and 20% of a population as being suspect. Those children who are suspect on first-stage screening should be scheduled for second-stage screening using the complete DDST. A child who receives other-than-normal results on the DDST (abnormal, questionable, or untestable) should be scheduled for further medical and developmental evaluation.

To use the DDST and its variations effectively, individual examiners must be trained to administer and interpret the tests

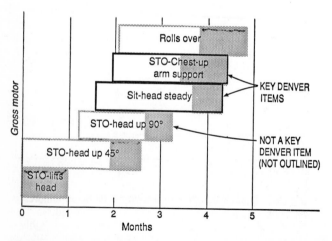

Figure 2–3. Key Denver Items.

properly. DDST training consists of an introductory videotape, the DDST training manual, a second videotape demonstrating correct and incorrect ways of administering the DDST items, a written proficiency test, practice testing, and administration of a DDST for a trained observer. Completion of this training ensures minimal false-positive and false-negative identifications. A free catalogue describing the training materials, the DDST (with key items), and the R-PDQ is available from Denver Developmental Materials, PO Box 20037, Denver, CO 80220–0037, (303) 355-4729.

PERSONALITY DEVELOPMENT

Personality development is a dynamic process, and no summary can give a complete picture of what takes place. The goal of the individual, both as a child and as an adult, is to be able to work, to play, to master personal problems, and to love and be loved in a manner that is creative, socially acceptable, and personally gratifying.

The development of personality is a complicated process involving all aspects of the individual and the environment. The process varies from one child to another, but, on the whole, all children pass through various phases of development of which the broad general outlines are essentially the same.

Each successive stage of development is characterized by definite problems the child must solve in order to proceed with confidence to the next stage. The highest degree of functional harmony will be achieved when the problems of each stage are met and solved at an orderly rate and in a normal sequence. On the other hand, it is important to remember that the successive personality gains the child makes are not rigidly established once and for all but may be reinforced or threatened throughout life. Even in adulthood, a reasonably healthy personality may be achieved in spite of previous misfortunes and defects in the developmental sequence.

It is important to remember that psychologic development takes place within a cultural milieu. Not only the form of large social institutions but also the framework of family life, the attitudes of parents, and the parents' practices in childrearing will be conditioned by the culture of the given period.

Psychologic development in childhood may be roughly divided into 5 stages: infancy (birth–18 months), early childhood (18 months–5 years), late childhood (5–12 years), early adolescence (12–16 years), and late adolescence (16 years–maturity). Early and late adolescence are discussed in Chapter 13.

Infancy

Much of the psychologic development that occurs during the first year is interrelated with physical development, ie, dependent upon the maturation of the body to the extent that the infant can discriminate self from nonself. Knowledge of the environment comes with increasing sharpening of the senses (from indiscriminate mouthing to coordinated eye–hand movements). Beginning of mastery over the environment comes with increasingly adept coordination, the development of locomotion, and the beginnings of speech. The realization of the self as an individual in relation to an environment that includes other individuals is the basis upon which interpersonal relationships are founded.

The newborn infant is at first aware only of bodily needs, ie, of the presence or absence of discomfort (cold, wet, etc). The pleasure of relief from discomfort gradually becomes associated with mothering and later (when perception is sufficient for recognition) with the mother. The infant derives a feeling of security when bodily needs are satisfied and from contact with the mother. The feeding situation provides the first opportunity for development of this feeling of security, and it is therefore important for the physician to ensure that this is a happy event.

The development of the first emotional relationship, then, comes through close contact with the mother. It develops from a meeting of the infant's physical needs into a sustained physical contact and emotional interaction with one person. Prolonged deprivation of this relationship, if no satisfactory substitute is provided, is damaging to the infant's personality. Permanent deprivation leads to restriction of personality development, even to pseudoretardation in all areas. Such behavior may also occur in a home situation, but it is more striking and more common in infants who remain for long periods of time in hospitals or in other institutions where adequate personalized and kindly attention is not given to each infant. The infant who is deprived of the security and affection necessary to produce a sense of trust may respond with listlessness, immobility, unresponsiveness, indifferent appetite, an appearance of unhappiness, and insomnia. In other cases, the continued deprivation of consistent care during infancy may not become apparent until later life, when the individual may feel no reason to trust people and thus lack a sense of responsibility toward others.

No particular techniques are necessary to develop an infant's feeling of security. The infant is not easily discouraged by an inexperienced mother's mistakes; rather, the infant seems to respond to the warmth of her feelings and her eagerness to keep trying. The feeling of security derived from satisfactory relationships during the first year is probably the most important single element in the personality. It makes it possible for the infant to accept restrictions without fearing that each restriction implies total loss of love.

Toward the end of the first year, other personal relationships also are developing, particularly with the father, who is now recognized as comparable in importance with the mother. Relationships perhaps are also forming with siblings.

Early Childhood

In early childhood, the child's horizon continues to widen. Increased body control makes possible the development of many physical skills. The very important development of speech permits extension of the social environment and increasing ability to understand and perfect social relationships.

Perhaps the central problem of early childhood is still, however, the development of control over the instinctive drives, particularly as they arise in relation to the parents. The acceptance of limitations on the need for bodily love (the realization that complete infantile dependency is not permitted or desirable) and the control of aggressive feelings are prime examples. This control of primitive feelings is largely accomplished through the psychologic process of "identification" with the parents—the desire in the child to be like the parents and to emulate them. With this desire come the beginnings of conscience as the moral values of the parents are incorporated into the child's own personality.

The child now begins to have a feeling of autonomy—of self-direction and initiative. The child 18 months to 2½ years of age is actively learning to exercise the power of "yes" and "no." The difficulty the 2-year-old has in deciding between the two often leads to parental misunderstanding; the child may say "no" but really mean "yes," as if compelled to exercise this new "will" even when it hurts.

At this period, parental "discipline" becomes very important. Discipline is an educative means by which the parent teaches the child how to become a self-respecting, likable, and socially responsible adult. Disciplinary measures have value chiefly as they serve this educative function; if used as an end in themselves, to establish the "authority" of the parent irrespective of the issues at hand, they usually lead only to warfare (open or surreptitious) between parent and child.

Ideally each child will develop the feeling of being a responsible human being without rejecting the help and guidance of others in important matters. The favorable result is self-control without loss of self-esteem. Adults must allow children increasingly wide latitude in undergoing experiences that permit them to make choices they are ready and able to make and yet must also teach them to accept restrictions when necessary.

The parents must be firm and consistent to protect the child against the consequences of immature judgment. Perhaps the most constructive rule a parent can follow is to decide which kinds of conformity are really important and then to clearly and consistently require obedience in these areas. Then "discipline" will have the positive goal of making the child able to live comfortably in society without feeling guilty about basic drives but will not stifle the need for some expression of independence.

Late Childhood

In this period, children achieve a rapid intellectual growth and actively begin to establish themselves as members of society. Psychiatrists call this the latency period, because the force of the primitive drives has been fairly successfully controlled, expressed in a socially acceptable way, or repressed. The energy derived from the instinctive drives whose direct expression society does not permit is diverted into the great drive for knowledge—a process of "sublimation." At no time in life does the individual learn more avidly and quickly. Reading and writing (the intellectual skills) and a vast body of information are quickly assimilated. The preoccupation with fantasy gradually subsides, and the child wants to be engaged in real tasks that can be carried through to completion. Even in play activities, the emphasis is on developing mental and bodily skills through interest in sports and games.

Late childhood is also a period of conformity to the group. The environment enlarges to include school and, particularly, other children. Much of the emotional satisfaction previously derived from the parents now comes from the child's relationships with peers. The need to become a member of this larger group of equals tends to encourage the qualities of cooperation and obedience to the will of the group (elements of democracy). It also paves the way for questioning parental values where these differ from those of the group—a direct impact of broader cultural values upon the environment of the home.

GROWTH

General Considerations

    A. Fetal Growth: During fetal life, the rate of growth is extremely rapid. During the early months, the fetal rate of gain in length is greater than the rate of gain in weight when expressed as percentage of value at birth. By the eighth month, the fetus has achieved 80% of the birth length and only 50% of the birth weight (Table 2–1).

    B. Organs: At birth, the proportion of the weight of the pancreas and the musculature to that of the entire body is less in the infant than in the adult; that of the skeleton, lungs, and stomach is the same; and that of other organs is greater in the infant than in the adult. Major types of postnatal growth of various parts and organs of the body are shown in Fig 2–4.

    C. Trunk–Leg Ratio: At birth, the ratio of the lower to the upper segment of the body (as measured from the pubis) is approximately 1:1.7. The legs grow more rapidly than does the trunk; by age 10–12 years, the segments are approximately equal.

    D. Height: Rate of growth is generally more important than actual size. For more accurate comparisons, data should be recorded both as absolute figures and as a percentile for that particular age, and the rate of growth should be determined. Birth length is doubled by approximately age 4 years and tripled by age 13 years. The average child grows approximately 10 inches (25 cm) in the first year of life, 5 inches (12.5 cm) in the second, 3–4 inches (7.5–10 cm) in the third, and approximately 2–3 inches (5–7.5 cm) per year thereafter until the growth spurt of puberty appears (Fig 2–5).

    E. Weight: Body weight is probably the best index of nutrition and growth. The average infant weighs approximately 7 lb 5 oz (3.33 kg) at birth. Within the first few days of life, the newborn loses up to 10% of the birth weight. Birth weight is doubled between the fourth and fifth months of age, tripled by the end of the first year, and quadrupled by the end of the second year. Between ages 2 and 9 years, the annual increment in weight averages about 5 lb (2.25 kg) per year (Fig 2–6).

    F. Growth at Puberty: Although children pass through the phase of accelerated growth associated with pubescence at different chronologic ages, the pattern or sequence of pubescent growth tends to be similar in all children. Children destined to mature sexually at an early age tend to be tall and have an

Table 2–1. Fetal and newborn dimensions and weights of the body and its organs.

Fetal Age (wk)†	Crown-heel (cm)	Crown-rump (cm)	Head Circumference (cm)	Body Weight (g)	Adrenal (g)	Brain (g)	Heart (g)	Kidney (g)	Liver (g)	Lungs (g)	Pancreas (g)	Pituitary (g)	Spleen (g)	Thymus (g)	Thyroid (g)
Prenatal and Newborn															
12	9.0	7.5	7.4	18.6	0.087	2.32	0.098	0.163	0.097	0.69	0.013		0.006	0.010	0.026
16	16.7	12.8	12.6	100	0.417	14.40	0.662	0.962	5.94	3.23	0.095	0.011	0.086	0.122	0.133
20	24.2	17.7	17.6	310	1.07	43	2.08	2.77	16.8	8.18	0.314	0.024	0.41	0.553	0.352
24	31.1	21.9	22.3	670	2.02	91	4.47	5.69	34.5	15.2	0.695	0.040	1.16	1.53	0.684
28	37.1	25.5	26.3	1150	3.16	153	7.70	9.43	57.4	23.7	1.22	0.058	2.43	3.14	1.08
30	39.8	27.1	28.1	1400	3.78	189	9.78	11.5	70.3	28.2	1.53	0.067	3.26	4.18	1.33
32	42.4	28.5	29.9	1700	4.44	228	11.6	13.8	84.3	33.0	1.88	0.076	4.25	5.41	1.54
34	44.8	29.9	31.5	2000	5.11	268	13.7	16.2	100.0	37.8	2.24	0.085	5.36	6.77	1.78
36	47.0	31.2	33.1	2450	5.77	309	15.9	18.6	113.0	42.7	2.61	0.094	6.55	8.22	2.01
38	49.1	32.4	34.4	2900	6.45	352	18.2	21.0	129.0	47.5	3.01	0.103	7.86	9.82	2.26
40	51.0	33.5	35.7	3150	7.10	394	20.6	23.5	143.5	52.5	3.40	0.111	9.22	11.5	2.50
Postnatal															
Age (yr)															
1		See Inside Back Cover			4	875	43	62	350	160		0.15	30	23	
5					5	1250	90	110	575	305		0.23	55	28	
10					6	1325	145	150	825	450		0.33	77	31	
15					8	1340	245	220	1275	675		0.48	125	27	
Adult‡															
Male					6	1375	300	320	1600	1000			165	14	
Female					6	1280	250	280	1500	750			150	14	

* Adapted from Edith Boyd. See also Inside Back Cover. † Time from first day of last menstrual period. ‡ Adapted from several sources.

advanced bone age (Fig 2–7); late-maturing children are short and show epiphyseal retardation in childhood.

G. Variations in Growth: Obese children are usually taller and have an advanced bone age. Children from high socioeco-

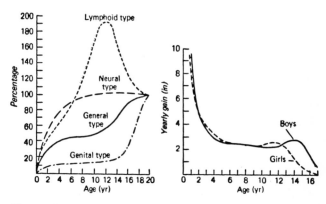

Figure 2–4. Major types of postnatal growth of various parts and organs of the body.

Figure 2–5. Yearly gain in height.

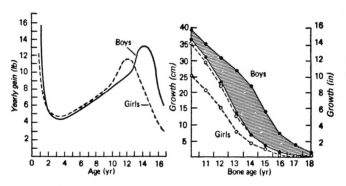

Figure 2–6. Yearly gain in weight.

Figure 2–7. Growth expectancy at bone ages indicated.

Figures 2–4 through 2–7 are redrawn and reproduced, with permission, from Holt LE, McIntosh R, Barnett HL: *Pediatrics,* 13th ed. Appleton-Century-Crofts, 1962, as redrawn from Harris JA et al: *Measurement of Man.* University of Minnesota Press, 1930.

nomic groups are larger than those from lower socioeconomic groups in the same area.

Head & Skull

At birth, the head is approximately three-fourths of its total mature size, whereas the rest of the body is only one-fourth its adult size.

Six fontanelles (anterior, posterior, 2 sphenoid, and 2 mastoid) are usually present at birth. The anterior fontanelle normally closes between 10 and 14 months of age but may be closed by age 3 months or remain open until age 18 months. The posterior fontanelle usually closes by age 2 months but in some children may not be palpable even at birth.

Cranial sutures do not ossify completely until later childhood.

While the averages of head and chest circumference in children during the first 4 years of life are approximately equal, during this period the head circumference may normally be from 5 cm larger to 7 cm smaller than that of the chest. Growth of the skull, as determined by increasing head circumference, is a much more accurate index of brain growth than is the presence or size of the fontanelle.

Sinuses

Maxillary and ethmoid sinuses are present at birth but are usually not aerated for approximately 6 months. The sphenoid sinuses are usually not pneumatized (or visible on x-ray) until after the third year of life. Frontal sinuses usually become visible by x-ray between 7 and 9 years of age, seldom before age 5.

The mastoid process at birth is relatively large and has a relatively wide communication with the middle ear. Its cellular structure appears gradually between birth and age 3 years.

Eyes

The eyes can follow, even at birth, and the ability to fixate is usually well developed by age 2–3 months. Strabismus normally may be present for the first 4–6 months of life.

Respiration & Heart Rate

The respiratory rate decreases steadily during childhood, averaging approximately 30 breaths per minute during the first year of life, 25 during the second year, 20 during the eighth year, and 18 by the 15th year.

The heart rate falls steadily throughout childhood, averaging about 150 beats per minute in utero, 130 at birth, 105 during the second year of life, 90 during the fourth year, 80 during the sixth year, and 70 during the tenth year.

Abdomen

The abdomen tends to be prominent in infants and toddlers. In the infant, the ascending and descending portions of the colon are short compared with the transverse colon, and the sigmoid extends higher in the abdomen than during later life.

Gas may be visualized roentgenographically almost immediately after birth in the stomach, within 2 hours in the ileum, and, on the average, in 3 or 4 hours in the rectum.

Muscle

At birth, muscle constitutes 25% of total body weight, as compared with 43% in the adult.

Ossification Centers

At birth, the average full-term infant has 5 ossification centers demonstrable by x-ray: distal end of femur, proximal end of tibia, calcaneus, talus, and cuboid.

The clavicle is the first bone to calcify in utero, calcification beginning during the fifth fetal week.

Epiphyseal development of girls is consistently ahead of that of boys during all of childhood.

Puberty

Sexual maturation is more closely correlated with bone maturation than with chronologic age. The maximal yearly increase in height occurs during the year before menarche in most girls. Climate apparently has little effect on sexual development. Nigerian girls and Eskimo girls have their menarche at approximately the same age. If environmental and nutritional factors are similar, girls of different races tend to have their menarche at approximately the same age.

During the first 1–2 years following menarche, the menstrual periods of most girls are anovulatory and often irregular, and the interval between periods may be longer or shorter than is characteristic during later life.

Girls who mature late are taller (on the average) when final stature is attained.

Some degree of breast hypertrophy (gynecomastia) is relatively common in boys at puberty.

Senses

At birth, the newborn infant has mature sensory receptors for pressure, pain, and temperature over the entire body surface, in the mouth, and in the external genitalia; there are also mature pain receptors in the viscera and proprioceptive receptors in muscles, joints, and tendons.

A. Taste: The ability to taste is present in the newborn infant, who is capable of distinguishing the 4 basic tastes.

B. Olfaction: The human infant is born with fully mature receptors for olfaction.

C. Hearing: Normal infants can hear almost immediately after birth, but they respond to sounds at a subcortical level.

D. Vision: About 80% of newborn infants are hyperopic; the eyeball grows rapidly during the first 8 years of life. Thus, hyperopia should be expected during the preschool and early school years. Strabismus normally may present for the first 4–6 months of life. Mature adult function of the eye muscles is usually reached by the end of the first year.

At birth, the infant demonstrates an awareness of light and dark, possesses peripheral vision, and is capable of rudimentary fixation on near objects. Other visual functions are deficient. At age 4 months, vision is 20/300–20/200 (6/90–6/60); at age 10 months, 20/200 (6/60); and at age 2 years, 20/40 (6/12). Vision becomes 20/20 (6/6) by age 4 years.

Water Content

The water content of the body is approximately 95% of weight during early fetal life, 65–75% at birth, and 55–60% at maturity.

Blood

If the umbilical cord is not clamped for 2–3 minutes after delivery of the infant, 75–135mL of blood will be transferred from the placenta to the infant. Late clamping will produce a red blood cell count approximately 1 million/μL higher, a hemoglobin level approximately 2.5 g/dL higher, and a hematocrit count 7% higher than if early clamping were carried out.

At birth, 5% of all red blood cells may be reticulocytes; this percentage drops to less than 1% after the second week of life. Nucleated red cells (up to 5% as a percentage of the total number of nucleated cells) and immature lymphocytes may be present in the newborn but disappear within the first week of life. Fetal hemoglobin accounts for 80% of total hemoglobin at birth (cord blood), 75% of the total at age 2 weeks, and 55% at age 5 weeks; it falls to 5% by age 20 weeks.

Table 2-2. Dental growth and development.

Primary or Deciduous Teeth

	Calcification		Eruption		Shedding	
	Begins At	Complete At	Maxillary	Mandibular	Maxillary	Mandibular
Central incisors	4th fetal mo	18–24 mo	6–10 mo	5–8 mo	7–8 yr	6–7 yr
Lateral incisors	5th fetal mo	18–24 mo	8–12 mo	7–10 mo	8–9 yr	7–8 yr
Cuspids	6th fetal mo	30–39 mo	16–20 mo	16–20 mo	11–12 yr	9–11 yr
First molars	5th fetal mo	24–30 mo	11–18 mo	11–18 mo	9–11 yr	10–12 yr
Second molars	6th fetal mo	36 mo	20–30 mo	20–30 mo	9–12 yr	11–13 yr

Secondary or Permanent Teeth

	Calcification		Eruption*	
	Begins At	Complete At	Maxillary	Mandibular
Central incisors	3–4 mo	9–10 yr	7–8 yr (3)	6–7 yr (2)
Lateral incisors	Maxilla 10–12 mo Mandible 3–4 mo	10–11 yr	8–9 yr (5)	7–8 yr (4)
Cuspids	4–5 mo	12–15 yr	11–12 yr (11)	9–11 yr (6)
First premolars	18–24 mo	12–13 yr	10–11 yr (7)	10–12 yr (8)
Second premolars	24–30 mo	12–14 yr	10–12 yr (9)	11–13 yr (10)
First molars	Birth	9–10 yr	5½–7 yr (1)	5½–7 yr (1a)
Second molars	30–36 mo	14–16 yr	12–14 yr (12)	12–13 yr (12a)
Third molars	Maxilla 7–9 yr Mandible 8–10 yr	18–25 yr	17–30 yr (13)	17–30 yr (13a)

* Figures in parentheses indicate order of eruption. Many otherwise normal infants do not conform strictly to the stated schedule.

The leukocyte count is high at birth, rises slightly during the first 48 hours after birth, falls for the next 2 or 3 weeks, and then rises again. In some infants, it reaches its highest level in life sometime before the seventh month. The lymphocyte count is highest during the first year of life and then falls progressively during the remainder of childhood.

Children have a higher sedimentation rate than do adults.

Urine

The average infant secretes 15–50 mL of urine per 24 hours during the first 2 days of life, 50–300 mL/d during the next week, and 400–500 mL/d by the latter half of the first year. There is subsequently a gradual increase in urinary output; 700–1500mL/d is secreted between ages 8 and 14 years.

Tears

Tears can be produced during the early weeks of life.

Teeth

Stages of dental growth and development are shown in Table 2–2.

Ambulatory Pediatrics | 3

Barton D. Schmitt, MD

HEALTH MAINTENANCE VISITS

Health maintenance or health supervision visits are the key to preventive pediatrics. The visit has several purposes: responding to the parent's or child's current concerns, presenting age-appropriate anticipatory guidance, assessing growth and development (Chapter 2), performing a physical examination (Chapter 1), obtaining laboratory screening tests, and administering immunizations (Chapter 9).

PARENTAL CONCERNS

The first part of each well-child visit should be directed toward dealing with the current concerns of the parent, usually the mother. Most expectant mothers have many questions that should be discussed with their pediatrician several weeks prior to delivery. The most frequent concerns include arguments for and against breast-feeding and circumcision, preparation of the breasts if breast-feeding is to be used, hospital policies about rooming-in and parent–infant contact in the delivery room, essential baby equipment, separation problems with other children during the mother's confinement, and ways of decreasing sibling jealousy. It has been traditional for the first newborn office visit to take place at 6 weeks, probably because 6 weeks is the traditional time for the mother's first postdelivery obstetric visit. However, most mothers—particularly primiparas—have many questions and concerns well before this traditional interval after birth. A 2-week postpartal office visit is much more logical.

A health maintenance visit without parental concerns is uncommon. Some mothers bring a list of questions, "How much should babies cry?" "How do I know he's getting enough to eat?" "Can I spoil her by picking her up too much?" "Is it all

right to spank children?" "How old should Johnny be before I let
him cross the street alone?" Many of the questions have no
clear-cut answers. The seasoned pediatrician usually enjoys the
challenge of these discussions and the satisfaction that comes
with reassuring an anxious parent.

ANTICIPATORY GUIDANCE

Anticipatory guidance usually includes nutritional counseling, accident prevention, behavioral counseling, suggestions
for developmental stimulation, sex education, dental recommendations, medical information, etc. Special counseling is in order
for adolescents (see Chapter 13). A list of suggested topics to be
discussed at particular ages is found on the health maintenance
forms presented in Figure 3–1. A blank space or line on these
forms indicates that a comment is required following that item.
All anticipatory guidance advice is followed by the optimal age
for discussion in parentheses. A check mark in the box that
follows each of these advice items indicates that this counseling
was done.

INJURY PREVENTION

Injuries kill more children than the 6 other leading causes of
childhood deaths combined. Between ages 1 and 14, over 50% of
deaths are due to injuries; between ages 15 and 23, over 80% are
due to injuries. Each year 100,000 children under 15 years of age
are left with permanent disabilities owing to injuries. During the
first 3 years of life, children have little sense of danger or self-
preservation. They are totally dependent on adults to look after
their safety.

Injury prevention advice should be an integral part of medical care provided for all infants and children. Several years ago,
the American Academy of Pediatrics put together The Injury
Prevention Program (TIPP), which includes parent questionnaires for assessing risk and information sheets to prevent accidents. The main thrust of the program was to advise parents in
the 5 following areas:

(1) Approved child car restraints.
(2) Smoke detectors.
(3) Hot water heater set to less than 130 °F.
(4) Guards for windows and gates for stairways.
(5) Syrup of Ipecac.

Motor Vehicle Crashes

The number one killer and crippler of children in the United States is motor vehicle crashes. Proper use of car safety seats can reduce fatalities and hospitalizations by at least 70%. Laws have been passed in all 50 states that require children to be sitting in an approved safety seat. The type of safety seat depends on the child's weight. In general, the smaller seats are more protective and should be used as long as they are appropriate. The following are guidelines for selecting a seat based on weight: less than 20 pounds, rear-facing infant seat; 20 to 40 pounds: forward-facing toddler seat; 40 to 60 pounds: booster seat; over 60 pounds: regular lap belt; over 48 inches (4 feet): the shoulder strap can be safely used.

Prevention of Burns

(1) Never drink anything hot while holding a baby.

(2) Keep hot substances away from the edge of a table or stove.

(3) Don't let your child turn the faucet handles in the bathtub.

(4) Set your hot water heater to less than 130 °F.

(5) Use flame-resistant sleepwear.

(6) Install smoke detectors in your home.

(7) Keep cigarette lighters and matches away from children.

(8) Keep electric cords unplugged or out of the reach of children.

Prevention of Choking

(1) Don't allow your children to have foods that are commonly aspirated into the lungs until they are old enough to chew them (usually 4 years of age): nuts of any kind, sunflower seeds, orange seeds, cherry pits, raw carrots, raw peas, raw celery.

(2) Carefully chop up any foods that might block the windpipe, such as hot dogs, grapes, and caramels.

(3) Warn babysitters and siblings not to share these foods with small children.

(4) Don't allow children to run or play with food in their mouth.

(5) Avoid toys with small detachable parts that could enter the windpipe.

(6) Dispose of button batteries carefully.

Prevention of Drowning

(1) Never leave a child less than 3 years old unattended in the bathtub or a wading pool.

PEDIATRIC HEALTH MAINTENANCE
Birth through 3 months

Parent's concerns

Newborn data base
  Birth weight .... Gestational age ....
  Pregnancy or delivery problems   Neonatal problems

Growth (comment on growth curve)

Feeding advice
  Formula .... oz/24 hours ....
  Breast-feeding: Frequency .... min/feeding ....
  Vitamins .... Iron ....
  Solids .... Fluoride drops ....
  Feeding problems ....
  Advice: Introduce bottle in breast fed (2w) ❏; Introduce fluids other than milk (2m) ❏

Developmental status
  Stimulation advice: Hold baby (2w) ❏ Talk to baby (2m) ❏

Childrearing advice
  Sleep pattern ....
  Crying or colic ....
  Mother-child interaction ....
  Sibling rivalry (2w) ....

Family status
  Advice: Paternal involvement, family planning (2w) ❏ Utilize sitter (2m) ❏

Accident prevention advice
  Car seat, crib safety (2w) ❏ Rolling over (2m) ❏ Smoke detector ❏

Medical advice
  Demonstrate use of bulb syringe for nose (2w)❏ Foreskin or circumcision care ♂ (2w) ❏
  Temperature taking, Tylenol and fever handout (2m)❏ Discuss when to call doctor (2m) ❏

Intercurrent illness

Figure 3–1. Pediatric health maintenance record.

PEDIATRIC HEALTH MAINTENANCE
4 months through 14 months

Parent's concerns

Growth (comment on growth curve)

Feeding advice
Formula ———————————————— oz/24 hours ————————————————
Breast feeding: Frequency ———————— min/feeding ————————————
Vitamins ————————————————————— Iron ————————————————
Solids ————————————————————— Fluoride drops ————————————
Feeding problems ——————————————
Advice: No bottles in bed; introduce solids, spoon, cup (4m) ❑
Confirm intake of iron-rich solids (6m) ❑
Introduce finger foods, confirm on 3 meals/day (9m) ❑
Entirely on table foods. Phase out bottle by 18 mo (12m) ❑

Developmental status
Stimulation advice: Toys for reaching (4m) ❑ Avoid confining baby equipment (6m) ❑
Repeat baby's sounds (9m) ❑ Name objects and pictures for baby (12m) ❑

Child rearing advice
Sleep pattern ——————————————————————————————
Behavior problems ————————————————————————————
Advice: Sleeps through the night (4m) ❑ Normal separation anxiety (6m) ❑
Discipline: Use negative voice and eye contact rather than physical punishment (9m) ❑
Don't punish for normal exploratory behavior, discuss positive strokes for good behavior
(12m) ❑

Family status

Accident prevention advice
Safe toys (4m) ❑ Stairs and gates, drowning in bathtub (9m) ❑
Electrical cords (6m) ❑ Ipecac and poison talk (12m) ❑

Medical advice
Teething myths (6m) ❑ Avoid expensive shoes (9m) ❑ Use of 911 (12m) ❑

Intercurrent illness

Figure 3–1. Pediatric health maintenance record. (*Continued*)

PEDIATRIC HEALTH MAINTENANCE
15 months through 3 years

Parent's concerns

Growth (comment on growth curve)

Diet
Milk _____ oz/24 hours
Eating problems _____
Advice: Entirely on table foods, off all bottles (18m) ❑
Normal decreased appetite, iron intake (2y) ❑

Developmental status
Advice: Read to child (1½, 2) ❑   Listen to child (2) ❑   TV rules (3) ❑

Childrearing advice
Sleep problems _____
Behavior problems _____
Frequency of spanking _____
Advice: Don't punish for normal negativism, ignore temper tantrums (1½) ❑
Discuss toilet training and readiness (1½, 2, 3) ❑
Discuss positive "strokes" for good behavior (2) ❑
Emphasize consistency in discipline and use of time-out room (2, 3) ❑

Family status

Injury prevention advice
Scalds, aspiration foods (1½) ❑   Street/garage safety (2) ❑
Drowning in ditch and pools (3) ❑

Dental advice
Brushing frequency _____   Fluoride intake _____
Advice: Avoid snacks that cause cavities (1½) ❑   Benefits of fluoride toothpaste (2) ❑
Brushing techniques (3) ❑

Intercurrent illness

Figure 3–1. Pediatric health maintenance record. (*Continued*)

PEDIATRIC HEALTH MAINTENANCE
4 years through 5 years

To be completed by parent	Check correct answer	
School readiness:		
1. Does your child pay attention when being read to?	Yes	No
2. Can your child play quietly alone for over ½ hour?	Yes	No
3. Does your child mind adults and follow instructions?	Yes	No
4. Does your child speak clearly enough for others to understand?	Yes	No
5. Does your child object to being left with a sitter?	No	Yes
6. Can your child dress without help?	Yes	No
7. Does your child ever wet or soil him/herself during the day?	No	Yes

To be completed by physician or nurse

Parent's concerns

Growth (comment on growth curve)

Diet

School readiness
  Problems detected by above questions _____
  Development: PDQ (4, 5) Score _____ Weak category _____
    DDST (If fails PDQ) Result _____
  Articulation: DASE (4) Score _____ Percentile _____
  Advice: Preschool if any problems (4) ❑

Injury prevention advice
  Adult seat belts, petting dogs (4) ❑ Crossing street, trampoline (5) ❑

Dental advice
  No daytime thumb-sucking (4) ❑ No nighttime thumb-sucking (5) ❑
  Frequency of brushing _____ Type of toothpaste _____ Fluoride intake _____

Intercurrent illness

Figure 3–1. Pediatric health maintenance record. (*Continued*)

PEDIATRIC HEALTH MAINTENANCE
6 years through 11 years

Parent's concerns

Diet

School
Name of school ——————————— Grade ————————————
Academic performance ————————————————————————
Attendance ————————————————————————————————
Behavior ————————————————————————————————————
Advice: Child's responsibility for schoolwork (6) ❑
Adult at home before and after school (6–10) ❑

Behavior
Behavior problems ——————————————————————————————
Chores ——————————————————————————————————————
Friends ——————————————————————————————————————
Advice: TV less than 2 h/d (6) ❑ Understanding of death (6) ❑
One sport or club (8–10) ❑ Smoking (10) ❑

Family status

Sex education
Discuss puberty and menarche before junior high school (10) ❑
Menstrual status (10 ♀) ——————————————————————————

Injury prevention advice
Bicycle safety (6) ❑ Swimming lessons (8) ❑
Fires, matches (10) ❑

Dental advice
Frequency of brushing ———— Type of toothpaste ———— Fluoride intake ————
Dental referral (6) ❑

Intercurrent illness

Figure 3–1. Pediatric health maintenance record. (*Continued*)

PEDIATRIC HEALTH MAINTENANCE
12 years through 18 years

Parent's concerns

Adolescent's concerns

Growth (comment on growth curve)

Diet

School
Name of school ————————— Grade ——————————
Academic performance ——————————————————————
Attendance ——————————————————————————
Behavior ——————————————————————————
Career plans ——————————————————————————

Behavior
Free time/friends ——————————————————————
Chores/job ——————————————————————————
Person to confide in ——————————————————————
Predominant mood ——————————————————————
Advice: Discuss values of babysitting (12) ❑ Discuss drugs and alcohol (12–16) ❑
Discuss smoking (14) ❑

Family status
Advice: Discuss independence and parent's trust (16) ❑

Sex education
Dating, masturbation (14) ❑ Marriage (18) ❑
Sexual activity, preventing pregnancy, STD (14, 16, 18) ——————————

Injury prevention advice
Firearms (12) ❑ Cycling safety (14) ❑ Driving safety, water safety (16) ❑
Motorcycles, seat belts (18) ❑

Dental advice
Frequency of brushing ——————————— Type of toothpaste ——————————

Medical advice
Acne ❑ Personal hygiene (14) ❑ Teach self-examination of breasts (16 ♀) ❑

Intercurrent illness

Figure 3–1. Pediatric health maintenance record. (*Continued*)

(2) Never leave children who can't swim unattended near a swimming pool—more children drown in backyard swimming pools than at beaches or public pools.

(3) Remember that infant water programs are for fun, not for learning how to swim. (Children cannot be made water safe before age 3.)

(4) Try to arrange swimming lessons for your child between ages 3 and 8.

Prevention of Head Trauma

(1) Never leave an infant of any age alone on a high place.

(2) Always leave the side rails on the crib up.

(3) Avoid bunk beds.

(4) Avoid baby walkers. (Over 35% of infants using them have an accident requiring emergency care. The most serious accidents occur when children fall down a stairway in a walker. Keep a sturdy gate at the top of all stairways.)

(5) Teach your child how to cross the street safely at age 4 or 5.

(6) Don't teach your child to ride a bicycle until age 7 or 8.

(7) Forbid trampolines.

Prevention of Poisoning

(1) Keep chemicals and drugs locked up and out of reach. Drain cleaners, furniture polish, and insecticides are the most dangerous of the common household poisons.

(2) Use the safety cap on all drug containers.

(3) Have some syrup of Ipecac handy.

(4) Know the telephone number of your nearest poison control center.

PHYSICAL EXAMINATION

A complete physical examination should be performed during most health maintenance visits (see Chapter 1). Height, weight, and head circumference should be measured and plotted on growth curves (see Chapter 2). During childhood, most chronic diseases will affect growth. Although physical examinations are usually normal, they serve as a point of reference in evaluating future illnesses. Therefore, the extent of the examination should be carefully recorded. To save time, the checklist shown in Table 3–1 can be used. Elaboration is required only for the abnormal findings.

Some physical findings are silent—ie, they are not notice-

Table 3–1. Checklist for physical examination.

	Normal	Abnormal
1. GENERAL APPEARANCE: well nourished, hydrated, alert		
2. SKIN: color, rash, swelling, hair, nails		
3. HEAD: shape, anterior fontanelle		
4. EYES: conjunctiva, cornea, pupils, extraocular movement		
5. EARS: pinnae, canals; tympanic membrane appearance, mobility		
6. NOSE: nares, turbinates		
7. MOUTH: tongue, teeth, oral mucosa, tonsils, pharynx		
8. NECK: thyroid, range of motion		
9. NODES: cervical, axillary, inguinal, other		
10. CHEST: symmetry, expansion, breasts		
11. LUNGS: rate, auscultation, percussion		
12. HEART: rate, rhythm, S_1, S_2, murmur, femoral pulses		
13. ABDOMEN: contour; palpation of liver, spleen, and kidney; mass; tenderness		
14. GENITALIA: ♀ external; ♂ penis, meatus, testes, hernia		
15. SPINE: curvature (scoliosis), sacral area		
16. EXTREMITIES: range of motion, tenderness, edema, clubbing		
17. NEUROLOGIC (SCREEN): cranial nerves 3, 4, 6, 7, and 12; gait; cerebellar function; motor system (strength, tone)		
18. NEUROLOGIC (COMPLETE): above plus other cranial nerves: sensory and motor systems (deep tendon reflexes, clonus)		

able to parents and cause few if any symptoms. Of greatest concern are disorders that are treatable if detected early but potentially serious when not detected. A routine examination will diagnose most such conditions (eg, congenital heart disease). A few conditions are detected only by a detailed examination (eg, retinoblastoma [red fundus reflection test], strabismus [corneal light reflection test], congenital hip dislocation [Ortolani maneuver, or restricted abduction], scoliosis, coarctation of the aorta [femoral pulses], hypertension, lower urinary tract obstruction [inquire about urine stream], imperforate hymen, and labial adhesions). Visual deficits (eg, refractive errors or color blindness) and hearing deficits can also be missed if appropriate testing is not included. Dental caries may be overlooked by physicians who assume, not always rightly, that their patients are receiving periodic dental examinations. Early cancer detection can be improved by teaching self-examination of the breasts or testes.

THE SCHOOL READINESS EXAMINATION

The preschool examination of the 4- or 5-year-old child should be designed to answer the basic question, "Is the child ready for school?" Auscultation of the heart and lungs at this time is probably far less important than noting any abnormalities of speech, hearing, or vision and determining if developmental age is commensurate with chronologic age, if attention span is adequate for learning, and if parents have adequately prepared the child for separation when entering school. These problems should also be investigated earlier, but they are of greatest significance at the preschool examination. A school readiness screening questionnaire is included in Figure 3–1.

Vision

Five to 10% of preschool children have some kind of visual impairment. The illiterate E chart, Snellen chart, STYCAR test, or Allen picture cards can be used for checking visual acuity, and each eye should be tested separately. Testing should be attempted at age 3. The 5-year-old child should have a visual acuity of 20/30 (6/9) or better in both eyes, and there should be no more than a 1-line difference between the 2 eyes. Suppression amblyopia affects 2–5% of children and must be detected early before permanent loss of vision occurs. Amblyopia is often secondary to strabismus, which can be detected by noting the position where light is reflected off both corneas or by the cover test. Alignment can be tested by 6 months of age.

Hearing

Hearing deficits occur in approximately 1% of young school children, and in 10% the loss is profound and bilateral. Most children with hearing loss have recurrent purulent otitis media or serious otitis media. Even children with a single episode of otitis media may have some degree of hearing impairment for 3–6 months after the acute episode. Although the losses are generally not too severe, if they occur at an inopportune time they may be sufficient to prevent an early school-age child from learning phonics; hence, the effect of the loss may be carried on and magnified throughout much of the school years (see Chapter 20). If such losses are detected before entry into school, some of the learning, behavior, and discipline problems that occur secondary to poor attention might be averted. Detection of such problems is as much a part of preventive pediatrics as is the immunization routine. Audiologic screening tests can be performed by nonprofessional technicians and should be a part of the preschool examination.

Speech

The child entering school should be able to speak distinctly and clearly without difficulty; should be able to answer questions; and, after a period of getting acquainted, should be able to carry on a conversation with the physician about recent events. Poor speech may impair performance in school. An easily administered screening articulation test—the Early Language Milestone Scale—has been developed to identify children who should be referred to a speech pathologist for definitive evaluation.

Emotional Development & Behavior

The assessment of emotional development and behavior is an important part of the preschool examination. In one study, 42 physicians were observed conducting 673 well-child clinic visits. On the average, they said fewer than 2 sentences per visit to the mother that were relevant to child behavior. Yet, when given the opportunity to respond to a questionnaire about behavior, 85% of mothers of preschool children (ages 1½–6 years) indicated one or more such concerns (mean of 3.5 concerns per child). A simple self-administered questionnaire is an effective and efficient device which not only indicates to the parent that the physician is interested in discussing behavioral problems and emotional growth but also helps the physician to concentrate on areas of guidance most relevant to the parent's concerns. The pediatric health maintenance forms (see Fig 3–1) stress anticipatory guidance and counseling for behavioral aspects of pediatrics. Developmental screening is discussed in Chapter 2.

LABORATORY SCREENING TESTS

A health maintenance flow sheet (Fig 3–2) is a helpful reminder to the nurse and physician that certain procedures, laboratory tests, developmental evaluations, and immunizations need to be done. All these items can be initiated by the nurse or aide if the physician establishes the routine to be followed.

Blood

Iron deficiency anemia (see Chapter 23) is found more often in lower socioeconomic populations and has its highest incidence in infants between 9 and 24 months of age. A routine hemoglobin or hematocrit is recommended in this age group and is particularly important in the child whose diet is low in iron-containing foods.

Children with sickle cell disease (see Chapter 23) must be diagnosed before 6 months of age to prevent death due to sepsis or splenic sequestration (10–20% mortality rate). Do not wait for the routine hematocrit at age 9 months. Prophylactic antibiotics should be started by 3 months of age. It is strongly recommended that all black newborns have hemoglobin electrophoresis performed on cord blood or in conjunction with heel-stick testing for phenylketonuria. If it is not done then, the test should be performed at the 2-month check-up.

All states now require screening for phenylketonuria (see Chapter 10) by blood test in the hospital nursery prior to the infant's discharge. An infant with this disorder who failed to ingest sufficient milk protein may have a negative test in the first few days of life. Therefore, most centers recommend a repeat test at 10–14 days of age if the first test was performed before 48 hours of age. Screening newborns for other treatable causes of mental retardation, congenital hypothyroidism, and galactosemia is required in most states and should be performed in all newborns regardless of the state law. A T_4 or TSH assay can be done by using cord blood.

Screening for lead poisoning (see Chapter 7) is extremely important in areas where the child has access to lead-based paint or soil contaminated by lead. Children living in such neighborhoods should have a routine blood lead level performed at 18–24 months of age. This test should be repeated at 6-month intervals until age 3 years in children with pica or where there is an index case in their building.

Routine cholesterol testing of all children is controversial. For now, the AAP recommends testing of those children who have a family history of hyperlipidemia or early myocardial infarction (< 50 years of age in men and < 60 in women). Since these criteria miss 50% of children with elevated cholesterol, all children may need screening. Testing should be performed at 2 to 3 years of age.

Urine

Routine urinalysis has a low yield in the asymptomatic patient. In contrast to the adult population, it is unusual for a child to have asymptomatic diabetes, and proteinuria is a rare presenting sign for renal abnormality in an asymptomatic child. Transient orthostatic proteinuria is common in adolescents but benign. While many physicians recommend that the urine dipstick test be performed only on symptomatic children, testing once at age 3 or 4 is not unreasonable.

In screening for asymptomatic urinary tract infection, microscopic examination of the urinary sediment is time-consuming and not reliable. Several inexpensive methods are available to screen a first-morning specimen for bacteriuria (eg, nitrite or glucose detection strips), followed by a urine culture if the dipstick test is positive. Since untreated asymptomatic bacteriuria usually clears spontaneously and does not lead to renal damage, screening should be reserved for high-risk groups (eg, children with diabetes). On the other hand, the clinician must not hesitate to check the urine for bacilluria in any child with unexplained fevers, unexplained abdominal pain, enuresis, foul-smelling urine, or other vague symptoms.

Teenage girls who are sexually active will benefit from annual gonococcal cultures, chlamydia cultures, and Papanicolaou smears. Birth control counseling and sexuality counseling can also be offered at this time.

IMMUNIZATIONS

A child's immunization status can be easily monitored on the health maintenance flow sheet (see Fig 3–2). A record of the child's immunizations should also be given to the parents and updated by the nurse as additional immunizations are given. The details of routine immunization of children are presented in Chapter 9.

Title: _____

Name: _____   Hosp. No.: _____   Date of Birth: _____

Directions: Record date only for all immunizations.
Record value for head circumference, height, weight, BP, and Hct.
Record N (normal) or ABN (abnormal) for all other items.

	NB	2 wk	2 mo	4 mo	6 mo	9 mo	12 mo	15 mo	18 mo	2 yr	3 yr	4 yr	5 yr	6 yr	8 yr	10 yr	12 yr	14 yr	16 yr	18 yr
Today's date																				
Head circumference																				
Height (cm)																				
Weight (kg)																				
BP																				
Dental caries screen																				
DTP (Td after 6 years)																				
OPV																				
Measles, mumps, rubella																				
Haemophilus influenzae type b conjugated vaccine																				

TB test[6]																				
PDQ or DDST = R[7]																				
Speech (ELM)																				
Hearing[1]																				
Vision[2]																				
Biochemical screen[3]																				
Hct																				
Sickle cell test for black patients[4]																				
Pap smear/GC[5]																				

LEGEND:

[1]High-risk inquiry (NB)
Listens to soft sounds (2m)
Turns to sound (6m)
Audiometrics (4y and thereafter)

[2]Red reflex (NB or 2w)
Regards smiling face (2m)
Follows past midline (4m)
Corneal light reflections test (6m)
Visual acuity (3y and thereafter)
Color vision once (6y)

[3]PKU, thyroid, galactosemia (newborn nursery)
PKU retest (2w) if first test done before 48 hours

[4]If not performed in newborn, perform at 2 months of age

[5]Sexually active patients

[6]High risk groups; TB test yearly

[7]Screen with PDQ if high school graduate. Screen with DDST=Revised if parent did not complete high school. If child fails PDQ or DDST=R, perform complete DDST.

Figure 3–2. Health maintenance flow sheet.

ACUTE ILLNESS VISITS

ASSESSING ACUTE ILLNESS

Optimal management of an acute illness mainly includes telephone triaging, office triaging, diagnosis, assessment of the need for hospitalization, home therapy, and a follow-up plan.

1. TELEPHONE TRIAGING & ADVICE

Does the Patient Need to Be Seen?

The physician is the person best qualified to give medical advice, both in the office and over the phone. However, because talking with parents on the phone may take up too much of the physician's time, this function is usually delegated to another member of the office team. Most of the questions are routine ones that require only routine answers. An office nurse specifically trained for the role is probably the best person to take routine calls. Office policies about medical advice over the phone should be standardized. Routine instructions for handling minor infections, minor injuries, reactions to immunizations, infant feeding problems, newborn care, and prescription refills are easy to communicate to parents if they are written down in an office protocol book. The protocol book should also specify the point at which each problem requires an office visit. This decision depends on (1) the type of symptom, (2) the duration of the symptom, (3) the age of the patient, (4) whether or not the patient acts "very sick," (5) an assessment of the parents' anxiety, and (6) the presence of any underlying chronic disease. (For example, most patients under 1 year of age with diarrhea and vomiting need to be examined.) After telephone baseline data are gathered, the nurse must be able to decide whether the child needs an appointment or not; the nurse should err on the side of giving an appointment when in doubt. For patients not seen, any pertinent telephone data should be entered on a temporary log sheet. If an office visit later becomes necessary, the data should be transferred to the patient's chart.

2. OFFICE TRIAGING & PROCEDURES

How Sick Is the Patient?

The nurse should screen all sick patients as soon as possible after they arrive at the office. They can be thought of in terms of 3 general groups: emergency, contagious, and minor illness. Most patients have a minor illness (eg, cold, accident, earache) and can be seen at their appointed time. Some patients are contagious until proved otherwise and should quickly be moved from the waiting room to an isolated examining room (eg, febrile illnesses with rashes, lice, jaundice, possible pertussis). An attempt should be made to keep children with bronchiolitis or croup away from infants. When an office emergency (eg, febrile seizures, respiratory distress) is recognized by the nurse, the physician should be notified immediately. The physician can take appropriate emergency action, stabilize the patient, and arrange for transfer to the hospital if necessary (eg, an acidotic, dehydrated infant).

Preparation of the Patient for the Physician

The office aide can record the sick patient's temperature, height, and weight. The office nurse can record the chief complaint. Depending upon the symptom, the nurse can take vital signs and initiate the office's standing orders on laboratory procedures and symptomatic treatment listed below.

Initial Treatment & Laboratory Workup

Steps in initial management are listed below. Details of procedures are outlined elsewhere in the text.

A. Abdominal Pain: Take samples for urinalysis and urine culture; save stool specimen for occult blood testing.

B. Animal Bite: Wash out immediately with benzalkonium chloride for 10 minutes. Initiate the official reporting form, and call the county health department. Delay irrigation if the wound is infected and a culture is needed.

C. Cough: If present over 1 month, apply a tuberculin skin test.

D. Diarrhea: Take a sample for stool culture if the stool contains blood or mucus or if diarrhea has persisted for more than 1 week at any age. For children under age 2, give 180 mL (6 oz) of an oral electrolyte solution, and record the naked weight on each visit. If a child appears dehydrated, collect urine for specific gravity.

E. Earache: Give acetaminophen if in obvious pain. If there is a possibility of mumps, isolate the patient.

F. Eye Injury: Test visual acuity if child is over age 3. Place eye tray in the examining room.

G. Fever: In children, the degree of fever may not reflect the severity of the disease process. Extremes of temperature may occur without relation to the significance of the infection. A small infant may have a very serious illness with normal or subnormal temperatures, whereas a 2- to 5-year-old child may have a fever above 40°C (104°F) with a minor respiratory infection. In children over age 8 years, temperature response is similar to that in adults.

Some children with high temperatures may convulse ("febrile convulsions"). Rapid elevation of temperature should therefore receive prompt care in the form of antipyretic therapy. Fever and convulsions may be the presenting findings of a central nervous system infection, and the patient may require a spinal tap for diagnostic evaluation. In general, fever as high as 41°C (105.8°F) is not in itself harmful.

For a fever over 39°C (102.2°F), give acetaminophen at 15 mg/kg per dose. Put the child in an examining room and assist with undressing. Give a sponge bath if the temperature exceeds 40°C (104°F) despite drugs and if the child is uncomfortable. Provide a bag for urine if the child is not toilet trained, and save urine in refrigerator for analysis and culture. If unexplained fever has been present over 24 hours, order a white count and differential. If the infant is under 2 months of age, notify the physician immediately.

H. Fractures: Notify physician immediately, obtain equipment to immobilize the site, and fill out the x-ray request.

I. Head Injury: Record vital signs and level of consciousness, and check pupils for equal size and reaction to light.

J. Infectious Hepatitis Exposure: Record weights of persons who have had intimate contact with the patient, and anticipate giving immune globulin, 0.03 mL/kg intramuscularly.

K. Lacerations: Wash thoroughly for at least 10 minutes. Check date of last tetanus shot and record. (The physician must decide whether tetanus booster or antitoxin is needed.) Shave around the wound edges if necessary (but never shave eyebrows). Have parents sign consent for suturing.

L. Nosebleed: Instruct the parent or child on how to compress the bleeding site for 10 minutes. Check blood pressure and perform fingerstick for hematocrit.

M. Painful Urination (Burning or Frequency): Take sample for urinalysis, urine culture, nitrite dipstick, and a gram-stained smear of unspun drop.

N. Pinworms: Record the approximate weights of all family members if the infection is a recurrent one (see Chapter 16).

O. Sore Throat: Take material for throat culture (contraindicated if the patient has croup).

P. Streptococcal Sore Throat (Culture Positive): Inquire about penicillin allergy and record. Arrange for symptomatic family contacts to have throat cultures taken.

Q. Vomiting: Record exact weight. Give patient emesis basin and sips of ice water while waiting. If patient appears dehydrated, collect urine for specific gravity.

3. THE WORKING DIAGNOSIS

The physician makes the final decision about the diagnosis and the severity of the disease. Emergency conditions (eg, shock or meningitis) may be noted and emergency intervention begun. History taking can be modified to emphasize the chief complaint. A history of recent contact with persons with contagious diseases is often important. Severity can be partially assessed by inquiries about playfulness, energy, ability to sleep, and the parent's feelings about how sick the child is this time compared with other times. If a family of sick children is brought in, the physician should ask the mother which children she considers the sickest. The physical examination should be mainly directed toward the chief complaint. A patient with a dog bite does not require a complete examination, but a patient with an earache must be checked for mastoid swelling and meningeal signs in addition to otoscopic examination.

Utilizing the conventional techniques of history, physical examination, and laboratory tests, the physician will correctly diagnose most acute chief complaints. However, a vigilant clinical mind is necessary in order not to miss a diagnosis of septicemia. Septic children usually present with unexplained fever, but (unlike children with acute viral fevers) they often will not smile or play, even with their parents. They frequently are physically exhausted and too weak to resist the physical examination, constantly irritable and unable to sleep, and respond paradoxically to cuddling by the mother. Irritability usually stems from pain or hypoxia. A less common finding in the toxic child is constant lethargy or sleepiness. This is difficult to assess because most sick children sleep more than normally. A child with suspected septicemia requires an intensive workup and therapy in a hospital setting. These more complicated acute illness evaluations can be expedited if the physician has studied appropriate decision-making algorithms.

4. INDICATIONS FOR HOSPITALIZATION

For every acute problem, the physician must decide whether to treat the child at home or in the hospital.

The 3 major indications for hospitalization are major emergencies, potentially life-threatening illnesses, and psychosocial problems.

Major Emergencies

Some examples of obvious life-threatening conditions are shock, severe dehydration, coma, meningitis (bacterial or of unknown cause), respiratory distress, congestive heart failure, symptomatic hypertension, acute renal failure, status epilepticus, and surgical emergencies.

Potentially Life-Threatening or Crippling Illnesses

Some patients are not in critical condition when first seen but require hospitalization because their problem may be rapidly progressive during treatment. If deterioration occurs in the hospital, emergency therapy can be rapidly instituted. Most of the entities in this group are caused by infection or trauma. Endogenous diseases rarely change this rapidly. Although absolute rules cannot be formulated for every situation, the following guidelines can be applied to most cases of acute illness. Obviously, these rules will have some exceptions, such as when the emergency room has an 8-hour observation area.

The following sections list problems that may require hospitalization, according to body systems:

A. Skin:
1. Cellulitis if the patient is less than 2 months old; if there is buccal involvement or the cavernous sinus drainage area is involved; if underlying sinusitis or osteomyelitis is suspected; if cellulitis is secondary to a puncture wound in the foot; or if there is no response after 2 days of therapy.
2. Erysipelas, toxic epidermal necrolysis, or acute necrotizing fasciitis. Omphalitis if the patient is less than 2 months old.
3. Suspected thrombophlebitis.
4. Burns (second- or third-degree) involving more than 10% of surface area (> 15% if the patient is more than 1 year old); burns of perineal area, hand, or face if they might need grafting; all inhalation burns; and most electrical burns.
5. Pupura with fever, without fever but unexplained, or without fever but progressive.

B. Eyes:
1. Gonococcal conjunctivitis or bacterial keratitis.
2. Eye injury if visual acuity is decreased.
3. Papilledema.

C. Ears, Nose, and Throat:
1. Acute otitis media if the patient is less than 1 month old

with fever, systemic symptoms, or no response after 2 days of therapy.
2. Mastoiditis.
3. Sinusitis if overlying redness or edema is present.
4. Nasal obstruction if the patient is less than 6 months old and an apneic episode has occurred.
5. Epistaxis if uncontrolled; if hypertension is present; if there is bleeding elsewhere; or if severe anemia is present.
6. Fluctuant tonsillar abscess.
7. Retropharyngeal abscess.
8. Diphtheria (any symptoms at any age).
9. Cervical adenitis if the patient is toxic, dehydrated, dysphagic, dyspneic, or less than 6 months old and needs treatment by incision and drainage.

D. Respiratory System:
1. Epiglottitis (all cases).
2. Viral laryngitis if there is stridor at rest, dyspnea, or drooling; if the child has repeatedly awakened from sleep with stridor; if there is a history of a previous bout with rapid progression; if there are apneic or cyanotic episodes; or if the patient is less than 1 year old and the stridor is easily provoked (eg, occurs with any crying).
3. Pertussis if symptomatic and the patient is less than 1 year old; pertussis at any age if accompanied by apnea, respiratory distress, a whoop, or weight loss.
4. Bronchiolitis if the patient is dyspneic, has a resting respiratory rate greater than 60, has apneic or cyanotic episodes ($P_{O_2} < 50$), has poor fluid intake, or is unable to sleep.
5. Asthma if respiratory distress persists after 2 injections of epinephrine or 2 nebulized doses of a beta-agonist.
6. Pneumonia if the patient is less than 1 month old; if bacterial pneumonia is suspected and the patient is less than 6 months old; if there is a history of dyspnea (any age); if there is pleural effusion; if staphylococcal pneumonia is suspected (any age); if aspiration pneumonia is present; if fluid intake is poor; if there is underlying cystic fibrosis or congenital heart disease; or if there is no response after 2 days of therapy.
7. Suspected foreign body of the airway.
8. Hemoptysis if unexplained; if there is bleeding elsewhere; or if anemia is present.
9. Apnea in all cases except periodic breathing, breath-holding spells, or mild choking on food.

E. Cardiovascular System:
1. Suspected subacute bacterial endocarditis.
2. Any myocarditis or pericarditis.
3. Acute hypertension or shock.
4. Unexplained dysrhythmias.

F. Gastrointestinal System:
1. Vomiting with dehydration, delirium, or persistent abdominal pain.
2. Hematemesis if documented and not caused by swallowed blood.
3. Diarrhea if explosive in character; if accompanied by abdominal distention or associated Kussmaul respirations; if typhoid fever is suspected in a patient of any age; if acute *Shigella* infection is suspected in a patient less than 1 year old; or in a patient who has moderate or mild dehydration with vomiting or fluid refusal.
4. Melena or unexplained bright-red blood mixed in the stools.
5. Suspected appendicitis, peritonitis, or intussusception.
6. Abdominal trauma if penetrating injury has occurred or if damage to the spleen, liver, kidneys, pancreas, or intestines is suspected.
7. Toxic ileus.

G. Urinary System:
1. Pyelonephritis if the patient is less than 2 months old, toxic, or unimproved after 2 days of therapy; if gram-negative sepsis is suspected; if underlying renal disease is present; or if recurrences have been frequent.
2. Acute edema, oliguria, or azotemia.
3. Hematuria with symptoms listed in (2), renal colic, and unexplained or posttraumatic gross hematuria.
4. Acute urinary retention.

H. Genitalia:
1. Vaginitis if associated with salpingitis.
2. Vaginal injury with sharp object.
3. Suspected testicular torsion.
4. Priapism.

I. Skeletal System:
1. Suspected osteomyelitis.
2. Arthritis if possibly septic or acute rheumatic fever.
3. Wringer injury if above the elbow; if a hematoma or avulsed skin is present; if a fracture or nerve injury is present; or if the peripheral pulse is diminished.

J. Nervous System:
1. Aseptic meningitis if the level of consciousness is depressed or there is a motor deficit.

2. Suspected tetanus.
3. Suspected epidural spinal abscess or brain abscess.
4. Febrile or afebrile seizures if they continue more than 30 minutes; if there are persistent neurologic signs; if the level of consciousness is decreased; or if serious underlying disease cannot be ruled out.
5. Head injury if the patient has been unconscious longer than 5 minutes; if there are persistent neurologic signs; if the level of consciousness is decreased; if a seizure has occurred; if cerebrospinal fluid rhinorrhea or otorrhea is present; if there is significant swelling over the middle meningeal artery; if there are retinal hemorrhages or progressive headaches; or if abnormal or irregular vital signs are present.
6. Skull fractures that are depressed or compound (ie, into air sinuses or overlying scalp laceration), fractures across the middle meningeal artery or venous sinus, occipital fracture into the rim of the foramen magnum, or any fracture with an underlying bleeding disorder.
7. Suspected spinal cord trauma.
8. Acute muscle weakness.
9. Acute cognitive deterioration, including delirium that is unexplained or persists longer than 2 hours.
10. Suspected increased intracranial pressure.

K. General:
1. Fever if the patient is less than 2 months old; if toxicity is evident and serious underlying disease cannot be ruled out; or if fever is due to heat stroke.
2. Poisoning if the patient is symptomatic (eg, respirations slow or irregular, drowsiness, etc); the agent or dosage is unknown; or the dosage is a potentially fatal one.
3. Suspected lead poisoning.
4. Unexplained mass.
5. Failure to thrive if severe or unexplained or if serious neglect is suspected.
6. Unexplained hypoglycemia.
7. Suspected anaphylactic reaction with laryngeal reaction, bronchospasm, hypotension, or dysrhythmias.

Psychosocial Problems

Patients with acute psychosocial problems now comprise a larger proportion of hospitalized children than was formerly the case. In many cities, the child can be placed in an emergency receiving home or an acute psychiatric ward. Sometimes the child can temporarily stay with a relative. Psychosocial indications for hospitalization fall into 3 general groups: parent, child, and disease problems.

A. Parent Problems:

1. Child abuse (eg, battering, failure to thrive secondary to neglect, or incest).
2. Incipient battering (eg, the parent has made a homicidal threat against a child).
3. Absent parents (eg, abandonment, emancipated minors without caretakers, or the parents themselves are hospitalized).
4. Physically exhausted parents (eg, no sleep for 2 nights).
5. Severely overanxious parents (eg, if the parents remain immobilized and extremely anxious after a careful explanation of their child's illness).
6. Neglectful parents who seem uninterested in their child's illness or therapy (eg, neglected eczema). This is a rare situation compared with overly anxious parents.
7. Intellectually incompetent parents (eg, a mentally retarded mother who cannot reliably follow verbal or written instructions).
8. Emotionally disturbed parents who need psychiatric hospitalization and treatment for their own problems (eg, a floridly psychotic mother).
9. Parent who is an alcoholic or drug abuser.

B Child Problems:

1. Suicide attempt—a short hospital admission allows time for the mental health worker to make an evaluation and for the family to look seriously at their problems.
2. A destructive, dangerous child can be held on a pediatric ward pending placement. A dangerous adolescent will require a psychiatric care facility.
3. An incapacitating emotional symptom (eg, a severe conversion reaction such as paraplegia or blindness).

C. Disease Problems:

1. An incapacitating (but not life-threatening) physical disease (eg, severe Syndenham's chorea).
2. Initial diagnosis of a disease with a complex treatment regimen. The parents and patient deserve a careful, unhurried, and organized introduction to the complex home management of some chronic diseases (eg, diabetes mellitus).
3. Initial diagnosis of a fetal disease—this gives the family time to work through the impact phase (eg, leukemia).
4. Terminal care if the family does not want the child to die at home.

5. Chronic diseases that are exacerbated by family conflicts (eg, ulcerative colitis).
6. Hazardous home (eg, carbon monoxide or lead poisoning).

Emotional Aspects of Hospitalization

Hospitalization nearly always involves some degree of psychic trauma, especially in a young child; the need for hospital care must therefore be balanced against the possible emotional consequences. The physician, parents, and hospital staff must try to minimize the psychologic effect of the hospital stay and the procedures involved during the time of the child's hospitalization. Above all, the child must be made to understand the parents' attitude. Candor and reassurance are never more important to a child than at this time. The physician can help by seeing to it that the practical affairs of running a hospital interfere as little as possible with the parents' visits.

Hospital personnel must be brought to a sympathetic awareness of the ill child's emotional needs. The child should be given a reasonable and candid explanation of what is likely to happen. If surgery is to be performed, children should be told how anesthesia will be administered and how they will feel and where they will be after surgery. Explanation and forewarning can make significant modifications in the emotional sequelae of hospitalization, whereas failure to prepare the child may have far-reaching psychologic consequences.

The emotional state of the parents must also be considered. It should be recognized that they may have a sense of guilt for the child's illness and that this reaction may be aggravated when hospitalization is necessary. Their defense mechanisms may be manifested by an inclination to blame others, including the physician.

5. TREATMENT OF THE NONHOSPITALIZED PATIENT

Words are as necessary as drugs in the treatment of a sick child. The parents expect to be told their child's diagnosis and its causes, prognosis, and treatment. They also need to have their special concerns acknowledged and clarified. If this communication does not take place, the parents will often be dissatisfied with the quality of care being given, and their compliance with regard to medications, advice, and follow-up will probably be less than optimal.

If the child has a mild acute illness (eg, viral nasopharyngitis), the parent would be reassured by the following general types of comment.

Diagnosis

"David has a cold." The diagnosis should be conveyed in plain English, not in medical jargon. If the physician does not specifically state the diagnosis, the parents may assume none has been arrived at.

Etiology

"It's due to a virus." This means to most parents that the infection is not serious. Some parents need an added statement that there was nothing they could have done to prevent it—eg, "Everyone is coming down with this."

Parents' Concerns

Mothers often do not listen to their physician's instructions until their own main concerns have been discussed. These concerns are easily elicited by Korsch's 3 questions: (1) "Why did you bring David to the clinic today?" (2) "What worried you most about him?" (3) "Why did that worry you?" After these concerns are out in the open, the physician is in a position to clarify misconceptions. Reassurance can be specific—eg, "He doesn't have meningitis," or, "It won't turn into leukemia."

Treatment

In self-limited disease, the goal of medication is to keep the patient comfortable. A list of useful approaches to management (sometimes overlooked) is as follows: (1) An antipyretic is useful if the patient's fever causes discomfort. (2) Dextromethorphan can be used for acute cough that interferes with sleep. (3) Teaching the parent how to suction the nose properly can turn a restless baby into a sleeping one. (4) Advice about diet and bed rest (see below) is also appreciated by the parent. (5) Isolation within the family structure is rarely indicated, since exposure has usually preceded the diagnosis. (6) Parents can be reassured about temporary moodiness and emotional regression during an acute illness. A return to the previous level of maturity need not be encouraged until good health returns.

A. Rest and Activity During Illness: During most acute illnesses, children may be allowed to establish their own limits of activity, since attempts to enforce bed rest often do more harm than good. Enforced bed rest often results in a crying and resentful child.

The ill child requires a great deal of reassurance and should be spared knowledge of the concern others may feel. It is important to minimize the child's anxiety by discussion and explanation and to avoid the detrimental effects of restlessness and unhappiness that result from overzealous limitations.

In convalescence from a serious illness, consideration should be given to properly controlled occupational and play therapy, a home teaching program for the school-age child, and extra periods of rest until the child is strong enough to do without them.

B. Nutrition During Illness: In the severely ill infant, breast-feeding may have to be temporarily discontinued. Regular emptying of the mother's breasts, manually or with a pump, may allow prompt reinstitution of breast-feeding when the child can again nurse. However, breast-feeding can be continued during most illnesses.

Acutely ill infants have a decreased ability to utilize fat and may have increased requirements for carbohydrates, water, and electrolytes to compensate for increased losses.

Acutely ill children, especially those with pain and fever, are generally anorexic and irritable. Often one cannot supply optimal food requirements during the acute phase of the illness but should provide the 3 items most needed: water, electrolytes, and sugar, especially to avoid ketosis. It is not unusual to give for several days a diet consisting only of such items as sweetened carbonated beverages, gelatin desserts, ice cream, sherbet, and applesauce.

Parents should be cautioned to avoid a struggle in feeding the ill child. In general, free choice and frequent small feedings at intervals of 1–2 hours are sufficient to maintain optimal water, electrolyte, and sugar intake during the acute phase of the illness. Requirements for protein should be met in the immediate convalescent period.

When the acute phase has passed, easily digestible solids that the child enjoys may be introduced. Hamburger patty, buttered toast, strained fruits and vegetables, and mashed potatoes with a small amount of butter are successful foods during this period.

Supplemental vitamin intake should be added through the convalescent period.

Prognosis

"David will probably feel better in 2 or 3 days. This is not a serious infection. If his fever lasts over 3 days or he gets worse, give me a call." Nothing is gained by mentioning all the possible complications. Without promoting anxiety, the door to additional medical evaluation is quietly left open for any new problems that might arise.

Closing

"You're doing a fine job with David. Just hold the fort and he will be his old self in a few days." The visit should close on a positive note, even a compliment if possible. If David is older, an attempt can be made to boost his morale as well—eg, "This won't keep *you* out of action for long."

6. FOLLOW-UP OF THE NONHOSPITALIZED PATIENT

Many children seen in an emergency room have conditions that require following (eg, asthma, bronchiolitis, croup, pneumonia, otitis media, burns, and seizures). If a child has an ambiguous diagnosis (eg, high fever of unknown origin) or an unpredictable course (eg, vomiting), daily follow-up is necessary. This protects both the patient and the physician. Follow-up can be accomplished by revisits, telephone calls, or a visiting nurse.

Revisits

Daily office visits are the best approach to the more serious problem. The weight of an infant with diarrhea and the degree of respiratory distress in a child with croup cannot be estimated over the phone. If a scheduled appointment is not kept, the office clerk should immediately notify the physician, and a phone call or home visit should be made on that same day. If transportation is a problem for the parent, a community service agency can usually help. If the late results of laboratory tests indicate that an illness is quite serious (eg, stool culture growing *Salmonella* in a 2-month-old infant) and reasonable attempts to locate the parents fail, the police may be asked to find and bring the patient to the clinic or office.

Telephone Calls

A daily telephone call will suffice for milder problems when only historical follow-up data are needed (eg, vomiting or lethargy). Since these calls are essential to proper management, the physician or nurse should make them. A daily telephone list can be kept and the charts pulled prior to calling. If the follow-up is felt to be important, parents should not be depended upon to initiate these calls. Telephone calls become the realistic choice of follow-up when long distances and cost are a factor.

MEDICOLEGAL PROBLEMS

The management of acute illness offers the greatest potential for malpractice litigation in pediatrics. Physicians are legally liable for damage proximately caused not only by their own mistakes but by the mistakes of their employees as well. Errors can be made in any of the areas previously discussed. An error in telephone triaging can result in a delay in diagnosis (eg, calling meningococcemia a viral exanthem, or arranging an appointment for the next day for scrotal pain that turns out to be a testicular torsion). An error in underhospitalization can lead to death (eg, epiglottitis being treated on an outpatient basis). Errors in therapy may result in sciatic nerve palsy if an injection is given into an inappropriate quadrant of the buttocks or may result in acute rheumatic fever if penicillin is not given for streptococcal sore throat because it was not cultured. Errors in follow-up can result in undiagnosed abdominal pain silently progressing to ruptured appendix. Consultation should be sought whenever a physician is uncertain about what is happening with an acutely and perhaps seriously ill patient.

MEDICAL CARE COMPLIANCE

Correct diagnoses and optimal therapeutic recommendations can be ensured by the voluntary type of peer review. An aspect of the quality of care not easy to assess by chart review but which needs to be borne in mind is patient compliance. Superb recommendations do not guarantee anything. Medical care does not become effective until the parent accepts the diagnosis and carries out the therapeutic recommendations. Compliance is improved by providing written instructions, including the parent in treatment planning, simplifying the treatment regimen, linking medication-taking with daily routines, explaining the reason for each treatment, and clarifying misconceptions. Strong parent–physician rapport also enhances compliance. The physician must make an effort to find out why appointments are not kept, medications are not given, etc; otherwise, even the best-conceived therapeutic goals will often not be achieved.

4 | Nutrition & Feeding

K. Michael Hambidge, MD, ScD

The act of feeding is important to the young child not only because of the nutritive substances obtained from the food but also because of the emotional and psychologic benefits derived. Drinking and eating are intense experiences to an infant and can and should be sources of great satisfaction. From these experiences and from the persons who feed them, infants obtain many of their early ideas about the nature of life and people.

Parents must be made to understand that there is much individual variation in the nutritional needs and desires of infants and that differences occur in the same child at various times.

The feeding of children is constantly being made more flexible and simple as knowledge of their nutritional requirements increases; however, certain basic information and data are necessary for a practical understanding of the subject.

Neither strict adherence to a time schedule nor feeding when the infant cries is necessary for successful and satisfactory feeding. For most parents and infants, a flexible schedule with reasonable regularity is most satisfactory, but in some cases either a strict routine or complete "demand" feeding gives better results.

BREAST-FEEDING

Advantages & Disadvantages

Apart from considerations of economy and convenience (temperature, asepsis, automatic adjustment in most instances to infant's needs), breast-feeding is superior to bottle-feeding because the composition of breast milk is ideal for nearly all infants; because breast milk has specific antibacterial and antiviral activities that protect infants from gastrointestinal disease; because breast-feeding produces less infantile allergy; and because breast-feeding can be psychologically beneficial to both mother and infant.

In the past decade, breast-feeding has been reestablished as the predominant mode of feeding the young infant in the United States. Unfortunately, breast-feeding rates remain low among several subpopulations of women, including low-income, minority, and young mothers. Many mothers face unique obstacles to maintaining lactation once they return to work. Skilled use of the breast pump may help to maintain lactation in this circumstance.

Breast-feeding may be temporarily impossible for a weak, ill, or premature infant or one with a cleft palate, although in such cases breast milk may be expressed and fed in another way.

Absolute contraindications to breast-feeding (eg, galactosemia) are rare. Maternal infection with human immunodeficiency virus and untreated tuberculosis are other contraindications.

Infants weighing less than 1500 g are likely to benefit from the addition of an infant milk fortifier to increase the density of energy, protein, calcium, and phosphorus. Some breast-fed infants with cystic fibrosis also will need a supplement.

Menstruation is not a contraindication to breast-feeding.

Transmission of Drugs & Toxins in Breast Milk

Virtually all drugs consumed by the mother will appear in her milk to some degree, usually in homeopathic amounts. Drug excretion into milk is affected by the drug's ionization, lipid solubility, protein binding, and molecular size, as well as other factors. Effects on the infant also depend upon the route of administration, the dosage, and the mother's timing in taking the drugs as well as the drug's metabolites and whether it is absorbed in the gastrointestinal tract. It is believed that the amount of drugs present in breast milk is least just before the mother takes medications.

Maternal use of illicit or recreational drugs is a contraindication to breast-feeding.

While it is wise to observe carefully a nursing infant whose mother is taking medications, very few drugs are actually contraindicated. Those that are include radioactive compounds, antimetabolites, lithium, diazepam (Valium), chloramphenicol, and tetracycline. A regional drug center should be consulted for up-to-date information on which drugs are contraindicated. When a course of therapy of a potentially hazardous drug will be brief, the mother can temporarily interrupt breast-feeding and maintain her supply by expressing and discarding her milk.

Composition of Breast Milk (Table 4–1)

Favorable features of human milk include an optimal amino acid and protein content for the normal infant; a generous, but not excessive, quantity of essential fatty acids; an adequate but

Table 4–1. Composition of milk and commercial formula (per 100 ml).*

Component	Unit	Human Milk	Typical Commercial Formula	Whole Cow's Milk
Osmolality	mosm/kg water	282	290	275
Energy	kcal	67	67	61
Carbohydrate (lactose)	g	7.3	7.2	4.7
Fat	g	4.2	3.8	3.3
Minerals				
Calcium	mg	25	51	119
Chloride	mg (meq)	40 (1.1)	53 (1.5)	102 (2.9)
Copper	µg	35	41	30
Fluorine	µg	7	20	15
Iodine	µg	7	10	5
Iron	µg	40	150 (1200 w/Fe)	50
Magnesium	mg	3	41	13
Manganese	µg	0.4	3	2–4
Phosphorus	mg	15	39	93
Potassium	mg (meq)	58 (1.5)	78 (2)	152 (3.9)

	mg (meq)	15 (0.8)	25 (1.1)	49 (2.1)
Sodium	µg			
Zinc		100–300	500	300
Proteins				
Casein	mg	187	1185	2700
Lactalbumin	mg	161	52	400
Total proteins	g	0.9	1.5	3.3
Vitamins				
A (retinol equivalents)	µg (IU)	47 (155)	75 (250)	31 (126)
B_6 (pyridoxine)	µg	28	40	42
B_{12} (cyanocobalamin)	ng	26	150	357
C (ascorbic acid)	mg	4	5.5	0.9
D	µg (IU)	0.04 (1.6)	1 (40)	1 (42)
E (total tocopherols)	µg (IU)	315 (0.32)	1700 (1.7)	80 (0.08)
K	µg	0.21	3	6
Folic acid	µg	5.2	5	5
Niacin	µg	200	790	84
Pantothenic acid	µg	225	300	314
Riboflavin	µg	35	100	162
Thiamine	µg	16	65	30

* Adapted from various sources.

relatively low sodium content; a low solute load compared with cow's milk; and very favorable absorption of iron, calcium, and zinc, which results in the provision of adequate quantities of these nutrients to the infant fully breast-fed for 4–6 months.

Breast-fed infants do require standard neonatal prophylactic vitamin K and may require vitamin D supplements if not exposed to any sunlight or if maternal vitamin D status is suboptimal. Breast milk will be low in vitamin B_{12} if the mother is an unsupplemented vegetarian; low in thiamine if the mother abuses alcohol; and low in folate if the mother is generally malnourished.

Management of Breast-feeding

Because today's grandmothers predominantly bottle-fed their children, the "art" of breast-feeding is no longer automatically passed from mother to daughter. Hence, the role of the health professional in supporting and promoting breast-feeding is of utmost importance.

Perinatal hospital routines and follow-up pediatric care have a great impact on the successful initiation of breast-feeding. Breast-feeding is promoted by prenatal and postpartum education, frequent mother/baby contact after delivery, one-on-one advice about breast-feeding technique, demand feeding, rooming in, avoidance of bottle supplements, early follow-up after delivery, maternal confidence, family support, adequate maternity leave, and accurate advice for common problems such as sore nipples. Breast-feeding is undermined by mother and baby separations, feeding babies in the nursery at night, routinely offering supplemental bottles, conflicting advice from staff, incorrect infant positioning and latch-on, scheduled feedings, lack of maternal confidence or support, delayed follow-up, early return to employment, and inaccurate advice for common breast-feeding difficulties.

Before discharge, individualized assessment should identify those mother/baby pairs needing additional support. In all such cases, there should be early follow-up after discharge. The onset of copious milk secretion between the second and fourth postpartum day is a critical time in the establishment of lactation.

A. Prelactation (Colostrum) Phase: Colostrum is an alkaline, yellow, breast secretion that may be produced during the last few months of pregnancy and for the first 2–4 days after delivery. It has a higher specific gravity (1.040–1.060); a higher content of protein, fat-soluble vitamins, and minerals; and a lower content of carbohydrate and fat than does breast milk.

Colostrum contains secretory IgA, leukocytes, and other

immune substances that play a part in the immune defenses of the newborn. Colostrum has a natural laxative action and is an ideal starter food.

Although the milk may not "come in" until 2–4 days after delivery, prelactation nursing is very important because of the value of colostrum, the effect of the nursing stimulus to increase milk supply and lessen engorgement, and the opportunity nursing provides for the mother and infant to become accustomed to one another. While some infants nurse irregularly the first few days, others demand feeding as often as every 2 hours. Nursing is commonly limited to 5 minutes per breast per feeding the first day, 10 minutes per breast per feeding the second day, and 15 minutes or longer per breast per feeding thereafter.

There is no need for routine supplementation for the full-term, healthy infant who appears satisfied, but when the infant is persistently hungry or has an underlying condition (eg, hypoglycemia) requiring increased caloric intake, then formula may be offered after nursing until the milk comes in. Once milk is in, further supplements should not be given.

B. Lactation Phase: Forty-eight to 96 hours postpartum, the mother's breasts change from soft to firm and full as engorgement (lactogenesis) occurs. The infant may be fed at each hungry period, day and night, which is usually every 2–3 hours during the first month with longer intervals (4–5 hours) at night. The infant should nurse at the first breast for approximately 10 minutes and then be put to the other breast and allowed to suckle as long as required (unless the nipples are sore). At the next feeding, the last breast nursed should be offered first. During the early weeks of lactation, the milk supply seems to be more sensitive to negative stimuli such as maternal fatigue, anxiety, and lack of suckling. The infant will usually have frequent, somewhat loose bowel movements (often with each feeding) during this period.

The let-down reflex, by which milk is actively ejected through the duct system for easy access ro the infant, is usually conditioned and evident by 2 weeks. The mother feels "tightening," "stinging," "tingling,"or "burning" circumferentially in both breasts shortly after the infant begins nursing. The nursing mother should eat a well-balanced diet with additional intake of protein, calcium, and fluids. Drinking a glass of liquid with each nursing is helpful. Additional rest, with several naps each day, should be encouraged.

"Frequency days," or "appetite spurts" when infants desire to nurse more often than their established routine, typically occur for several days at approximately 3 weeks, 6 weeks, 3 months, and 6 months of age. Increased frequency of nursing increases the milk supply and allows resumption of the former nursing schedule.

A woman with activities outside the home should feel free to take her nursing infant with her and breast-feed discreetly when the infant is hungry.

Problems with Breast-feeding

A. Failure to Thrive: Some breast-fed infants fail to thrive. The most common cause of early failure to thrive is poorly managed mammary engorgement, which will rapidly decrease milk supply. Unrelieved engorgement can result from inappropriately long intervals between feeding, improper infant suckling, a nondemanding infant, sore nipples, maternal or infant illness, nursing from only one breast, and latching difficulties. Poor maternal knowledge and lack of maternal fluids and rest can all be factors. Some infants are too sleepy to do well on an ad libitum regimen and, in particular, may need waking to feed at night. Primary lactation failure is rare but does occur. Some decline in weight for age percentiles after 3 months should not necessarily be taken as an indication of inadequate nutrition, since the commonly used percentile charts have been constructed from data on infants who have been primarily formula-fed. However, if there is a decline in weight-for-length of more than 20 percentile points, solids should be introduced earlier than may otherwise be intended and formula supplement may be indicated for individual infants.

B. Breast-feeding Jaundice: Breast-feeding jaundice is exaggerated physiological jaundice associated with inadequate intake of breast milk, infrequent stooling, and unsatisfactory weight gain. Where possible, this condition should be managed by increasing the frequency of nursing and, if necessary, augmenting the infant's suckling with regular breast pumping. Supplemental feedings may be necessary but care should be taken not to decrease breast-milk production further.

C. Breast-milk Jaundice: In a small percentage of breast-fed infants, breast-milk jaundice occurs as the result of an unidentified property of the milk that inhibits conjugation of bilirubin or deconjugates bile in the lumen of the small intestine. In severe cases, interruption of breast-feeding for 24–36 hours may be necessary. The mother's breast should be emptied with an electric breast pump during this period.

D. Sore Nipples: Mild nipple tenderness requires attention to proper positioning of the infant and correct latch-on. Ancillary measures include nursing for shorter periods, beginning feeds on the less sore side, air drying the nipples after nursing, and the application of lanolin cream. Severe nipple pain and cracking usually indicate improper infant attachment. Temporary pumping, which is well tolerated, may be needed.

E. Mastitis: Maternal mastitis should be suspected when a nursing mother complains of a "flu-like" illness, with local breast tenderness. Antibiotic therapy providing coverage against beta-lactamase–producing organisms should be given for 10 days. Analgesics may be necessary but breast-feeding should be continued. Breast pumping may be a helpful adjunctive therapy.

FORMULA FEEDING

The standard milk-based infant formulas (Table 4–2) contain heat-treated protein (at reduced concentration), lactose and minerals from cow's milk, vegetable oils, minerals, and vitamin additives. Iron-fortified formulas are recommended after 2 months. Standard formulas contain 20 kcal/oz and 0.45 g protein/oz.

Evaporated milk formula can be used as an alternative to proprietary infant formulas. It is prepared as follows: To make 32 oz of formula, mix 1 can (13 oz) of whole evaporated milk, 1½ cans (19 oz) of water, and 2 tablespoons of corn syrup. To make 5 oz, mix 2 oz of evaporated milk, 3 oz of water, and 1 teaspoon of corn syrup.

Infants should be fed formula for a minimum of 6 months—or, ideally, for the entire first year of life. Low-fat and skimmed milk are inappropriate for use in the first year of life.

Lactose intolerance is the main indicator for a soy-based formula, which may be used for a period of 2–4 weeks during recovery from acute gastroenteritis. Semi-elemental formulas have a wide range of uses in intestinal disease, including malabsorption syndromes, chronic diarrhea, and short-bowel syndrome. They are also used in infants who are intolerant of cow's protein and soy protein. Elemental formulas also find some applications in infancy, for example, when continuous drip feeding is indicated in infants with cystic fibrosis. Special formulas are marketed for several inborn metabolic diseases and for a variety of disease states. The latter should be used only for specific clinical indications in individual subjects. Polycose and medium-chain triglycerides are used as formula supplements. Increasing the concentration of the formulas to provide > 24 kcal/oz is preferable if the aim is an overall increase in nutrient density.

Table 4–2. Selected normal and special infant formulas.*

Product	Protein Source, Amount	CHO Source, Amount	Fat Source, Amount	Indications for Use	Comments (Nutritional Adequacy)
Milk-based formulas					
Enfamil (Mead Johnson)†	Nonfat cow's milk, reduced mineral whey, 1.5 g/dl	Lactose, 6.9 g/dl	Coconut, soy oils, 3.8 g/dl	For full-term and premature infants with no special nutritional requirements	Available fortified with iron, 12 mg/L; whey:casein ratio 60:40
Similac (Ross)†	Nonfat cow's milk, 1.5 g/dl	Lactose, 7.2 g/dl	Coconut, soy oils, 3.6 g/dl	Same as Enfamil	Available fortified with iron, 12 mg/L
SMA (Wyeth)†	Nonfat cow's milk, demineralized whey, 1.5 g/dl	Lactose, 7.2 g/dl	Oleo, coconut, safflower, soy oils, 3.6 g/dl	Same as Enfamil	Supplemented with iron, 12 mg/L; whey:casein ratio 60:40
Soy-protein formulas					
Isomil (Ross)	Soy, 1.8 g/dl	Sucrose, corn sugar,‡ 6.8 g/dl	Coconut, soy oils, 3.7 g/dl	For infants with lactose intolerance or milk-protein allergy	
Nursoy (Wyeth)	Soy protein isolate, 2.1 g/dl	Sucrose, 6.9 g/dl	Oleo, coconut, safflower, soy oils, 3.6 g/dl	Same as Isomil	

Product	Protein source	Carbohydrate source	Fat source	Indications	Comments
ProSoBee (Mead Johnson)	Soy protein isolate with added L-methionine, 2.0 g/dl	Corn syrup solids, 6.6 g/dl	Soy, coconut oils, 3.5 g/dl	Same as Isomil	
Products for premature infants					
Enfamil Premature Formula (Mead Johnson)	Nonfat cow's milk demineralized whey, 2.4 g/dl	Lactose, corn syrup solids, 8.9 g/dl	MCTs (coconut source), corn, coconut oils, 4.1 g/dl	For rapidly growing low-birth-weight infants	Protein, 3 g/100 kcal; Ca:P ratio, 2:1; E:PUFA ratio ‖, 1.7:1. Supplemental vitamin E is recommended
Preemie SMA (Wyeth)	Nonfat cow's milk, whey protein concentrate, 2.0 g/dl	Lactose, glucose polymers, 8.6 g/dl	MCTs, oleo, oleic, soy, coconut oils, 4.4 g/dl	Same as Enfamil Premature Formula	Protein, 2.5 g/100 kcal; osmolality, 268 mosm/kg water
Similac 24 Special Care (Ross)	Cow's milk, 2.2 g/dl	Lactose, glucose polymers, 8.5 g/dl	MCTs, coconut, soy oils, 4.3 g/dl	Same as Enfamil Premature Formula	Protein, 2.7 g/100 kcal; E:PUFA ratio ‖ 2:1; osmolality, 300 mosm/kg water
Partially demineralized whey formulas					
Similac PM 60/40 (Ross)	Whey, casein, 1.6 g/dl	Lactose, 6.8 g/dl	Coconut, corn oils, 3.7 g/dl	For newborns predisposed to hypocalcemia and infants with renal or heart disease	Ca:PO$_4$ ratio, 2:1; low phosphorus; relatively low solute load; Na = 7 meq/l

(continued)

Table 4–2. (Continued)

Product	Protein Source, Amount	CHO Source, Amount	Fat Source, Amount	Indications for Use	Comments (Nutritional Adequacy)
Semi-elemental formulas					
Nutramigen (Mead Johnson)	Casein hydrolysate, 1.9 g/dl	Modified corn starch, corn syrup solids, 9.0 mg/dl	Corn oil, 2.6 g/dl	For infants and children intolerant of food proteins and for galactosemic patients	
Pregestamil (Mead Johnson)	Casein hydrolysate, 70% amino acids, 30% peptides, 1.9 g/dl	Corn syrup solids, 6.9 g/dl	60% MCTs, 20% corn oil, 20% high oleic safflower, 3.8 g/dl	For infants with malabsorption syndromes	Contains added iron and vitamins
Other formulas for malabsorption syndromes					
Alimentum (Ross)	Casein hydrolysate, 1.8 g/dl	71% sucrose, 29% modified tapioca starch, 6.5 g/dl	50% MCTs, 40% safflower oil, 10% soy oil	Same as Pregestamil	
Portagen (Mead Johnson)	Sodium caseinate, 2.3 g/dl	Sucrose, corn syrup solids, 7.7 g/dl	MCTs (coconut source), corn oil, 3.2 g/dl	For management of chyluria, intestinal lymphangiectasia, various forms of steatorrhea, biliary atresia	88% MCTs, oil

	Protein source	Carbohydrate source	Fat source	Indications	Comments
Elemental formula					
Tolerex (Norwich Eaton)	Free amino acids, 2.1 g/dl	Glucose, oligosaccharides, 22.6 g/dl	Safflower oil, 0.5 g/dl	Use limited in infants; eg, nocturnal tube feeding in cystic fibrosis	Osmolality 550 mosm/kg water at 1 kcal/ml. Use at ≤ 2/3 strength for infants
Products for infants with inborn errors					
Lofenalac (Mead Johnson)	Casein hydrolysate, L-amino acids	Corn syrup solids, modified tapioca starch	Corn oil	For infants and children with phenylketonuria	Must be supplemented with other foods to provide minimal phenylalanine
MSUD Diet (Mead Johnson)	L-Amino acids	Corn syrup solids, modified tapioca starch	Corn oil	For children with branched-chain ketoaciduria	Leucine-, isoleucine-, and valine-free; must be supplemented
Phenyl-Free (Mead Johnson)	L-Amino acids	Sucrose, corn syrup solids, modified tapioca starch	Corn oil	For children over 1 year of age with phenylketonuria	Phenylalanine-free. Permits increased supplementation with normal foods

(continued)

Table 4-2. (*Continued*)

Product	Protein Source, Amount	CHO Source, Amount	Fat Source, Amount	Indications for Use	Comments (Nutritional Adequacy)
Product 3232A (Mead Johnson)	Enzymatically treated casein	Modified tapioca starch	MCT,§ corn oil	Protein hydrolysate formula base for use in diagnosis and nutritional management of infants with disaccharidase deficiencies	Monosaccharide- and disaccharide-free powder
Product 80056 (Mead Johnson)	None	Corn syrup solids, modified tapioca starch	Corn oil	For formulation of special diets for infants requiring specific mixtures of amino acids	Protein-free; carbohydrate, fat, vitamin, and mineral mix

* Committee on Nutrition, American Academy of Pediatrics: Commentary on breast feeding and infant formulas including proposed standards for formulas. *Pediatrics* 1976;**57**:278. Committee on Nutrition, American Academy of Pediatrics: Nutritional needs of low-birthweight infants. *Pediatrics* 1977;**60**:519.
† Ready-to-use, concentrated liquid, and powder forms.
‡ Composed of glucose, maltose, and dextrins.
§ Medium-chain triglycerides (MCT).
‖ Ratio of vitamin E (E) to polyunsaturated fatty acids (PUFA).

Preparation of the Formula

(1) The formula should be mixed correctly. *No* water is added to ready-to-feed preparations. Most concentrated formulas are mixed 1:1 with water. Most powdered formulas are mixed in proportions of 1 scoop (which comes in the can) to 2 oz of water.

(2) Sterilization of formula, water, bottles, and nipples is not required if the equipment is washed well with hot soapy water and a hygienic water supply is available. It is best to prepare only one bottle of formula at a time. If bottles of formula must be stored before being used, they must be sterilized.

(3) If the nipple holes are the right size, a drop of milk will form on the end of the nipple when the cool bottle is turned upside down and will drop off with little shaking of the bottle.

Feeding the Infant

(1) The bottle should be held, not propped.

(2) More water may be added to the formula if the infant consistently finishes each bottle and caloric intake is adequate.

(3) The infant need not empty every bottle.

(4) The infant should be "burped" during and at the end of feeding.

(5) After feeding, the infant should be placed on the side (preferably the right side) or prone.

(6) A few ounces of water may be offered between feedings once or twice a day, especially during excessively hot weather or during febrile illnesses.

Vitamin Supplements

Infants who are fed most complete proprietary infant formulas require no additional vitamin supplements. Those fed evaporated milk formula should have daily supplements of vitamins C and D. Supplemental vitamin D, generally recommended for breast-fed infants, is most conveniently given as a multivitamin liquid preparation.

Supplemental vitamins are usually unnecessary for the older child who is eating a relatively well balanced diet. Ingestion of more than the daily dietary requirement of vitamins is unnecessary and potentially harmful.

Night Feedings

Infants will "sleep through the night" (8-hour interval between feedings) at an average age of approximately 6 weeks (range, newborn to 15 months). There is no correlation between the interval between feedings at night and such things as the infant's age when solids are added to the diet, type of milk offered, or caloric intake.

Weaning

Small amounts of fluid may be offered from a cup when the infant is about age 6 months. The infant should not be allowed to nurse from the bottle throughout the night, because this is associated with "bottle-mouth caries." Weaning from the bottle is best done gradually and may not be completed until the child is over 1 year old.

"SOLID" FOODS

(1) Solid foods can be introduced gradually starting at age 4–6 months. Solids should not be introduced until the infant can sit with support and show good control of the head and neck. The infant should be able to indicate a desire for food by opening the mouth and leaning forward and to indicate disinterest by leaning back and turning away.

Start with an iron-fortified cereal, preferably rice. This may be followed by pureed vegetables, fruits, strained meat, and egg yolks. Junior-type foods can be introduced at age 7–8 months.

(2) There is no exact order for starting solid foods. The first physiologic requirement for foods other than milk occurs at about age 4–6 months, when a need for iron develops. When solid foods are started, they should initially be given in small amounts for several consecutive days to determine the infant's reaction and any adverse response. The amount should be gradually increased if the food is well tolerated. If the infant continues to refuse a food, another food may be tried; if that is also rejected, discontinue the attempt for 1–2 weeks before trying again. Foods prepared commercially have no nutritional advantage over those prepared at home, provided that the foods prepared at home are not seasoned.

(3) Many infants can learn to take semisolid food from a small spoon by age 4 months. If the infant cannot master spoon-feeding, postpone the attempt for a few weeks; otherwise, undesirable behavior may result and may make spoon-feeding difficult for months.

(4) The transition from strained to chopped foods should be gradual and may be started when the infant begins to make chewing motions.

(5) Egg white, wheat, orange juice, corn, and other allergenic foods should not be given (especially when there is a family predisposition to allergy) until the child is in the latter part of the first year of life.

(6) Infants should be allowed to feed themselves with fingers or a spoon when they wish to do so.

(7) Avoid feeding nuts, popcorn, and other foods that are easily aspirated to all children under age 4 years.

NUTRIENT REQUIREMENTS

Recent estimates of energy requirements for infants, based on measurements of energy expenditure and energy intakes of breast-fed infants, are lower than earlier figures (Table 4–3). The components of energy expenditure are given in Table 4–4. There are wide individual variations in energy requirements. In general, appetite and, especially, growth provide useful guides. Protein requirements for infants are also given in Table 4–3. These have also recently undergone downward revision. Infants require 43% and children 36% of their protein as essential amino acids. Cysteine, tyrosine, and taurine are considered partially essential in the premature infant.

Infants should receive 45–50% of their calories as fat until age 2 years, after which fat consumption should be reduced to < 30% of calories. At least 2% of calories should be provided as essential fatty acids of the $\omega 6$ series, and up to 1% as the $\omega 3$ series.

Medium-chain triglycerides (MCTs), energy density 7.6 kcal/g, are not essential in the normal diet but are invaluable in malabsorption syndromes. MCTs are especially useful when bile secretion is diminished or absorption and transport of long-chain fatty acids is impaired by other mechanisms. MCTs are very readily absorbed without mycelle formation and are transported via the portal circulation directly to the liver where they undergo rapid beta-oxidation (without the need for carnitine) or ketogenesis.

Recommended dietary allowances (RDAs), which exceed the actual requirements of most individuals, are given in Table 4–5. The utility of the RDAs is especially limited for young infants because recommendations cover a wide age range at a time when physiological changes are occurring rapidly. It should be emphasized that the RDAs are not designed to provide guidelines for individual requirements.

Table 4–3. Guide to protein, energy, and fluid requirements of infants and frequency of feeds.*

Age (mo)†	0	1	2	3	4	5	6	7	8	9	10	11	12
Calories (kcal/kg/d)	120	115	105		95				90				
Protein (g/kg/day)		2.25 0–3 months		2.0 3–4 months		1.7 4–6 months					1.5 6–12 months		
Fluid		130–200 mL/kg/d (2–3 oz/lb/d)				130–165 mL/kg/d (2–2.5 oz/lb/d)					130 mL/kg/d (2 oz/lb/d)		
Number of feedings (per day)	6–7			5–7	4–5				3–4				3
Amount (oz) per feeding	2.5–4	3.5–5	4–6	5–7	6–8					7–9			

* Some prepared milk formulas may be deficient in vitamins C and D and need to be supplemented with vitamins (25–50 mg of vitamin C and 400 units of vitamin D daily). Iron supplementation of formulas is recommended after 2 months.
† Underweight or overweight infants generally have the same food requirements as do infants of the same age with a normal weight. Undiluted whole milk or formulas of equal parts of evaporated milk and water should not be used for young infants, since their kidneys do not have a range of safety in the event of high environmental or body temperature.

Table 4–4. Approximate daily expenditure of calories during the first year of life.

Use	Amount (kcal/kg/d)
Basal metabolism	50
Thermic effect of foods	5
Caloric loss in the excreta	10
Allowance for bodily activity*	2–20
Growth	50 → 10
Total	120 → 90

* Range is for infants up to 1 month old to those 6–12 months old.

NUTRIENT DEFICIENCIES AND EXCESSES

Failure to Thrive

Failure to thrive (FTT) is a term that is commonly applied to mild or moderate undernutrition. Errors in diet or feeding technique (eg, wrong dilution of formula, inadequate breast-feeding, too-small holes in bottle nipples) account for about 20% of cases of FTT. Thirty percent are secondary to organic disease, and 50% result from nutritional deprivation. Whatever the primary event, malnutrition is the final common pathway and the pattern of impaired growth is "wasting," that is, a low weight-for-length percentile with the weight-age declining earlier and more severely than the length-age. However, the end result, if not effectively treated at an early stage, is "stunting," which is characterized by a low height-for-age percentile and relatively normal weight-for-height percentile. "Stunting" of nutritional origin is usually seen only after infancy in the United States but frequently occurs before 6 months of age in less developed countries. Stunting must be distinguished from endocrinopathy and structural dystrophia. If the head circumference is severely affected the differential diagnosis includes primary central nervous system disease, severe intrauterine growth retardation, or very severe and early FTT.

For malnourished infants, requirements can be based on ideal body weight (ie, 50th percentile weight-for-height age) or by calculating energy required for the desired "catch-up" growth (5 kcal/g new tissue). Protein requirements also increase during "catch-up" growth (0.2 g protein/g new tissue). Weight velocity during rehabilitation of wasted infants is up to 20 times normal but in stunting does not exceed 3 times normal.

Table 4–5a. Recommended allowances of reference protein, U.S. dietary protein, and fat-soluble vitamins.[1]

Category	Age (years) or Condition	Weight (kg)	Derived Allowance of Reference Protein[2] (g/kg)[7]	Derived Allowance of Reference Protein[2] (g/day)	Recommended Dietary Allowance (g/kg)[3]	Recommended Dietary Allowance (g/day)	Fat-Soluble Vitamins Vitamin A (μgRE)[4]	Fat-Soluble Vitamins Vitamin D (μg)[5]	Fat-Soluble Vitamins Vitamin E (mg α-TE)[6]	Fat-Soluble Vitamins Vitamin K (μ)
Both sexes	0–0.5	6	2.20		2.2	13	375	7.5	3	5
	0.5–1	9	1.56		1.6	14	375	10	4	10
	1–3	13	1.14		1.2	16	400	10	6	15
	4–6	20	1.03		1.1	24	500	10	7	20
	7–10	28	1.00		1.0	28	700	10	7	30
Males	11–14	45	0.98		1.0	45	1,000	10	10	45
	15–18	66	0.86		0.9	59	1,000	10	10	65
	19–24	72	0.75		0.8	58	1,000	10	10	70
	25–50	79	0.75		0.8	63	1,000	5	10	80
	51+	77	0.75		0.8	63	1,000	5	10	80
Females	11–14	46	0.94		1.0	46	800	10	8	45

15–18	55	0.81	0.8	44	800	10	8	55
19–24	58	0.75	0.8	46	800	10	8	60
25–50	63	0.75	0.8	50	800	5	8	65
51+	65	0.75	0.8	50	800	5	8	65
Pregnancy 1st trimester		+1.3		+10	800	10	10	65
2nd trimester		+6.1		+10	800	10	10	65
3rd trimester		+10.7		+10	800	10	10	65
Lactation 1st 6 months		+14.7		+15	1,300	10	12	65
2nd 6 months		+11.8		+12	1,200	10	11	65

[1] Modified and reproduced, with permission, from Subcommittee on the Tenth Edition of RDAs, Food and Nutrition Board, Commission on Life Sciences, National Research Council: *Recommended Dietary Allowances*, 10th ed. National Academy Press, 1989.

[2] Data from WHO (1985).

[3] Amino acid score of typical USA diet is 100 for all age groups, except young infants. Digestibility is equal to reference proteins. Values have been rounded upward to 0.1 g/kg.

[4] Retinol equivalents. 1 retinal equivalent = 1 μg retinol or 6 μg β-carotene.

[5] As cholecalciferol. 10 ug cholecalciferol = 400 IU of vitamin D.

[6] α-Tocopherol equivalents. 1 mg d-α tocopherol = 1 α-TE.

[7] For infants 0 to 3 months of age, breast-feeding that meets energy needs also meets protein needs. Formula substitutes should have the same amount and amino acid composition as human milk, corrected for digestibility if appropriate.

85

Table 4–5b. Recommended daily dietary allowances.*† (Water-soluble vitamins.)

								Water-Soluble Vitamins				
Category	Age (years) or Condition	Weight‡ (kg)	(lb)	Height‡ (cm)	(in)	Vitamin C (mg)	Thiamin (mg)	Riboflavin (mg)	Niacin (mg NE)§	Vitamin B^6 (mg)	Folate (μg)	Vitamin B^{12} (μg)
Infants	0.0–0.5	6	13	60	24	30	0.3	0.4	5	0.3	25	0.3
	0.5–1.0	9	20	71	28	35	0.4	0.5	6	0.6	35	0.5
Children	1–3	13	29	90	35	40	0.7	0.8	9	1.0	50	0.7
	4–6	20	44	112	44	45	0.9	1.1	12	1.1	75	1.0
	7–10	28	62	132	52	45	1.0	1.2	13	1.4	100	1.4
Males	11–14	45	99	157	62	50	1.3	1.5	17	1.7	150	2.0
	15–18	66	145	176	69	60	1.5	1.8	20	2.0	200	2.0
	19–24	72	160	177	70	60	1.5	1.7	19	2.0	200	2.0
	25–50	79	174	176	70	60	1.5	1.7	19	2.0	200	2.0
	51+	77	170	173	68	60	1.2	1.4	15	2.0	200	2.0

Females	11–14	46	101	157	62	50	1.1	1.3	15	1.4	150	2.0
	15–18	55	120	163	64	60	1.1	1.3	15	1.5	180	2.0
	19–24	58	128	164	65	60	1.1	1.3	15	1.6	180	2.0
	25–50	63	138	163	64	60	1.1	1.3	15	1.6	180	2.0
	51+	65	143	160	63	60	1.0	1.2	13	1.6	180	2.0
Pregnant						70	1.5	1.6	17	2.2	400	2.2
Lactating	1st 6 months					95	1.6	1.8	20	2.1	280	2.6
	2nd 6 months					90	1.6	1.7	20	2.1	280	2.6

* Modified and reproduced, with permission, from Subcommittee on the Tenth Edition of RDAs, Food and Nutrition Board, Commission on Life Sciences, National Research Council: *Recommended Dietary Allowances*, 10th ed. National Academy Press, 1989.

† The allowances, expressed as average daily intakes over time, are intended to provide for individual variations among most normal persons as they live in the United States under usual environmental stresses. Diets should be based on a variety of common foods in order to provide other nutrients for which human requirements have been less well defined.

‡ Weights and heights of Reference Adults are actual medians of the USA population of the designated age as reported by NHANES II. The median weights and heights of those under 19 years of age, were taken from Hamill et al. (1979). The use of these figures does not imply that the height-to-weight ratios are ideal.

§ NE (niacin equivalent) is equal to 1 mg of niacin or 60 mg of dietary tryptophan.

Table 4-5c. Recommended daily dietary allowances.*† (Minerals.)

Category	Age (years) or Condition	Weight‡ (kg)	Weight‡ (lb)	Height‡ (cm)	Height‡ (in)	Minerals						
						Calcium (mg)	Phosphorus (mg)	Magnesium (mg)	Iron (mg)	Zinc (mg)	Iodine (μg)	Selenium (μg)
Infants	0.0–0.5	6	13	60	24	400	300	40	6	5	40	10
	0.5–1.0	9	20	71	28	600	500	60	10	5	50	15
Children	1–3	13	29	90	35	800	800	80	10	10	70	20
	4–6	20	44	112	44	800	800	120	10	10	90	20
	7–10	28	62	132	52	800	800	170	10	10	120	30
Males	11–14	45	99	157	62	1,200	1,200	270	12	15	150	40
	15–18	66	145	176	69	1,200	1,200	400	12	15	150	50
	19–24	72	160	177	70	1,200	1,200	350	10	15	150	70
	25–50	79	174	176	70	800	800	350	10	15	150	70
	51+	77	170	173	68	800	800	350	10	15	150	70

88

Females	11–14	46	101	157	62	1,200	1,200	280	15	12	150	45
	15–18	55	120	163	64	1,200	1,200	280	15	12	150	50
	19–24	58	128	164	65	1,200	1,200	280	15	12	150	55
	25–50	63	138	163	64	800	800	280	15	12	150	55
	52+	65	143	160	63	800	800	280	10	12	150	55
Pregnant						1,200	1,200	320	30	15	175	65
Lactating	1st 6 months					1,200	1,200	355	15	19	200	75
	2nd 6 months					1,200	1,200	340	15	16	200	75

* Modified and reproduced, with permission, from Subcommittee on the Tenth Edition of RDAs, Food and Nutrition Board, Commission on Life Sciences, National Research Council: *Recommended Dietary Allowances*, 10th ed. National Academy Press, 1989.

† The allowances, expressed as average daily intakes over time, are intended to provide for individual variations among most normal persons as they live in the United States under usual environmental stresses. Diets should be based on a variety of common foods in order to provide other nutrients for which human requirements have been less well defined.

‡ Weights and heights of Reference Adults are actual medians for the USA population of the designated age, as reported by NHANES II. The median weights and heights of those under 19 years of age were taken from Hamill et al. (1979). The use of these figures does not imply that the height-to-weight ratios are ideal.

Table 4–5d. SUMMARY TABLE. Estimated safe and adequate daily dietary intakes of selected vitamins and minerals.*†

Category	Age (years)	Vitamins	
		Biotin (μg)	Pantothenic Acid (mg)
Infants	0–0.5	10	2
	0.5–1	15	3
Children and adolescents	1–3	20	3
	4–6	25	3–4
	7–10	30	4–5
	11+	30–100	4–7
Adults		30–100	4–7

Trace Elements‡

Category	Age (years)	Copper (mg)	Manganese (mg)	Fluoride (mg)	Chromium (μg)	Molybdenum (μg)
Infants	0–0.5	0.4–0.6	0.3–0.6	0.1–0.5	10–40	15–30
	0.5–1	0.6–0.7	0.6–1.0	0.2–1.0	20–60	20–40
Children and	1–3	0.7–1.0	1.0–1.5	0.5–1.5	20–80	25–50
adolescents	4–6	1.0–1.5	1.5–2.0	1.0–2.5	30–120	30–75
	7–10	1.0–2.0	2.0–3.0	1.5–2.5	50–200	50–150
	11+	1.5–2.5	2.0–5.0	1.5–2.5	50–200	75–250
Adults		1.5–3.0	2.0–5.0	1.5–4.0	50–200	75–250

* Modified and reproduced, with permission, from Subcommittee on the Tenth Edition of RDAs, Food and Nutrition Board, Commission on Life Sciences, National Research Council: *Recommended Dietary Allowances*, 10th ed. National Academy Press, 1989.

† Because there is less information on which to base allowances, these figures are not given in the main table of RDA and are provided here in the form of ranges of recommended intakes.

‡ Since the toxic levels for many trace elements may be only several times usual intakes, the upper levels for the trace elements given in this table should not be habitually exceeded.

Marasmus & Kwashiorkor

Marasmus is the end result of severe undernutrition in which there has been successful adaptation to prolonged lack of energy and nutrients. Body weight is less than 60% median for age.

Kwashiorkor is edematous malnutrition with body weight 60–80% median for age. In kwashiorkor, hepatic protein synthesis is depressed at an early stage. Adaptation to malnutrition is poor, and a life-threatening disease develops despite the presence of some energy reserves and skeletal muscle. The etiology of this complex state of malnutrition remains controversial. Lack of protein in the diet appears to be a contributory factor in at least some cases. The features of kwashiorkor and marasmus are compared in Table 4–6.

Whereas FTT can be managed with aggressive nutritional rehabilitation from the outset, great care and patience are required in the initial management of kwashiorkor. Small, frequent, oral feeds should be given to avoid hypoglycemia. During the acute phase, provide only maintenance energy (95 kcal/kg/d) and protein (less than 1.5 g/kg/d), a very generous supply of potassium to replace intracellular losses, and a minimal amount of sodium (avoiding intravenous sodium completely). (Intracellular sodium levels and total body sodium are abnormally high.) Infections must be treated agressively. Initial progress over the

Table 4–6. Comparison of clinical and laboratory features of marasmus and kwashiorkor.

Clinical Features	Marasmus	Kwashiorkor
Weight loss	++++	++
Loss of muscle	++++	+
Loss of fat	++++	+
Edema	―――	++++
Psychological impairment	++	++++
Anorexia	+	++++
Hepatomegaly	―――	++
Associated infections	++	++++
Diarrhea	+++	+++
Skin lesions	―――	++
Hair changes	+	++
Laboratory Features		
Anemia	+	+++
Low serum albumin, transferrin, etc	+	++++
Impaired sodium homeostasis	+	++++
Total body potassium deficiency	++	++++
Prothrombin time	Normal	Prolonged
Immune system	Depressed	Depressed

first 1–2 weeks is characterized by loss of weight as the edema resolves. During the recovery phase provide 3.5 g protein and 150–200 kcal/kg/d with abundant minerals, vitamins, and trace elements.

Obesity

Obesity is a rapidly increasing problem in the United States; weight problems are evident in children as young as 6 years of age. Obesity results from an imbalance between energy intake and expenditure. However, it frequently involves more than simply overeating. For example, energy expenditure is probably low in preobese and definitely low in postobese states, such that an unusually low intake is necessary to avoid obesity or to maintain weight reduction. Intervention is likely to be successful only if the family has sought guidance.

For nutritional management, obtain a diet history and focus on reducing or eliminating specific items. For example, encourage intake of skim milk, nonsugared cereals, and diet soda, and avoidance of high-energy snacks, mayonnaise, and salad dressing. Even without counting calories, these measures are likely to reduce energy intake by about one-third. A reduction of 500 kcal/d will result in the loss of 1 pound of fat per week, provided the same rate of energy expenditure is maintained as weight is lost. Exercise and behavioral modification are important components of weight management.

Essential Fatty Acids

Clinical features of $\omega6$ deficiency include growth failure, abnormal scaliness of the skin, erythematous skin lesions, decreased capillary resistance, increased fragility of erythrocytes, thrombocytopenia, poor wound healing, and increased susceptibility to infection. Deficiency of $\omega3$ fatty acids (linolenic) has been less clearly documented but recent evidence shows that visual acuity is compromised by feeding premature infants formulas that lack docosohexanoic acid (22:6 $\omega3$). Excess $\omega6$ fatty acids may lead to an undesirable increase in the production of leukotrienes and thromboxane.

Carbohydrates

A high intake of complex carbohydrates (more than 55–60% of calories) and of fiber is a key feature of the diet now recommended for children more than 2 years of age. Ketosis develops with diets containing less than 10% carbohydrates. Glucose enhances the absorption of sodium and thus of water, which provides a theoretical basis for the composition of oral dehydration solutions in the management of acute diarrhea.

Sucrose is currently consumed in large quantities by children and adolescents in North America in such items as soda, candy, syrups, and sweetened breakfast cereals. The average consumption of sugar by adolescents is 210 pounds per year. A high intake of sucrose predisposes to obesity and is a major risk factor for dental caries.

Calcium (Ca)

Calcium deficiency can occur in very premature infants fed human milk or a relatively low calcium formula; in lactating adolescents who do not have a good intake of dairy products; and in patients with steatorrhea. The principal effect of calcium deficiency is a decrease in bone density, possibly progressing to rickets. Hypocalcemic tetany occurred historically in neonates fed unmodified cow's milk, which has a high phosphorus:calcium ratio.

Phosphorus (P)

Nutritional phosphorus deficiency is rare but can occur in very premature infants fed human milk, in whom it can cause osteoporosis and rickets, and in patients recovering from protein energy malnutrition. One nonnutritional cause of phosphorus depletion is the use of phosphorus-binding antacids. Severe hypophosphatemia results from phosphorus deficiency together with an acute extracellular-to-intracellular shift in phosphorus. This shift can be triggered by a glucose load, insulin, or nutritional rehabilitation. Phosphorus deficiency affects most organ systems, including muscle (weakness, progressing to rhabdomyolysis); bone (pain, rickets, osteomalacia); central nervous system; gastrointestinal system; and cellular components of blood. Respiratory insufficiency may result from weakness of the diaphragm. Phosphorus depletion in the premature infant can cause hypercalcemia; while phosphorus retention (such as can occur in chronic renal disease) leads to metabolic bone disease.

Magnesium (Mg)

Because of very powerful homeostatic control of magnesium by the kidney, dietary magnesium deficiency is not recognized except as a component of protein energy malnutrition. Magnesium depletion may occur secondary to renal disease or intestinal malabsorption. Effects include neuromuscular excitability, muscle tremors, personality changes, neurological abnormalities, and depression of S–T segment and T waves. Magnesium excess can cause respiratory depression, lethargy, and coma.

Sodium (Na) & Chloride (Cl)

Despite a trend toward dietary reductions, sodium and chloride intakes still tend to be generous in North America. Sodium deficiency occurs most commonly as a result of diarrhea and vomiting; it causes dehydration. Chloride deficiency has occurred in infants fed formulas low in chloride and as a result of vomiting, diarrhea, diuretic therapy and Bartter's syndrome. Chronic sodium and chloride deficiency can occur in cystic fibrosis, resulting in anorexia, failure to thrive, vomiting, and mental apathy.

Potassium (K)

Potassium deficiency occurs in patients with protein energy malnutrition, in whom it can be a cause of sudden death from cardiac failure. Excessive loss of potassium occurs in any catabolic state. Causes of potassium deficiency include acidosis, diarrhea, and diuretic therapy. Effects of potassium deficiency are muscle weakness, mental confusion, and sudden death from arrhythmias.

Iron (Fe)

Nutritional iron deficiency is effectively prevented by the use of an iron-supplemented formula after 2 months of age and the use of iron-fortified infant cereals later in the first year. It is necessary for the toddler to eat a diet containing enough iron, to avoid deficiency in the second year. Iron deficiency can cause some impairment of cognitive development even when insufficiently severe to cause anemia. The federal government's WIC program appears to have been effective in reducing the incidence of iron-deficiency anemia in the United States.

Zinc (Zn)

Causes of zinc deficiency are diets low in available zinc during periods of rapid growth in infancy and childhood, synthetic diets lacking adequate zinc, diseases causing impaired absorption, or excessive losses and inborn errors of zinc metabolism. Effects of mild zinc deficiency include failure to thrive, poor appetite, and abnormalities of the immune system. Severe zinc deficiency is characterized by an acro-orifacial skin rash, together with diarrhea, alopecia, increased susceptibility to infection, irritability, and lethargy. Treat dietary zinc deficiency with 1 mg zinc per kilogram per day for 3 months.

Copper (Cu)

Copper deficiency may occur in premature infants fed a formula low in copper, in generalized malnutrition states, during intravenous nutrition, and secondary to intestinal malabsorption or prolonged diarrhea. Features include osteoporosis progressing to more severe bone lesions, neutropenia, and a microcytic anemia. Treat copper deficiency in infants with a 1% solution of copper sulphate (2 mg of salt or 0.5 mg of elemental copper per day).

Selenium (Se)

Severe selenium deficiency can cause a severe skeletal myopathy or fatal cardiomyopathy. Macrocytosis and poor hair growth may result from mild selenium deficiency. Deficiency of this element is endemic in certain areas of China. In North America, it has been documented in patients on long-term intravenous nutrition; it also may be a common problem in very-low-birth-weight premature infants, in whom selenium provides one of the body's defenses against oxygen toxicity.

Iodide (I)

Endemic goiter due to iodide deficiency has been eradicated from North America. However, it continues to be a major health problem in several developing countries. The neurologic form of endemic cretinism is seen most frequently. This condition is characterized by severe mental retardation, deaf-mutism, spastic dyplegia, and strabismus. "Myxedematous" endemic cretinism predominates in some Central African countries. Signs of congenital hypothyroidism are seen in this type of cretinism. Milder neurologic damage occurs in many other cases of endemic neonatal goiter. Muscular depot injection of iodized oil or use of iodized salt are widely used to prevent iodide deficiency.

Fluoride (Fl)

Small doses of fluoride are of major value in the prevention of dental caries. Fluoride is most effective when provided in the early posteruptive period but may also have some effect prior to eruption. In areas where the water is not fluoridated (1 mg Fl/L), fluoride supplements are recommended at a level of 0.25 mg/d from ages 2 weeks to 2 years; 0.5 mg/d from 2–3 years, and 1 mg/d from 3–16 years.

Carnitine

Synthesis of carnitine may be inadequate in premature infants fed unsupplemented soy formula or fed intravenously; in dialysis patients; in patients with inherited defects of carnitine synthesis or organic acidemias; and with the therapeutic use of valproic acid. Effects of carnitine deficiency include increased serum triglycerides and free fatty acids, decreased ketones, fatty liver, and hypoglycemia. In genetic forms, there may be progressive muscle weakness or cardiomyopathy or hypoglycemia. Treat these inborn errors of metabolism and organic acidemias with 50–300 mg carnitine/kg/d.

Fat-Soluble Vitamins

A. Vitamin A: Vitamin A deficiency can occur in premature infants, in association with intravenous nutrition, and in protein-energy malnutrition; manifestations are frequently made more severe by measles. Other causes of vitamin A deficiency are cultural factors and fat malabsorption syndromes. Classic features of vitamin A deficiency are related to the eyes and vision. Night blindness progresses to dryness of the cornea and conjunctiva, clouding and softening of the cornea, ulceration and perforation with prolapse of the lens and iris, and eventual blindness. Vitamin A deficiency is the leading cause of irreversible blindness in children worldwide. Other features include follicular hyperkeratosis, pruritus, growth retardation, increased susceptibility to infection, anemia, and hepatosplenomegaly. In the premature neonate, vitamin A deficiency may contribute to the onset of bronchopulmonary dysplasia. Serum levels of retinol below 20 mg/dl are low; those below 10 are indicative of deficiency. In fat-malabsorption syndromes, provide a vitamin A supplement of 2500–5000 IU/day (800–1600 μg/d). Higher doses may be needed. Provide as aquasol A (1 mL = 50,000 IU). Therapy of eye lesions requires 50,000–100,000 IU orally or intramuscularly.

Vitamin A toxicity can result from chronic ingestion of more than 20,000 IU/d. Features of toxicity include vomiting, pseudotumor cerebri, irritability, headaches, insomnia, emotional instability, dry desquamating skin, myalagia, arthralgia, abdominal pain, hepatosplenomegaly, and cortical thickening of hands and feet. Some families may be genetically susceptible to toxicity of vitamin A at lower doses.

B. Vitamin D: Vitamin D deficiency results from the lack of adequate sunlight coupled with a low dietary intake. An infant requires only half an hour total body exposure or 2-hour head exposure to the sun per week to maintain adequate vitamin D status. In the United States, cow's milk and infant formulas are routinely supplemented with vitamin D. Occasional rickets may occur in older infants and children who are not exposed to the sun and who do not take a vitamin-D fortified milk or in breast-fed infants not exposed to the sun and whose mother's vitamin D status is suboptimal. Vitamin D deficiency also occurs in fat malabsorption syndromes. Hydroxylation of vitamin D may be impaired by hepatic and renal disease, by inborn errors of metabolism, and by use of P_{450}-stimulating drugs. End-organ unresponsiveness to calcitriol may also occur. Effects of vitamin D deficiency are osteomalacia in adults and rickets in children. There is accumulation in bone of osteoid (matrix) with reduced calcification. Clinical features include craniotabes, rachitic rosary, pigeon breast, bowed legs, delayed eruption of teeth and enamel defects, Harrison's groove, scoliosis, kyphosis, dwarfism, painful bones, fractures, anorexia, and weakness. X-ray findings include cupping, fraying, and flaring of metaphyses and loss of sharp definition of bone trabeculae leading to a general decrease in skeletal radiodensity. Serum phosphorus is low and serum alkaline phosphatase and parathormone levels are elevated. The diagnosis can be confirmed by a finding of low serum 25-OH vitamin D.

Rickets is treated with 1,600–5000 IU/d vitamin D_3 (1 IU = 0.25 ug). If this is poorly absorbed give 25-OH vitamin D, 2 μg/kg/d or 1, 25-OH_2 vitamin D, 0. 05–0.2 μg/kg/d. Treat renal osteodystrophy with 1,25-OH_2 vitamin D.

Vitamin D intake of 40,000 IU/d or more are toxic and will lead to hypercalcemia, vomiting, constipation, and nephrocalcinosis. Some subjects are genetically susceptible to toxicity from much lower doses of vitamin D.

C. Vitamin E: Vitamin E deficiency may occur in the premature infant and in patients with cholestatic liver disease, pancreatic insufficiency (including cystic fibrosis), abetalipoproteinemia, short bowel syndrome, an isolated inborn error of metabolism, and possibly as a result of increased utilization due to oxidant stress. One of the effects of deficiency is hemolytic anemia; chronic vitamin E deficiency causes a progressive neurological disorder. Laboratory findings of vitamin E deficiency include a serum vitamin E level of less than 3 μg/ml and a vitamin E : total serum lipid ratio less than 0.8 mg/g. Large oral doses (up to 100 IU/kg/d) correct deficiency resulting from most malabsorption syndromes. Intramuscular injections (5–7 mg/kg/wk) may be necessary in some cases of cholestatic liver disease.

Excess vitamin E may be hepatotoxic in the premature infant.

D. Vitamin K: Vitamin K deficiency occurs in newborns who do not receive vitamin K prophylaxis after delivery and results in hemorrhagic disease. Later vitamin K deficiency may result from fat malabsorption syndromes and the use of nonabsorbed antibiotics and anticoagulant drugs. Clinical features of deficiency are hemorrhage into the skin (purpura), gastrointestinal tract, genitourinary tract, gingiva, lungs, joints, and central nervous systems. Vitamin K status is assessed with plasma levels of PIVKA or the prothrombin time. The prophylactic dose of vitamin K (lipid-soluble only) is 0.5–1.0 mg. Later vitamin K deficiency is treated with 3.0–10.0 mg of parenteral vitamin K.

Water-Soluble Vitamins

With the exception of cobalamin, water-soluble vitamins are not stored in the body; thus, a regular (though not necessarily daily) intake is required (Table 4–7). Substantial quantities of biotin are synthesized by intestinal bacteria. While classic water-soluble vitamin deficiency diseases are very rare in developed countries, deficiencies may occur in several special circumstances (Table 4–8). Many children and adults have excess intakes of water-soluble vitamins. Though concern about toxicity is not as great as with excess intake of fat-soluble vitamins, a number of cases of water-soluble vitamin toxicity have been reported (Table 4–9).

A. Thiamine (B_1): Thiamine deficiency has been described in 2- to 5-month-old infants breast-fed by mothers with alcoholism or poor diet, as a complication of long-term total parenteral nutrition (TPN) use, with protein-energy malnutrition, and in preterm infants. The clinical syndrome of beriberi is characterized by anorexia, listlessness, irritability, vomiting, constipation, and edema. Progression is marked by cardiac symptoms (dyspnea, tachycardia, heart failure), CNS signs (peripheral neuritis, loss of deep tendon reflexes, paresthesias, meningismus, coma), and psychic disturbances. Diagnosis is confirmed by whole blood thiamine/erythrocyte transketolase.

Table 4–7. Major dietary sources of vitamins.

Thiamin	Cereals (including fortification), all foods
Riboflavin	Leafy vegetables, fish, meat
Pyridoxine	All foods
Niacin	Meats, fish, wheat, all foods except fats
Pantothenic acid	Ubiquitous
Biotin	Yeasts, liver, kidneys
Folic acid	Leafy vegetables (lost in cooking)
Cobalamin	Small quantities in animal products (none in plants)
Vitamin C	Fresh fruit and vegetables, dairy products

Table 4–8. Circumstances in which the possibility of vitamin deficiencies merit particular consideration.

Prematurity	All vitamins
Breast-feeding	B_1*, folate†, B_{12}‡, D, K
Protein-energy malnutrition	B_1, B_2, folate, A
Fat malabsorption syndromes	Fat-soluble vitamins
Synthetic diets, including TPN	All vitamins
Inherited disorders	Folate, B_{12}, D
Vitamin–drug interactions	B_6, biotin, folate, B_{12}, fat-soluble vitamins

* Alcoholic or malnourished mother.
† Mother folate deficient.
‡ Mother vegetarian.

B. Riboflavin (Vitamin B_2): Deficiency of riboflavin is seen with general undernutrition, in preterm infants, and with long-term TPN use (inactivated by light exposure). Clinical features include cheilosis, angular stomatitis, glossitis, soreness and burning of lips and mouth, dermatitis of the nasolabial folds and genitals, and ocular signs (photophobia, indistinct vision). Diagnosis is confirmed by serum riboflavin/erythrocyte glutathione reductase.

C. Pyridoxine (Vitamin B_6): Pyridoxine deficiency is seen in preterm infants (who may not convert pyridoxine to pyridoxal-

Table 4–9. Toxicity of water-soluble vitamins.

Thiamin (rare)	Anaphylaxis, respiratory depression
Riboflavin	None
Pyridoxine (rare)	Sensory neuropathy
Niacin	Histamine release, cutaneous vasodilation, cardiac arrythmias, cholestatic jaundice, gastrointestinal disturbance, hyperuricemia, glucose intolerance
Pantothenic acid	Diarrhea
Biotin	None
Folate	None (except masking B_{12} deficiency)
Cobalamin	None
Vitamin C	Maternal excess in pregnancy may lead to infantile scurvy, poor copper absorption, decreased tolerance to hypoxia, increased oxalic acid excretion

5-phostate), in B_6 dependency syndromes, and associated with drug use (eg, isoniazid). Clinical features include failure to thrive, listlessness, irritability, seizures, gastrointestinal disturbances, anemia, cheilosis, and glossitis. Diagnosis is confirmed by plasma pyridoxine/erythrocyte GOT.

D. Niacin: Deficiency of this vitamin (pellagra) is seen with maize or millet diets (high leucine intake) and in preterm infants. Clinical features of pellagra include weakness, lassitude, dermatitis of exposed areas, gastrointestinal disturbances, and dementia. Diagnosis is confirmed by whole blood niacin.

E. Biotin: Biotin deficiency is seen in patients with suppressed intestinal flora and impaired intestinal absorption. Clinical features include a scaly dermatitis, alopecia, irritability, and lethargy. Diagnosis is confirmed with a serum biotin determination.

F. Folic Acid: Folic acid deficiency is seen in preterm infants (though it is rarely clinically significant), term breast-fed infants whose mothers are folate-deficient, and term infants fed unsupplemented processed cow's milk or goat's milk. Folate deficiency can also be seen with kwashiorkor, chronic hemolytic anemias, diarrhea, malignancies, hypermetabolic states, infections, extensive skin disease, cirrhosis, malabsorption, drug therapy (eg, phenytoin and sulfasalazine), and with chronic overcooking of food. Clinical features include megaloblastic anemia, neutropenia, thrombocytopenia, growth failure, delayed CNS maturation in infants, diarrhea, mucosal ulcerations, glossitis, jaundice, and mild splenomegaly. Diagnosis can be confirmed by determination of serum or erythrocyte folate levels.

G. Cobalamin (Vitamin B_{12}): Cobalamin deficiency is very rare, but can be seen in breast-fed infants of mothers who have latent pernicious anemia or who are on strict vegatarian diets. B_{12} deficiency is also seen associated with absence of luminal proteases and with congenital malabsorption. The clinical syndrome is that of megaloblastic anemia; diagnosis is confirmed with a serum B_{12} level.

H. Ascorbic Acid (Vitamin C): Ascorbic acid deficiency is seen in breast-fed infants of mothers with vitamin C deficiency and in infants fed a diet of unsupplemented cow's milk. Clinical features of scurvy include anorexia; irritability; apathy; pallor; fever; tachycardia; diarrhea; failure to thrive; increased susceptibility to infection; hemorrhages under skin, mucous membranes, into joints, and under periostium; long-bone pain; immobility; and costochondral beading. Diagnosis confirmed by determination of serum or leukocyte ascorbate levels.

INTRAVENOUS NUTRITION

Indications

The principal indication for total parenteral nutrition (TPN) is loss of ability to absorb nutrients from the gastrointestinal tract. If it is apparent in a newborn that the loss is permanent, TPN should not be started. Supplemental intravenous nutrition, which can be administered via a peripheral vein, is useful as a temporary measure in the premature neonate or, for example, in the malnourished postoperative surgical patient.

Catheter Selection & Placement

The Broviac is the catheter of choice. Use a double-line catheter if required for multiple purposes. If TPN will be needed for less than a month, a Perq catheter can be inserted into a peripheral vein. The tip of the central venous catheter should be located in the superior vena cava or right atrium. Check placement radiologically before using.

Complications

Because of the cost and the risk of complications, TPN should be used only with adequate indication. Complications include mechanical complications that result from problems with insertion; thrombosis of a major vessel; metabolic complications including TPN liver disease and bone disease; and, most commonly, septic complications. The latter, in particular, underlie the need for rigid protocols for nurses and physicians and the advantage of an effective nutrition support team.

Central catheters may be lost owing to sepsis; lack of response to therapy; thrombosis; composition of the infusate (excessive concentrations of calcium and phosphorus); incompatible medications administered with the infusate; or slipping, kinking, or breaking of the catheter. Most breaks are exterior to the skin and can be repaired with kits, which must be kept readily available. Urokinase is effective in dissolving recently formed clots in the catheter.

Nutrient Requirements & Administration

Energy requirements are approximately 10% lower than those for enteral feeding. At least 60% of energy is provided as dextrose monohydrate (3.4 kcal/g). Dextrose concentrations greater than 12.5% (630 mosm/kg water) cannot be administered via peripheral vein. With a central catheter start with D10 and advance by approximately 2.5% per day as tolerance (owing to decreased endogenous glucose production) increases, up to 20% or higher if needed. The rate of advance and final concentration will depend on flow rates.

Tolerance to IV dextrose is especially limited in premature infants and hypermetabolic ICU patients. Excess administration of dextrose will cause hyperglycemia, osmotic diuresis, fatty liver and elevated Pa_{co2}. If unexpected hyperglycemia occurs check for error in dextrose concentration, uneven flow rate, sepsis, stress, or pancreatitis. Intravenous insulin may not be metabolically desirable. When the infusate is discontinued either temporarily or during cyclic IV feeding, taper glucose delivery over at least 2 hours to avoid hypoglycemia. A minimum of about 5% of total calories per week should be provided as an intravenous fat emulsion (2.7% calories as essential fatty acids) to avoid risk of essential fatty acid deficiency; there are potential advantages in providing up to 40% of calories as lipid according to individual tolerance. Advantages include the high energy density, low osmolality, low CO_2 production, and negligible energy cost of storage. However, administration of fat emulsions beyond tolerance will impair leukocyte function, cause coagulation defects, decrease pulmonary oxygen diffusion, and compete with bilirubin and drugs for albumin binding sites. Commence fat emulsion with 1 g/kg/day and, as tolerated, advance by 0.5 g/kg/d up to a maximum of 3 g/kg/d.

Provide nitrogen (one g N = 6.25 g protein) as an amino acid solution, usually 1–3% depending on flow rate and requirements (the same as for enteral feeding). Trophamine (McGaw) may currently be the best source of nitrogen for the premature infant with added cysteine (40 mg/g trophamine). Optimal N (g):kcal ratios are usually 1:150–300. When energy intake is low, administration of nitrogen will improve but not correct negative nitrogen balance. When nitrogen intake is low, provision of energy (< 70 kcal/kg/day in an infant) will improve negative nitrogen balance.

One vial (5 mL) of MVI Pediatric (Armour) meets the vitamin guidelines for term infants. Administer 2 mL (40% of a single-dose vial) per kg to premature infants. Additional supplements of vitamins A (250 μg) and E (10 mg) may be beneficial.

Mineral and trace element recommendations are given in Figure 4–1.

Ordering

See sample order form in Figure 4–1. Orders should be reviewed each morning.

PEDIATRIC PARENTERAL NUTRITION (PN) ORDER FORM

Imprint Patient Plate

Weight of patient _____ kg   Central line _____   Peripheral line _____

Rate _____

	Standard Order	Modifications To Standard Order	*Adjustments for Neonates and Premature Infants (Circle these when required and cross out corresponding items* under "standard order").
Protein (as amino acid)*	g%		*Use trophamine and cysteine for patients in level II and III nurseries who have a central line or are on day 6 of peripheral therapy.
Dextrose	g%		
Na .... 30 meq/L			
K .... 25 meq/L			
Cl .... 20 meq/L			
Acetate .... 45 meq/L			
Ca (as gluconate) (10 mM Ca/L) .... 20 meq/L			
Mg (as sulfate) .... 3 meq/L			

P .... 10 mM/L
MVI Pediatric .... *5.0 mL/d
Zinc .... *1.0 mg/L   *2 mL/kg/d for patients < 2.5 kg
Copper .... 200 µg/L   *Zn: 400 µg/kg/d < 2 kg body weight
Manganese .... 5.0 µg/L   250 µg/kg/d others < 3 mo old
Chromium .... 2.0 µg/L
Selenium .... 20.0 µg/L
Iodide .... 10 µg/L
Heparin .... 1000 Units/L
Cysteine (40 mg/g trophamine)* .... _____ mg/L   *Use only with trophamine

Pharmacy will automatically account for electrolytes provided in amino acid preparation.
Changes in Na or K to be made as: Cl only ___, or Acetate only ___, or Cl: Acetate 1:1 ___, or other
Cl: Acetate ratio (specify _____).

Date: _____ Signature: _____ M.D.

Figure 4–1. Pediatric parenteral nutrition (PN) order form. (Modified from the pediatric parenteral nutrition order form of the University of Colorado Health Sciences Center Department of Pharmacy.)

Monitoring

Maintain PN flow chart at bedside or in hospital chart.

(1) Weight daily; height and head circumference weekly.

(2) Urine glucose, specific gravity: Dipstick once each shift while changing concentrations of dextrose.

(3) Blood glucose: Four hours after starting or changing infusion rate or changing glucose concentration; then daily for 2 days; then every third day.

(4) Serum Na-K-Cl-CO_2-BUN: Daily for 2 days after starting or changing infusion rate or changing composition of infusate; then every third day.

(5) Serum Ca-Mg-P: Every third day initially then once weekly when flow rate and composition of infusate are stabilized.

(6) Total protein, albumin, bilirubin, AST, GGT, alkaline phosphatase, CBC: Initially and then weekly. Zinc and copper: Initially, then monthly.

(7) Serum triglycerides (monitor if IV fat emulsion is used): One day after starting or changing quantity of fat, then weekly. (Draw level just prior to starting daily infusion of fat emulsion.)

Note: These assays will have to be performed more frequently in some patients according to their clinical status and the results of previous assays.

Fluid & Electrolyte Disorders | 5

Michael R. Clemmons, MD

Children are different from adults and so are their fluid and electrolyte requirements. Specifically, children have a greater percentage of total body weight that is water, a higher basal metabolic rate, and a higher body surface area:weight ratio.

All these features lead to increased water turnover per kilogram of body weight when compared with adults.

Fluid and electrolyte therapy for children may be approached by considering three major components: maintenance requirements, rehydration therapy, and replacement of ongoing losses.

MAINTENANCE REQUIREMENTS

Fluid and electrolyte needs are most closely related to the body's metabolic demand. Once caloric (metabolic) needs are known, water and salt requirements can be easily calculated. Table 5–1 shows approximate caloric requirements based upon body weight. Approximately 1 mL of water is required for every Kcal burned. A 10-kg child therefore requires 100 mL/kg/d × 10 kg = 1000 mL water per day. A 70-kg adult would need 1000 mL for the first 10 kg, 500 mL for the next 10 kg, and 1000 ml for the next 50 kg, for a total of 2500 mL.

Sodium, potassium, and chloride needs are also based on the body's metabolic demand. Losses occur primarily through the urine, though smaller amounts are lost through the skin and in stool. Because these electrolyte needs are paralleled by water requirements, maintenance electrolytes can be expressed as meq/100 mL water per day (Table 5–2).

When administering fluid intravenously for short periods of time, enough glucose should be provided in the solution to prevent ketosis and minimize protein breakdown. In most instances a 5% dextrose solution will suffice.

Table 5-1. Caloric and water requirements based upon body weight.

Body Weight	kcal/kg/d	mL H_2O/kg/d
<10 kg*	100	100
10–20 kg	50	50
>20 kg	20	20

* Requirements for neonates often differ. The normal term infant needs 60 mL/kg/d on day 1, increasing to 100 mL/kg by day 3 or 4. Water requirements are higher in preterm infants due to increased insensible water losses (through immature skin) and increased renal water losses (poor concentrating ability).

Summary of Daily Maintenance Requirements

(1) Water: 100 mL/kg for < 10 kg; 50 mL/kg for 10–20 kg; 20 mL/kg for > 20 kg.

(2) Sodium: 3 meq/100 mL water required.

(3) Potassium: 2 meq/100 mL water required.

(4) Chloride: 3 meq/100 mL water required.

(5) Glucose: 5 g/100 mL water required.

An ideal maintenance solution would therefore be D_5W ¼ NS with 20 meq KCl/L.

Special Considerations

The guidelines listed above are simply that—guidelines. Maintenance requirements may need to be adjusted up or down depending on the clinical situation. Maintenance requirements may need to be adjusted upward for the following reasons: low-birth-weight infants, fever (increase water by 12% per 1 °C rise), sweating, respiratory distress, skin disease, diabetes insipidus, high-output renal failure, and phototherapy.

Requirements need to be adjusted downward for syndrome of inappropriate ADH secretion, increased intracranial pressure, congestive heart failure, and oliguric renal failure.

Table 5-2. Maintenance electrolyte requirements.

Electrolyte	meq/100 mL H_2O/d
Sodium	3–4
Potassium	2–3
Chloride	3–4

DEHYDRATION

General Considerations

Children are at high risk for the development of dehydration. The reasons for this are many. (1) Children have an increased incidence of gastrointestinal (GI) disease, especially gastroenteritis. (2) GI symptoms occur with many nongastrointestinal diseases. (3) Children suffer relatively greater GI losses than do adults. (4) Infants cannot respond to thirst independently.

All sick children, not merely those with gastroenteritis, should be assessed for their hydration status. Evaluation of a child for dehydration includes obtaining appropriate historical data, performing a physical examination, and obtaining laboratory data.

History

A detailed history should be taken to determine the child's fluid intake and output, especially for the previous 24 hours. Information about intake should include the type of fluid, quantity, and frequency of intake. Information about output should include vomiting (frequency, presence of bile or blood, amount), diarrhea (frequency, consistency, volume, presence of blood or mucus), and urine output (frequency and amount). Associated symptoms (eg, fever), weight changes, medications given, and previous medical conditions should also be noted.

Types of Dehydration

By convention, the type of dehydration is based on the serum sodium concentration.

A. Isotonic: Isotonic dehydration is characterized by a serum sodium concentration of 130–150 meq/L. This is the most common form of dehydration, with the most straightforward management (see below).

B. Hypertonic: Hypertonic dehydration is defined by a serum sodium of > 150 meq/L. This serious medical condition is often secondary to administration of hypertonic fluids. Despite the increased serum sodium, total body sodium is actually low. Due to the hypernatremic state, the degree of dehydration is often clinically underestimated (patients are drier than they look). A doughy quality to the skin and neurologic symptomatology are suggestive of this type of dehydration. The hypertonic state should be corrected slowly to avoid the genesis of cerebral edema and seizures.

C. Hypotonic: Hypotonic dehydration is characterized by a serum sodium < 130 meq/L. This form of dehydration is often secondary to administration of hypotonic fluids. Due to the hyponatremic state, the degree of dehydration is often overestimated (patients are not as dry as they look). Treatment with hypertonic saline is rarely indicated, as the correction of water and sodium deficits is usually fairly straightforward.

Physical Examination and Laboratory Findings

Table 5–3 presents clinical and laboratory information valuable for estimating the degree of dehydration in infants and children. Determining severity requires estimating the percent of body weight lost.

Calculating Deficits

Once the severity of dehydration has been determined, water and electrolyte deficits may be calculated using Tables 5–4 and 5–5.

Treatment

Intravenous rehydration is usually carried out in 3 phases.

Table 5–3. Estimating the severity of dehydration.*

Physical Signs	Mild	Moderate	Severe
Weight loss			
Infant	5%	10%	15%
Older child	3%	6%	9%
Vital Signs			
Pulse	± ↑	↑	↑ ↑
Blood pressure	normal	normal	normal or ↓
Eyes	± tearing	↓ tearing ± sunken	↓ tearing sunken
Mucous membranes	± tacky	tacky/dry	parched
Skin			
Turgor	± ↓	↓	↓ ↓
Perfusion	normal	± mottled	poor/mottled
Laboratory Findings			
Urine output	↓	↓ ↓	↓ ↓ ↓
Urine specific gravity	↑	↑	↑
BUN	normal	± ↑	↑
CO_2	↓	↓ ↓	↓ ↓ ↓

* Adapted from Barkin RM (editor): *Emergency Pediatrics*, Mosby, 1986, p 44.

Table 5–4. Estimation of water deficits
in dehydration.

Degree of Dehydration	Infant (mL/kg)	Child ≥ 1 yr (mL/kg)
Mild	50	30
Moderate	100	60
Severe	150	90

Phase 1–Rapid volume expansion (for all types of dehydration).
   Goal: To restore circulating volume and adequate perfusion.
   Rate: 20–40 ml/kg over 30–60 minutes. Repeat as necessary until perfusion is improved.
   Fluid: Isotonic solutions (normal saline, Ringer's lactate, 5% albumin).

Phase 2–Rapid repletion phase (for isotonic and hypotonic dehydration).
   Goal: Replenish intracellular deficits.
   Rate: ½ of deficit along with maintenance fluid and ongoing losses; over 8 hours.
   Fluid: Usually D_5W ½ NS with added potassium.

Phase 3–Slow repletion phase (for isotonic and hypotonic dehydration).
   Goal: Complete correction of deficits.
   Rate: ½ of deficit along with maintenance fluid and ongoing losses; over 16 hours.
   Fluid: Usually D_5W ¼ NS or ⅓ NS with added potassium.

Fluids and electrolytes given during rapid volume expansion should be subtracted from the calculated deficit used to determine fluid administration in phases 2 and 3. Potassium should be added only after urine output has been established. The progress of rehydration should be followed with careful monitoring of

Table 5–5. Electrolyte deficits with different types of dehydration

Type of Dehydration	Sodium (meq/kg)	Potassium (meq/kg)	Chloride (meq/kg)
Hypotonic	10–12	10–12	8–10
Isotonic	8–10	8–10	8–10
Hypertonic	2–4	—	0–4

input, output, urine specific gravity, serum electrolytes, and body weights.

A. Hypertonic Dehydration: Volume expansion to restore circulation in hypertonic dehydration is done the same as that for isotonic and hypotonic dehydration. The use of hypotonic fluid is not indicated. Further correction should proceed *slowly*. The aim is to correct the serum sodium at a rate of ½–1 meq/L/h. The higher the initial sodium concentration, the slower should be the rate of decrease. The water and electrolyte deficit correction should take place over 48 hours. The fluid used after phase 1 is usually D_5W ¼ NS with added potassium. Again, maintenance fluids and ongoing losses need to be considered.

B. Replacement of Ongoing Losses: The electrolyte composition of gastrointestinal secretions and diarrhea stools can be roughly estimated for purposes of replacement (Table 5–6). When the child's condition is tenuous or when GI losses are voluminous, secretions may be sent for determination of the exact electrolyte concentrations. Replacement fluids are usually administered on a milliliter for milliliter basis calculated every 8 hours. Examples of some replacement fluids are: nasogastric suction fluid may be replaced with D_5W ½ NS with 20 meq/L KCl; and diarrhea stools may be replaced with D_5W ⅓ NS with 40 meq/L KCl.

Sodium bicarbonate may be substituted for a portion of the sodium chloride if significant acidosis is present.

SPECIFIC ELECTROLYTE DISTURBANCES

1. HYPERKALEMIA

Clinical Findings

Causes of hyperkalemia include renal disease, hemolysis/rhabdomyolysis, shock, adrenal insufficiency, and excess administration (usually IV).

Table 5–6. Composition of gastrointestinal secretions.

	H^+ (meq/L)	Na^+ (meq/L)	K^+ (meq/L)	Cl^- (meq/L)	HCO_3 (meq/L)
Gastric	40–60	20–80	5–20	80–150	—
Biliary	—	120–140	5–15	80–120	30–50
Pancreatic	—	120–140	5–15	40–80	70–110
Small bowel	—	100–140	5–15	90–130	20–40
Stool (diarrhea)	—	40–65	25–50	25–55	—

Physical findings relate to the neuromuscular effects of increased extracellular potassium and include listlessness, confusion, parasthesias, peripheral vascular collapse, bradycardia, and asystole. The most important clinical effect of hyperkalemia is on the myocardium. Electrocardiographic changes, including peaked T waves, widened QRS complex, increased P–R interval, irregular rhythm, heart block, and ventricular tachycardia or fibrillation, should be sought. Laboratory diagnosis is defined by a serum potassium greater than 6 meq/L in a nonhemolyzed specimen. Symptoms often will not be manifest until the potassium rises above 7 meq/L.

Treatment

The major principles of treatment of all types of hyperkalemia include the following.

(1) Continuously monitor ECG.

(2) Withhold all potassium.

(3) If the serum potassium is less than 7 meq/L, give Kayexalate exchange resin, 1 g/kg PR or PO.

(4) If serum potassium is greater than 7 meq/L or cardiovascular instability is present give

Acute: A. Calcium gluconate 10% 1.0–1.5 mL/kg IV slowly. This is the treatment of choice since it acts directly on the myocardium.

B. Sodium bicarbonate 1–2 meq/kg IV. This transiently moves potassium intracellularly.

Chronic: C. Glucose 0.5 g/kg/h and insulin 1 U regular for each 3 g glucose.

D. Kayexalate as above

E. Dialysis is indicated for refractory hyperkalemia in the face of renal dysfunction

F. Treat the underlying condition

2. HYPOKALEMIA

Clinical Findings

Causes of hypokalemia include: vomiting, diarrhea, nasogastric suction, inadequate intake, diuretics, correction of metabolic acidosis, and primary renal disease (renal tubular acidosis).

The physical findings relate to decreased neuromuscular excitability and include weakness, hypotonia, decreased deep tendon reflexes, and ileus. ECG changes consistent with hypokalemia include flattened T waves, the presence of U waves, S–T segment depression, and arrhythmias (extrasystole, AV block). Arrhythmias may be exacerbated if the patient is taking digitalis.

Treatment

(1) Obtain serum and urine electrolytes, urinalysis, ECG.

(2) Establish adequate urine output before giving potassium.

(3) Correct if serum potassium is less than 3.5 meq/L.

(4) Parenteral correction can be done with 20–40 meq/L potassium peripherally. Higher concentrations require a central venous line and ICU monitoring. A rapid infusion up to 0.3 meq/kg/h can be done with ECG monitoring. Total dose is usually 3 meq/kg/d plus maintenance needs. Correct slowly unless life-threatening complications are present.

(5) Correction with 3 meq/kg/d can also be done orally. Potassium irritates the GI tract and should be given on a full stomach.

3. HYPONATREMIA

Clinical Findings

The differential diagnosis of hyponatremia is based on total volume status and urine sodium concentration (Table 5–7). Keep in mind that pseudohyponatremia may be seen with hyperglycemia, hyperlipidemia, and hyperproteinemia. The symptoms and signs of hyponatremia include nausea, vomiting, muscular twitching, lethargy, obtundation, seizures, and coma.

Table 5–7. Differential diagnosis of hyponatremia.

Urine sodium	High (> 20 meq/L)	Low (< 20 meq/L)
Circulating Volume		
Normal or increased	SIADH* Renal failure Polydipsia	Nephrotic syndrome Cirrhosis Cardiac failure
Decreased	Adrenal insufficiency Salt-wasting renal disease Diuretics (early)	GI losses Diuretics (late) Burns

* SIADH = syndrome of inappropriate antidiuretic hormone secretion.
Adapted from Perkin, RM, Levin, DL: Common fluid and electrolyte problems in the pediatric intensive care unit. *Pediatr Clin North Am* 1980; **27**:573.

Treatment

If the volume status is low, replace fluid and salt; consider steroids. If the volume status is normal or increased, restrict fluid and salt, treat the underlying condition, and consider diuretics.

4. HYPERNATREMIA WITHOUT DEHYDRATION

Hypernatremia without dehydration (salt poisoning) often occurs accidentally. Symptoms include pulmonary edema, CNS bleeds, and increased blood pressure. As with hypernatremic dehydration, correction should proceed slowly. Specific treatment includes diuretics if renal function is good and peritoneal dialysis if renal function is impaired. Serum sodium and osmolality should be monitored carefully during correction.

5. ACID–BASE DISTURBANCES

The normal pH range is 7.38–7.42. pH changes 0.15 units for every 10 meq/L change in serum bicarbonate and 0.08 units for every 10 torr change in P_{CO_2}.

The laboratory findings in acute acid–base disturbances are given in Table 5–8.

Metabolic Acidosis

Metabolic acidosis is caused by a gain in hydrogen ion or a loss of bicarbonate. Calculation of the anion gap can help determine the cause (Table 5–9). Anion gap = $Na - (Cl + HCO_3)$. A normal anion gap is 8–16 meq/L. An increased anion gap suggests accumulation of organic acids (ketones, lactic acid, toxins, etc).

Treatment of acidosis involves identification of the underlying cause. Bicarbonate therapy is usually indicated only if the serum HCO_3 is less than 10–12 meq/L or the pH is less than 7.20.

Table 5–8. Laboratory findings in acute acid–base disturbances.

	pH	P_{CO_2}	HCO_3
Metabolic acidosis	↓	↓	↓
Respiratory acidosis	↓	↑	Normal or ↑
Metabolic alkalosis	↑	↑	↑
Respiratory alkalosis	↑	↓	Normal or ↓

Table 5–9. Causes of metabolic acidosis.
Normal anion gap
GI losses: diarrhea, enterostomies, fistulas
Renal tubular acidosis
Acid ingestion (NH_4Cl, arginine Cl)
Hyperalimentation
Increased anion gap
Lactic acidosis
Diabetic ketoacidosis
Inborn errors of metabolism
Uremia
Acid ingestion (ethanol, methanol, ethylene glycol, salicylates)

The dose of bicarbonate is calculated as weight (kg) × base deficit × 0.6. The base deficit is the desired HCO_3—the measured HCO_3. Half the calculated dose can be given immediately with the remainder given over the next 1–2 hours.

Respiratory Acidosis

Respiratory acidosis occurs as a result of hypoventilation due to pulmonary parenchymal disease or central respiratory depression. Treatment involves adequate ventilation; bicarbonate therapy is not indicated.

Metabolic Alkalosis

This condition results from loss of hydrogen ion (vomiting), excess intake of bicarbonate, or as compensation for excess renal loss of chloride (diuretics). The underlying cause must be treated and adequate chloride supplements provided.

Respiratory Alkalosis

The presence of a respiratory alkalosis suggests hyperventilation, salicylate intoxication, and hyperammonemia. Treatment involves identification of the underlying cause. Adequate potassium and calcium must also be provided.

ORAL REHYDRATION THERAPY

Oral rehydration should be considered for pediatric patients with mild to moderate dehydration secondary to gastroenteritis. Vomiting is not an absolute contraindication to oral rehydration;

in fact, many children with a history of vomiting will tolerate oral rehydration solutions quite well.

An oral glucose–electrolyte solution containing 50–90 meq of sodium per liter and 20–25 grams of glucose per liter should be used. Small aliquots are given ad libitum to provide approximately 50 mL/kg over a 4-hour period to the child with mild dehydration. For moderate dehydration, the dose should be increased to 100 mL/kg over 6 hours.

Inability to tolerate oral rehydration suggests the need for intravenous therapy.

6 | Pediatric Emergencies

Roger M. Barkin, MD, MPH

Most pediatric medical emergencies other than poisoning are associated with coma, convulsion, dyspnea or respiratory failure, or cardiopulmonary arrest. Other emergencies include trauma, disorders due to heat or cold, electric shock, and drowning. Tables 6–1 through 6–4 outline procedures for management of coma, status epilepticus, febrile seizures, and respiratory distress.

Adequate professional help must be promptly mobilized to manage the emergency efficiently. Resuscitation should involve a team of physicians, nurses, and other support personnel, with one member designated as the team leader.

Emergency Measures—The ABCs

(1) Assess the adequacy of the **airway, breathing,** and **circulation.** Basic life-support measures should be rapidly supplemented with advanced measures.

(2) Clear the airway of debris, vomitus, and foreign bodies. Position the patient's head. Perform intubation if the airway passage is not adequate or there is no air movement. Rarely, surgical intervention (cricothyrotomy or tracheostomy) is needed. Consider possible cervical spine injury if there is preceding trauma.

(3) Give oxygen in high concentrations immediately and continue giving oxygen during history taking, physical examination, and diagnostic procedures.

(4) Establish active breathing if the patient is not ventilating or is hypoventilating.

(5) Initiate closed chest massage if the circulation is inadequate and there is no pulse or blood pressure is low.

(6) After the airway and ventilation are stabilized and cardiac support is initiated, establish an intravenous line for administration of drugs and fluids and treatment of shock.

Table 6–1. Items to consider in the assessment and management of coma.

Immediate treatment
  (1) Stabilize airway, breathing, and circulation.
  (2) Give glucose, 0.5–1 g/kg IV.
  (3) Give naloxone, 0.1 mg/kg (maximum, 2 mg) IV, if there is any suggestion of poisoning.

Evaluation
  (1) History:
    Infection (eg, meningitis, encephalitis)
    Head trauma
    Ingestion of a toxic substance
    Endocrine and metabolic disorders (eg, diabetes, renal or hepatic failure)
    Seizure
    Vascular accident
  (2) Physical examination:
    Respiratory pattern (Cheyne–Stokes breathing, hyperventilation, or ataxia)
    Position (decorticate or decerebrate)
    Pupils (size; fixed or reactive)
    Eye movement (response to doll's eye maneuver and caloric testing; conjugate or asymmetric movement; nerve palsy)
    Blood pressure (hypo- or hypertensive)
    Nuchal rigidity
    Other clues to cause of coma (eg, evidence of trauma, icterus, acetone on breath)
  (3) Laboratory tests:
    Serum electrolytes
    Blood glucose
    Blood urea nitrogen
    Serum creatinine
    Urinalysis
    Toxicologic screen
  (4) Other procedures:
    Skull x-ray and CT scan if trauma or if an anatomic or mass lesion is suspected
    Lumbar puncture if there is no evidence of increased intracranial pressure or mass lesion, as determined by clinical or CT scan findings

Further management
  (1) Continued support of vital functions.
  (2) Specific therapy as indicated by findings.
  (3) Further diagnostic workup as necessary.

Table 6–2. Items to consider in the assessment and management of status epilepticus.*

Immediate treatment
(1) Stabilize airway, breathing, and circulation.
(2) Give glucose, 0.5–1 g/kg IV.
(3) Consider giving naloxone, 0.1 mg/kg (maximum, 2 mg) IV, if there is any suggestion of poisoning.

Evaluation
(1) History:
   Previous episodes of seizures
   Compliance with prescribed anticonvulsant therapy (if any)
   Head trauma
   Infection (eg, meningitis, encephalitis)
   Ingestion of a toxic substance
   Endocrine and metabolic disorders (eg, diabetes, sodium or calcium abnormalities, hypoglycemia)
   Vascular accident
(2) Physical examination:
   Focal or generalized seizures
   Level of consciousness
   Fecal or urinary incontinence
   Pupils and gaze (upward deviation of eyes)
   Other clues to cause of status epilepticus: eg, evidence of trauma or infection
(3) Laboratory tests (as indicated):
   Serum electrolytes
   Serum calcium
   Blood glucose
   Anticonvulsant drug levels
   Blood urea nitrogen
   Serum creatinine
   Toxicologic screen
(4) Other procedures:
   CT scan if there is any suggestion of trauma or anatomic or mass lesion
   Lumbar puncture if there is any suggestion of infection

Further managment
(1) Continued support of vital functions.
(2) Use of anticonvulsants for grand mal or tonic-clonic seizures†:
   (a) Initially, give diazepam (Valium), 0.2–0.3 mg/kg IV; repeat in 5–10 min if no response; monitor respiration. Lorazepam (Ativan) can be given as an alternative. If intravenous access cannot be achieved, consider rectal administration of diazepam.
   (b) Begin phenobarbital, 10–15 mg/kg IV given slowly (maximum, 100 mg IV every 20 minutes during the first hour); maintenance dose for patients not previoussly taking anticonvulsants is 3–5 mg/kg/24 h IV or orally.†
   (c) Further diagnostic workup as necessary and specific therapy as indicated by findings.

---

* Status epilepticus is defined as continuous seizures for over a 20-min period or more than 2 seizures without an intervening lucid period.
† Reference to alternative anticonvulsants include phenytoin (Dilantin), valproic acid, or Carbamazepine (Tegretol).

Table 6–3. Items to consider in the assessment and management of febrile seizures.*

Immediate treatment
  (1) Stabilize airway, breathing, and circulation.
  (2) Give glucose, 0.5–1 g/kg IV.
  (3) Consider giving naloxone, 0.1 mg/kg (maximum 2 mg) IV, if there is any suggestion of poisoning.

Evaluation
  (1) History:
      Infection (meningitis, encephalitis, roseola infantum, shigellosis, urinary tract infection)
      Ingestion of a toxic substance (eg, salicylates)
      Family history of febrile or afebrile seizures
  (2) Physical examination:
      Focal or generalized seizures
      Length of seizures
      Foci of infection
      Temperature
      Neurologic responses
  (3) Laboratory tests and other procedures:
      Blood glucose
      Lumbar puncture if there is any suggestion of meningitis and if there is no evidence of increased intracranial pressure, as determined by clinical findings
      Other studies as indicated by specific underlying disease considerations

Further management
  (1) Continued support of vital functions.
  (2) Use of antipyretics.
  (3) Use of anticonvulsants should be considered if the patient is under 12 months of age or if 2 or more of the following criteria are met:
      (a) Abnormal neurologic findings were present before the seizure occurred.
      (b) The seizure was complex (focal seizure lasted longer than 15 min or 2 seizures occurred within a 24-hr period).
      (c) There is a family history of afebrile seizures.
  (4) Parental education.

* For management of status epilepticus, see Table 6–2.

Diagnostic Measures

A. History: An essential case history must be obtained before rational treatment is possible. Among other items, the history should include the following:

1. Time and nature of onset.

a. In cases of trauma, the mechanism of injury and time interval since injury was sustained are crucial factors.

Table 6–4. Items to consider in the assessment and management of respiratory distress.

Immediate treatment
    Stabilize airway, breathing, and circulation.

Evaluation
    History and physical examination should assist in differentiating lower and upper airway disease.
        The **presence** of stridor indicates upper airway disease:

Usually due to–	Occasionally due to–
Epiglottitis	Laryngomalacia
Croup	Cord paralysis
Foreign body	
Bacterial tracheitis	

        The **absence** of stridor indicates lower airway disease:

Usually due to–	Occasionally due to–
Pneumonia	Congestive heart failure
Asthma	Trauma with flail chest
Bronchiolitis	Pulmonary edema
Foreign body	Cystic fibrosis
	Acidosis
	Anemia

    If upper airway disease, consider visualizing the epiglottis; do not visualize unless prepared to intubate or provide surgical airway.
    If lower airway disease is suspected, chest x-ray is essential.

Further management
    Specific therapy is indicated by findings.

  b. In cases of suspected poisoning (see Chapter 7), details of exposure are crucial; if possible, obtain and examine the container of the ingested substance, noting the list of contents and manufacturer's name and address.
  2. Previous occurrence and method of treatment, if any.
  3. History of preexisting disease or recent illness.
  4. History of drug therapy, including insulin, penicillin, etc.
  5. History of drug allergies.
  B. Physical Examination:
  1. General evaluation of state of consciousness, vital signs (including orthostatic blood pressure, pulse, respiration, temperature), hydration status, etc.
  2. Estimation of cardiorespiratory function, including electrocardiography if indicated.
  3. Examination of chest for respiratory pattern, retractions, dullness, and rales, including chest x-ray if indicated.
  4. Careful neurologic examination.

5. Examination of abdomen for size of liver, masses, tenderness, guarding, and rebound tenderness.

6. Examination of skin and musculoskeletal system for evidence of trauma.

7. Complete physical examination after the patient's condition has stabilized.

8. Frequent reassessment of the patient's status.

C. Laboratory Studies:

1. Determination of the hematocrit and a complete blood count. A sample of blood for typing and cross-matching should be obtained on admission to the hospital in anticipation of future transfusions.

2. Urinalysis for determination of glucose and acetone levels, microscopic examination, and specific gravity. Hematuria may be due to trauma or associated with an acute medical problem (eg, Henoch–Schölein purpura). An indwelling catheter may be needed.

3. Blood chemistries, including serum electrolytes, blood glucose, blood urea nitrogen, and those indicated by a specific condition. (See Tables 6–1 through 6–4.)

4. Cultures and x-ray examinations as indicated.

CARDIOPULMONARY ARREST

In children, cardiac arrest is usually secondary to respiratory insufficiency or arrest. Therefore, it is crucial to focus efforts on establishing an airway and adequate ventilation.

Basic Life Support

(1) Establish patency of the airway. In patients without cervical trauma, this may be achieved by use of the head tilt–neck lift technique. Place one hand under the patient's neck and the other hand on the forehead. Lift the neck gently, and push the head backward by gentle pressure on the forehead.

(2) Evaluate the patient's ventilatory status. If inadequate, begin mouth-to-mouth resuscitation, use a mechanical resuscitator, or deliver oxygen with a self-inflating bag (if available).

(3) Assess circulation by measuring pulse and, if possible, blood pressure. If decreased, institute external cardiac compression in conjunction with ventilatory support. In the infant, compression should be done midsternum; in the child, just above the xiphoid process. The rate of compression should be 100/min in

the infant and 80/min in the older child. The ratio of compression to respirations should be 5:1.

Advanced Life Support

Central to the initiation of advanced life support is the coordination of personnel and access to appropriate equipment and drugs. One member of the team must assume leadership.

(1) Give 100% oxygen to all patients.

(2) Assure patency of the airway. In the nontraumatized patient, positioning may be helpful. Suction and clear debris. An oropharyngeal or nasopharyngeal airway may be useful. Perform endotracheal or nasotracheal intubation, if appropriate and safe. The size of the endotracheal tube varies with the patient's age. The following sizes are recommended: under 6 months (newborns), 3 mm; 6 months, 3.5 mm; 18 months, 4 mm; 3 years, 4.5 mm; 5 years, 5–6 mm; 6–8 years, 6–6.5 mm; 8–12 years, 6.5–7 mm; and over 12 years, 7–9 mm.

(3) Establish adequate ventilation. A positive-pressure bag is often used. Oxygen content may be maximized by using a self-inflating rebreathing bag.

(4) Establish an intravenous line for administration of drugs. If unable to achieve venous access, consider placing an intraosseous line into the tibia.

(5) Correct acidosis. Acidosis has a negative effect on cardiac function and the efficacy of adrenergic drugs. Following cardiac arrest, the reduction of the Pa_{co2} may partially reduce acidosis. Correction of the metabolic component requires use of sodium bicarbonate at an initial dose of 1–2 meq/kg given over 1–5 minutes if the arrest has lasted longer than 10 minutes. Subsequent infusions should reflect arterial blood gas determinations.

(6) Control bradycardia and hypotension. Sympathomimetic drugs stimulate the β-adrenergic receptors; their effects vary, depending on the relative balance of stimulation achieved. The primary effect of α-adrenergic drugs is vasoconstriction; β_1-adrenergic drugs, tachycardia and increased myocardial contraction; and β_2-adrenergic drugs, vasodilatation and bronchodilatation. The following drugs are commonly utilized:

(a) Atropine–This drug has vagolytic action, with increased sinoatrial node discharges and increased atrioventricular node conduction, and is useful in cases of symptomatic severe bradycardia. The dose is 0.01–0.03 mg/kg (minimum, 0.1 mg; maximum, 0.6 mg per dose).

(b) Epinephrine–Epinephrine stimulates both α- and β-adrenergic receptors and increases heart rate, force of myocardial contraction, and vascular resistance. It is utilized in cases of ventricular standstill or fine ventricular fibrillation to convert the latter to coarse fibrillation. The dose of epinephrine (1:10,000 solution) is 0.1 mL/kg; it may be repeated every 5–10 minutes.

(c) Dopamine–Dopamine stimulates α- and β-adrenergic receptors as well as specific dopaminergic receptors that maintain renal and mesenteric blood vessel dilatation at low doses (< 5 μg/kg/min). It is particularly helpful in cases of shock and hypotension (5–20 mg/kg/min). Mix 200 mg of dopamine in 500 mL of 5% dextrose in water (400 μg/mL). Begin with an infusion of 2 μg/kg/min and increase slowly up to 20 μg/kg/min.

(d) Isoproterenol–This pure β-adrenergic drug increases heart rate and myocardial contraction and produces vasodilatation. The blood pressure is usually maintained by the greater cardiac output. It is particularly useful in cases of bradycardia unresponsive to atropine until pacemaker support is available. Mix 1 mg of isoproterenol in 100 mL of 5% dextrose in water (10 μg/mL). Begin with a continuous infusion of 0.1 μg/kg/min and increase up to 1.5 μg/kg/min.

(7) Control ventricular dysrhythmia, if present (rare in children). Treatment with lidocaine should be initiated when there are more than 5 premature beats per minute and beats are multifocal or come in bursts of 2 or more in rapid succession. An initial dose of 1 mg/kg is infused rapidly; if the patient responds, give a continuous infusion of 30 μg/kg/min. If the patient does not respond, give bretylium, 5 mg/kg intravenously. Defibrillation, employing an initial shock of 2 joules (watt-seconds) per kilogram, is indicated in the presence of ventricular fibrillation.

SHOCK

Shock is a clinical syndrome characterized by prostration and hypotension resulting from profound depression of cell functions associated with or secondary to poor perfusion of vital tissue. If cell function is not improved, shock becomes irreversible and death will ensue even if the initiating cause is corrected.

Clinical Findings

Early signs of shock are agitation, confusion, and thirst. As shock progresses, the patient will become increasingly unresponsive and eventually comatose.

The skin is pale, wet, and cold. The nail beds are cyanotic.

Local and peripheral edema may be present. Capillary filling is poor, and skin turgor is decreased. Tachycardia and tachypnea are present.

Newborns in shock appear pale and slightly gray, with poor capillary filling and decreased skin turgor. In late shock, there may be a decrease in skin temperature, particularly of the extremities.

Emergency Treatment

A. Position Patient: Lay the patient flat. Elevation of the legs is helpful except in respiratory distress, when it is contraindicated. In older children, use of military antishock trousers (MAST suits) may be helpful.

B. Support Life: Establish a patent upper airway, administer oxygen, and support circulation and ventilation. Follow the principles of basic life support outlined above. Prepare to institute advanced life support.

C. Establish Intravenous Access: Establish 1 or 2 intravenous lines with a large-bore catheter. Intraosseous access may be considered as an alternative.

D. Administer Fluids: Initiate fluid therapy with lactated Ringer's injection or isotonic saline solution given intravenously at a rate of 20 mL/kg over the first 30 minutes. Thereafter, administer fluids at a rate sufficient to replace and maintain blood volume while maintaining urine flow.

E. Monitor Central Venous Pressure: Establish a central venous pressure monitor if shock is not easily reversible following initial administration of fluids.

Evaluation of Emergency Treatment

The patient must be observed constantly. The pulse, blood pressure (including orthostatic, as appropriate), respiratory rate, and temperature should be taken immediately and monitored every 15 minutes until vital signs stabilize. Determine hematocrit count (this should be done in the emergency department), and send blood for white blood cell count, measurement of electrolytes and glucose level, and typing and cross-matching.

An indwelling catheter should be placed to monitor urine flow. The minimum acceptable urine output is 1 mL/kg/h; the optimal output is 2–3 mL/kg/h.

If response to fluid therapy is unsatisfactory, further vigorous antishock therapy should be instituted.

Treatment of Specific Types of Shock

A. Hypovolemic Shock: Hypovolemic shock is characterized by reduction in the effective size of the vascular compartment, with falling blood pressure, poor capillary filling, and a low central venous pressure. Treatment consists of prevention of further fluid loss and replacement of existing volume losses. Vasopressors are not useful. The type of fluid used as a volume expander depends on the cause of the hypovolemia.

1. Blood loss–Blood is the replacement fluid of choice for shock due to hemorrhage. Whenever circumstances permit, type-specific (and, optimally, cross-matched) blood should be used. Unmatched type O Rh-negative blood may be used, especially in the trauma arrest situation.

The rate of blood replacement is determined by the patient's vital signs, the rate of continuing blood loss, the response to the infusion, and the amount of crystalloid solution previously infused.

2. Dehydration–For hypovolemic shock due to dehydration, give lactated Ringer's injection or isotonic saline with 5% dextrose until electrolyte determinations have been obtained. Begin intravenous infusion of fluid at a rate of 20 mL/kg over the first 30 minutes; thereafter, administer fluid at a rate calculated to replace the deficit and maintain blood volume.

B. Cardiogenic Shock: This type of shock results from decreased cardiac output, which may be due to cardiac tamponade, myocarditis, abnormal heart rate and rhythm, or biochemical abnormalities.

1. Cardiac tamponade secondary to fluid collection in the pericardial space or constrictive pericarditis is treated by pericardiocentesis or by surgery. Limited intravenous infusion of crystalloid solution may increase venous pressure enough to allow a delay before more definitive treatment is instituted.

2. Abnormal heart rate and rhythm may cause decreased cardiac output.

a. Marked sinus bradycardia can occur during anesthesia, particularly during surgery of the neck and thorax. Sinus bradycardia can be blocked with atropine, 0.01 mg/kg as a single intravenous dose. The minimum dose of atropine for newborns is 0.1 mg regardless of weight. The maximum dose for older children is 0.6 mg, up to a total of 2 mg administered as 3–4 doses.

b. Atrioventricular block may be secondary to inflammatory disease, surgical trauma, or ischemic injury to the conduction system. If use of atropine is unsuccessful, the ventricular rate may be increased with isoproterenol, pending use of a pacemaker.

c. Ventricular arrhythmias may be secondary to hypoxia, acidosis, or myocarditis. If no specific abnormality can be found or if an abnormality is not immediately correctable, lidocaine, bretylium, or another antiarrhythmia drug may be useful in correcting the arrhythmia.

3. Biochemical disturbances, including acidosis, hypoxia, and hyperkalemia, can result in decreased cardiac output.

C. Vasogenic (Distributive) Shock:

1. Bacteremic (septic) shock–This is the most common type of vascular shock; it occurs when overwhelming sepsis and circulating bacterial toxins produce peripheral vascular collapse. Clinical recognition is based upon the toxic appearance of the patient, who often has purpura, splinter hemorrhages, hepatosplenomegaly, and jaundice.

Adequate treatment of bacteremic shock depends on supportive care of the patient and proper antibiotic treatment of the primary infection. If sepsis is likely but no specific etiologic agent can be defined immediately, take appropriate specimens for culture and then give a third-generation cephalosporin (cefotaxime, ceftriaxone, etc).

Supportive measures include the following:

a. Fluids–Replace fluids as necessary.

b. Vasopressors–Vasopressor agents may be useful.

c. Heparin–Heparin may be of value when bacterial infections are complicated by disseminated intravascular coagulation.

2. Anaphylactic shock–This is an extreme form of allergy or hypersensitivity to a foreign substance and is characterized by very low peripheral resistance. The diagnosis is established by a history of exposure to an antigen followed almost immediately by clinical signs of respiratory distress and circulatory collapse. Urticaria and angioneurotic edema are often present.

a. Tourniquet–If the shock was precipitated by a drug given intramuscularly, apply a tourniquet proximal to the site of injection. The tourniquet should be tight enough to restrict venous return but should not interrupt arterial flow.

b. β-Agonist agents–Give nembulized albuterol (0.25–0.50 mL/dose) to patients with respiratory distress, wheezing, or bronchoconstriction (see Chapters 21 and 30).

c. Corticosteroids–Give hydrocortisone sodium succinate in a dose of 4–5 mg/kg intravenously.

d. Aminophylline–For treatment of respiratory distress or wheezing, give aminophylline, 6–7 mg/kg intravenously as a loading dose, followed by a maintenance dose of 16 mg/kg/d.

e. Diphenhydramine–Diphenhydramine, 5 mg/kg/d intravenously in 4 divided doses, is a useful antihistaminic adjunct.

f. Airway–Secretions should be suctioned to maintain a clear airway. Repeated bronchoscopy may be required. Laryngeal edema may necessitate tracheal intubation followed by tracheostomy.

3. Neurogenic shock–There is usually a history of exposure to anesthetic agents, spinal cord injury, or ingestion of barbiturates, narcotics, or tranquilizers. Examination reveals abnormal reflexes and muscle tone, tachycardia and tachypnea, and low blood pressure. The pathophysiologic mechanism is loss of vessel tone with subsequent expansion of the vascular compartment, resulting in relative hypovolemia. Many anesthetic agents have a direct effect on the myocardium, causing a decreased cardiac output.

a. Underlying problem–Treat the underlying neurologic problem. Head trauma does not produce shock in the absence of involvement of other organ systems unless there is major scalp injury or an open and full fontanelle.

b. Fluids–When head trauma is not present, fluid therapy may stabilize vital signs.

3. Vasopressors–Use of vasopressor drugs may be indicated until definitive treatment has been given.

4. Shock due to miscellaneous causes–

a. Due to pulmonary embolism–Pulmonary embolism may be present if there is a fracture or significant soft tissue injury followed by symptoms of chest pain, dyspnea, hemoptysis, cyanosis, and signs of right heart failure. Treatment of shock is supportive, with oxygen and analgesics. If hypotension occurs, isoproterenol is the drug of choice, since it provides a bronchodilator effect. If right heart failure develops, a rapid-acting digitalis preparation such as digoxin should be given.

b. Due to respiratory disease–Respiratory disease due to any cause can result in sufficient hypoxia to cause shock. Shock of this nature is reversible only to the extent that the underlying disease is reversible, and treatment should be directed toward the primary pulmonary disorder. Treatment with oxygen and alkalies will only temporarily improve the patient's condition.

c. Metabolic shock–Shock may be secondary to a number of metabolic conditions, eg, adrenocortical insufficiency and diabetic acidosis.

SUDDEN INFANT DEATH SYNDROME (SIDS)

The incidence of sudden infant death syndrome (SIDS) is approximately 2–3 deaths per 1000 live births. SIDS accounts for one-third of deaths in infants between 1 month and 1 year of age. The peak incidence is between 1 and 4 months of age. In SIDS, the death is not correlated with a history of illness or disease, and a thorough postmortem examination fails to demonstrate a definitive cause of death. There are probably multiple contributing factors, including respiratory obstruction and central apnea.

When a child has died of SIDS, it is crucial for the health care provider to help the family members deal with their sense of guilt and grief. Families should be advised of support services in the community that may be useful in adjusting to their loss.

TRAUMA

The traumatized patient requires expert medical care combined with reassurance and a special sensitivity to the emotional support needed by the child and family. Establishment of appropriate treatment priorities is crucial to the management of such patients.

An aggressive and deliberate approach must be the basis for caring for the patient and should be individualized to reflect the extent of injury. Victims of major accidents should be considered to be seriously injured until their condition is proved stable. Treatment must often be initiated on the basis of clinical findings and cannot await diagnostic confirmation. The assessment and management must be individualized, but the multiply traumatized patient will benefit from the following approach.

Primary Assessment

Primary assessment must focus on the airway, ventilation, adequacy of circulation and perfusion, and management of cervical spine injury or exsanguinating hemorrhage.

A. Airway: Assure patency of the airway by clearing debris (especially chewing gum) and positioning the head to minimize any obstruction. In all patients with head trauma or multiple injuries, specific attention must be directed toward stabilizing the cervical spine to avoid further injury.

B. Ventilation: Ventilation must be assessed to determine its adequacy and ensure that breath sounds are symmetric, with consideration given to the presence of pneumothorax, hemothorax, flail chest, or pulmonary contusion. Evaluate for evidence of respiratory distress, cyanosis, tracheal deviation, and bony crepitus.

C. Circulation: Circulation may be rapidly assessed by determining adequacy of perfusion and by measuring blood pressure. Up to 25% of blood volume may be lost before hypotension is detected in patients in the supine position. Orthostatic changes occur early. In the absence of external trauma, the major body cavities that require evaluation are the chest, abdomen, and retroperitoneum.

Major blood loss may occur secondary to orthopedic injuries.

Head trauma does not cause shock unless bleeding is massive with spreading of sutures in the infant or avulsion of the scalp. Other causes of posttraumatic shock to consider are cardiac contusion or rupture, lacerations, vascular injury, and underlying disease; these causes should be detectable on physical examination.

D. Cervical Spine Injuries: Cervical spine injuries should be considered in all multiply traumatized patients as well as those with head injuries or impaired sensorium. If there is any question of injury, the head should be immobilized with sandbags and secured in position until a series of x-rays of the cervical spine can be completed. A cross-table lateral neck film will detect 80–90% of injuries.

Initial Resuscitation

Initial management must focus on eliminating life-threatening conditions and ensuring that a number of technical activities are completed as appropriate.

(1) Oxygen should be administered to all patients. If there is any question of airway patency, the patient should be intubated. Nasotracheal intubation is preferred if cervical spine injury is suspected and there are no facial injuries. If there is no evidence of spinal injury or if the cross-table lateral x-ray shows negative results, oral intubation may be attempted. Cricothyroidotomy is rarely indicated.

(2) Active intervention may be necessary to control ventilation following stabilization of the airway. If there is evidence of pneumothorax or hemothorax, a chest tube should be inserted, often on the basis of clinical examination of the unstable patient.

(3) External hemorrhage must be controlled, usually by direct pressure. Be careful of pressure over the neck or eyes, since pressure may cause an increase in vagal tone.

(4) An intravenous line must be placed; the number and size of lines should reflect the severity of the injury. If shock is present, a bolus of normal saline solution or lactated Ringer's injection (20 mL/kg) should be given intravenously as rapidly as possible. Subsequent administration of crystalloid and blood must reflect the response to this initial infusion. In general, once a total of 40–50 mL of crystalloid per kilogram has been given,

blood is required if hypovolemic shock is still present. Type- and cross-matched blood should be given if possible.

(5) If significant shock is present, pediatric pneumatic anti-shock trousers should be inflated after the lower extremities, back, and abdomen have been examined for injury. Once inflated, pneumatic trousers should not be removed until some stability has been achieved. At that time, the compartments of the trousers should be deflated one at a time, starting with the abdomen, and vital signs and acid–base status should be carefully monitored.

(6) If blood is present at the urethral meatus, immediate urologic consultation is necessary and radiologic examination required. Urinary catheters should usually be inserted after ensuring that there is no blood at the urethral meatus. Dipstick tests should be done; if positive, a microscopic examination should follow.

(7) A nasogastric tube should be inserted after the cervical spine is proved stable. Aspirate should be obtained and tested for blood.

(8) Cardiac monitoring should be initiated and an ECG done.

(9) Immediately after intravenous catheters are placed, blood should be drawn for hematocrit, complete blood count, typing and cross-matching, and arterial blood gas measurements. Electrolyte, glucose, and blood urea nitrogen determinations and urine and serum toxicology screens should be ordered if appropriate.

(10) X-rays should include a complete series of cervical spine films as well as chest and pelvic films. X-rays of the abdomen and extremities may be done, if indicated, after the patient's condition is stable. Portable films are useful in the unstable patient.

(11) All of the patient's clothing should be removed so that the patient can be examined thoroughly. This prevents overlooking an injury. A complete examination is necessary; do not stop the examination when one major injury has been detected.

(12) The initial history must be sufficient to determine the nature of the injury, with particular attention to measures of severity (eg, in the case of an accident, the extent of damage to the automobile and its speed) as well as the time elapsed since the accident. Past medical problems, allergies, use of medications, and other relevant medical data should be ascertained rapidly.

(13) Once the priority areas have been evaluated and treatment initiated, the patient should be reassessed. If no further immediate therapy is required, a more complete secondary examination can be initiated and detailed history obtained.

Secondary Assessment & Treatment

The secondary assessment must include a systematic examination and initiation of appropriate therapeutic procedures.

A. Head and Nerve Injuries: A rapid but complete neurologic examination should be performed, with assessment of the following:

1. Level of consciousness.

2. Movement of the body–Determine symmetry, position, and posturing.

3. Pupils–Dilated fixed pupils are a reliable sign of the site of the lesion unless drug ingestion has occurred. For example, in cerebral mass lesions, there is ipsilateral dilatation of the pupil with contralateral hemiparesis.

4. Extraocular movement–A hemispheric lesion will cause the eyes to deviate toward the lesion, but a brainstem lesion will cause the eyes to deviate away from the lesion.

5. Reflexes

6. Tympanic membrane and nose–Determine if hematotympanum or otorrhea is present.

7. Rectal examination–Determine muscle tone. Absence of rectal tone in a comatose patient may be the only evidence of spinal cord injury.

8. Head and scalp–Frequent serial examinations of neurologic function are indicated to determine progression of deficits.

Diagnostic procedures include cervical spine x-rays, as discussed above. The cross-table lateral spine x-ray is an excellent screening mechanism that detects 80–90% of injuries. It is indicated in any patient with decreased sensorium, neck trauma, or tenderness of the neck following trauma, as well as in patients with major trauma and an unknown or unreliable medical history.

Skull x-rays are indicated in patients with an abnormal sensorium following trauma if there was a significant loss of consciousness, a neurologic defect, or increasing or persistent headache; in patients with head trauma, especially trauma due to a depressing force, such as a shoe or hammer; and in cases in which CT scans are necessary and a delay in obtaining their results is anticipated.

CT scan is the definitive test and should be done following trauma if there is a localized neurologic defect, deteriorating neurologic status, evidence of skull depression on x-ray or clinical examination, or any evidence of increased intracranial pressure.

B. Face and Mouth Injuries: The patient should be assessed for lacerations, fractures, malocclusion, and loose teeth.

Most linear lacerations or punctures of the buccal mucosa, tonsillar pillars, or posterior pharynx in children result from falling with a lollipop stick, pencil, ruler, or other object in the mouth. These injuries usually require no therapy beyond antibiotics. They heal as well without sutures as they do with them. The specific indications for examination and possible suturing under anesthesia are (1) deep puncture of the soft palate, (2) the presence of a flap of mucoperiosteum lifted off the hard palate, and (3) crepitus of the neck, indicating deep puncture.

Tongue lacerations usually result from penetration by the incisors. These, too, will heal without sutures in most cases. Lacerations through the edge of the tongue, producing a triangular flap, are best sutured with an absorbable suture.

Treatment of traumatic injuries to the teeth must reflect the degree of displacement or mobility and whether primary or secondary teeth are involved. In general, displacement or evulsion of a permanent tooth requires emergency care after the patient's condition is stable. The tooth should be reinserted and held in place until a dentist can see the patient. Injuries to primary teeth should be seen but on a less urgent basis.

C. Neck Injuries: The patient should be assessed for tracheal deviation, vein distention, ecchymosis, and evidence of penetrating injuries. Injuries may be indicative of chest disorders or cervical spine damage. Lesions that penetrate the platysma usually require surgical exploration.

D. Chest Injuries: The chest should be reexamined more thoroughly, and response to initial measures for stabilization should be evaluated. Chest x-ray and determination of arterial blood gases may be indicated if the patient is stable and findings on examination remain equivocal.

1. Rib fracture–Pleuritic pain (sharp pain exacerbated with breathing), localized severe pain with pressure at the fracture site, crepitus with respiration, pain with compression of the sternum or lateral chest, or pleural friction rub may be present. Patients should be examined for hemothorax or pneumothorax. Rib fractures are unusual in younger children and indicate a severe traumatic injury. Fractures of ribs 1 and 2 may be associated with a vascular injury. Fractures of ribs 10–12 often accompany abdominal injuries.

2. Flail chest–If 3 or more adjacent ribs are fractured at 2 points, the chest may move paradoxically with respiration—ie, the chest moves inward with inspiration and outward with expiration. Flail chest is characterized by pain, dyspnea, and respiratory distress. The respiratory distress is primarily due to the underlying pulmonary injury. Stabilization of the flail chest is necessary, often by mechanical means. Intubation may be required if respiratory distress is present or there are massive injuries with accompanying pathologic disorders. Positive pressure ventilation will stabilize the chest.

3. Pulmonary contusion–This results when there is lung parenchymal damage. Chest trauma causes hemorrhage over the contused area of lung, often with a rapid deceleration injury. Respiratory distress develops with significant hypoxia, usually within 4–6 hours of the injury. Increased pulmonary shunting leads to a progressive rise in a Pa_{CO2} and fall in Pa_{O2} levels. Chest x-ray demonstrates alveolar infiltrates progressing on occasion to consolidation. The findings may be delayed.

Patients with pulmonary contusion require oxygen by mask and pulmonary support. Intubation and ventilation may be necessary, with accompanying use of positive end-expiratory pressure.

4. Pneumothorax–Pneumothorax is classically characterized by dyspnea, cyanosis, and absence of breath and voice sounds on the involved side. In cases of tension pneumothorax, pulsus paradoxus is seen.

a. Spontaneous pneumothorax–In older children, there is usually rupture of a bleb, with leakage of air into the pleural cavity; the source of the leak usually heals spontaneously. Spontaneous pneumothorax is characterized by the sudden onset of dyspnea, pleuritic pain, hyperresonance, and absent breath and voice sounds over the involved lobe. Symptoms and signs do not progress. The condition may complicate an asthmatic attack or cystic fibrosis.

b. Tension pneumothorax–Failure of the lung leak to seal may produce a one-way valve effect leading to an increase of air in the pleural space with each breath. This results in mediastinal shift, rapidly progressive dyspnea and cyanosis, and typical physical findings. Tension pneumothorax may result from trauma such as a penetrating or blunt injury or may accompany spontaneous pneumothorax. This is a life-threatening condition and requires immediate decompression by needle or chest tube (usually preceding chest x-ray).

c. Open pneumothorax–Open pneumothorax is characterized by the presence of an open wound and severe respiratory distress with cyanosis and audible sucking sounds. The opening should be closed at once and covered with an occlusive dressing (eg, petrolatum gauze). A chest tube is required.

5. Hemothorax–Signs of pleural fluid include absent fremitus, loss of resonance, absent breath and voice sounds, and tracheal shift, together with evidence of hemorrhage into the chest. Hemothorax is often associated with pneumothorax. Use of a chest tube is definitive therapy and should follow chest x-ray if the patient is stable.

6. Penetrating wounds of the chest–

a. Closed wounds–A minute point of entry may be associated with extensive intrathoracic damage. The patient should be assessed for pneumothorax, hemothorax, subcutaneous or mediastinal emphysema, cardiac contusion, or cardiac tamponade and treated appropriately on the basis of findings.

b. Open wounds–Open wounds inevitably produce critical pneumothorax (see above).

E. Cardiac Injuries: Patients should be examined for evidence of anterior chest wall trauma, which may be the only evidence of cardiac contusion. Tachycardia may also be present, consistent with cardiac contusion or evidence of ischemia. Fullness of the jugular vein should be ascertained and the point of maximal impulse determined.

1. Cardiac contusion–Cardiac contusion results from blunt trauma to the anterior mid chest. Chest pain may be present initially or may be delayed. Findings on ECG demonstrate tachycardia or nonspecific ST–T wave changes. Dysrhythmia may be present.

2. Pericardial tamponade–This results from penetrating wounds of the chest and accumulation of blood in the pericardial sac, progressing to limitation of diastolic filling of the heart and subsequent narrowing of pulse pressure, increased pulse rate, paradoxic pulse, engorged neck veins with high central venous pressure, and hypotension. Pericardiocentesis is the treatment of choice.

F. Abdominal Injuries: In children, abdominal injuries are primarily blunt in origin. The ability to obtain an accurate history is often compromised by the clinical condition of the patient, the age of the child, the presence of intracranial injuries, or drug or alcohol use. Tenderness is usually present in patients with abdominal disorders and alert mental status. It may be localized or diffuse. Bowel sounds may be absent, and distention may develop. After consultation and with the advice and assistance of a surgical consultant, peritoneal lavage should be performed if indicated. A modified open technique is usually preferred. Helpful x-ray studies that may be done, depending upon the stability of the patient, include plain films, contrast studies, a liver–spleen scan, and a CT scan.

1. Nonpenetrating abdominal injuries–Injuries with significant hypotension and cardiovascular collapse usually require immediate laparotomy. Stable patients with equivocal results of examination may be observed or undergo peritoneal lavage, depending upon the condition of the child and the facilities and expertise available to care for the patient.

a. Splenic rupture–Manifestations are due to hemorrhage and shock. Splenic rupture is characterized by a history of injury followed immediately or with some delay (subcapsular hemorrhage) by left upper quadrant and shoulder pain, rebound tenderness, muscle rigidity, signs of bleeding, a mass in the left upper quadrant, and shock. Spontaneous rupture may occur with leukemia, infectious mononucleosis, or malaria.

b. Liver rupture–Manifestations are due to hemorrhage, shock, and possibly bile peritonitis. Liver rupture is characterized by a history of injury followed immediately or after a few hours by right upper quadrant pain, tenderness, and signs of hemorrhage. Shock and rapid exsanguination may occur.

c. Pancreatic and duodenal injuries–Because these organs are retroperitoneal, signs and symptoms are often obscure and delayed. Pancreatic injuries may be associated with diffuse midepigastric, abdominal, or back pain. Amylase levels may be elevated. Pancreatic pseudocysts may develop. Intramural duodenal hematomas cause proximal intestinal obstruction.

d. Intestinal rupture–Manifestations are due to localized peritonitis, anemia, or gangrene of the bowel following injury or mesenteric tear and impairment of blood supply. Upright x-rays show free air under the diaphragm and ileus and free fluid in the abdomen. Amylase levels may be elevated.

e. Kidney rupture–Manifestations are due to perirenal bleeding and urinary extravasation or intrarenal bleeding. Kidney rupture is characterized by a history of bleeding or injury followed by flank pain, hematuria, local costovertebral angle tenderness, swelling, muscle spasms, a palpable mass, nonshifting flank dullness, shock, and ecchymoses. An intravenous urogram is important for confirmation and determination of the extent of injury. Hematuria may not be present with renal vascular thrombosis, renal pedicle injury, or complete transection of the ureter.

f. Bladder rupture–Bladder rupture occurs from blunt trauma and may be intraperitoneal or extraperitoneal, thereby determining the nature of the signs and symptoms. The trauma usually occurs when the patient has a full bladder. Patients develop persistent pain, suprapubic tenderness, ileus, and inability to void. Signs of free fluid in the peritoneal cavity may be present, and a boggy suprapubic mass may be felt if the diagnosis is delayed. Radiologic examination is the most dependable test for bladder injury and should include a pelvic x-ray to rule out concurrent fractures.

g. Urethral rupture–Manifestations depend upon the segment of the urethra involved. Urine or blood extravasates around the bladder, prostate, or perineum or in the anterior perineal wall. An abdominal or perineal injury followed by pain, blood at the urethral meatus, difficulty in voiding, and signs of extravasation requires immediate evaluation. Urologic consultation should be obtained immediately (before inserting a urinary catheter).

2. Penetrating abdominal injuries–Penetrating injuries must be explored locally and the patient examined thoroughly. Minute wounds may mask extensive internal damage. If there is any evidence of intraperitoneal penetration on local wound exploration, peritoneal lavage should be performed if the patient is stable; laparotomy should be performed if the patient is deteriorating.

G. Perineal Injuries: Perineal injuries most often result from falls on a bicycle (impact of the bicycle seat), falls in a bath tub, or sexual assault.

Injuries to the labia often cause bruising, edema, and urinary retention. Have the child attempt to urinate while sitting in a tub of warm water. Catheterization is rarely necessary.

Vaginal injuries in the young child require examination under sedation or anesthesia.

Penile, scrotal, and testicular injuries will reflect the nature of the insult. A urologist should usually be consulted. Superficial lacerations may be closed with absorbable suture. Deeper wounds require operative exploration.

H. Orthopedic Injuries: See Chapter 26.

ACUTE HEAD INJURIES

Head injuries may be classified as open or closed. Both types are often seen in the same patient and may require consideration jointly. Attention should always be given to the possibility of injury elsewhere, particularly to the cervical spine.

SEVERE CLOSED WOUNDS OF THE HEAD

The chief dangers of closed head injuries are from immediate destruction of brain tissue (contusions, lacerations); mass effect, compression (subdural, epidural), and progressive secondary damage due to anoxia; and cerebral compression due to intracranial hemorrhage or edema.

Anoxia is one of the most frequent causes of death from head injuries. It is induced by (1) respiratory tract obstruction or involvement, which leads to hypoxia, or (2) a decrease in the capacity of the contused brain to utilize oxygen.

The single best indicator of progressive intracranial bleeding is a change in the level of consciousness. The appearance of focal signs such as seizures or weakness is an important diagnostic aid.

Treatment

A. Emergency Measures:

1. Maintain an adequate airway to minimize hypoxia due to mechanical respiratory obstruction. Elevate the head (if possible) to maximize venous drainage of the head. Do *not* elevate the head if secretions are a problem. Surgical management of the airway is indicated if there is major facial trauma and endotracheal or nasotracheal intubation is contraindicated.

2. Immobilize the cervical spine.

3. Give oxygen. Hypoxia of the brain may exist in the absence of noticeable peripheral cyanosis. The most satisfactory route for oxygen administration is by nasal catheter, but this may be difficult in a small child. Stabilize ventilation.

4. Treat shock if present. Shock does not occur with closed head trauma unless there is major scalp injury and bleeding or unless the sutures are open, in which case extensive intracranial bleeding may occur. If shock is present, look for other injuries.

5. In patients with severe head trauma and altered mental status, monitor and control intracranial pressure. Initially, patients may be hyperventilated following intubation and establishment of an airway. Elevate the patient's head and administer diuretics as follows: mannitol, 0.5 mg/kg intravenously over 10–15 minutes every 3–4 hours as needed, or furosemide (Lasix), 1 mg/kg intravenously every 4–6 hours. In severe cases, intracranial monitoring with institution of prolonged barbiturate-induced coma in an intensive care unit may be indicated.

6. Treat hyperthermia promptly. Hyperthermia indicates a disturbed temperature-regulating mechanism. It increases the metabolic and oxygen requirements of tissues that already suffer from lack of oxygen, and it may result in peripheral vascular collapse and may further increase brain hypoxia.

B. General Measures:

1. Perform x-rays of the skull in cases of major head trauma and in patients with neurologic deficits, loss of consciousness for

more than 5 minutes, accompanying seizures, or a worrisome or inconsistent history. Skull x-rays may often be omitted in favor of doing an emergent CT scan as the *primary* diagnostic study.

2. Perform CT scans in all cases of severe injury and in patients with neurologic deficits, especially those with progressive, altered, or deteriorating neurologic status. This may substitute initially for skull x-rays if bone windows are done.

3. Correct fluid imbalance by parenteral administration of fluids that are designed to provide maintenance sodium requirements and to replace losses through vomiting or via lungs, kidneys, or skin. Do not flood the patient with excessive amounts of fluid. Maintenance fluids should be two-thirds to three-fourths of normal levels to assist in decreasing cerebral edema.

4. Institute gastric feeding of a high-protein diet by nasal catheter in cases of prolonged coma. Tracheostomized patients can more readily be maintained in this fashion, because the danger of aspiration of vomitus is decreased. Small gastric tubes are less likely to contribute to the formation of tracheoesophageal fistula in the presence of a tracheostomy. Intravenous hyperalimentation may also be utilized.

5. Avoid the use of sedatives. If sedation is required in a restless, apprehensive patient, the patient's condition should be monitored by CT scanning.

6. Avoid the use of morphine and codeine. They may depress respiration and may cause edema of the larynx, and the attendant alteration of pupil size is undesirable for diagnostic reasons.

C. Ongoing Measures: Clinical response in the first few hours will generally indicate whether urgent surgical intervention is necessary.

1. Take pulse and respiration every 15 minutes, temperature every 30 minutes, and blood pressure every hour.

2. Test the level of consciousness by ability to respond.

3. Install an indwelling urinary catheter if indicated (usually necessary).

4. Continue oxygen inhalation. A free airway should be maintained and the patient suctioned when necessary.

5. Use restraints if necessary (not usually indicated).

6. Look for signs of worsening of the child's condition. Patients with signs of progressive stupor, convulsions, focal paralysis, and disturbance of vital signs (such as alterations of pulse, respiration, and blood pressure) require neurosurgical intervention as a lifesaving measure.

7. Do not institute hypothermia therapy. This is contrain-

dicated, since the oxygen requirements at 34 °C (93 °F) are much greater than at the isothermic temperature of 37 °C (98.6 °F). True hypothermia of 28–30 °C (82–84 °F) is of questionable value in this situation.

8. Always consider the possibility of an inflicted head injury, including injury resulting from violent shaking of a small child.

OPEN WOUNDS OF THE HEAD
(Lacerations)

Treatment

The measures described here represent treatment for lacerations and extensive wounds. They are performed after stabilization of the airway, breathing, and circulation, and may lead directly to a neurosurgical procedure. Measures should be instituted as the child's general condition permits.

A. Emergency Measures:

1. Apply a compression bandage to control bleeding.

2. Shave the scalp widely around the wound.

3. Cleanse the wound with soap and water and irrigate it thoroughly.

4. Infiltrate margins of the wound with procaine or lidocaine.

5. Debride the wound thoroughly.

6. Gently explore the outer table of the skull for fracture. If no fracture is found, close the wound snugly in one or 2 layers with interrupted sutures of nonabsorbable material.

B. General Measures:

1. Give a tetanus toxoid booster if the patient has been immunized previously. Give 500–3000 units of tetanus immune globulin if a history of immunization cannot be obtained.

2. Give broad-spectrum antibiotics in massive doses only if the wound is dirty.

3. Suture and close appropriately.

C. Surgical Measures: Treatment of associated extensive brain injury requires prompt neurosurgical consultation as well as special equipment. Leakage of cerebrospinal fluid from the nose or ears poses a special problem of incipient bacterial meningitis. Prompt use of massive antibiotic prophylaxis is justified to prevent this serious complication. The child should be kept in a sitting position. Leakage usually improves spontaneously within 10 days.

DISORDERS DUE TO HEAT

BURNS

Burns are tissue injuries due to heat and may be graded as follows:

(1) Classification by depth–In first-degree burns, there is erythema without blistering; in second-degree burns, erythema with blistering; and in third-degree burns, destruction of deeper tissues.

(2) Classification by extent–Minor burns involve less than 10% of the body surface (Fig 6–1) and are usually first-degree burns. Extensive, major burns involve over 20% of the body surface with second-degree burns or over 10% of the body surface with third-degree burns. A smaller burn with significant involvement of the hands, face, feet, or genitalia qualifies as a major burn because of the difficulty in caring for such injuries.

1. MINOR (FIRST-DEGREE) BURNS

Local application of ice for 30–60 minutes markedly decreases the development of the burn and may produce relief of pain. Blebs should be protected or, if open, debrided under sterile conditions. Debrided blebs may either be left open or treated with silver sulfadiazine.

2. EXTENSIVE (SECOND- & THIRD-DEGREE) BURNS

When tissues are burned, plasma is lost into the burned area and from the surface of the burn. This leads to hypoproteinemia, which remains as long as a granulating surface is present. In turn, the granulating surface heals poorly as long as there is hypoproteinemia. The loss of plasma results in a reduced blood volume, hemoconcentration, low cardiac output, decreased blood flow, oliguria, elevated nonprotein nitrogen level, and leukocytosis. Although anemia due to hemolysis may occur in the first 2–4 days, it more commonly becomes apparent on about the fifth day. Secondary infection frequently occurs and must be treated promptly. Death may result in an adult when 30% or more of the body surface is involved. In an infant, involvement of 10% may be associated with very severe effects.

The course of a severe burn is usually as follows: (1) neu-

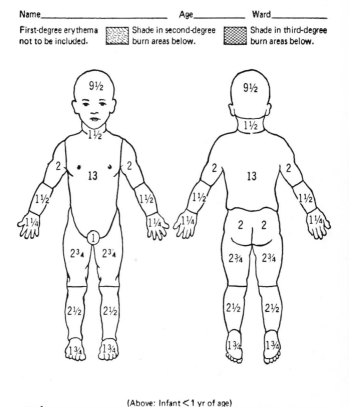

Figure 6–1. Lund and Browder modification of Berkow's scale for estimating extent of burns.

rogenic shock (immediate), (2) burn shock (first 48 hours), (3) toxemia (occurring on about the third day), (4) sepsis (also about the third day), and (5) healing and restoration of function.

Treatment

A. Emergency Measures:

1. Promptly hospitalize patients with major or extensive burns.

2. Give meperidine (Demerol) or morphine intravenously if analgesia is indicated.

3. Administer oxygen by mask or catheter. Active airway management is rarely indicated.

4. Begin treatment for shock if present. Aggressive fluid administration is essential. Hypotension is usually delayed in onset.

5. Promptly cool the affected part (eg, by immersion in cool water or application of ice or cool compresses).

6. Obtain surgical consultation early for moderate and severe burns.

B. General Measures:

1. Determine levels of hemoglobin or hematocrit and electrolytes.

2. Determine the surface area involved, utilizing Figure 6–1.

3. Determine the urine output. Flow should be maintained at a level of at least 1 mL/kg/h and optimally 2–3 mL/kg/h. Use of a catheter is often indicated.

4. Carefully debride and cleanse all second- and third-degree burns prior to application of topical creams or dressings.

5. Use topical creams or dressings as indicated. Individualization of treatment is essential for each patient. Silver sulfadiazine (Silvadene), 1% cream, is applied topically to most second- and third-degree burns; the frequency of secondary infection is reduced. The approach to dressings is determined by the degree of burns, the areas involved, and the expertise of the health care team. Many prefer to leave burns open, allowing them to air dry. This works particularly well for small burns and in those areas that are difficult to cover (eg, face, genitalia). Some health care teams recommend that large burns be covered with topical creams and dressings or with material such as pig skin.

6. Replace fluid loss. Electrolyte solutions should be given rapidly intravenously, using large-bore catheters. Lactated Ringer's injection should be initiated at a rate of 4 mL/kg body weight times the percentage of body surface area burned. Half the calculated replacement volume should be given during the first 8 hours

after the burn and the remainder over the next 16 hours. Maintenance therapy is given in addition to replacement therapy. The adequacy of fluid therapy is monitored by urinary flow.

7. Give a tetanus toxoid booster if the child is immunized, or give tetanus immune globulin if the child is unimmunized. The dosage for infants is 500 units intramuscularly, and that for older children and adults is 500–3000 units intramuscularly.

8. Maintain the nutritional status in patients with burns. Efforts should be made to maintain normal caloric intake.

9. Use antibiotics only if infection is present. The choice of drugs depends on the demonstration of the etiologic agent by cultures of blood and exudate from the burned area.

HEAT EXHAUSTION

Heat exhaustion is caused by sustained exposure to heat and is characterized by volume depletion and collapse of peripheral circulation, accompanied by salt depletion and dehydration.

Clinical Findings

A. Symptoms and Signs: Findings include weakness, dizziness, and stupor; headache; profuse perspiration; cool, pale skin; oliguria; and tachycardia. There are no muscle cramps.

B. Laboratory Findings: Findings include hemoconcentration and salt depletion. In some instances, serum sodium levels are not strikingly low.

Treatment

A. Emergency Measures: Treat shock when present. Give saline solution, 20 mL/kg over 30 minutes intravenously. Replace fluid deficits.

B. General Measures: Place the child at rest in a cool, shady place. Elevate the feet and massage the legs.

HEAT STROKE
(Sunstroke)

Heat stroke is caused by prolonged exposure to high temperatures and is characterized by failure of the heat-regulating mechanism. A number of factors increase the risk of experiencing heat stroke; these include drug ingestion (phenothiazines), extremes of age (infancy or old age), and excessive excercise or manual labor.

Clinical Findings

A. Symptoms and Signs: Findings include sudden loss of consciousness; hyperpyrexia; hot, flushed, and dry skin; rapid, irregular, and weak pulse; and cessation of sweating (an index of the failure of the heat-regulating mechanism). There may be premonitory headache, dizziness, nausea, and visual disturbances. Rectal temperatures may be as high as 42.2–43.3 °C (108–110 °F).

B. Laboratory Findings: Hydration and the salt content of the body are normal.

Treatment

A. Emergency Measures: Treatment is aimed at reducing high temperature.

1. Place the child in a cool, shady place and remove all of the child's clothing. Cool the child by fanning after sprinkling with water. Immerse in tepid water or sponge thoroughly to reduce body temperature. *Caution:* Discontinue all antipyretic measures when a temperature of 39 °C (102 °F) is reached.

2. Avoid sedation (unless the child is having convulsions, in which case diazepam may be used). Use of sedation further disturbs the heat-regulating mechanism.

3. Monitor fluid and electrolyte levels. Replace losses if indicated.

B. General Measures: Avoid immediate reexposure to heat. Inability to tolerate high temperatures may remain for a long time.

DISORDERS DUE TO COLD

Keeping the child warm and dry will prevent most disorders due to cold. Children in cold climates should be taught to exercise the extremities (including fingers and toes) to maintain circulation and warmth.

FROSTBITE

Frostbite, an injury of the superficial tissues, is caused by freezing. There are 3 grades of severity: In first-degree frostbite, there is freezing without blistering or peeling; in second-degree, freezing with blistering or peeling; and in third-degree, freezing with necrosis of the skin or deeper tissues (or both).

Mild cases of frostbite are characterized by numbness, prickling, and itching. More severe degrees of frostbite may produce paresthesia and stiffness. As the body part thaws, tenderness and burning pain become severe. The skin is white or yellow, and the involved joints are stiff. Hyperemia, edema, blisters, and necrosis may appear. Localized frostbite may prove difficult to diagnose. The most common areas are on the face under hat straps and buckles.

Treatment

A. Emergency Measures: Treatment is best instituted during the stage of reactive hyperemia, as thawing begins. Rewarming should be done only once. If there is any possibility that the injured part may experience refreezing en route to definitive therapy, rewarming should be delayed.

1. Do *not* rub or massage parts or apply ice, snow, or heat.

2. Protect the injured part from trauma and secondary infection and loosen all constricting garments.

3. Remove the patient to a warm environment.

a. In mild cases, warm the exposed part with natural body heat (eg, place the patient's hands in his or her axillae, next to the abdomen, or in the groin).

b. In severe cases, keep the affected parts uncovered at room temperature (23–27 °C [74–80 °F]). Fairly rapid thawing at temperatures slightly above that of body heat may lessen the extent of necrosis.

4. Elevate the affected part.

5. Give sedation if necessary.

B. General Measures: If indicated, give a tetanus toxoid booster (for immunized child) or tetanus immune globulin (for unimmunized child). Antibiotics should be used only when specific infection is present. The use of heparin is controversial, and its effects are not well documented in cases of frostbite.

C. Surgical Measures: The need for amputation should be carefully evaluated; necrosis and gangrene may be very superficial, and the tissue may heal well. Sympathetic and paravertebral block are contraindicated.

DROWNING & ELECTRIC SHOCK

DROWNING

Contrary to some published reports, there is no essential clinical difference between near drowning in salt water or fresh water, and the treatment is the same for both. Differences may arise in the amounts of fresh or sea water absorbed from the stomach. The basic problems are hypoxemia, acidemia, and severe laryngospasm associated with pulmonary edema.

Treatment
A. Emergency Measures:
1. Clear the upper respiratory tract and pull the tongue forward.

2. Begin artificial respiration (resuscitation) immediately if required. Resuscitation replaces spontaneous respiration and provides needed oxygen to the tissues until the paralyzed respiratory center can resume its normal function.

3. Continue artificial respiration for many hours, even in the absence of any signs of life. Only absolute signs of death (ie, rigor mortis and persistent hypothermia) justify discontinuing efforts.
B. General Measures:
1. Administer oxygen during manual artificial respiration if possible. It is necessary only to maintain a free flow of oxygen close to the mouth and nose.

2. Give external cardiac massage.

3. Empty stomach contents to minimize aspiration.

4. Aggressively treat metabolic and respiratory acidosis, which may both develop. Closely monitor blood gas determinations.

5. Treat shock and respiratory distress associated with the onset of pulmonary edema. Often, ventilator support with positive end-expiratory pressure (PEEP) is necessary, as well as diuretics.

6. Give morphine as necessary to control agitation but only if ventilation is being controlled. (Stimulants and corticosteroids are not useful.)

7. Give antibiotics only if signs of infection appear. Direct culturing is recommended if near drowning occurs in contaminated water.

ELECTRIC SHOCK

Direct current is much less dangerous than alternating current. Alternating current of high frequency or high voltage is less dangerous than alternating current of low frequency or low voltage. With alternating currents of 25–300 Hz, low voltages tend to produce ventricular fibrillation; high voltages (> 1000 Hz), respiratory failure; and intermediate voltages (220–1000 Hz), both.

Clinical Findings

A. Symptoms: Electric burns are usually small, round or oval, sharply demarcated, painless gray areas without associated inflammatory reaction. Little happens to them for several weeks; sloughing then occurs slowly and in a fairly wide area. Electric shock may produce loss of consciousness, which may be momentary or prolonged. With recovery, there may be muscular pain, fatigue, headache, and nervous irritability (the so-called postshock psychosis).

B. Signs: The physical signs are often misleading in that the small entry and exit wounds may be associated with major muscle injury (similar to a crush injury), electrolyte imbalance, renal failure, and cardiac dysrhythmias. Over a period of days, there may be intravascular thrombosis resulting in necrosis of muscle fibers. In cases of ventricular fibrillation, the patient is unconscious; no heart sounds or pulse can be found; and the respirations continue for a few minutes, becoming exaggerated as asphyxia occurs and then ceasing as death intervenes. In cases of respiratory failure, the patient is unconscious; respirations are absent; the pulse can be felt, although there is a marked fall in blood pressure; and the skin is cold and cyanotic.

Treatment

A. Emergency Measures:

1. Interrupt the current.

2. Give artificial respiration (mouth-to-mouth) and administer oxygen if available.

3. Give external cardiac massage.

4. Treat shock promptly.

5. Treat cardiac dysrhythmias.

6. Monitor electrolytes (especially potassium) and renal function.

B. General Measures:

1. Treat simple burns, if indicated, by local therapy to affected areas of skin and mucous membrane.

2. Treat severe burns conservatively. Infection is usually not present early. Granulation tissue should be well established before surgery is attempted. Hemorrhage may occur late and may be severe. Debridement may be necessary and should be left to the surgeon.

BITES

DOG BITES

Perhaps the greatest service the physician can render to the patient who has been bitten by a dog is to ensure the patient has not been exposed to rabies. This may be done by ascertaining the local epidemiologic pattern of rabies and (if there is a risk) having the dog impounded by the local health department so that it may be observed for the development of clinical signs of rabies. The dog must never be destroyed, except in self-defense or to prevent its escape. The examination of the dog's brain by a department of health or university medical center may allow a histologic and immunologic diagnosis of rabies to be made or ruled out.

Treatment
    A. Emergency Measures: Rabies vaccine and rabies immune globulin are discussed in Chapter 9.
    B. General Measures:
    1. Cleanse the wound thoroughly with soap and water, using a syringe to force water into the wound.
    2. Debride the wound to remove dead tissue and dirt.
    3. Give tetanus toxoid booster if the patient has been immunized previously. Give tetanus immune globulin if immunization has not taken place.
    4. Give antibiotics if wounds are on the face, hand, or feet or if wounds are extensive. Penicillin or a cephalosporin is preferred.
    5. Avoid suturing minor dog bites; the potential for infection is tremendous if sutures are used. If suturing is done for cosmetic reasons, give antibiotics in large doses.

HUMAN BITES

Minimal abrasions of the skin resulting from bites among children require only local care and generally heal promptly.

However, penetrating bites cause some of the most severe of all infections because of the wide variety of pathogenic organisms present in the human mouth. Prompt and vigorous treatment is necessary to prevent prolonged infections.

Treatment

A. Emergency Measures: Give antibiotics if wounds are on the face, hand or feet or if wounds are extensive. Ampicillin, a cephalosporin, or a combination of both may be given.

B. General Measures:

1. Cleanse the wound thoroughly with soap and water, using a syringe to force water into the wound.

2. Debride the wound as indicated.

7 | Poisons & Toxins

Barry H. Rumack, MD, &
David G. Spoerke, MS, RPh

At least 1.2 million cases of poisoning were reported to the American Association of Poison Control Centers in 1987, and approximately 60% of those were in children under 6 years of age. The most frequent causes of poisoning (each accounting for about 8–9% of the total) were cleaning substances, plants, and analgesics.

Accidents involving household poisons, especially in children under the age of 5, can be attributed to 4 main factors: improper storage, failure to return a poison to its proper place, failure to read the label properly, and failure to recognize the substance as poisonous. It is clearly the responsibility of a parent to create a safe environment for the child.

Although many common exposures do not result in serious symptoms, the child who survives the ingestion of a highly toxic poison may be permanently disabled. Disabilities may include esophageal stricture after ingestion of lye, permanent liver or kidney damage after ingestion of poisons such as chlorinated hydrocarbons, or bone marrow depression after benzene poisoning.

GENERAL MANAGEMENT OF POISONINGS

Prophylaxis

Instructions in poison prevention and poison-proofing of homes should be given to the parents prior to or during the child's 6-month checkup. As the child grows, further areas of discussion should be raised with the parents. For example, when the child begins climbing or walking, the danger of storing pharmaceuticals in the medicine cabinet should be discussed, and other areas of storage should also be investigated. Parents should be asked about the contents of such areas as under the sink (drain cleaners), kitchen pantries (cleaning supplies), bathroom cabinets (medicines, antiseptics), basements and utility rooms (paints, thinners, salt), garage (antifreeze, automotive supplies), storage sheds (pesticides, herbicides), and laundry rooms (detergents, ammonia, fabric softeners).

Following the discussion of these areas, other general concepts of poison-proofing the house should be discussed. Sample questions would include: Has there been ample provision for locked storage? How should medicines and products be disposed of safely? How should containers be labeled, especially if the product is taken from its original container? What are the best methods of dealing with a child's normal investigation of the environment that may lead to tasting or handling toxic substances?

Treatment issues should also be discussed. Do the parents know of the use of such substances as activated charcoal and syrup of ipecac? If possible, they should be given the phone number of the local poison control center, and urged to obtain any poison prevention literature that the center may be distributing. The physician should provide (or prescribe) a 1-oz bottle of syrup of ipecac for the parent.

Poison prevention is important. The peak age of accidental poisoning is 2 years. If a child ingests a poison, there is a 56% chance of a repeat poisoning in the family within 1 year, and a 25% chance of a repeat poisoning in the same child. If adequate prevention has been discussed, the risk of repeat poisonings is reduced. When poison prevention appears to be adequate, but there are repeated exposures to toxic substances, child battering or neglect should be considered.

Diagnosis

Most childhood exposures are not intentional ingestions. Rather, the child "textures" and "tastes" the poison using its mouth as a sensitive organ. Ninety-five percent of all childhood exposures do not result in serious symptoms, most probably because the amount ingested is quite small. In the absence of a definite history of ingestion or of contact with a toxic substance, the diagnosis of poisoning versus another childhood illness presents many difficulties. Most of the symptoms of poisoning are not diagnostic, but certain clues to the presence of an unsuspected poisoning are included below.

A. History: The child is frequently found near the source of the poison shortly after having eaten it. Product containers should be brought to the office or hospital, since the ingredients are often listed on the labels, and sometimes antidotes are given. The physician should call the nearest poison control center or manufacturer in cases of exposure, since product formulation and treatment may have changed since the time the label was printed. Poison centers can also be of help if the label does not have specific ingredients, or if it has been obliterated. Unfortunately, the initial history correlates with the actual agent ingested less than half the time. It is best to compare the clinical condition of the patient with the probable signs and symptoms of poisoning using a recognized reference, such as the computer-updated POISINDEX Information System.

B. Symptoms and Signs: The signs and symptoms may vary greatly, depending upon what toxic substances are involved in the exposure. Symptoms may be gastrointestinal, respiratory, cardiovascular, neurologic, or metabolic. Table 7–1 gives a few examples of common symptoms seen with various toxic agents.

C. Laboratory Findings: Evidence may be obtained from the appearance, smell, or chemical analysis of blood, urine, vomitus, gastric washings, or fat obtained by biopsy. Occasionally, characteristic odors of poisons may be detected on the patient's breath. Blood in vomitus or stool may suggest the ingestion of a strong irritant or corrosive. Other specialized tests include urinary porphyrins (lead), red cell stippling (lead), cholinesterase levels (organophosphates), and salicylate levels. The use of ferric chloride or Phenistix may be helpful in initial urine testing for salicylates and phenothiazines, but should always be followed by more specific quantitative or qualitative laboratory tests.

D. X-Ray Findings: Various x-rays may be helpful in evaluating poison exposures. Just a few examples would include location of swallowed coins or other radiopaque pharmaceuticals and foreign objects, x-rays of bones to evaluate chronic lead and bismuth poisoning, and evaluation of pulmonary edema from aspiration of hydrocarbons.

EMERGENCY TREATMENT
(See Table 7–2.)

Specific types of poisoning are discussed on the following pages. Emergency care should be supervised by a physician and not left to other office personnel. Much of this care is best done in a hospital, where complete facilities and antidotal substances are available. The immediate management of acute poisoning in children should include the measures outlined below.

Table 7–1. Symptoms and signs of acute poisoning by various substances.*

Symptoms and Signs	Substance or Other Cause
Albuminuria	Arsenic, mercury, phosphorus.
Alopecia	Thallium, arsenic, selenium, radiation sickness.
Blood changes Anemia	Lead, naphthalene, chlorates, favism, solanine and other plant poisons, snake venom.
Cherry-red blood	Cyanide. (The lips in carbon monoxide poisoning are usually dusky and not cherry-red.)
Hematuria or hemoglobinuria	Heavy metals, naphthalene, nitrates, chlorates, favism, solanine, and other plant poisons.
Hemorrhage	Warfarin, thallium.
Methemoglobinemia	Nitrates, nitrites, aniline dyes, methylene blue, chlorates, pyridium.
Breath odors Bitter almond	Cyanide (Odor only detected by 40% of people.)
Garlic	Arsenic, phosphorus, organic phosphate, selenium.
Oysters	DMSO.
Burns of skin and mucous membranes	Lye, hypochlorite, phenol, sodium bisulfate, etc.
Cardiovascular collapse	Arsenic, boric acid, iron, phosphorus, food poisoning, nitrates.
Cyanosis	Barbiturates, opiates, nitrites, aniline dyes, chlorates.
Eye manifestations Lacrimation	Organic phosphates, nicotine, mushrooms, riot agents.

(continued)

Table 7–1. *(cont'd).*

Symptoms and Signs	Substance or Other Cause
Ptosis	Botulism, thallium.
Pupillary constriction	Opiates, parathion and other organic phosphates, mushrooms and some other plant poisons.
Pupillary dilatation	Atropine, nicotine, antihistamines, phenylephrine, mushrooms, thallium, oleander.
Strabismus	Botulism, thallium.
Visual disturbances	Atropine, parathion and other organic phosphates, botulism.
Fever	Atropine, salicylates, food poisoning, antihistamines, tranquilizers, camphor.
Flushing	Atropine, antihistamines, tranquilizers.
Gastrointestinal tract symptoms Abdominal cramps	Corrosive substances, food poisoning, lead, arsenic, black widow spider bite, boric acid, carbon tetrachloride, organic phosphates, phosphorus, nicotine, castor beans, fluorides, thallium.
Diarrhea	Food poisoning, iron, organic phosphates, arsenic, naphthalene, castor beans, mercury, boric acid, thallium, nicotine, nitrates, solanine and other plant poisons, mushrooms.
Dry mouth	Atropine, antihistamines, ephedrine, furosemide.
Hematemesis	Corrosive substances, warfarin, aminophyline, fluorides.
Stomatitis	Corrosive substances, thallium.
Vomiting	Aminophyline, food poisoning, organic phosphates, nicotine, digitalis, arsenic, boric acid, lead, mercury, iron, phosphorus,

	thallium, DDT, dieldrin, nitrates, castor beans, mushrooms, oleander, naphthalene.
Headache	Carbon monoxide, organic phosphates, atropine, lead, dieldrin, carbon tetrachloride.
Heart abnormalities Bradycardia	Digitalis, mushrooms, organic phosphates.
Tachycardia	Atropine, tricyclic antidepressants.
Other irregularities of rhythm	Nitrates, oleander.
Jaundice	Phosphorus, chlordane, favism, mushrooms, acetaminophen.
Muscle involvement Cramps	Lead, black widow spider bite.
Spasm or dystonia	Phenothiazines.
Nervous system involvement Ataxia	Lead, organic phosphates, antihistamines, thallium.
Coma	Barbiturates, carbon monoxide, cyanide, opiates, ethyl alcohol, salicylates, hydrocarbons, parathion and other organic phosphates, lead, mercury, boric acid, antihistamines, digitalis, mushrooms.
Convulsions	Aminophyline, amphetamine and other stimulants, atropine, camphor, boric acid, lead mercury, parathion and other organic phosphates, nicotine, phenothiazines, antihistamines, arsenic, DDT, dieldrin, kerosene, fluorides, nitrates, barbiturates, digitalis, salicylates, solanine and other plant poisons, thallium.
Delirium	Aminophyline, antihistamines, atropine, salicylates, lead, barbiturates, boric acid.

(continued)

Table 7–1. *(cont'd).*

Symptoms and Signs	Substance or Other Cause
Depression	Barbiturates, kerosene, tranquilizers, arsenic, lead, boric acid, DDT, naphthalene.
Mental confusion	Alcohol, barbiturates, atropine, nicotine, antihistamines, carbon tetrachloride, mercury, digitalis, mushrooms.
Paresthesias	Lead, thallium, DDT.
Weakness	Organic phosphates, arsenic, lead, nicotine, thallium, nitrates, fluorides, botulism.
Pallor	Lead, naphthalene, chlorates, favism, solanine and other plant poisons, fluorides.
Proteinuria	Arsenic, mercury, phosphorus.
Respiratory tract symptoms Aspiration pneumonia	Kerosene.
Cough	Hydrocarbons, mercury vapor.
Respiratory difficulty	Barbiturates, opiates, salicylates, ethyl alcohol, organic phosphates, dieldrin.
Respiratory failure	Cyanide, carbon monoxide, antihistamines, thallium, fluorides.
Respiratory stimulation	Salicylates, amphetamine and other stimulants, atropine, mushrooms.
Salivation and sweating	Parathion and other organic phosphates, muscarine and other mushroom poisoning, nicotine.
Shock	Food poisoning, iron, arsenic, fluorides.
Skin erythema	Boric acid.

* Adapted from Arena JM: The clinical diagnosis of poisoning. *Pediatr Clin North Am* 1970:**17**:477.

Table 7–2. Emergency treatment for poisoning.

Ingested Poisons
1. Syrup of ipecac may be useful in all cases except corrosives, coma, or seizures.
2. Lavage only if semiconscious or in coma. Endotracheal tube is inserted in larger children.
3. Activated charcoal.
4. Dilute ingested chemicals with water. *Do not* give fluids to dilute ingested medications.

Inhaled irritants
1. Oxygen therapy.
2. Mouth-to-mouth resuscitation.
3. Humidity.
4. Observe for pneumonitis and pulmonary edema.

Local Irritants
1. Copious water irrigation.
2. Careful eye examination.
3. No chemical ''antidotes.''

Available Consultants
1. Poison control centers.
2. State health departments.
3. Medical center consultants.
4. Pharmaceutical houses.
5. US agricultural office.
6. Medical examiner (coroner's office, toxicologist).

Specific ''Antidote'' Treatment Available
1. Amphetamines (see p 165).
2. Arsenic (see p 166).
3. Belladonna derivatives (see p 168).
4. Carbon monoxide (see p 170).
5. Cyanide (see p 171).
6. Ferrous sulfate (see p 172).
7. Mercury (see p 177).
8. Narcotics (see p 180).
9. Nitrites and nitrates (see p 181).
10. Phosphates, organic (see p 184).
11. Snake bites (see p 187).
12. Spider bites (see p 188).
13. Tranquilizers (see p 188).
14. Tricyclic antidepressants (see p 190).

Ingested Poisons

Speed is essential for effective therapy. The choice of which method to use is not always clear. Induced vomiting is much more effective than lavage with a small-bore nasogastric tube; however, a large-bore nasogastric tube is more effective than emesis.

A. Emesis in the Home: Contraindications to emesis include absent gag reflex, coma, convulsions, and ingestion of strong acids or strong bases. In making a recommendation to induce emesis, one should be cognizant of not only the patient's current condition but also the potential symptoms that may be seen 15–60 minutes from the time of your recommendation.

Since the induction of emesis may be delayed 30 minutes or more, it is important to instruct the parents on the use of ipecac as early as possible. Syrup of ipecac can be used to induce emesis at a dose of 30 mL for a child 40–45 kg or greater, 15 mL for a child 1–12 years old, and 5–10 mL in a child 6–12 months old (consider administering this dose in a health care facility only). After the dose has been given, the child should be encouraged to drink 4–6 oz of clear fluid, and then should be ambulated. This dose may be repeated once if emesis does not occur within the first 30 minutes. *Do not* administer more than 30 mL of syrup of ipecac to a young child. *Do not* use mustard water, salt water, or gag a child with a spoon. Consult your local poison control center to determine whether or not it is necessary to send the child to a health care facility after emesis. In many cases it will be important to send the child to the hospital whether or not vomiting has occurred. If vomiting has occurred, have the parents recover the regurgitated vomitus in a pan for later analysis, and bring it to the hospital along with the remainder of the uningested poison and the original container.

B. Emesis in the Hospital: Administer syrup of ipecac and follow the same procedure as outlined above. The use of syrup of ipecac produces an average recovery of 30% of the ingested agent.

C. Lavage: The use of gastric lavage is recommended if performed soon after ingestion, or in comatose or convulsing patients. The patient's airway should be protected by placement in the Trendelenburg and left lateral decubitus position with suction available. In unconscious patients, cuffed, endotracheal intubation is recommended. In children over 5, lavage should be done with 150–200 mL of lukewarm tap water or saline per wash. In younger children, 50–100 mL of normal saline per wash is used. Lavage should continue until the return is clear. The amount of fluid returned in the lavage should approximate the amount of fluid given to avoid fluid–electrolyte imbalance.

D. Catharsis: The dose of the saline cathartics magnesium or sodium sulfate is 250 mg/kg, and the dose of magnesium citrate is 4 mL/kg up to 300 mL per dose. Usually only one dose of a saline cathartic is administered. Sorbitol is also used as a cathartic, both alone and combined with activated charcoal. In a child over 1 year of age, 1–1.5 g/kg per dose as a 35% solution may be administered up to a maximum of 50 g per dose. It is best to administer sorbitol in a health care facility so fluids and electrolyte status can be monitored.

E. Activated Charcoal: This adsorbent material has a large surface area on which to adsorb various toxins. Although additives such as cherry syrup, simple syrup, ice cream, ethanol, milk, and cocoa powder or chocolate milk have been recommended to increase the palatability of activated charcoal, most of these decrease the adsorbing capacity somewhat, and should only be used when there is no other way of getting the child to take the charcoal. In patients with a nasogastric tube in place, using the tube to place the charcoal in the child's stomach is preferable to mixing with these other agents. Sorbitol and bentonite do not appear to alter significantly the adsorptive capacity of charcoal.

The most common use of activated charcoal is as a single dose. The optimum dose in children is 15–30 g, with some authors suggesting that 1–2 g/kg be used as a rough guideline, especially in infants. The FDA suggests a minimal dilution of 240 mL of water per 20–30 g of activated charcoal given as an aqueous slurry. A maximum dose has not been recommended. For some poisons, a repeated oral dose of charcoal may enhance total body clearance. A saline cathartic or sorbitol can be given with the first dose, but the safety of administering multiple cathartic doses with the charcoal has not been established. Multiple doses of cathartic have caused life-threatening complications. Occasionally, when large doses are required and the patient is unable to hold the charcoal down, continuous nasogastric infusion of 0.25–0.5 g/kg/h may be successful in ameliorating the vomiting associated with charcoal administration.

Activated charcoal is not absorbed orally, but adverse reactions have occurred, including black stools, vomiting (12–16%), constipation, gastrointestinal obstruction, aspiration pneumonitis, and emphysema.

There are certain classes of toxins in which activated charcoal may not be a standard recommendation. When given with a corrosive, it may cause vomiting, which could cause further damage to esophageal mucous membranes. In addition, many corrosives are not well adsorbed by charcoal. When given with hydrocarbons, charcoal may cause vomiting, which could lead to aspiration.

Surface Poisons

Remove poisons by washing the area with large volumes of water or soap and water. In cases involving water-insoluble substances, the solubility of that compound in various solvents should be checked before recommending large areas of the skin be washed with alcohol or various hydrocarbons. These substances may defat the skin, and may present more hazard than the toxin itself. *Caution: Do not* use chemical antidotes. Neutralization with liberated heat during the reaction may actually increase the extent of injury.

Inhaled Poisons

Patients exposed to toxic inhalants should be removed from exposure to these compounds, monitored for respiratory distress, and given emergency airway support, 100% humidified supplemental oxygen with assisted ventilation, or both, as required. An Ambu bag or other positive-pressure device may be required.

MANAGEMENT OF SPECIFIC COMMON TYPES OF POISONING IN CHILDREN

ACETAMINOPHEN

In large overdose, this commonly used analgesic–antipyretic may produce hepatotoxicity. Because of differences in metabolism, children under age 12 are unlikely to suffer hepatotoxicity even if plasma levels of the drug are in the toxic range. Children over age 12 may develop hepatotoxicity if untreated and if plasma levels are in the toxic range (see Fig 7–1).

Initial symptoms during the first 24 hours may include nausea, vomiting, diaphoresis, and a feeling of general malaise. Coma and metabolic acidosis have been seen. If the patient is not treated, hepatotoxicity may be observed via laboratory tests at approximately 36 hours, with peak AST (SGOT), ALT (SGPT), bilirubin levels, and prothrombin time occurring by 3 days. This hepatotoxic event is transient, and even in children with AST levels as high as 20,000 IU/L, discharge from the hospital with no sequelae usually occurs by the seventh day.

The plasma drug level should be determined 4 or more hours after ingestion, when it will have reached its peak. This assumes there is no further absorption. If the level is in the toxic range, treatment with the antidote must be initiated.

Treatment

Emesis or lavage should be performed upon arrival at the emergency care facility. In general, activated charcoal should be administered in the first 4 hours to ensure the amount of acetaminophen absorbed is small. N-acetylcysteine (Mucomyst), which is antidotal for acetaminophen, should not be given with

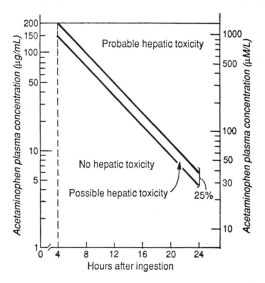

Figure 7–1. Semilogarithmic plot of plasma acetaminophen levels vs. time (Rumack-Matthew nomogram for acetaminophen poisoning). *Cautions for use of this chart:* (1) The time coordinates refer to time of ingestion. (2) Serum levels drawn before 4 hours may not represent peak levels. (3) The graph should be used only in relation to a single acute ingestion. (4) The lower solid line 25% below the standard nomogram is included to allow for possible errors in acetaminophen plasma assays and estimated time from ingestion of an overdose. (Adapted, with permission, from Rumack BH, Matthew H: Acetaminophen poisoning and toxicity. *Pediatrics* 1975;**55**:871. Copyright Midromedex Inc, 1974–1989.)

activated charcoal since there is some indication that it is adsorbed onto the charcoal. When both agents are to be given, they should be given at least 1 hour apart. N-acetylcysteine (NAC) should be administered in an oral loading dose of 140 mg/kg. It may be diluted in fruit juice or in cola beverage. Then 70 mg/kg every 4 hours must be administered for 17 additional doses. NAC is also available under an investigational protocol for use intravenously. AST, ALT, bilirubin levels, prothrombin times, and other evidence of liver failure should be monitored.

ACIDS, CORROSIVES

The strong mineral acids exert primarily a local corrosive effect on the skin and mucous membranes. Classically, acids cause oral and gastric burns, but seldom produce esophageal damage. The majority of these burns resolve. However, pyloric constriction with obstruction and vomiting may occur at 3 weeks. This response is thought to be due to pylorospasm occurring immediately after ingestion, which traps the acid in this area and produces a more significant burn.

Symptoms include severe pain in the throat and upper gastrointestinal tract; marked thirst; bloody vomitus; difficulty in swallowing, breathing, and speaking; discoloration and destruction of skin and mucous membranes in and around the mouth; collapse; and shock. Milder burns may result in fewer symptoms but serious sequelae are still possible.

Eye contact may produce severe pain, swelling, corneal erosions, and in some severe cases, blindness. Normally, brief exposures to acidic solutions with a pH of greater than 2 produce no injury to the corneal epithelium. Inhalation of acidic agents may produce dyspnea, chest pain, and pulmonary edema. Bronchospasm and hypoxemia may result.

Treatment

Do not give emetics or lavage. Dilute the acid immediately with 4–8 oz (not over 15 mL/kg) of water or milk. Avoid carbonates or bicarbonates internally, since they may form gas and cause distension of a perhaps weakened stomach wall. Do not administer other alkaline or neutralizing agents. Diagnostic endoscopy may be performed as indicated within the first 12 to 24 hours. This procedure may help grade the extent of damage and predict the necessity of further treatment. The use of steroids is debatable. They are extensively used by some surgeons in the same way as for alkaline burns. The dose of prednisone recommended is 1–2 mg/kg/d for 21 days.

ALCOHOL, ETHYL

Incoordination, slow reaction time, blurred vision, staggering gait, slurred speech, hypoglycemia, convulsions, and coma are the potential manifestations of overdosage. The diagnosis of alcoholic intoxication is commonly overlooked in children.

Treatment

Supportive treatment and aggressive management of any degree of hypoglycemia are usually the only treatments required. Although naloxone may antagonize the depressant effects found in ethanol overdose, the effect does not appear to be predictable or consistent. Fructose has been advocated as an accelerator of ethanol metabolism, but it is not commonly used in children.

AMPHETAMINES

Acute ingestion results in initial hypertension, hyperpyrexia, and hyperactivity. Extreme, unmanageable, hyperactivity and anxiety, as well as flushing, various cardiac arrhythmias, cardiac pain, and eventual circulatory collapse may be seen. Gastrointestinal complaints include nausea, vomiting, diarrhea, and abdominal pain.

Treatment

Standard gastric decontamination should be performed on children who ingest amphetamines. Activated charcoal effectively binds amphetamine, and the immediate administration of charcoal may be more effective than syrup of ipecac for the awake but symptomatic patient. Gastric lavage, which is followed by activated charcoal, may be the optimal decontamination regimen for patients who are exhibiting CNS effects.

The hyperactivity is generally managed with diazepam (0.25–0.4 mg/kg, up to a maximum of 5 mg in children 30 days to 5 years old and a maximum of 10 mg in children over 5 years; given intravenously over 2–3 minutes) unless severe hallucinations and agitation are present. In these cases, intravenous haloperidol or droperidol may be more effective. Clorpromazine is generally not recommended. Acid diuresis is not recommended because of potential dangers.

ANTIHISTAMINES

The effects of poisoning with these agents are variable, but anticholinergic or sympathomimetic effects are apparent in most cases. Atropinelike toxic effects such as dry mouth, fever, and dilated pupils may predominate. Signs of CNS toxicity include ataxia, hallucinations, and convulsions followed by coma and respiratory depression. Especially in older children, depression comparable to that seen with poisoning with tranquilizers may be prominent.

Prolonged toxic manifestations may be caused by sustained-action tablets. Most antihistamines are combined in products that also contain stimulants (phenylpropanolamine, ephedrine) and analgesics (aspirin, acetaminophen). These agents should be considered when treating antihistamines.

Treatment

Treatment consists of emesis or lavage, charcoal, and catharsis; the latter are important when sustained-action tablets have been ingested. Convulsions should be controlled with diazepam. Stimulants are contraindicated. Decrease fever with fluids and sponge baths as required. Avoid salicylates and acetaminophen, especially if found in a combination product. Physostigmine, 0.5–2 mg intravenously, slowly, will reverse coma, hallucinations, dysrhythmias, convulsions, and hypertension, but should only be used to reverse life-threatening manifestations. Repeat doses should be given only to reverse these toxic manifestations.

ARSENIC

Acute arsenic intoxication usually produces symptoms in 30 minutes. It is characterized by severe gastrointestinal symptoms and may be accompanied by a metallic taste, hoarseness, dysphagia, renal damage, shock, and fever. Increased capillary permeability, dehydration, protein depletion, garlicy odor on the breath, and hypotension may be noted. Chronic toxicity is characterized by peripheral neuritis, weight loss, and, sometimes, involvement of the skin, kidneys, and gastrointestinal tract. Laboratory determination of arsenic levels in vomitus, urine, and tissues is confirmatory. Blood levels below 1 μg/100 mL are within the normal range. Blood levels are generally only useful after acute exposures.

Treatment

Treatment consists of antishock therapy and specific therapy with penicillamine (Cuprimine), 100 mg/kg/d orally on an empty stomach, to a maximum of 1 g/d for 5 days. Penicillamine is an effective chelating agent when oral medication can be given. Use of dimercaprol (BAL), 2.5 mg/kg intramuscularly immediately and then 2 mg/kg intramuscularly every 4 hours, may be indicated. After 4–8 injections, give BAL twice daily for 5–10 days or until recovery. BAL produces a reaction similar to serum sickness in over 80% of patients.

BARBITURATES

There are two categories of barbiturate poisoning: (1) intoxication with short-acting drugs (eg, pentobarbital, secobarbital), which are detoxified in the liver; and (2) intoxication with long-acting drugs (eg, phenobarbital), which are cleared via the kidneys. The general symptoms are similar in both types and consist of drowsiness, ataxia, difficulty in thinking clearly, depression of spinal reflexes, respiratory depression, hypotension, and coma. Coma should be classified by the Reed classification (Table 7–3).

Treatment

Since histories are usually unreliable, treatment decisions based on an estimate of the amount of barbiturate ingested may be risky. Any amount in excess of 10–15 mg/kg for long-acting agents or 5–8 mg/kg for short-acting agents may produce more than therapeutic depression. Treatment measures are based on the type of barbiturate ingested (ie, short-acting or long-acting). Following suspected ingestion, close observation should be continued for a minimum of 4–6 hours.

A. Short-Acting Drugs:

1. Emesis, lavage, charcoal, and cathartics should be administered as under Emergency Treatment (see p 154). Emesis may be contraindicated because of the short time to CNS depression.

2. Analeptic agents (eg, doxapram, nikethamide, caffeine) are contraindicated in all cases.

3. Respiratory assistance should be provided, by respirator if necessary.

Table 7–3. Clinical classification of coma.*

Symptoms	Class
Asleep; can be aroused and can answer questions.	0
Comatose; does not withdraw from painful stimuli; reflexes intact.	1
Comatose; does not withdraw from painful stimuli; no respiratory or circulatory depression; most reflexes intact.	2
Comatose; no respiratory or circulatory depression; most or all reflexes absent.	3
Comatose; respiratory depression, with cyanosis; circulatory failure or shock (or both); reflexes absent.	4

* After Reed.

4. Hypotension is common and should be treated with fluids, plasma, etc. Vasopressors may be utilized if fluids are inadequate.

5. Shock lung with pulmonary edema may occur and may require positive end-expiratory pressure.

6. Forced diuresis is ineffective, since less than 3% of the drug is excreted via the kidneys. Fluids should be held to three-fourths of maintenance, since cerebral edema may be a complication, especially following anoxia. Hemodialysis and hemoperfusion may be helpful but should be reserved for severe cases.

7. Vital signs should be monitored continuously until the patient has been free of symptoms for 24 hours and charcoal stools have been passed.

8. Coma lasts approximately 10 hours for each milligram of barbiturate above the therapeutic level of 0.5–2 mg/dL.

B. Long-Acting Drugs:
1–5. As above.

6. Forced alkaline diuresis improves clearance by 3 times. Urine output should be 3–6 mL/kg/h, preferably 6 mL/kg/h. If the urine pH is less than 7.5, alkalinization may be performed with sodium bicarbonate.

7. Hemodialysis or charcoal perfusion may be useful if the patient is not responsive to the above measures. These procedures are rarely needed, and their use should not be based on blood levels but rather on deteriorating clinical condition.

8. Therapeutic levels of long-acting barbiturates are 2–4 mg/dL, but patients with tolerance may have considerably higher levels without toxicity. Correlate levels with clinical status before using them to classify severity of toxicity.

BELLADONNA DERIVATIVES
(Atropine, Scopolamine)

The belladonna alkaloids are parasympathetic depressants with variable CNS effects. The patient complains of dryness of mouth, thirst, difficulty in swallowing, and blurring of vision. The physical signs include dilated pupils, flushed skin, tachycardia, fever, delirium, delusions, weakness, and stupor. Symptoms are rapid in onset but may last for long periods, because gastric emptying time is slowed.

Treatment
Provide emergency emesis. Physostigmine, 0.5–2 mg intravenously slowly, dramatically reverses the central and periph-

eral effects of belladonna alkaloids. Physostigmine should be reserved for cases of severe toxicity. Seizures should respond to diazepam; if not, physostigmine may be used. Forced diuresis is ineffective with the synthetic alkaloids. Peritoneal and hemodialysis are ineffective; exchange transfusions may be helpful if very high doses have been taken.

BIRTH-CONTROL PILLS

The only toxic effects noted are nausea, vomiting, and vaginal bleeding. These effects are rare. The only treatments are prevention, by keeping all medications out of the reach of children, and fluid replacement when necessary.

BORIC ACID

Toxicity can result from ingestion of boric acid or absorption through inflamed skin. Manifestations include severe gastroenteritis, CNS signs such as irritability, restlessness, and seizures, and a firery red rash, called toxic epidermal necrolysis. Shock, coma, and death may be seen in more serious ingestions.

Note: There is no justification for keeping boric acid solution or powder where infants and children can be accidentally exposed to it. The drug has no medicinal value.

Treatment

Gastric lavage or induced emesis (or both) is the immediate therapy. Although it is commonly stated that boric acid is not adsorbed by activated charcoal, one study showed that 90 g of activated charcoal did adsorb 38% of a 3-g dose of boric acid. Very large doses of charcoal may be required. Good supportive care includes maintenance of fluid and electrolyte balance and treatment of hypotension with fluids and vasopressors as needed. Seizures may be treated with intravenous diazepam. Excretion of ingested or absorbed boric acid can be facilitated with exchange transfusion, hemodialysis, or peritoneal dialysis. Hemodialysis is more effective than peritoneal dialysis and is probably indicated in severely symptomatic patients with impaired renal function, and in patients with severe fluid–electrolyte abnormalities not amenable to conventional therapy.

CARBON MONOXIDE

Carbon monoxide combines with hemoglobin to form carboxyhemoglobin, which cannot carry oxygen and may result in tissue hypoxia. The cellular cytochrome systems may also be affected. Levels of carboxyhemoglobin can be measured easily, and they correlate well with the degree of toxicity. The patient is generally asymptomatic with levels of 10–20%; levels of 20–30% produce mild symptoms, 30–40% moderate symptoms, and 40–50% severe symptoms. Symptoms are more severe in patients who have exercised or taken alcohol or who reside at high altitudes. Symptoms consist of headache, lethargy, depressed sensorium, nausea, vomiting, and occasionally seizures. The heart is particularly sensitive to the hypoxia caused by carbon monoxide and clinical effects including tachycardia, hypotension, peripheral vasodilatation, cyanosis, shock, and cardiac arrest may be seen. Early cardiac arrhythmias are thought to be rare. Severe carbon monoxide intoxication may result in pulmonary edema. After prolonged exposure, psychotic behavior may be noted. Residual or delayed neurologic effects may occur after acute carbon monoxide poisoning. The incidence of sequelae appears to correlate directly with the level of consciousness and the duration of initial coma. Patients with normal CT scans appear to do better than similar patients with abnormal scans.

Treatment

Therapy consists of exposure to air and administration of oxygen. The half-life of carboxyhemoglobin is 40–90 minutes in 100% oxygen and 180–360 minutes in room air. The half-life is somewhat dependent on respiratory rate, age, pulmonary health, and physical activity. Hyperbaric oxygen is now considered to be the treatment of choice for symptomatic patients or for those with elevated carboxyhemoglobin levels. Hyperbaric oxygen increases the concentration of the oxygen dissolved in the plasma and displaces carbon monoxide from the hemoglobin. The necessity for hyperbaric oxygen therapy is more accurately assessed using neurologic, metabolic, and cardiovascular findings than by carboxyhemoglobin measurements. Severely symptomatic patients should be referred to a facility with a hyperbaric chamber. Symptoms considered severe include coma, dizziness, seizures, focal neurologic deficits, severe metabolic acidosis (pH less than 7.25), pulmonary edema, and other cardiovascular signs.

CYANIDE

Cyanide specifically inhibits the cytochrome oxidase system, causing cellular anoxia. The onset of symptoms after ingestion or inhalation is rapid. Symptoms include giddiness, hyperpnea, headache, palpitation, and unconsciousness. The breath may smell of bitter almonds. Death usually occurs in 15 minutes unless treatment is immediate.

Treatment

Immediately begin 100% oxygen. Obtain the Lilly Cyanide Antidote Kit and prepare it for use. Initially, inhalation of 1 ampule of amyl nitrate for 30 seconds of every minute produces 5% methemoglobinemia, which binds cyanide better than hemoglobin. Once the cyanide antidote kit is obtained, read the directions for therapy, noting that most of the doses are for adults and need to be modified for children. Intravenous sodium nitrite 3% is given first, followed by intravenous sodium thiosulfate (25%). A dosage chart for children is available on the POISINDEX Information System. The amount of sodium nitrite should not exceed that listed in the chart. Fatal methemoglobinemia may result. As an approximation only, the average child with 12 g of hemoglobin would be given 0.33 mL/kg of the 3% sodium nitrite at a rate of 2–5 mL/min. This should produce approximately 30% methemoglobinemia. The initial dose of sodium thiosulfate 25% is 1.65 mL/kg. If clinical response is inadequate, additional sodium nitrite, at half the amount of the initial dose, may be administered 30 minutes following the first dose. These antidotes should be used in significantly symptomatic patients such as those with seizures, unconsciousness, acidosis, or unstable vital signs.

DETERGENTS

Fatalities due to poisoning with anionic and nonanionic detergents have not been reported. The primary symptoms associated with these agents alone include nausea, vomiting, and diarrhea. Occasionally, these detergents may contain alkaline irritants that have the potential for causing alkaline burns.

Cationic detergents may also be found in the home, in products such as antiseptics and antistatic agents. Acute poisoning from these agents may cause gastroenteritis, convulsions, burns, and strictures. Insufficient data are available to determine the nontoxic amount of a cationic detergent or noncorrosive concentration (approximately 7.5%). Extrapolating from one adult fatality, a serious amount of a 1% solution in a child weighing 10 kg would be about 1 oz. Burns may occur with benzalkonium chloride in concentrations of 10% or greater. There is only one report involving a lesser concentration.

Treatment

Anionic and nonanionic detergents generally cause minimal effects and require only monitoring for excessive fluid loss if vomiting and diarrhea are extensive.

In cases involving cationic detergents, dilution with water or milk may be initiated first; there is some risk in inducing emesis or performing gastric lavage since many of these compounds are corrosive and if systemic effects occur, seizures and coma may be seen fairly rapidly. These agents are well adsorbed to charcoal and rapid administration of activated charcoal is recommended for large amounts of dilute solutions. With more concentrated solutions, esophagoscopy should be considered and performed within the first 24–48 hours. Definitive burn care may be required if burns are identified on esophagoscopy. Supportive care may be required for seizures, hypotension, and pulmonary edema.

FERROUS SULFATE

Accidental ingestion of ferrous sulfate (elemental iron) in amounts as low as 60 mg/kg may cause serious intoxication. Five phases of intoxication are described: (1) Hemorrhagic gastroenteritis occurs shortly after ingestion (30–120 minutes); shock due to blood loss may be present. (2) A recovery phase occurs and lasts from 2 to 12 hours after ingestion. (3) Delayed shock may occur 12–24 hours after ingestion and may be due to a vasodepressant action of ferritin or unbound ionic iron. (4) Liver damage occurs at 3–5 days. (5) Delayed gastric obstruction may occur, usually at 3 weeks after ingestion.

The history is the most important diagnostic clue. X-rays of the abdomen may show the radiopaque tablets in the gastrointestinal tract. Laboratory determination of serum iron and total iron-binding capacity allows calculation of free iron, an excess of which is diagnostic.

Treatment

Remove ferrous sulfate by induced vomiting and lavage with a large-bore tube. Lavage with sodium bicarbonate; Phosphasoda (Fleets), or deferoxamine is of questionable value. Supportive measures (blood, plasma, saline, and vasopressors as indicated) are imperative. Exchange transfusion may be useful if the patient does not respond to standard measures. Deferoxamine (Desferal) is useful in cases of severe intoxication. The dose is 15 mg/kg/h as a drip—not a push—during the first 12–24 hours. In general, as long as chelation occurs, the urine shows a reddish "vin rosé" color.

FLUORIDES

Fluorides are found in high concentrations in agricultural poisons and insecticides. Lower concentrations are found in such things as toothpaste and fluoride tablets used for prevention of dental caries. Clinical reactions produced by fluorides include nausea, vomiting, colicky abdominal pain, diarrhea, cyanosis, excitement, and convulsions. In most instances, gastrointestinal signs and symptoms predominate, but in fatal poisonings, death is usually a result of cardiac failure or respiratory paralysis. In serious poisonings, degeneration of the kidney may occur, as may hypocalcemia, hyperkalemia, and a variable skin rash. In general, ingestion of fluoride tablets used for dental care does not result in severe symptoms owing to their low concentration (1 mg per tablet).

Treatment

Calcium salts (chloride, carbonate, lactate) have been used orally as lavage solutions in concentrations of 5 mL/L of water or a 0.15% calcium hydroxide (lime water) solution. Most household exposures are treated with milk in large quantities (10–15 mL/kg orally). Vomiting may be induced or gastric lavage performed with a large-bore tube. Activated charcoal is not generally of use with fluoride ingestion. For a cathartic, sodium sulfate, sodium citrate, or sorbitol may be used. Monitor serum calcium and observe for clinical signs of hypocalcemia. If necessary, administer calcium gluconate (10%) slowly intravenously, and repeat as necessary. After the initial correction of hypocalcemia, a calcium gluconate infusion at a rate of 15 g/m^2 for 24 hours may be required to compensate for the slow release of fluoride ion from the bone.

GLUE

Toluene was once the most common solvent used in glue, but it has largely been replaced in products by less toxic substances. The most frequent symptoms following glue "sniffing" or "huffing" include weakness, fatigue, confusion, lacrimation, euphoria, headache, dizziness, muscular weakness, nausea, and dilated pupils. Chronic inhalers may develop muscular weakness syndromes, gastrointestinal syndromes, or neuropsychiatric syndromes. Death may occur from respiratory failure.

Treatment

Eliminate exposure to the solvent. Conservative management is indicated, but fluid–electrolyte status should be monitored, as should hepatic, renal, and hematologic parameters.

HALLUCINOGENS

Marijuana has stimulant, depressant, and hallucinogenic properties, but usually the depressant properties predominate. Euphoria, mood swings, and distortion of time and space commonly occur. Performance skills may be affected. Panic states or psychotic reactions are uncommon.

LSD (lysergic acid diethylamide) causes euphoria, mood swings, loss of inhibitions, and depersonalization. Flashbacks (recurrence of initial effects), panic states, and hallucinations occur in some individuals.

Mescaline typically produces mydriasis, salivation, tachypnea, headache, nausea and vomiting, flushing, and diaphoresis. Auditory, gustatory, olfactory, tactile, and visual hallucinations have all been seen with mescaline. These psychologic effects are generally mild in adults, but may be more pronounced in children; they rarely last longer than 6–12 hours.

PCP (phencyclidine) is a veterinary anesthetic that causes agitation, paranoid behavior, nystagmus, hypertension, muscle rigidity, respiratory depression, renal failure, "staring" coma, and occasionally self-destructive behavior. It is often mistakenly taken as or with LSD, mescaline, psilocybin, or marijuana.

Treatment

Treatment of hallucinogenic agents is primarily symptomatic and supportive. Patients should be placed in a low-stimulus environment and given reassurance by a parent, psychiatrist, or psychologist. Anxiety states can be reduced with diazepam (0.04–0.2 mg/kg per dose every 2–4 hours to a maximum of

0.6 mg over 8 hours). Seizures may also be treated with diazepam (0.2–0.5 mg/kg per dose, maximum 5 mg in children under 5 and 10 mg in children over 5). Management of PCP ingestion may include treatments for dystonias, renal failure due to rhabdomyolysis or myoglobinuria, hypoglycemia, and hypertension.

IBUPROFEN

Ibuprofen is a popular nonsteroidal anti-inflammatory that has been changed from prescription-only to over-the-counter status. Children who are exposed to mild overdoses of this agent generally don't have serious effects. One study states that children who ingest up to 2.4 grams remain asymptomatic. In cases where symptoms occur, abdominal pain, vomiting, drowsiness, and lethargy are seen most frequently. A few case reports, especially in young children, have reported apnea, seizures, metabolic acidosis, and CNS depression leading to coma.

Treatment

For children who have ingested less than 100 mg/kg, only dilution with milk or water, to soothe any potential gastrointestinal irritation, is required. Dilution should be with less than 4 oz of fluid in children. The use of the ibuprofen nomogram by Hall et al (Fig 7–2) may provide some guidelines for predicted toxicity. If more than 400 mg/kg have been ingested, there is a potential for seizures or CNS depression. In such cases, gastric lavage may be preferred to emesis. In cases where 100–400 mg/kg have been ingested, emesis may be of equal value. A cathartic combined with activated charcoal may also be of some use in adsorbing the material and removing it from the gastrointestinal tract. Multiple-dose activated charcoal has been suggested because of the possibility of enterohepatic circulation. Treatment is symptomatic and supportive—there is no specific antidote. Patients should be monitored for hypotension, seizures, acidosis, and gastrointestinal bleeding. Hemodialysis and alkalinization of the urine have not been shown to be of definitive advantage in treatment of ibuprofen poisoning.

LYE & BLEACHES

Ingestion of lye and bleaches may result in ulceration and perforation of the gastrointestinal tract and in long-term compli-

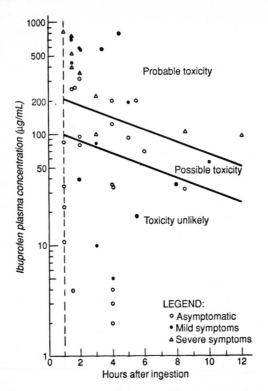

Figure 7–2. Nomogram for ibuprofen poisoning. (Adapted, with permission, from Hall AH et al: Ibuprofen overdose: 126 cases. *Ann Emerg Med* 1986;15:1308.)

cations such as esophageal stricture. Burns in the mouth indicate an absolute need for esophagoscopy, but many cases have been reported in which patients have not sustained oral burns but have developed esophageal burns. Alkaline corrosives in the eye may cause disruption of cellular membranes; loss of corneal, conjunctival, and lens epithelium; and, if the penetration is deeper, corneal edema and necrosis of the ciliary body and iris. Deep penetration may result in cataract formation.

Treatment

Avoid emetics. Dilute with water or milk. Do not exceed 15 mL/kg orally in a child (125–250 mL in an older patient or adult) as vomiting may occur with excessive fluids. Perform esophagoscopy after 12 hours but before 24 hours. Corticosteroids may be helpful and, if used, should be given early and continued for 3 weeks. Antibiotics are not indicated unless an infection is demonstrated. Give supportive therapy with sedation and analgesia as necessary. Intravenous nutrition and fluids may be necessary in the early stages of treatment. Early tracheostomy may be indicated in cases of severe ingestion.

MEPROBAMATE
(Equanil, Miltown)

Respiratory depression, coma, arrhythmias, lethargy, headache, hyperactive deep-tendon reflexes, increased heart rate, hypotension, and pulmonary edema may be noted. Death may occur from cardiac or respiratory failure.

Treatment
Emesis or gastric lavage with a large-bore tube may be performed. Although supportive treatment may be sufficient in mild intoxications, hemodialysis, hemoperfusion, and charcoal hemoperfusion may be indicated in severe cases. Forced diuresis is theoretically useful, but hypotension and the risk of pulmonary edema make this procedure difficult and potentially harmful. Peritoneal dialysis is not as effective as hemodialysis.

MERCURY

Acute symptoms of mercury poisonings include sudden, profound circulatory collapse, increased heart rate, peripheral vasoconstriction, vomiting, decreased blood pressure, and possibly bloody diarrhea. Kidney failure has been seen within 24 hours. Severe acidosis and leukocytosis may occur. Some symptoms may be delayed until after 12 hours, including a mercury gum line, lower nephron nephrosis, ulcerative colitis, hepatic damage, and shock. Chronic symptoms generally reported are those of gastrointestinal irritability, a blue-black gum line, salivation, stomatitis, nephrosis, and irritability. Acrodynia occurs in children following chronic exposure to small amounts of mercury, including topically applied mercury.

Treatment
For ingested mercury, consider emesis or gastric lavage. Inorganic mercury salts may produce gastric erosion, and the

possibility of perforation should be considered before using emesis or lavage in patients presenting some time after an ingestion. Abdominal x-rays may be helpful in determining whether lavage or emesis is required. Good supportive and symptomatic care should be given for symptoms such as seizures and hypotension. A timed, 24-hour baseline urinary mercury level is a good index of total body burden. For acute poisoning, extrapolating a collection of 2–12 hours is a good initial index. This should be followed by a 24-hour collection. Chelation can be performed with several agents. Penicillamine, 100 mg/kg/d orally in children, may be given, up to a maximum of 1 g/d in divided doses for 3–10 days. The urine should be monitored daily for urinary excretion of mercury. If the urine mercury decreases rapidly, the body burden is probably small. After waiting 10 days, a repeat baseline collection should be performed to determine whether rebound has occurred and rechelation is necessary. For those individuals who are sensitive to penicillamine, or cannot take oral medications, BAL may be used in doses of 3–5 mg/kg per dose every 4 hours given deep IM for the first 2 days, 2.5–3 mg/kg per dose IM every 6 hours for the next 2 days, then 2.5–3 mg/kg per dose every 12 hours for a week after that. Again, urine mercury levels should be monitored to assess the effects of therapy.

MUSHROOMS

Mushrooms are responsible for rare deaths and common nonfatal poisonings. A history of mushroom ingestion always arouses concern, which is intensified because some toxins present in mushrooms may not show their effects until many hours after ingestion and because it is often not known exactly what kind of fungus was ingested.

The most common intoxicating American species are delineated below. Almost 90% of cases of childhood accidental ingestions involve nontoxic puffballs or nontoxic "little brown mushrooms." The services of a mycologist must be obtained through a botanical garden or poison control center to identify the species.

Clinical Findings & Treatment

Clinical findings and treatment vary according to the type of mushroom ingested (Table 7–4).

A. Cyclopeptide-containing: These include *Amanita verna* (in the USA) and *Amanita phalloides* (in the USA and Europe). The toxins are cyclopeptides. Vomiting and severe diarrhea oc-

Table 7-4. Mushroom poisoning.

Class	Representatives	Clinical Effects	Treatment
Cyclopepides	*Amanita verna* *Amanita phalloides* *Galerina* species	Vomiting, diarrhea, delayed liver and kidney damage	Supportive care, penicillin, silibinin
Muscarinic	*Boletus satanas* *Clitocybe dealbata* *Inocybe* species	Salivation, bradycardia, miosis, increased peristalsis, hypotension, wheezing	If muscarinic, atropine, 50 μg/kg SC
Hydrazine	*Gyromitra* species	Vomiting, diarrhea, muscle cramps, fever, liver failure, seizures, coma	For CNS effects, pyridoxine
Psilocybin	*Psilocybe* species	Hallucinations	Treatment usually not necessary
Coprine	*Coprinus atramentarius*	Flushing, vomiting, tachycardia, vertigo	Usually symptomatic; for severe cases methylpyrazole (experimental)
Muscimol	*Amanita muscarid* *Amanita patherina*	Drowsiness, delirium, muscle spasms, seizures, coma	Supportive
Orellanine	*Cortinarius* species (some)	Delayed kidney damage	Supportive, hemoperfusion

cur after a latent period of 6–20 hours, followed by liver and kidney damage. Thioctic acid was once suggested as an antidote, but it is now believed not to be useful. High-dose penicillin and silibinin are being investigated as treatments. Good supportive care is required.

B. Muscarinic-containing: These include *Amanita muscaria* and *Amanita pantherina*. These fungi may contain muscarine that may cause parasympathomimetic manifestations. Some may cause an anticholinergic syndrome (see Belladonna Derivatives, above). Hallucinations may occur with ingestion of either type of mushroom. Atropine sulfate, 50 μg/kg subcutaneously immediately and then as required, should be used only if muscarinic signs appear. Discontinue if signs of atropine poisoning appear. If patients have severe atropinic signs, physostigmine may be tried (see above).

C. Hydrazine-containing: These are potentially toxic mushrooms that may cause nausea and vomiting, muscle cramps, abdominal pain, severe diarrhea, fever, liver failure, seizures, and coma. Hemolysis may be seen, as may methemoglobinemia. The toxin, which closely resembles monomethylhydrazine, may be removed or decreased by cooking or drying. Pyridoxine may be antidotal for neurologic symptoms, but there is limited experience with its use. The dose recommended in the literature is 25 mg/kg given as an infusion over 15–30 minutes. Repeat doses up to a maximum daily dose of 15–20 g may be administered for recurring neurologic signs such as seizures and coma. The maximum nontoxic dose of pyridoxine is unknown, but doses of 0.2–5 g/d for 2–40 months have caused neurologic symptoms such as ataxia and severe sensory nervous system dysfunctions. Methemoglobinemia can be treated with methylene blue in a dose of 1–2 mg/kg per dose (0.1–0.2 mL/kg per dose) given intravenously over a few minutes as needed every 4 hours. Additional doses may be required. Doses of greater than 15 mg/kg may cause hemolysis.

D. Psilocybin-containing: Psilocybin causes nausea, vomiting, headache, and hallucinations. Onset of symptoms is generally within 30–60 minutes, but may be as long as 3 hours. Most cases recover fully within 12 hours. Tonic–clonic seizures, usually intermittent, have occurred in children after ingestion of large quantities.

NARCOTICS
(Opiates)

Intoxication with narcotics (eg, morphine, codeine, and diphenoxylate [in Lomotil]) produces respiratory depression, hypotension, pinpoint pupils, skeletal muscle relaxation, decreased urinary output, and, occasionally, shock. Propoxyphene (Darvon) has been associated with convulsions in a high percentage of cases of overdosage. Diphenoxylate is especially known for its delayed-onset CNS and respiratory depression.

Treatment

Acute overdosage is treated similarly to barbiturate intoxication. Respiratory assistance and maintenance of adequate blood pressure are mandatory. Naloxone (Narcan) is an effective narcotic antagonist that does not cause respiratory depression and has no known toxicity even with relatively large doses. The dose of naloxone should be no less than 0.4 mg regardless of the patient's age. If there is no immediate response, 2–4 mg should be given rapidly intravenously. The use of doses based on a set ratio of dose per unit of weight (mg/kg) is frequently inaccurate, since the treatment goal of reversing binding cannot be achieved consistently with these doses. Patients who have had opiate reversal with naloxone should be observed carefully for continuation of CNS and respiratory depression.

NITRITES & NITRATES

Methemoglobinemia is produced by the administration of a nitrite compound or a nitrate that is converted to the nitrite in the large bowel. Sodium nitrite, food preservatives, phenacetin, home remedies such as spirits of nitrite, a high concentration of nitrites in water, as well as various inhalants (amyl, butyl, and isobutyl nitrate) may produce these effects. The onset may be gradual and symptoms may be deceiving. Ingestion of as little as 10 mL of isobutyl or amyl nitrate has produced severe methemoglobinemia and death in both adults and children. Clinical signs include hypertension, tachycardia, respiratory depression, methemoglobinemia, headache, nausea, vomiting, and diarrhea, and in severe cases, seizures may be seen. Symptoms depend on the amount of available hemoglobin to carry oxygen, but generally do not occur until approximately 30% of the hemoglobin has been converted to methemoglobin. A drop of the patient's blood dried on filter paper may appear brown if levels are 15% or greater.

Treatment

Intravenous methylene blue allows electron transfer to reverse methemoglobinemia. A 1% solution is administered in the amount of 0.1 mL/kg and may be repeated 30 minutes later to reverse symptoms. Persistence of methemoglobinemia at high levels in a symptomatic patient is an indication for exchange transfusion. Laboratory determinations for methemoglobin are available.

PETROLEUM DISTILLATES
(Charcoal Starter, Kerosene, Paint Thinner, Turpentine, & Related Products)

The petroleum distillates are mixtures of saturated and unsaturated hydrocarbons of the aliphatic and aromatic series. The following products are common causes of poisoning: kerosene, lamp oils, turpentine, other pine products, gasoline, lighter fluid, insecticides with petroleum distillate bases, benzene, naphtha, and mineral spirits.

Ingestion of petroleum distillates causes local irritation with a burning sensation in the mouth, esophagus, and stomach. Vomiting and occasionally diarrhea with blood-tinged stools may occur. Kerosene and similar products are likely to cause spontaneous emesis in 1 hour in about 90% of patients. It is essential to remember that just a few drops aspirated into the pulmonary tree can cause a severe and fatal pneumonia, a complication to which infants and children are particularly prone. Pulmonary complications are reported with greater frequency among children who ingest kerosene or mineral seal oil than in those who ingest other petroleum distillate products with higher viscosity. Pulmonary involvement is usually indicated by cyanosis, rapid breathing, tachycardia, and fever. Basilar rales may progress rapidly to massive pulmonary edema or hemorrhage, infiltration, and secondary infection.

In general, ingestion of more than 30 mL (1 oz) of a petroleum distillate is associated with a higher incidence of CNS complications such as lethargy, coma, seizures, confusion, disorientation, and peripheral neuropathy. CNS involvement is reported most frequently among patients who ingest lamp oils and kerosene. In severe poisonings, there may be cardiac dilatation, hepatosplenomegaly, proteinuria, formed elements in the urine, and cardiac dysfunction associated with congestive heart failure. In fatal poisonings, death usually occurs in 2–24 hours.

Treatment

Although controversial, induced emesis is useful in cases where systemic toxicity is predicted. The American Academy of

Pediatrics recommends emesis if more than 1 mL/kg has been ingested. Estimation of the amount ingested may be difficult in children. Gastric lavage should be performed only if a cuffed endotracheal tube is inserted, because there is no such thing as a "careful gastric lavage" in children. If the amount ingested is small, a saline cathartic is all that is necessary. For CNS depression, supportive care is indicated.

"Prophylactic" antibiotic therapy is of questionable value and does not speed resolution when pneumonia exists. Oxygen and mists are helpful. Corticosteroids have not been shown to be of benefit in treating hydrocarbon pneumonitis. Hospitalization is indicated only if the child has taken a large amount or is symptomatic. Fever and other symptoms may continue for as long as 10 days without infection, and pneumatoceles may develop 3–5 weeks after pneumonitis.

Withhold digestible fats, oil, and alcohol, which may promote absorption from the bowel or cause aspiration pneumonitis on their own.

The rapidity of recovery depends upon the degree of pulmonary involvement. Resolution may take as long as 4 weeks.

PHENOTHIAZINES

Phenothiazine compounds produce significant anticholinergic, alpha-adrenergic blocking, and extrapyramidal properties. The symptoms seen will depend on the class of the agent ingested, but may include extrapyramidal motor symptoms (opisthotonos, oculogyric crisis, torticollis, trismus, rigidity) and convulsions.

Treatment

Decontamination should be done either with emesis or gastric lavage depending on the potential for CNS depression and seizures. Activated charcoal and a cathartic will also be useful. Symptomatic measures should be used and blood pressure monitored. Phenytoin (2 mg/kg every 8 hours) may be useful in reversing the depressed intraventricular conductivity of the myocardium. Dystonic disorders may be treated with diphenhydramine at a dose of 1–2 mg/kg to a maximum of 50 mg intravenously. The malignant neuroleptic syndrome, sometimes seen with phenothiazines such as haloperidol and fluphenazine, may be treated successfully with oral dantrolene at a dose of 1 mg/kg orally every 12 hours up to 50 mg per dose.

PHOSPHATES, ORGANIC
(Diazinon, Disyston, Malathion, Parathion, etc)

Many insecticides contain organic phosphates. Parathion is one of the most toxic examples. All inhibit cholinesterase, resulting in parasympathetic and CNS stimulation. Symptoms include headache, dizziness, blurred vision, diarrhea, abdominal pain, dyspnea, chest pain, bronchial constriction, pulmonary edema, respiratory failure, convulsions, cyanosis, coma, loss of reflexes and sphincter control, sweating, salivation, miosis, tearing, muscle fasciculations, and even generalized collapse.

Lowered red cell cholinesterase activity helps to confirm the diagnosis.

Treatment

The patient who has been exposed dermally must be decontaminated with soap and water or tincture of green soap as soon as possible to prevent further absorption. For children who have ingested an organophosphate, lavage is probably safer than emesis because of the rapid onset of symptoms, which may include CNS depression and seizures. Many organophosphates are dissolved in a hydrocarbon solvent, which could lead to aspiration. Atropine is primarily useful for treatment of the muscarinic effects, and will not reverse nicotinic effects. Severely poisoned patients may require exceedingly large doses of atropine to achieve adequate atropinization (ie, drying up of secretions). Early, prompt, and adequate atropinization is of paramount importance in symptomatic patients. If anticholinergic findings occur following a diagnostic dose of atropine, the patient is probably not seriously poisoned. Begin with 50 μg/kg intravenously in a small child and 1–2 mg intravenously in an older child. Repeat every 15–30 minutes until dry mouth, mydriasis, and tachycardia appear. In addition, pralidoxime (2-PAM), 500 mg intravenously injected slowly over 5 minutes, should be given if symptoms are severe, but may be delayed until confirmation of red cell cholinesterase depression.

Supportive measures include oxygen, artificial respiration, postural drainage of secretions, and measures to combat shock and seizures.

RAUWOLFIA DERIVATIVES

Rauwolfia derivatives produce parasympathetic effects: nasal congestion, salivation, sweating, bradycardia, abdominal cramps, and diarrhea. Parkinsonian symptoms occasionally develop.

Treatment

Give supportive treatment and remove the poison by emesis and lavage. The effects of parkinsonism may be alleviated with anticholinergic agents such as atropine. This treatment should be reserved for severe cases. Atropine may also be useful to reverse the gastrointestinal effects. Digitalis derivatives should not be used to reverse cardiac failure. The combination has shown evidence of enhancing cardiac dysrhythmias.

RIOT-CONTROL DRUGS

Several riot-control drugs are now available. In general, they consist of a chemical and a hydrocarbon solvent such as kerosene, and in some cases a propellant such as freon gas. There are a number of chloroacetophenone derivatives as well as chloropicrin agents, dibenzoxazepine compounds, ortho-chlorobenzylidene malononitrile agents, and capsicum. The chemical agent typically causes lacrimation, photophobia, and in some instances nausea and vomiting. In lower concentration, these materials cause lacrimation and pain but no tissue damage. Skin sensitization and corneal scarring can occur, particularly when the chemical is released close enough to the victim's face or skin to create a high local concentration.

Treatment

The most effective treatment is prompt removal from the sprayed area and careful decontamination of the patient. After removing all clothes, the patient should shower carefully, using copious amounts of soap and water. An ophthalmologist should examine the eyes for possible corneal damage. Medical personnel involved in decontamination should wear surgical scrub suits and should also shower with copious amounts of soap and water when the decontamination is completed.

SALICYLATES

Although salicylates are not as commonly used in children as they once were, they are still frequently involved in pediatric exposures. Acute salicylate ingestion involves vomiting, tinnitus, hyperpnea, acid–base disturbances such as respiratory alkalosis and metabolic acidosis, electrolyte imbalances such as hypokalemia, fever, dehydration, lowered cerebrospinal fluid glucose levels, and pulmonary edema. Severe cases may involve hallucinations, seizures, coma, cerebral edema, and mild hepatotoxicity.

Salicyaltes stimulate the respiratory center, a property that may cause respiratory alkalosis. Bases are then compensatorily excreted. Salicylates also interfere with intermediary metabolism and allow the accumulation of organic acids. The two processes together produce a metabolic acidosis that is difficult to treat. In chronic cases, the initial alkalosis may not be evident.

Treatment

Emesis and lavage are useful methods for eliminating salicylates that have not been absorbed. The method used depends on such factors as the patient's condition (coma, seizures), dosage form (liquid vs tablet), and time since ingestion. Activated charcoal and cathartics are also useful.

Adequate hydration is important, usually with a hypotonic glucose solution such as 0.2–0.45 normal saline. In acidotic patients, administration of sodium bicarbonate (3–6 mL/kg/h of a solution containing 88 mEq/L) should be given.

Potassium supplementation may be required because sodium or potassium is excreted with the bicarbonate during the respiratory alkalosis stage. Depletion may be present even with normal serum potassium. Potassium supplements may be at levels of 10–20 mEq/L of fluid, depending on the patient's condition.

Treatment of tetany may require intravenous calcium. The dose depends on serum calcium levels. The pulmonary edema is *not* responsive to digoxin, diuretics, or tourniquets.

Alkalinizing the urine to a pH of 7–8 will enhance salicylate excretion but without proper potassium supplementation may be difficult to maintain. Carbonic anhydrase inhibitors such as Diamox should *not* be used to alkalinize the urine because of negative acid–base reactions.

SCORPION STINGS

The toxin of the less venomous species of scorpions causes only local pain, redness, and swelling; that of the more venomous species causes generalized muscular pains, convulsions, nausea, vomiting, variable CNS involvement, and collapse.

Treatment

Keep the patient recumbent and quiet. If the species is known to be one of those that does not cause systemic reactions, stings can be treated much as bee or wasp stings. For the toxic *Centruroides* species (found in extreme southwestern United States), treat the wound as for a snake bite, below. If absorption has occurred, and the patient is complaining of muscle spasms, consider administering 0.1 mL/kg of a 10% calcium gluconate or 0.1 mg/kg of diazepam. Provide adequate sedation and institute supportive measures. Symptomatic measures should be used for control of seizures, hypertension, and supraventricular tachycardia. Antivenin is of some value in cases involving *Centruroides* species.

SNAKE BITES

Snake venom may be neurotoxic, hemotoxic, or a combination of both. Neurotoxin (cobra, coral snake) causes respiratory paralysis; hemotoxin (rattlesnake, copperhead, moccasin, pit viper) causes hemolysis, tissue destruction, and damage to the endothelial lining of the blood vessels. Manifestations consist of local pain, thirst, nausea and vomiting, profuse perspiration, local swelling and redness, abdominal cramps, urticaria, dilated pupils, stimulation followed by depression, extravasation of blood, respiratory difficulty, muscle weakness, hemorrhage, and circulatory collapse.

Note: Thirty to 70% of snake bites do not result in envenomation. Crotalid bites can be expected to show local hemorrhage if envenomation occurred. In most cases, swelling and edema will appear. Swelling is usually seen around the injured area within 5 minutes of the bite and may progress rapidly, involving the entire extremity within 1 hour. Generally, however, edema spreads more slowly and will develop over a period of 8–36 hours.

Treatment

Keep the patient recumbent and quiet. Remove rings and other constrictive items. The injured part should be slightly immobilized and kept just below the heart level. Patients should be transported to a medical facility as soon as possible. At no time should the bite be packed in ice. Treat shock or respiratory failure with all available means. Tetanus and gas gangrene prophylaxis may be indicated. A tourniquet that occludes venous and lymphatic return might be applied, although its value is questionable. (If envenomation of the arterial tree is suspected or if prolonged delay in definitive treatment is unavoidable, the tourniquet should completely occlude arterial supply.) Incision for suction is probably useless, but a Sawyer extractor used over the bite area may be helpful if transport to the medical facility will take longer than 45 minutes. The Sawyer extractor must be used immediately. If a tourniquet is applied, it should probably remain until antivenin is available. There is a potential for release of large amounts of venom when the tourniquet is removed. Fasciotomy should rarely be used.

Administer antivenin as indicated. (The American Association of Poison Control Centers maintains an index of antiserum availability—contact your local poison control center for sources.) If the bite is major, give antivenin intravenously; be prepared to treat possible anaphylactic reactions. To be effective, treatment must be initiated immediately. Antivenin is efficacious when given within 4 hours of a bite, and is less effective if delayed for 8 hours. It is of questionable value if given 26 hours after envenomation. At the present time, it appears advisable to recommend its use up to 30 hours after envenomations and all severe cases of crotalid poisoning. A crystalloid solution such as lactated Ringer's or sodium chloride should be started. If shock or bleeding is present consider plasma or whole blood. The amount of antivenin to be used will depend on the species and size of snake, the site of envenomation, the size of the patient, and other factors. If the patient has a reaction to the antivenin, it should be discontinued for 5 minutes and the patient given diphenhydramine intravenously; the antivenin can then be reinstituted at a slower rate and the patient observed for further reaction. Should this reaction reoccur, the antivenin should be discontinued and an envenomation expert should be consulted. Steroids should not be used during the acute phase of poisoning, except in conditions of shock or severe allergic reactions.

SPIDER BITES

Black Widow Spider

The bite of a female black widow spider (*Latrodectus mactans*) causes pain at the site of injection. Clinical manifestations include generalized muscle pains with severe abdominal cramps, irritability, nausea and vomiting, variable CNS symptoms, profuse perspiration, labored breathing, and collapse. Convulsions may rarely occur in children. Examination reveals a small papule at the area of bite, board-like rigidity of the abdomen, restlessness, and hyperactive deep tendon reflexes.

Keep the patient recumbent and quiet with adequate sedation. No first aid measures have proven to be of value. Calcium gluconate in a dose of 50 mg/kg intravenously (up to 250 mg/kg per 24 hours) has been shown to be of some value in reducing the muscle spasms. Methocarbamol in a dose of 15 mg/kg every 6 hours has also been of some value. Antivenin (*Latrodectus mactans*) has been shown to be effective to reverse muscle cramping, CNS effects, and hypertension. This antivenin should be reserved for patients who display severe symptoms that are not relieved by other methods. Instructions for use are included in the package. Morphine or codeine may help control pain. A tetanus toxoid booster should be given to the previously immunized child (if a booster has not been given within 4 years) and tetanus immune globulin should be given to a nonimmunized child. Other methods to reduce muscle spasm and pain include diazepam and narcotics such as meperidine.

Brown Spider

The North American brown recluse spider (violin spider, *Loxosceles reclusa*) is most commonly seen in the central and Midwestern areas of the USA. Its bite characteristically produces a localized reaction with progressively more severe pain over 8 hours. The initial bleb on an erythematous ischemic base may occur before ulceration. Other symptoms may include cyanosis, a morbiliform rash, fever, shock, chills, malaise, weakness, nausea and vomiting, joint pains with hemoglobinuria, jaundice, and delirium.

There is no specific antivenin. Many bites require little treatment other than local care and an antitetanus agent. If there is severe itching, diphenhydramine, 5 mg/kg/d orally (maximum dosage 25–50 mg 4 times a day) may be used. The use of steroids is questionable. If given, the usual course is dexamethazone, 4 mg intramuscularly 4 times a day during the acute phase, and then a decreasing dose regimen. A polymorphonucular leukocyte inhibitor such as dapsone or colchicine may be helpful. Dapsone may cause hemolysis, which is also a complication of *Loxosceles* envenomation. Oxygen supplied to the bite area through an improvised face mask may also be of some value. Surgical intervention should be delayed until 6 or more weeks after the bite. In rare cases, platelets may be needed when thrombocytopenia is present. Hyperbaric oxygen is being investigated for the treatment of bites rated as class 3 or 4 (severe). Therapy was instituted 2–6 days after envenomations, and all cases healed properly without hospitalization, surgery, serious skin slough, or significant scarring. A *Loxosceles* antivenin is currently being investigated but is not yet available.

TRICYCLIC ANTIDEPRESSANTS
(Amitriptyline, Doxepin, Imipramine, Nortriptyline, etc)

Amitriptyline (Elavil), doxepin (Sinequan), imipramine (Tofranil), nortriptyline (Aventyl), and other tricyclic antidepressants characteristically cause cardiac dysrhythmias, CNS abnormalities (agitation, hallucinations, seizures, and coma), and other signs of atropinism such as dilated pupils, malar flushing, dry mouth, hyperpyrexia, and urinary retention. Some of the newer cyclic antidepressants such as amoxapine have less cardiovascular toxicity but still cause CNS toxicity, with subsequent convulsions.

Treatment
Emesis is not indicated after overdose since rapid neurologic deterioration may occur. Gastric lavage and activated charcoal and a cathartic may be of use. Multiple-dose activated charcoal may be effective with these agents. Prolonged PR intervals may respond to phenytoin. Lidocaine may be of some use as well. Use of sodium bicarbonate is also helpful in correcting and preventing recurrence of cardiac dysrhythmias. Good supportive care is required for control of seizures, hypertension, hypotension, respiratory depression, and pulmonary edema. Physostigmine should be used only to control convulsions, severe coma, hypertension, hallucinations, and dysrhythmias. Give 0.5 mg of physostigmine intravenously over 1 minute. This dose may be repeated every 5 minutes until a total dose of 2 mg has been given. Repeated doses at 20–30-minute intervals may be necessary because the drug is rapidly metabolized. The lowest effective dose should be given. Relative contraindications to physostigmine include gangrene, urinary obstruction, bowel obstruction, asthma, and diabetes. If it is deemed necessary to use it in these circumstances, have available atropine in half the physostigmine dosage being given; atropine will reverse toxic findings of physostigmine.

Drug Therapy | 8

Robert F. St. Peter, MD, & Brenda L. Huffman, MD

When treating children with medications, physicians must not only be aware of the correct dosages and current indications, but must also take into account other important factors such as the optimal route and frequency of administration. Other considerations are the rates of absorption, metabolism, and elimination, which may vary greatly at different ages and under different physiologic conditions. This chapter provides a brief discussion of the principles of drug therapy in children, followed by an updated formulary of drugs commonly used in pediatrics.

DETERMINATION OF DRUG DOSAGE

A standard dose, or choice of standard doses, is usually available when prescribing a medication for use in adults. Because of the great variability in size and physiologic maturity, determining appropriate drug dosages in children is more complicated.

Pediatric drug dosages are generally based on body weight (in kilograms), or on body surface area (in meters squared). Dosage based on body surface area is the more accurate method of estimating the dose for a child. Body surface area can be determined using a nomogram that utilizes the readily available parameters of body weight and height (see Fig 8–1). In most cases, however, body weight is used to calculate dosages and provides an accurate, safe, and effective regimen. In the formulary that follows, most doses are reported in mg/kg, ie, based on body weight, and only occasionally reported in mg/m^2, based on body surface area.

Some general considerations should be kept in mind when calculating pediatric drug dosages. When calculating a dosage based on body weight, older children should not receive a dose greater than the recommended adult dose. Adjustments in the dosage may have to be made for many clinical situations: liver or

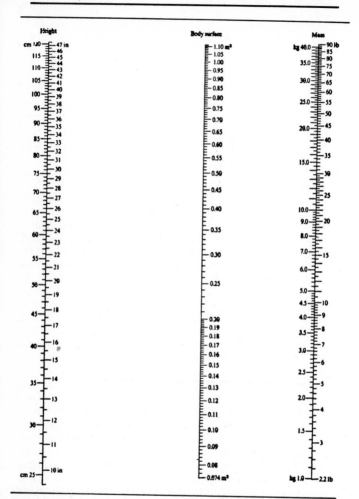

To determine the body surface area in a child, use a straight edge to connect the height and mass. The point of intersection on the body surface line gives the area in m².
From Lentner C (ed): Geigy Scientific Tables, ed 8. Basle, CIBA-GEIGY, 1981, vol 1, p 227.

Figure 8–1. Body surface area: Children. To determine the body surface area in a child, use a straight edge to connect the height and mass. The point of intersection on the body surface line gives the area in m². (Reproduced with permission, from *Geigy Scientific Tables,* 8th ed. Vol 1. Lentner C [editor]. CIBA-GEIGY, Basle, 1981.)

kidney disease, depending on the route of metabolism and elimination; edema and hypoproteinemia, depending on the drug's volume of distribution and protein binding properties; significant obesity; and in cases where drug interactions may occur.

In newborns, both full-term and premature, detoxifying enzymes may be deficient or absent; renal function relatively inefficient; and the blood–brain barrier and protein binding altered. Dosages have not been determined as accurately for newborn infants as for older children. Careful attention must be paid to the gestational age and metabolic status of each neonate being treated with pharmaceutic agents.

DETERMINATION OF ROUTE OF ADMINISTRATION

In addition to knowing what drug and what dose to give, you must also know how to give it. Oral administration is the most common route used. Infants and younger children usually receive liquid preparations (suspensions, elixirs, solutions). An accurate measuring device (a small syringe with the needle removed, or a graduated measuring spoon) makes administration of liquids relatively easy and accurate. Administration of medicines using kitchen spoons is notoriously inaccurate and should be discouraged. Liquids may be mixed with flavored syrups to make them more palatable. Tablets may be crushed and given with chocolate syrup, honey, jam or corn syrup. Special care should be given to keep all medications in a safe location, but especially those medications that are pleasant tasting. Older children may be able to take whole tablets or capsules. They or their parents should be asked whether they prefer liquids or tablets, if either is an acceptable alternative. Ease of administration is a major factor affecting compliance with a lengthy course of therapy.

Rectal administration of a medicine is often a good alternative to oral administration. In a patient who is vomiting, rectal administration may be the preferred route. The choice of which drug to use may be influenced by the different routes of administration available for otherwise comparable drugs. Many different drugs are available in pediatric suppository sizes.

Parenteral administration of drugs is usually limited to inpatient situations. Intravenous, intramuscular, and subcutaneous routes are frequently used. The volume of the injection should be considered when determining whether the IM or IV route is preferred.

Other routes of administration include **topical application,**

eye drops, ear drops, and **aerosol inhalation.** Careful details should be given to the parent and the patient concerning the appropriate use and administration of all medications in order to ensure maximum efficacy and safety.

MONITORING DRUG THERAPY

Determining the plasma levels of drugs can be extremely useful in monitoring therapy. For some drugs (eg, digoxin, theophylline, phenobarbital) the plasma level is well correlated with the drug's physiologic effect and is easier to determine than the physiologic effect itself. For other drugs (eg, antibiotics, anticoagulants, insulin) it is more important to measure the physiologic effect directly; serum bactericidal level, prothrombin time, blood glucose level, etc.

Therapeutic ranges have been determined for many commonly used drugs. The therapeutic range is the range of plasma levels for a given drug at which the majority of a treated population will receive the drug's intended therapeutic benefit without experiencing serious toxic side effects. Table 8–1 lists the therapeutic ranges of many commonly used pediatric drugs. Reported therapeutic ranges may vary between institutions, and should always be interpreted in light of the clinical situation.

Many factors contribute to the measured amount of a drug in the plasma. The time the sample is drawn in relation to the time of the last dose, the route of administration, the volume of distribution, and the rates of metabolism and elimination all affect the measured plasma levels.

CALCULATION OF LOADING DOSES

Following the intravenous administration of a drug, plasma levels will fall rapidly as the drug is distributed from the vascular compartment to the extracellular, intracellular, and other "compartments" of the body. The plasma level is determined by the dose given and the volume of distribution of that particular drug. This can be expressed mathematically in the equation:

Plasma level (mg/L) =
$$\frac{\text{Dose (mg/kg)}}{\text{Volume of distribution (L/kg)}}$$

Table 8–1. Therapeutic blood levels.

Drug	Therapeutic Levels*
Amikacin	(peak) 20–30 μg/mL
	(trough) 1–5 μg/mL
Caffeine	7–20 μg/mL
Carbamazepine	8–12 μg/mL
Chloramphenicol	(peak) 10–25 μg/mL
	(trough) 0–5 μg/mL
Cyclosporine	(trough) 50–150 μg/L
Digoxin	0.8–2.0 ng/mL
Gentamicin	(peak) 5–10 μg/mL
	(trough) 0.5–1.5 μg/mL
Phenobarbital	15–40 μg/mL
Phenytoin	10–20 μg/mL
Salicylate	
antipyretic	20–100 μg/mL
analgesic	20–100 μg/mL
anti-inflammatory	150–300 μg/mL
Theophylline	
asthma	10–20 μg/mL
apnea	5–10 μg/mL
Tobramycin	(peak) 5–10 μg/mL
	(trough) 1.0–2.0 μg/mL
Valproic acid	50–100 μg/mL
Vancomycin	(peak) 20–40 μg/mL
	(trough) 5–10 μg/mL

*Therapeutic levels may vary between institutions and should always be interpreted with regard to the individual clinical situation.

It follows that to reach a certain desired plasma level of a drug, you can calculate a loading dose using the following equation:

Dose (mg) = Desired plasma level (mg/L) × Patient weight (kg) × Volume of distribution (L/kg)

This equation is appropriate only for determining a loading dose; it is not for maintenance doses. Although the volumes of distribution are derived using intravenous administration of a given drug, it is generally applicable with oral or intramuscular administration as well. If absorption is complete, there is little difference between IM injection and slow IV infusion. The volume of distribution of a drug depends upon its solubility in body fluids and its tissue binding properties. Table 8–2 lists the volume of distribution of some commonly used drugs.

Table 8–2. Approximate volumes
of distribution (V_d).

Drug	V_d (L/kg)*
Acetaminophen	1.0
Aminoglycosides	0.3–0.5
Caffeine	0.9
Digoxin	7.5
Narcotics	> 5.0
Phenobarbital	0.75 (1.0)
Phenytoin	0.75 (1.0)
Salicylate†	0.2 (therapeutic doses)
	0.6 (toxic doses)
Theophylline	0.46 (0.69)

*Values in parentheses are for newborns.
†The V_d of salicylate increases with increasing dose owing to saturation of plasma-protein binding.

DRUGS & BREAST-FEEDING

Most drugs are excreted to some degree into breast milk, but the level of a drug in breast milk rarely exceeds the level in maternal plasma. Because of this, quantitative drug overdose of an infant via breast milk is virtually never a problem. However, certain drugs are toxic to infants in even trace amounts and these drugs should not be administered to breast-feeding women. Other drugs may be associated with idiosyncratic or allergic reactions that are not always dose related.

In general, radioactive compounds, antimetabolities, and chemotherapeutic agents should be avoided in breast-feeding mothers. Specific drugs that are contraindicated in lactating mothers are listed in Table 8–3.

Breast-feeding mothers may start oral contraceptives once their milk flow is well established, usually 3–6 weeks after delivery.

Commonly used nonprescription drugs, such as marijuana, nicotine, caffeine, and alcohol, are also excreted into breast milk. If used in excess, these drugs may cause changes in the child's behavior and state of wakefulness. There is a significant lack of knowledge concerning the long-term toxicity of these drugs in breast-fed infants, and lactating mothers should be encouraged to practice abstinence or prudent moderation.

General considerations for the use of drugs in lactating women include:

(1) Is the maternal drug therapy really necessary?

Table 8–3. Drugs that are contraindicated during breast-feeding.*

Bromocriptine
Cocaine
Clemastine
Cyclophosphamide
Cytosporine
Doxorubicin
Ergotamine
Methotrexate
Phencyclidine (PCP)
Phenindione
Thiouracil
Metronidazole (recommend discontinuation of breast-feeding for 12–24 hours to allow excretion of dose)
Radioactive compounds (recommend discontinuation of breast-feeding for variable periods of time depending on the specific agent)

*This list may not include all drugs that may be harmful if used in a breast-feeding mother. Individual consideration must be used when medicating a woman who is breast-feeding.
(Adapted from American Academy of Pediatrics, Committee on Drugs: The transfer of drugs and other chemicals into human breast milk. *Pediatrics* 1989;**84**:924–936)

(2) Is this the least toxic drug that is effective?

(3) Can the dosing schedule be arranged to minimize delivery of the drug to the infant?

(4) Are idiosyncratic or allergic reactions a particular concern for this infant?

(5) Are there known side effects? Are they easily recognized (eg, rash, drowsiness, etc)?

(6) Does the infant have a known medical problem (eg, hepatic or renal disease) that would diminish the drug's excretion and thereby allow it to accumulate in the infant?

Despite the discussion above, most drugs can be used safely in women who are breast-feeding, and it is a rare event when a course of therapy will have to be altered, or breast-feeding discontinued, because of the need for maternal medications.

ANTI-INFECTIVE CHEMOTHERAPEUTIC AGENTS & ANTIBIOTIC DRUGS

Effective treatment of bacterial, fungal, parasitic, and viral infections in pediatric patients depends on (1) knowledge of the antimicrobial, pharmaceutical, and toxic properties of the chemotherapeutic agents; (2) proper choice of one or more drugs that can inhibit, neutralize, counteract, or kill the organisms suspected or known to be the cause of infection (Table 8–4); and (3) initiation of treatment at the appropriate time and continuation of therapy for an appropriate duration.

The therapeutic efficacy of an agent is gauged by its ability to produce a desired effect with minimal or no toxicity. For most chemotherapeutic agents and antibiotics, dosages have been selected on the basis of the therapeutic index (ratio between effectiveness and toxicity). For a few, however, it is necessary to monitor drug levels either in the blood or at some peripheral site in order to adjust the dosage to the correct level for a given patient.

Toxicity of some agents is predictable and unavoidable, and use of such agents must take into account the ratio of risks to benefits. Toxicity of other agents is idiosyncratic and unpredictable, and these agents should be avoided if equally effective drugs are available. If not, the patient taking the potentially toxic drug should be carefully monitored for adverse reactions and the drug discontinued as soon as toxicity occurs.

Hypersensitivity reactions to antimicrobial agents can range from mild and transient skin rashes to life-threatening anaphylaxis. Therefore, a history of reactions to drugs (both tolerance and sensitivity) should always be elicited prior to therapy. If a hypersensitivity reaction occurs, this information should be prominently displayed in the patient's medical records.

Indications for Use

Antimicrobial therapy is indicated (1) if a clinical syndrome clearly identifies the most likely infectious agent, (2) if the pathogen can be isolated from a site that correlates with the clinical syndrome, or (3) if there is serologic or other laboratory evidence of a specific agent. In infants and children, these specific indications are not always present. For example, a very ill child may have high fever and no localizing findings, or a newborn infant may show signs of hypotonicity, pallor, and shock but have no specific evidence of infection. In circumstances such as these, large-scale studies have shown a predictable but wide range of possible infecting organisms. After obtaining appropriate specimens for specific microbiologic testing (eg, blood for culture), the clinician may employ one or several antibiotics expected to "cover" the range of possible organisms. Adjustment of the treatment regimen follows identification of the specific organisms involved; alternatively, therapy may be discontinued in the absence of any definite infectious agent.

Prophylactic use of antibiotics is seldom effective. In most circumstances, prophylactic use simply alters the flora in a sus-

Table 8–4. Choice of anti-infective agents.

Organism (Gram Reaction)	Drug(s) of First Choice	Drug(s) of Second Choice
Actinomyces (+)	Penicillin	Tetracyclines or sulfonamides
Bacillus anthracis (+)	Penicillin	Tetracyclines or erythromycin
Bacteroides (−)*	Chloramphenicol or clindamycin	Metronidazole, penicillin, cefoxitin, or imipenem
Bordetella pertussis (−)	Erythromycin	Ampicillin or TMP/SMX
Brucella (−)	Tetracyclines + streptomycin	Chloramphenicol, TMP/SMX, or rifampin
Candida albicans	Nystatin or amphotericin B	Flucytosine, ketoconazole, or clotrimazole
Chlamydiae	Erythromycin or tetracyclines	Chloramphenicol or sulfonamides
Clostridia (+)	Penicillin	Erythromycin, vancomycin, tetracyclines, or clindamycin
Corynebacterium diphtherisae (+)	Antitoxin + penicillin	Erythromycin
Erysipelothrix (+)	Penicillin	Tetracyclines or erythromycin
Francisella tularensis (−)	Streptomycin or gentamicin	Tetracyclines or chloramphenicol
Haemophilus influenzae (−)*	Chloramphenicol, cefotaxine, or ceftriaxone	TMP/SMX
Leptospira	Tetracyclines	Penicillin
Listeria monocytogenes (+)	Ampicillin + an aminoglycoside	TMP/SMX
Mycobacterium tuberculosis (+)*	Isoniazid + rifampin or Isoniazid + PAS + streptomycin or Isoniazid + ethambutol†	Pyrazinamide, cycloserine, or an aminoglycoside
Mycoplasma pneumoniae	Erythromycin	Tetracyclines
Neisseria gonorrhoeae (−)	Penicillin + probenecid or ceftriaxone	Ampicillin + probenecid, TMP/SMX, or spectinomycin

(continued)

Table 8–4. *(Continued)*

Organism (Gram Reaction)	Drug(s) of First Choice	Drug(s) of Second Choice
Neisseria meningitidis (−)	Penicillin	Ampicillin, chloramphenicol, cefotaxime, or ceftriaxone
Nocardia (+)*	Sulfonamides	Amikacin, TMP/SMX, cycloserine, or erythromycin
Proteus mirabilis (−)*	Ampicillin or penicillin	Kanamycin, gentamicin, or TMP/SMX
Pseudomonas aeruginosa (−)*	Tobramycin + either carbenicillin, ticarcillin, or piperacillin	Gentamicin, ceftazidime, or imipenem
Rickettsiae (−)	Tetracyclines	Chloramphenicol
Staphylococcus (+)* if sensitive to penicillin	Penicillin	Erythromycin or cephalexin
Staphylococcus (+)* if resistant to penicillin	Methicillin, nafcillin, oxacillin, dicloxacillin, or cloxacillin	Cefazolin, clindamycin, erythromycin, or vancomycin
Streptococcus (+)* (group A, group B, and non-enterococcal group D)	Penicillin	Erthromycin, ampicillin, clindamycin, vancomycin, or cephalosporins
Streptococcus faecalis (+)* (group D enterococci)	Penicillin + gentamicin or Ampicillin + an aminoglycoside	Vancomycin + an aminoglycoside
Streptococcus pneumoniae	Penicillin	Erythromycin, clindamycin, chloramphenicol, cephalosporins, or vancor
Treponema pallidum	Penicillin	Erythromycin, tetracyclines, or cephalosporins
Yersinia pestis (−)	Streptomycin + tetracycline or chloramphenicol	TMP/SMX or an aminoglycoside

*Sensitivity test usually indicated.
†Ethambutol should be used with caution in children too young to complain of or be tested for changes in visual acuity.

ceptible patient, thereby allowing a resistant organism to become predominant and making subsequent therapy more difficult. Among the legitimate and effective uses of prophylactic therapy are prevention of streptococcal infections in patients with rheumatic heart disease, prevention of endocarditis in patients with some types of acquired or congenital heart diseases, prevention of *Pneumocystis carinii* infection in certain susceptible hosts, and prevention of recurrences of otitis media or urinary tract infections in selected patients.

Resistance

Resistance tends to develop in some populations of organisms because of the selective pressure caused by the use of a specific antibiotic. For example, among the bowel flora, there may be some strains of *Escherichia coli* that are sensitive to ampicillin and a few that are resistant. Administration of ampicillin will reduce or eliminate the sensitive strains, thereby permitting overgrowth of the resistant ones. If infection ensues, it will be caused by a strain that is now resistant to ampicillin. In some populations of organisms, spontaneous mutation to a resistant strain may occur as a chance event; subsequent antibiotic use may encourage the persistence of that organism. Some organisms acquire resistance by exchange of genetic material in the cytoplasm (plasmids); for example, salmonellae and shigellae have rapidly become resistant by such genetic transfer.

To prevent the emergence of resistant strains, (1) use antibiotics only when they are indicated; (2) choose the most effective agent with the narrowest spectrum of activity; (3) administer the proper dosage and continue treatment for the proper duration; and (4) when appropriate, use 2 antibiotics that have different inhibitory effects on the organism.

Dosages in Newborn & Premature Infants (Table 8–5)

The term ''newborn'' usually refers to an infant in the first 7 days of life. In premature and full-term newborn infants, caution is necessary to prevent overdosage and avoid causing serious and permanent damage. However, undertreatment is a definite risk if doses are not adjusted as the infant's renal function matures. Failure to recognize that there is a marked increase in excretion of drugs such as penicillin G, methicillin, ampicillin, gentamicin, and kanamycin by the second week of life—and failure to increase drug dosages at this time—will result in unsatisfactory blood levels as well as clinical failure. The need for higher drug dosages in infants 8 or more days of age is especially important if therapy of gram-negative infections, including men-

Table 8–5. Suggested doses for newborn and premature infants.

Antibiotic	Preferred Route	Dosage and Frequency*	
		0–7 Days	8–30 Days
Amikacin	IV, IM	PI: 7.5–10 mg/kg every 24 h TI: 7.5 mg/kg every 12 h	PI: 7.5–10 mg/kg every 12–24 h TI: 7.5 mg/kg every 8 h
Ampicillin	IV	50–100 mg/kg every 8–12 h	50–100 mg/kg every 8–12 h
Cefotaxime	IV, IM	50 mg/kg every 12 h	50 mg/kg every 8 h
Chloramphenicol[†]	IV	PI: 2.5 mg/kg every 6 h TI: 5 mg/kg every 6 h	PI: 2.5 mg/kg every 6 h TI: 12.5 mg/kg every 6 h
Clindamycin	IV, IM, oral	PI: 5 mg/kg every 8 h TI: 5 mg/kg every 6 h	5 mg/kg every 6 h
Erythromycin estolate	Oral	10 mg/kg every 12 h	10 mg/kg every 6 h
Gentamicin	IM, IV	PI: 2.5 mg/kg every 24 h TI: 2.5 mg/kg every 12 h	PI: 2.5 mg/kg every 12–24 h TI: 2.5 mg/kg every 8 h
Kanamycin	IM	PI: 7.5 mg/kg every 12 h TI: 7.5–10 mg/kg every 12 h	PI: 7.5–10 mg/kg every 12 h TI: 7.5–10 mg/kg every 8 h
Methicillin (or nafcillin or oxacillin)	IV, IM	25–50 mg/kg every 12 h	25–50 mg/kg every 6–8 h
Meziocillin	IV, IM	75 mg/kg every 12 h	75 mg/kg every 8 h
Penicillin G	IV, IM	25,000–50,000 units/kg every 8–12 h	25,000–50,000 units/kg every 6–8 h
Ticarcillin	IV, IM	PI: 75 mg/kg every 12 h TI: 75 mg/kg every 8 h	75 mg/kg every 6–8 h

(continued)

Table 8–5. *(Continued)*

Antibiotic	Preferred Route	Dosage and Frequency*	
		0–7 Days	**8–30 Days**
Tobramycin	IV, IM	PI: 2.5 mg/kg every 24 h TI: 2.5 mg/kg every 12 h	PI: 2.5 mg/kg every 12–24 h TI: 2.5 mg/kg every 8 h
Vancomycin	IV	15 mg/kg every 12 h	15 mg/kg every 8 h

*PI = premature infant (<35 weeks postconceptional age); TI = term infant (≥35 weeks postconceptional age).
†Chloramphenicol must be used with extreme caution. Start with a loading dose of 20 mg/kg, and then follow schedule in table. Serum levels should be carefully monitored to adjust dosage (therapeutic serum levels are 5–10 μg/mL for troughs and 10–25 μg/mL for peaks; toxic level is probably >40 μg/mL).

ingitis, is to be successful. Whatever the age of the child, about 30 times as much ampicillin is required in blood or cerebrospinal fluid to kill a sensitive *E coli* strain as is required to kill a sensitive *Haemophilus influenzae* strain. Some strains of group B streptococci are 50 times more resistant to penicillin G than are group A strains. Marginal penicillin levels in the cerebrospinal fluid will result if the infant's increasing ability to excrete penicillin is not taken into account.

The small, sick, premature infant who is neither "just born" nor old enough in conceptual age to be considered "term" remains in no-man's-land, and drug dosages should be intermediate between those used for premature infants who are less than 3 days of age and those used for term infants who are more than 7 days of age.

Precautions in Oliguric Children

Regular drug dosages and intervals may result in drug levels that are too high in children with reduced renal function. Dosage and time schedules must be adjusted to renal output in the case of the more toxic agents (amikacin, gentamicin, kanamycin, tobramycin, and vancomycin), and serum half-lives should be carefully estimated as a basis for individual dosing. The usual dosing interval is every 3 half-lives for patients with significant renal failure. Subsequent doses are one-half to two-thirds of the initial loading dose. Patients on dialysis will need an additional dose at the end of each procedure if a significant amount of drug is removed (Table 8–6). In patients being treated with aminogly-

Table 8-6. Use of anti-infective agents in patients with renal failure.*

| Adjustment Needed | Drug | Approximate Half-Life in Serum (Hours) | | Usual Initial Dose | Significant Removal by: | |
		Normal	Renal Failure		Hemodialysis	Peritoneal Dialysis
Major	Amikacin	2	44–86	7.5 mg/kg	Yes	Small amount
	Flucytosine	3–6	70	30 mg/kg	Yes	Yes
	Gentamicin	2.5	72–96	2 mg/kg	Yes	Small amount
	Kanamycin	3	72–97	7.5–10 mg/kg	Yes	Small amount
	Streptomycin	2.5	72–96	10 mg/kg	Yes	Small amount
	Tubramycin	2.5	48–72	2 mg/kg	Yes	Small amount
	Vancomycin	6	>96	10 mg/kg	No	No
Moderate	Carbenicillin	0.5–1	12	75 mg/kg	Yes	No
	Cefazolin	2	32	35 mg/kg	Yes	No

	0.5	10	70,000 units/kg	No	No
Penicillin G					
Sulfamethoxazole	9	27	20–40 mg/kg	Yes	Small amount
Ticarcillin	1	13	50 mg/kg	Yes	No
Trimethoprim	11	25	5–10 mg/kg	Yes	Small amount
Amoxicillin	1	16	25 mg/kg	Yes	No
Ampicillin	0.5–1	8–20	50 mg/kg	Yes	No
Cefotaxime	1.5	3	50 mg/kg	Yes	No
Ceftriaxone	4–7	12–15	50 mg/kg	?	?
Chloramphenicol	3	4	30 mg/kg	No	No
Clindamycin	4	8	5 mg/kg	No	No
Cloxacillin	0.5	0.8	25–50 mg/kg	No	No
Erythromycin	1.5	5	20 mg/kg	No	No
Isoniazid	2	4	5 mg/kg	Yes	Yes
Rifampin	2–3	2–5	10 mg/kg	No	No

Minor or none

*This table should be used only as a guide. Renal failure is considered here to be marked by a creatinine clearance of 10 mL/min or less. Sources of data include the following: Bennett WM et al: *Ann Intern Med* 1980;**93**:62. Moellering RC: *Ann Intern Med* 1981;**94**:343. Nelson JD: *1985 Pocketbook of Pediatric Antimicrobial Therapy,* Williams & Wilkins, 1985.

cosides during continuous peritoneal dialysis, it may be convenient to merely adjust antibiotic doses in the dialysate.

AVERAGE DRUG DOSES FOR CHILDREN

The dosage recommendations that follow should be regarded only as approximations; careful clinical observation and the use of pertinent laboratory aids are necessary. All drugs should be used with caution in children, and dosage should be individualized. Whenever possible, reference should be made to the printed literature supplied by the manufacturer or to other recent sources.

FORMULARY (excludes anti-infectives and antibiotics see p 225)

Acetaminophen (many trade names) How supplied: tabs: 80, 325, 500 mg; caplets: 160 mg; liquid: 50 mg/15 mL; syrup: 160 mg/5 mL; drops: 80 mg/0.8 mL; suppository: 120, 125, 130, 300, 325, 500, 600, 650 mg. Dose: based on wt: 10–15 mg/kg/dose PO, PR Q4–6H; based on age: 1–2 yrs, 120 mg/dose; 2–3 yrs, 160 mg/dose; 4–5 yrs, 240 mg/dose; 6–8 yrs, 320 mg/dose; 9–10 yrs, 400 mg/dose; 11–12 yrs, 480 mg/dose; adult, 325–1000 mg/dose.

Acetazolamide (Diamox) How supplied: tabs: 125, 250 mg; caps (sustained release): 500 mg; injection: 500 mg/5 mL. Dose: 5–30 mg/kg/day PO or IV Q6–8H; adult: 250–1000 mg/day PO or IV Q6H–QOD.

Acetylcysteine (Mucomyst) How supplied: vials: 10% and 20% in 4, 10, and 30 mL vials. Dose: nebulization: 20%: 3–5 mL (diluted with equal volume of NS) 3–4 times/d; 10%: 6–10 mL 3–4 times/d. Direct instillation: 1–2 mL dose up to Q1H; acetaminophen overdose: 140 mg/kg loading dose PO or NG, then 70 mg/kg/dose PO or NG Q4H for a total of 17 doses (dilute 1:4 in water or soft drink).

ACTH (Acthar, Cortrophin-Zinc, Cortrosyn, HP-Acthar) How supplied: gel: 40, 80 USP/mL in 1, 5 mL vials; aqueous: 25, 40 USP/vial. Dose: gel: 0.8 USP/kg/d IM or SC Q12–24H; aqueous: 1.6 USP/kg/d IV, IM, or SC Q6–8H.

Albumin How supplied: injection: 5% in 50, 250, 500, 1000 mL vials; 25% in 20, 50, 100 mL vials. Dose: 0.5–1.0 gm/kg/dose IV as needed.

Albuterol (Proventil, Ventolin) How supplied: tabs: 2, 4 mg;

syrup: 2 mg/5 mL; solution for nebulization: 5 mg/mL; inhaler: 90 μg/puff, approx 200 puffs/inhaler. Dose: oral: children, 0.1 mg/kg/dose Q8H; adult, 2–4 mg Q8H; inhalation: 1–2 puffs Q4–6H; nebulization: 0.1 mg/kg/dose; max 2.5 mg/dose, diluted in 2–3 mL of NS, usually 2–4 times daily but may be repeated prn.

Allopurinol (Lopurin, Zyloprim) How supplied: tabs: 100, 300 mg. Dose: < 6 yr: 150 mg/d PO Q8H; 6–10 yr: 300 mg/d PO Q8H; adult: 200–600 mg/d PO Q8H (max dose 800 mg/d).

Aluminum Hydroxide (Amphojel, AlternaGel, others) How supplied: tabs: 320, 640 mg; suspension: 320, 600 mg/5 mL. Dose: 1–2 tsp PO 4–6 times/day.

Aminocaproic Acid (Amicar) How supplied: tabs: 500 mg; syrup: 250 mg/1 mL; injection: 250 mg/1 mL. Dose: adult: initial dose of 5 gm PO or IV once, then 1.0–1.25 gm PO or IV Q1H (max dose 30 gm in 24 hr); children: initial dose 3 gms/m^2/dose IV once, then 1 gm/m^2/dose IV Q1H.

Aminophylline How supplied: (see also theophylline) tabs: 100, 200 mg (79% theo); syrup: 105 mg/5 mL (86% theo, 90 mg theo/5 mL); injection: 25 mg/1 mL (79% theo, 20 mg theo/ 1 mL). Dose: oral: 1 yr–9 yr, 20 mg/kg/d Q6H; 9 yr–16 yr, 16 mg/kg/d Q6H; > 16 yr, 12 mg/kg/d Q6H; intravenous: loading: 2–6 mg/kg IV; maintenance (IV drip): neonates, 0.2 mg/kg/h; 1 mo–1 yr, 0.2–0.9 mg/kg/h; 1–9 yr, 1.0–1.2 mg/kg/h; 9–16 yr, 0.8–1.0 mg/kg/h; young adult smokers, 0.8–1.0 mg/kg/h; nonsmoking adults, 0.5–0.7 mg/kg/h.

Amitriptyline (Elavil, Endep, others) How supplied: tabs: 10, 25, 50, 75, 100, 150 mg; injection: 10 mg/1 mL. Dose: < 12 yr, 40–150 mg/d PO Q6–24H; > 12 yr, 20–30 mg/dose IM QID.

Ammonium Chloride How supplied: tabs: 300, 500, 1000 mg; caps: 300, 500 mg; syrup: 500 mg/5 mL; injection: 0.4, 4.0, 5.0 mEq/1 mL. Dose: urine acidification: 60–75 mg/kg/dose PO or IV Q6H (max dose 4–6 gm/d).

Aspirin How supplied: tabs: 65, 75, 200, 300, 325, 500, 600, 650 mg; caps: 325 mg; suppositories: 60, 65, 130, 150, 195, 200, 300, 325, 600, 1200 mg. Dose: antipyretic, analgesic: 10–15 mg/kg/dose PO or PR Q4h; adult, 325–650 mg/dose Q4H (max 4–6 doses/d); antirheumatic: 65–100 mg/kg/d PO Q4H.

Atropine Sulfate How supplied: tabs: 0.3, 0.4, 0.6 mg; injection: 0.1, 0.4, 1.0 mg/1 mL. Dose: oral: 0.01 mg/kg/dose PO Q4H; adult, 0.5 mg/dose; nebulization: 0.05–0.075 mg/kg/dose in 2 mL of NS (max dose 1.0–2.5 mg); cardiac arrest: 0.01–0.03 mg/kg/dose ET or IV Q2–5 min (min dose 0.1 mg); adult, 0.5–2.0 mg/dose.

Azathioprine (Imuran) How supplied: tabs: 50 mg; injection: 100 mg/20 mL. Dose: 1–5 mg/kg/d PO or IV.

Baclofen (Lioresal) How supplied: tabs: 10, 20 mg. Dose: 5 mg/dose PO TID and gradually increase as needed to max dose of 20 mg/dose QID.

Beclomethasone (Beclovent, Beconase, Vanceril) How supplied: oral inhaler: 42 μg/puff, approx 200 puffs/inhaler; nasal inhaler: 42 μg/puff; nasal spray: 42 μg/spray. Dose: 6–12 yr, 1–2 inhalations Q6–12H (max 10 inhalations/d); > 12 yr, 2 inhalations Q6–12H (max 20 inhalations/d).

Bethanechol (Urecholine, others) How supplied: tabs: 5, 10, 25, 50 mg; vials: 5 mg/1 mL. Dose: 0.6 mg/kg/d PO Q6–8H; adult, 30–120 mg/d TID–QID; 0.15–0.2 mg/kg/d SC Q6–8H; adult, 2.5–5.0 mg/d SC Q6–8H.

Bisacodyl (Dulcolax) How supplied: tabs: 5 mg; suppository: 10 mg. Dose: oral: 0.3 mg/kg/dose; adult, 1–15 mg/dose; rectally: < 2 yr, 5 mg/dose; > 2 yr, 10 mg/dose.

Bretylium How supplied: 50 mg/1 mL. Dose: NOT APPROVED FOR USE IN CHILDREN; cardiac arrest: 5–10 mg/kg/dose IV Q1–2H; maintenance: 5–10 mg/kg/dose IV Q6H or a constant infusion of 1–2 mg/min.

Caffeine How supplied: (as citrate) solution: 10 mg/1 mL; injection: 10 mg/1 mL. Dose: 20 mg/kg/dose PO or IV loading dose, then 10 mg/kg/d PO or IV QD.

Calcium Chloride (27% calcium) How supplied: solution: 10% or 100 mg/1 mL (1.4 mEq CA^{2+}/1 mL). Dose: children, 200–300 mg/kg/d PO as 2% solution Q6H; adult, 4–8 gm/d PO as 2% solution Q6H; cardiac arrest: 20 mg/kg/dose IV Q10 min; adult, 250–500 mg/dose IV Q10/min.

Calcium Gluconate (9% calcium) How supplied: tabs: 500, 650, 1000 mg; solution: 10% or 100 mg/mL (0.47 mEq Ca^{2+}/1 mL). Dose: infants, 200–500 mg/d added to IV fluids or 400–800 mg/kg/d PO Q6H; children, 200–500 mg/kg/d PO Q6H; adult, 5–15 gm/d PO Q6H; cardiac arrest: 100 mg/kg/dose IV Q10 min prn (max 10 mL/dose).

Calcium Lactate (13% calcium) How supplied: tabs: 325, 650 mg. Dose: children, 400–500 mg/kg/d PO Q6–8H; adult, 2–4 gm/kg/d PO TID.

Captopril (Capoten) How supplied: 12.5, 25, 50, 100 mg. Dose: infants, 1 mg/kg/d PO TID initially and increase as tolerated up to 6 mg/kg/d PO TID; children, 25 mg/d PO Q12H; adult,

25 mg/dose PO Q8–12H initially and increase as tolerated up to max of 450 mg/d.

Carbamazepine (Tegretol) How supplied: tabs: 200 mg; chewable tabs: 100 mg; suspension: 100 mg/5 mL. Dose: 6–12 yr, initial: 100 mg/dose PO BID; increment: weekly increases of 100 mg/d PO TID–QID; maintenance: 400–800 mg/d PO TID–QID (max dose 1000 mg/d); > 12 yr, initial: 200 mg/dose PO BID; increment: weekly increases of 200 mg/d PO TID–QID; maintenance: 800–1200 mg/d PO TID–QID (max dose 1200 mg/d).

Charcoal, activated How supplied: 25, 50 gm bottles. Dose: 0.5 gm/kg/dose PO or NG Q4H PRN (usual adult dose 50 gm).

Chloral Hydrate How supplied: tabs: 250, 500 mg; syrup: 500 mg/10 mL, 1000 mg/10 mL; suppository: 325, 500, 650 mg. Dose: children: 25–100 mg/kg/dose PO, NG, PR; adult: 250–2000 mg/dose PO, NG, PR.

Chlordiazepoxide (Librium) How supplied: tabs: 5, 10, 25 mg; caps: 5, 10, 25 mg; injection: 100 mg/5 mL. Dose: oral: > 6 yr, 5 mg/dose PO BID–QID; adult, 5–25 mg/dose PO BID–QID; injection: > 12 yr, 25–100 mg/dose IM or IV Q2–4H PRN.

Chlorothiazide (Diuril) How supplied: tabs: 250, 500 mg; suspension: 250 mg/5 mL; injection: 500 mg/20 mL. Dose: oral: children, 20 mg/kg/d PO Q12H; adult, 500–2000 mg/d PO Q12–24H; intravenous: adult, 500–2000 mg/d IV Q12–24H.

Chlorpheniramine (many trade names) How supplied: tabs: 4 mg; caps, timed release: 8, 12, mg; syrup: 2 mg/5 mL; injection: 10 mg/1 mL. Dose: 0.35 mg/kg/d PO or SC QID; adult, 2–4 mg/dose TID–QID.

Chlorpromazine (Thorazine) How supplied: tabs: 10, 25, 50, 100, 200 mg; caps: 30, 75, 150, 200, 300 mg; syrup: 10 mg/5 mL; suppository: 25, 100 mg; injection: 25 mg/1 mL. Dose: oral: 0.5 mg/kg/dose PO Q4–6H; adult, 10–50 mg/dose; rectal: 1–2 mg/kg/dose PR Q6–8H; adult, 10–50 mg/dose; injection: 0.5 mg/kg/dose IM or IV Q6–8H; adult, 25–100 mg/dose (maximum doses: < 5 yr, 40 mg/d; 5–12 yr, 75 mg/d; adult, 1–2 gm/d).

Cholestyramine (Questran) How supplied: powder: 9 gm/packet, 9 gm/tin. Dose: > 6 yr, 240 mg/kg/d PO TID; adult, 4 gm/dose PO TID–QID.

Cimetidine (Tagamet) How supplied: tabs: 200, 300, 400, 800 mg; syrup: 300 mg/5 mL; injection: 150 mg/1 mL. Dose: 20–40 mg/kg/d PO or IV Q6H; adult, 300 mg/dose PO or IV Q6H.

Citrate (Polycitra, Polycitra K, Bicitra) How supplied: Polycitra: 1 mEq Na, 1 mEq K, 2 mEq bicarbonate/1 mL; Polycitra K: 0 mEq Na, 2 mEq K, 2 mEq bicarbonate/1 mL; Bicitra: 1 mEq Na, 0 mEq K, 1 mEq bicarbonate/1 mL. Dose: 5–15 mL/dose PO Q6–8H; adult, 10–30 mL/dose PO Q6–8H.

Clemastine (Tavist) How supplied: tabs: 1.34, 2.68 mg; syrup: 0.5 mg/5 mL. Dose: 6–12 yr: 0.5–1.0 mg/dose PO BID (max dose 3 mg/d); > 12 yr: 1–2 mg/dose PO BID (max dose 6 mg/d).

Clonazepam (Clonopin) How supplied: tabs: 0.5, 1.0, 2.0 mg. Dose: < 10 yr: initial 0.01–0.03 mg/kg/d PO Q8–12H; increments of 0.25–0.50 mg every 3rd day to max maintenance dose of 0.1–0.2 mg/kg/d Q8–12H; adult: initial 1.5 mg/day PO TID; increments of 0.5–1.0 mg every 3rd day to max maintenance dose of 20 mg/d PO TID.

Codeine How supplied: tabs: 15, 30, 60, mg (sulfate); injection: 30, 60 mg/1 mL (phosphate). Dose: analgesic: children, 0.5–1.5 mg/kg/dose PO or IV Q4–6H; adult, 30–60 mg/dose PO or IV Q4–6H; antitussive: children, 0.2–0.5 mg/kg/dose PO Q4–6H; adult, 15–30 mg/kg/dose PO Q4–6H.

Cortisone Acetate (Cortone) How supplied: tabs: 25 mg; injection: 25 50 mg/1 mL. Dose: physiologic replacement: oral, approx 25 mg/m^2/day PO TID; IM, approx 15 mg/m^2/d QD; stress: 2–4 times physiologic replacement dose.

Cromolyn Sodium (Intal, Nasalcrom, Opticrom) How supplied: inhaler: 800 μg/puff, approx 200 puffs/inhaler; liquid for nebulization: 20 mg/2 mL; nasal spray: 5.2 mg/spray, 100 sprays/13 mL container; eye drops: 40 mg/1 mL (4%), 10 mL container. Dose: inhalation: 2 puffs QID; nebulization: 20 mg/dose TID–QID; nasal: 1 spray each nostril 3–4 times/d; eyes: 1–2 drops each eye 4–6 times/d.

Cyproheptadine (Periactin) How supplied: tabs: 4 mg; syrup: 2 mg/5 mL. Dose: 0.25 mg/kg/d PO Q8–12H (max dose 0.5 mg/kg/d).

Dantrolene (Dantrium) How supplied: caps: 25, 50, 100 mg; injection: 20 mg/70 mL. Dose: malignant hyperthermia: prophylaxis, 4–8 mg/kg/d PO Q6–8H starting 1–2 days before anesthesia; treatment, 1 mg/kg IV repeated prn up to max of 10 mg/kg.

Deferoxamine Mesylate (Desferal) How supplied: 500 mg/vial. Dose: diagnostic challenge: 1 gm IM once; therapeutic: 15 mg/kg/h IV by continuous infusion; 90 mg/kg/dose IM Q4–12H (max 500 mg/dose except 1000 mg/dose for first dose only).

Desmopressin Acetate (DDAVP) How supplied: nasal solution:

0.1 mg/1 mL; injection: 4 μg/1 mL. Dose: diabetes insipidus: children, 5–30 μg/d Q12–24H intranasally; adult, 10–40 μg/d Q8–24H intranasally; *or* 2–4 μg/day IV or SC Q12–24H; coagulopathy: 0.3 μg/kg/dose IV.

Dexamethasone (Decadron, others) How supplied: tabs: 0.25, 0.5, 0.75, 1.5, 4, 6 mg; elixir: 0.5 mg/5 mL; injection: 4, 24 mg/1 mL. Dose: increased intracranial pressure: initial: 0.5–1.5 mg/kg/dose IV or IM; adults, 10 mg/dose IV or IM; maintenance: 0.2–0.5 mg/kg/d IV or IM Q6H; adults, 4 mg/dose IV or IM Q6H, then taper slowly; airway edema: 0.25–0.5 mg/kg/dose PO, IV, or IM Q6H for 4–6 doses.

Dextroamphetamine (Dexedrine, others) How supplied: tabs: 5, 10 mg; caps: 5, 10, 15 mg; elixir: 5 mg/5 mL. Dose: attention deficit disorder: 3–5 yr: 2.5 mg/d PO initially then increments of 2.5 mg at weekly intervals; daily dose BID–TID; > 5 yr: 5.0 mg/d PO initially then increments of 5.0 mg at weekly intervals; daily dose BID–TID, max dose 40 mg/d.

Dextromethorphan (many trade names) How supplied: available in many preparations. Dose: 0.5–1 mg/kg/d PO Q6–24H.

Diazepam (Valium) How supplied: tabs: 2, 5, 10 mg; injection: 5 mg/1 mL. Dose: sedation: children, oral: 0.1–0.8 mg/kg/d PO Q6–8H; injection: 0.04–0.2 mg/kg/dose IV Q2–4H; adult, oral: 2–10 mg/dose PO Q6–8H; injection: 2–10 mg/dose IV Q3–4H; seizures: children: < 5 yr, 0.2–0.5 mg/kg/dose IV Q2–5 min; total max 5 mg; > 5 yr, 1 mg/dose IV Q2–5 min; total max 10 mg, repeat Q2–4H prn.

Diazoxide (Hyperstat, Proglycem) How supplied: caps: 50 mg; liquid: 50 mg/1 mL; injection: 15 mg/1 mL. Dose: hypertension: children, 3–5 mg/kg/dose IV rapid bolus, may repeat in 30 min then dose Q3–10H; adult, 1–3 mg/kg/dose IV rapid bolus, repeat Q5–15 min, then Q4–24H; hypoglycemia: infants, 8–15 mg/kg/d PO or IV Q8–12H; children and adults, 3–8 mg/kg/d PO or IV Q8–12H.

Digoxin How supplied: tabs: 125, 250, 500 μg (bioavailability 60–80%); caps: 50, 100, 200 μg (bioavailability 90–100%); elixir: 50 μg/1 mL (bioavailability 70–85%); injection: 100, 250 mg/1 mL (IV bioavailibility 100%). Dose: tabs or elixir: premature, 20–30 μg/kg PO digitalizing dose; maintenance dose is 20–30% of oral digitalizing dose, BID; full term, 25–35 μg/kg PO digitalizing dose*; 1–24 mo, 35–60 μg/kg PO digitalizing dose*; 2–5 yr, 30–40 μg/kg PO digitalizing dose*; 5–10 yr, 20–35 μg/kg PO digitalizing dose*; > 10 yr,

---

* IV: digitalizing doses are 80% of the oral digitalizing doses. Maintenance doses are based on the same percentages of the loading doses as above.

10–15 μg/kg PO digitalizing dose*; then maintenance dose is 25–35% of oral digitalizing dose, divided BID*; in < 10 yr digitalizing doses given as ½ the total digitalizing dose initially then ¼ the total digitalizing dose Q8–18H × 2.

Dimenhydrinate (Dramamine, others) How supplied: tabs: 50 mg; syrup: 15 mg/5 mL; injection: 50 mg/1 mL. Dose: < 12 yr: 5 mg/kg/d PO or IM Q6H (max 300 mg/d); > 12 yr: 50–100 mg/dose PO or IM Q4H (max 400 mg/d).

Dimercaprol (BAL) How supplied: oil for injection 100 mg/1 mL. Dose: lead poisoning: 3–4 mg/kg/dose IM Q4H for 2–7 days; arsenic poisoning: 2.5 mg/kg/dose IM Q4–6H for 2 days then decrease dose over next few days.

Diphenhydramine (Benadryl, others) How supplied: tabs: 50; caps: 25, 50 mg; elixir: 12.5 mg/5 mL; injection: 10, 50 mg/1 mL. Dose: children, 5 mg/kg/d PO, IV, or IM Q6–8H (max dose 300 mg/d); adult, 10–50 mg/kg/dose PO, IV, or IM Q6–8H (max dose 400 mg/d).

Diphenoxylate (Lomotil) How supplied: tabs: 2.5 mg; liquid: 2.5 mg/5 mL. Dose: > 2 yr, 0.3–0.4 mg/kg/d PO QID; adult, 5 mg/dose PO TID–QID.

Disopyramide phosphate (Norpace) How supplied: caps: 100, 150 mg; extended release caps: 100, 150 mg. Dose: < 1 yr, 10–30 mg/kg/d PO Q6H; 1–4 yr, 10–20 mg/kg/d PO Q6H; 4–12 yr, 10–15 mg/kg/d PO Q6H; 12–18 yr, 6–15 mg/kg/d PO Q6H; adult, 400–800 mg/d PO Q6H.

Dobutamine (Dobutrex) How supplied: injection: 12.5 mg/1 mL. Dose: IV infusion: 2.5–15 μg/kg/min (max dose 40 μg/kg/min).

Docusate Sodium (Colace, others) How supplied: caps: 50, 100, 150 mg; liquid: 10 mg/1 mL; syrup: 20 mg/5 mL, 50 mg/15 mL. Dose: < 3 yr, 10–40 mg/d PO QD–QID; 3–6 yr, 20–60 mg/d PO QD–QID; 6–12 yr, 40–120 mg/d PO QD–QID; > 12 yr, 50–200 mg/d PO QD–QID.

Dopamine (Intropin) How supplied: injection: 40, 80, 160 mg/1 mL. Dose: IV infusion: 2–20 μg/kg/min (max dose 20–50 μg/kg/min).

Edrophonium (Tensilon) How supplied: injection: 10 mg/1 mL. Dose: use in the diagnosis of myasthenia gravis; infants, 0.5 mg/dose IV or IM; < 75 lb, 1 mg/dose IV repeated Q30–45 sec up to max dose of 5 mg; > 75 lb, 2 mg/dose IV, may repeat 1 mg/dose Q30–45 sec up to max dose of 10 mg.

Enalapril Maleate (Vasotec) How supplied: tabs: 2.5, 5, 10, 20 mg. Dose: adult, 5 mg/dose PO QD initially then increase up to 40 mg/day PO QD–BID.

Epinephrine (Adrenalin, others) How supplied: inhalation: 0.16, 0.22 mg/puff; injection: 1:200 (5 mg/1 mL, Sus-phrine); 1:1000 (1 mg/ 1 mL; 1:10,000 (0.1 mg/1 mL). Dose: asthma, inhalation, 1–2 puffs Q4H; 1:200 (Sus-phrine): children, 0.005 mL/kg/dose SC Q6H (max dose 0.15 mL) adults, 0.1–0.3 mL/dose SC Q6H; 1:1000 concentration: 0.01 mL/ kg/dose SC, may repeat Q15 min 4 times; max dose 0.3 mL; cardiac arrest: 1:10,000 concentration: 0.1 mL/kg/dose IV or ET Q3–5 min prn; IV infusion: 0.1–1.0 μg/kg/min.

Epinephrine, racemic How supplied: solution: 2.25%. Dose: 0.5 mL diluted with 3 mL NS as nebulization; may repeat Q2H.

Ergocalciferol, Vitamin D₂ (Calciferol) How supplied: tabs: 1.25 mg (50,000 USP); solution: 0.2 mg/1 mL (8,000 USP); injection: 12.5 mg/1 mL (500,000 USP). Dose: maintenance: 400 IU/d; renal osteodystrophy: 25,000–250,000 IU/d PO; vit D–resistant rickets: 50,000–500,000 IU/d PO; vit D–dependent rickets: 5,000–15,000 IU/d PO; nutritional rickets: 10,000 IU/d PO.

Ethacrynic Acid (Edecrin) How supplied: tabs: 25, 50 mg. Dose: older children, 25 mg/dose PO initially then slowly increase in 25 mg/dose increments.

Ethosuximide (Zarontin) How supplied: caps: 250 mg; syrup: 250 mg/5 mL. Dose: (optimal dose usually 20 mg/kg/d) 3–6 yr, 250 mg/d PO initially then increase slowly by 250 mg/d increments Q4–7 days, daily dose divided Q12–24H; > 6 yr, 500 mg/day PO initially then increase slowly by 250 mg/d increments Q4–7 days, daily dose divided Q12–24H (max dose 1.5 gm/d).

Fentanyl (Sublimaze) How supplied: injection: 50 μg/1 mL. Dose: 2–10 μg/kg/dose IV or IM.

Flunisolide (Nasalide) How supplied: nasal spray (0.25%): 25 μg/spray, 200 sprays/bottle. Dose: 6–14 yrs, 1 spray each nostril TID or 2 sprays each nostril BID; adult, 2 sprays each nostril BID–TID (max dose 8 sprays/nostril/d).

Fluoride How supplied: tabs: 0.25, 0.5, 1.0 mg; liquid: 0.5, 2, 4 mg/1 mL. Dose: 2 wk–2 yr, 0.25 mg/d; 2–3 yr, 0.25–0.5 mg/d; 3–16 yr, 0.5–1.0 mg/d.

9-alpha Fluorocortisol (Florinef) How supplied: tabs: 0.1 mg. Dose: 0.05–0.15 mg/d PO.

Flurazepam (Dalmane) How supplied: caps: 15, 30 mg. Dose: > 15 yr, 15–30 mg/dose PO PHS.

Folic Acid How supplied: tabs: 1 mg. Dose: 0.2–1.0 mg/d PO; adult, 10–15 mg/d.

Furosemide (Lasix, others) How supplied: tabs: 20, 40, 80 mg;

syrup: 10 mg/1 mL; injection: 10 mg/1 mL. Dose: children, 1–2 mg/kg/dose PO, IV, or IM Q6–12H; adult, 20–80 mg/dose PO, IV, or IM Q12–24H (max 600 mg/d).

Gamma Benzene Hexachloride (Kwell, Scabene) How supplied: 1% cream, lotion, and shampoo. Dose: skin: a thin layer applied from the neck down, left on the skin for 8–12H then washed off, usually only one treatment is necessary, an adult usually uses 60 mL; hair: 30–60 mL per application, worked thoroughly into dry hair, stand for 4 mins, lather with water, rinse thoroughly, remove nits with comb provided.

Glucagon How supplied: injection: 1 mg/1 mL. Dose: 0.5–1.0 mg/dose SC, IM, or IV Q10–25 min (max 2 mg/dose).

Haloperidol (Haldol) How supplied: tabs: 0.5, 1, 2, 5, 10, 20 mg; syrup: 2 mg/1 mL; injection: 5 mg/1 mL. Dose: 3–12 yr, agitation: 0.5–1.0 mg/dose PO; pyschosis: 0.05–0.15 mg/kg/d PO BID–TID; Tourettes: 0.05–0.075 mg/kg/d PO BID–TID; > 12 yr, agitation: 0.5–5 mg/dose PO or IM Q1–8H prn.

Heparin Sodium How supplied: injection: 10, 100, 1,000, 2,500, 5,000, 7,500, 10,000, 15,000, 20,000, 40,000 U/1 mL. Dose: children, 50 U/kg IV bolus once, then 10–25 U/kg/hr as continuous infusion, or 100 U/kg/dose IV Q4H; adult, 10,000 U/dose IV bolus once, then 5,000–10,000 U/dose IV Q4–6H.

Hydralazine (Apresoline) How supplied: tabs: 10, 25, 50, 100 mg; injection: 20 mg/1 mL. Dose: oral: children, 0.75–3.0 mg/kg/d PO Q6–12H; adult, 10–50 mg/dose PO QID; injection: children, 0.1–0.5 mg/kg/dose IM or IV Q4–6H; adult, 20–40 mg/dose IM or IV Q4–6H.

Hydrochlorothiazide (Esidrix, HydroDiuril, others) How supplied: tabs: 25, 50, 100 mg. Dose: children, 2–3 mg/kg/d PO BID; adult, 25–100 mg/dose PO QD–BID (max 200 mg/d).

Hydrocortisone (Solu–cortef) How supplied: tabs: 10, 20 mg; injection: 50, 125, 250, 500 mg/1 mL (as sodium succinate). Dose: physiologic replacement: approx. 12.5 mg/m^2/d IM or IV QD, or approx 25 mg/m^2/d PO Q8H; asthma: children, initial dose 4–8 mg/kg/dose IV once then 8 mg/kg/d IV Q6H; adult, 100–500 mg/dose IV Q2–6H.

Hydroxyzine (Atarax, Vistaril) How supplied: tabs: 10, 25, 50, 100 mg (as HCl); caps: 25, 50, 100 mg (as pamoate); syrup: 10 mg/5 mL (as HCl); suspension: 25 mg/5 mL (as pamoate); injection: 25, 50 mg/1 mL (as HCl). Dose: oral: children, 1–2 mg/kg/d PO TID–QID; adult, 25–100 mg/dose PO QID; injection: children, 1 mg/kg/d IM; adult, 25–100 mg/dose IM.

Ibuprofen (Advil, Medipren, Motrin, Nuprin, others) How supplied: tabs: 200, 300, 400, 600, 800 mg; caps: 200, 300, 400, 600, 800 mg. NOT APPROVED FOR USE IN CHILDREN. Dose: 1200–3200 mg/d PO Q4–6H.

Imipramine (Tofranil) How supplied: tabs: 10, 25, 50 mg; caps: 75, 100, 125, 150 mg; injection: 12.5 mg/1 mL. Dose: depression: adolescents, initially 30–40 mg/d PO BID–TID, then gradually increase to maintenance of max 100 mg/d PO QD–BID; adult, initially 75–100 mg/d PO BID then gradually increase to maintenance of 50–300 mg/d PO QD–BID; enuresis: 25 mg/dose 1 hr before bedtime may increase to 50 mg/dose for 6–12 yr; 75 mg/dose for > 12 yr (max dose 2.5 mg/kg/d).

Indomethacin (Indocin) How supplied: caps: 25, 50 mg; suspension: 25 mg/5 mL; injection: 1 mg/vial. Dose: patent ductus closure:

age at first dose	dose:	(dose in mg/kg) # 1	# 2	# 3
< 48 hr		0.2	0.1	0.1
2–7 d		0.2	0.2	0.2
> 7 d		0.2	0.25	0.25

doses given 12–24 hr apart, total of 3 doses anti-inflammatory: < 14 yr, 1–3 mg/kg/d PO TID–QID; adult, 50–200 mg/d PO BID–QID.

Insulin How supplied: many formulations are available including human, pork, and beef products; some are rapid-onset (regular, Semilente), intermediate-onset (Lente, NPH) and delayed-onset (Ultralente); there are many considerations in deciding which type of insulin is optimal. Dose: DKA: usual dose 0.1 U/kg/hr IV of regular insulin given as continuous IV infusion; maintenance: usual dose range is 0.5–1.0 U/kg/d given in divided doses SC.

Ipecac Syrup How supplied: 7% syrup in 15 and 30 mL bottles. Dose: 6–12 mos: 10 mL PO once, followed by clear liquids; 1–12 yr: 15–30 mL PO once, followed by clear liquids; > 12 yr: 30–60 mL PO once, followed by clear liquids; may repeat dose once if no emesis occurs.

Iron Dextran How supplied: injection: 50 mg of elemental iron/1 mL. Dose: calculated using the following formulas: dose in mL: wt (kg) × 0.0476 × (normal Hgb − patient Hgb); dose in mg of iron: wt (kg) × 2.4 × (normal Hgb − patient Hgb); add 1 mL/5 kg (50 mg iron/5 kg) of body weight to the dose calculated above to replenish ironstores, up to max 14 mL;

max IV dose is 2 mL/d; max IM daily dose is based on weight:

< 5 kg	0.5 mL
5–10 kg	1.0 mL
> 10 kg	2.0 mL
adult	5.0 mL.

Iron Supplements How supplied: ferrous sulfate (Fer-In-Sol):

	ferrous sulfate	elemental iron
caps:	190 mg	60 mg
drops:	75 mg/0.6 mL	15 mg/0.6 mL
syrup:	90 mg/5 mL	18 mg/5 mL

ferrous gluconate (Fergon):

	ferrous gluconate	elemental iron
tabs:	320 mg	35 mg
caps:	435 mg	50 mg
elixir:	300 mg/5 mL	34 mg/5 mL

Dose: dietary supplement (in mg of elemental iron): premature infant, 1–2 mg/kg/d PO QD–TID; term infants, 1 mg/kg/d PO QD–TID; (US RDA for > 4 yr = 18 mg/d); iron deficiency (in mg of elemental iron): 6 mg/kg/d PO TID.

Isoetharine (Bronkometer, Bronkosol) How supplied: nebulization: 1% (10 mg/1 mL); inhaler: 340 μg/puff, 20 puffs/1 mL, in 10, 15 mL vials. Dose: nebulization: 0.25–0.5 mL in 2 mL of NS Q4H prn; inhaler: 1–2 puffs Q4H prn.

Isoproterenol (Isuprel) How supplied: injection (1:5000): 0.2mg/1 mL. Dose: cardiac arrest: 0.1–1.0 μg/kg/min as continuous IV infusion.

Isotretinoin (Accutane) How supplied: caps: 10, 20, 40 mg. Dose: 0.5–1.0 mg/kg/d PO BID (max dose 2 mg/kg/d).

Lactulose (Cephulac, others) How supplied: syrup: 10 gm/15 mL. Dose: infants: 2.5–10 mL/d PO TID–QID; older children and adolescents: 40–90 mL/d PO TID–QID; adult: 30–45 mL/dose PO TID–QID.

Levothyroxine (Synthroid) How supplied: tabs: 25, 50, 75, 100, 112, 125, 150, 175, 200, 300 μg; injection: 20, 50 μg/1 mL. Dose: children, 0–6 mo: 8–10 μg/kg/d PO (25–50 μg/d); 6–12 mo: 6–8 μg/kg/d PO (50–75 μg/d); 1–5 yr: 5–6 μg/kg/d PO (75–100 μg/d); 6–12 yr: 4–5 μg/kg/d PO (100–150 μg/d); adult, initially 25–50 μg/d PO then increase in increments of 25 μg Q2–3 wks to maintenance of 100–200 μg/d. (IV dose is approx 50% of PO dose.)

Lidocaine (Xylocaine) How supplied: (1% = 10 mg/1 mL); injection: 0.5%, 1.0%, 1.5%, 2.0% and also 50 mg/5 mL, 100 mg/5 mL prefilled syringes; ointment: 2.5%, 5.0%; oral spray: 10%; viscous: 2%. Dose: local anesthesia: 3–4.5 mg/kg max total dose; intravenous for cardiac arrhythmias: 1 mg/kg IV bolus Q5 min × 3, may be given as continuous IV infusion of 20–50 μg/kg/min.

Lindane (see Gamma Benzene Hexachloride)

Loperamide (Imodium, Imodium A-D) How supplied: caps: 2 mg; syrup: 1 mg/5 mL. Dose: initial daily dose: 2–5 yr: 1 mg/dose PO TID (3 mg/d); 6–8 yr: 2 mg/dose PO BID (4 mg/d); 8–12 yr: 2 mg/dose PO TID (6 mg/d); subsequent daily dose: 1 mg/10 kg weight/dose with each subsequent loose stool, max daily dose as listed above; adult: 4 mg/dose PO once, then 2 mg/dose with each subsequent loose stool (max 16 mg/d).

Lorazepam (Ativan) How supplied: tabs: 0.5, 1, 2 mg; injection: 2, 4 mg/1 mL. Dose: intravenous: 0.05–0.1 mg/kg/dose IV Q6H (adults 2–4 mg/dose max); oral: adults 2–6 mg/d PO Q8–12H (max 10 mg/d).

Lypressin (Diapid) How supplied: nasal spray: 2 USP/spray, 50 USP/1 mL, 8 mL bottle. Dose: diabetes insipidus: 1–2 sprays in each nostril QID, a QHS dose may be needed also.

Magnesium Citrate How supplied: solution: 300 mL bottles. Dose: 4 mL/kg/dose PO, max 200 mL dose.

Magnesium Hydroxide (Milk of Magnesia) How supplied: tabs: 311 mg; suspension: 405 mg/5 mL. Dose: children: 0.5–1.0 mL/kg/dose PO prn; adult: 15–60 mL/dose PO prn (1 mL = approx 80 mg).

Magnesium Sulfate How supplied: solution: 50% (500 mg/1 mL). Dose: cathartic: child, 250 mg/kg/dose PO; adult, 10–30 gm/dose PO.

Mannitol How supplied: injection: 50, 100, 150, 200, 250 mg/1 mL. Dose: oliguria: test dose of 0.2 gm/kg/dose IV; cerebral edema: 0.5–1.0 gm/kg/dose IV prn.

Meclizine (Antivert, Bonine) How supplied: tabs: 12.5, 25, 50 mg. Dose: vertigo: 25–100 mg/d PO Q6–12H; motion sickness: 25–50 mg/d PO 1 h prior to travel.

Meperidine (Demerol) How supplied: tabs: 50, 100 mg; syrup: 50 mg/5 mL; injection: 25, 50, 75, 100 mg/1 mL. Dose: children: 1–1.5 mg/kg/dose PO, SC, or IM Q3–4H prn; adult: 50–150 mg/dose PO, SC, or IM Q3–4H prn.

Metaproterenol (Alupent, Metaprel) How supplied: tabs: 10, 20 mg; syrup: 10 mg/5 mL; inhaler: 0.65 mg/puff, 300 puffs/inhaler; solution for nebulization: 5% (50 mg/1 mL). Dose: oral: < 6 yr, 1.3–2.6 mg/kg/d PO TID–QID; 6–9 yr, 10 mg/

dose PO TID–QID; > 9 yr, 20 mg/dose PO TID–QID; inhalation: 2–3 puffs at Q3–4H, max 12 puffs/d; nebulization: 0.2–0.3 mL/dose in 2.5 mL NS Q1–6H prn.

Methadone How supplied: tabs: 5, 10 mg; liquid: 5, 10 mg/5 mL; injection: 10 mg/1 mL. Dose: analgesic: children, 0.7 mg/kg/d PO, SC, or IM Q4–6H; adult, 2.5–10 mg/dose PO, SC, or IM Q3–4H.

Methimazole (Tapazole) How supplied: tabs: 5, 10 mg. Dose: children, initially 0.4–0.7 mg/kg/d PO Q8H then 50% of initial dose as maintenance; adult, initially 15–60 mg/d PO Q8H then 5–30 mg/d PO TID.

Methsuximide (Celontin) How supplied: caps: 150, 300 mg. Dose: 300 mg/d PO for 1 wk, then increase by 300 mg/d every 1 wk for 3 wk up to max 1200 mg/d, usual maintenance dose is 10–20 mg/kg/d PO.

Methyldopa (Aldomet) How supplied: tabs: 125, 250, 500 mg; suspension: 250 mg/5 mL; injection: 50 mg/1 mL. Dose: children, oral: 10 mg/kg/d PO Q6–12H, increase at 2-day intervals to max 65 mg/kg/d or 3 gm/d, whichever is less; intravenous (for hypertensive crisis): 20–40 mg/kg/d IV Q6H (max 65 mg/kg/d or 3 gm/d, whichever is less); adult, oral: 250 mg/dose PO BID–TID, increase at 2-day intervals to max 3 gm/d, usual maintenance dose is 500–2000 mg/d PO BID–QID; intravenous (for hypertensive crisis): 250–500 mg/dose IV Q6H, max 1 gm Q6H.

Methylene Blue How supplied: solution: 1% (10 mg/1 mL). Dose: 1–2 mg/kg/dose slowly IV.

Methylphenidate (Ritalin) How supplied: tabs: 5, 10, 20 mg; slow-release caps: 20 mg. Dose (> 6 yr): 5 mg/dose PO BID (before breakfast and lunch), increase gradually 5–10 mg/wk to max 60 mg/d.

Methylprednisolone (DepoMedrol, Medrol, Solumedrol) How supplied: tabs: 2, 4, 8, 16, 24, 32 mg; injection (Solu-Medrol, as succinate for IV, IM): 40, 125, 500, 1000, 2000 mg/vials; injection (Depo-Medrol, as acetate for IM repository): 20, 40, 80 mg/1 mL. Dose: asthma: initially 1–2 mg/kg/dose IV once, then 1–2 mg/kg/d IV Q6H; anti-inflammatory: 0.4–1.6 mg/kg/d PO or IV Q6–12H.

Metoclopramide (Reglan) How supplied: tabs: 5, 10 mg; syrup: 5 mg/5 mL; injection: 5, 10 mg/1 mL. Dose: GE reflux: 1–6 yr, 0.1 mg/kg/dose PO or IV QID; 6–12 yr, 2.5–5 mg/dose PO or IV QID; adult, 10–15 mg/dose PO or IV QID; antiemetic: 1–2 mg/kg/dose IV Q2–3H prn.

Midazolam (Versed) How supplied: injection: 1, 5 mg/1 mL. Dose: 0.07–0.08 mg/kg/dose IM, usual adult dose 5 mg/dose; 0.1–0.2 mg/kg/dose IV, usual adult dose 1–5 mg/dose.

Mineral Oil How supplied: plain and flavored preparations, 4.2 gm mineral oil/15 mL. Dose: 0.5 mL/kg/dose PO QD–QID, adults 15–30 mL/dose, titrate dose based on stools.

Morphine Sulfate How supplied: tabs: 10, 15, 30 mg; elixir: 2, 4, 20 mg/1 mL; suppository: 5, 10, 20 mg; injection: 8, 10, 15 mg/1 mL. Dose: children, 0.1–0.2 mg/kg/dose SC, IM, or IV Q2–4H prn; adult, 10–30 mg/dose PO Q4H prn, or 2–10 mg/dose IV Q2–4H prn.

Naloxone (Narcan) How supplied: injection: 0.02, 0.4, 1.0 mg/1 mL. Dose: children, 0.01 mg/kg/dose IV once, may repeat dose of 0.1 mg/kg if needed, SC and IM route acceptable; adult, 0.4–2 mg/dose IV once, may repeat Q2–3 min; max dose usually 10 mg, SC and IM optional.

Neomycin Sulfate How supplied: tabs: 500 mg; suspension: 500 mg/5 mL. Dose: hepatic encephalopathy: initially 2.5–7 gm/m^2/d PO Q6H for 5–7 days, then 2.5 gm/m^2 day PO Q6H.

Neostigmine (Prostigmin) How supplied: tabs: 15 mg; injection: 0.25, 0.5, 1 mg/1 mL. Dose: myasthenia gravis: test dose: children, 0.04 mg/kg/dose IM, 0.02 mg/kg/dose IV; adult, 0.02 mg/kg/dose IM; treatment: children: 0.01–0.04 mg/kg/dose SC, IM, or IV Q2–3H prn; 2 mg/kg/d PO prn; adult: 0.5 mg/dose SC, IM, or IV Q3–4H prn (max 10 mg/day); 15–375 mg/d PO prn.

Nifedipine (Adalat, Procardia) How supplied: caps: 10, 20 mg. Dose: children (not FDA approved): 0.25–0.5 mg/kg/dose PO or sublingual Q6–8H, not to exceed adult doses; adult: 10–20 mg/dose PO TID, max 30 mg/dose and 180 mg/d.

Nitroglycerine How supplied: injection: 0.8, 5, 10 mg/1 mL. Dose: 0.5–20 μg/kg/min as continuous IV infusion.

Nitroprusside (Nipride) How supplied: injection: 50 mg/5 mL. Dose: 0.5–10 μg/kg/min as continuous IV infusion.

Norepinephrine (Levophed) How supplied: injection: 1 mg/1 mL. Dose: begin at 0.05 μg/kg/min as continuous IV infusion.

Oxtriphylline (Choledyl) How supplied: (contains 64% theophylline) tabs: 100, 200 mg; sustained-release tabs: 400, 600 mg; elixir: 100 mg/5 mL. Dose: see Theophylline and convert using equivalent dosages.

Pancreatic Enzymes (Cotazym, Creon, Pancrease, Viokase, others) How supplied: powder: Cotazym (in caps), Viokase; enteric-coated spheres: Cotazym-S, Creon, Pancrease; non-enteric coated tabs: Viokase. Dose: 1–3 caps or tabs, or ¼ tsp of powder, with each meal, adjusted for each patient prn.

Pancuronium (Pavulon) How supplied: injection: 1, 2 mg/1 mL.

Dose: 0.03–0.1 mg/kg/dose IV Q½–2H prn, titrate dose based on patient's response.

Paraldehyde How supplied: solution: 1 gm/1 mL; injection 1 gm/1 mL. Dose: seizures: rectal, 0.3–0.6 mL/kg/dose in oil Q4–6H (adult 16–32 mL); IM, 0.1–0.15 mL/kg/dose (adult 4–10 mL); IV, 0.02 mL/kg/dose slow IV (adult 1–2 mL), or continuous IV infusion of 0.1–0.15 mL/kg/hr.

Paregoric How supplied: solution: 0.4 mg morphine/1 mL. Dose: opiate withdrawal in newborns: 0.2–0.5 mL/dose PO Q3–4H prn, max 0.7 mL/kg/dose; analgesia: 0.25–0.5 mL/kg/dose PO QD–QID, max 10 mL/dose.

Pemoline (Cylert) How supplied: tabs: 18.75, 37.5, 75 mg; chewable tabs: 37.5 mg. Dose: initially 37.5 mg/d PO QAM, increase by 18.75 mg/d at weekly intervals prn (max dose 112.5 mg/d).

Penicillamine (Cuprimine) How supplied: tabs: 250 mg; caps: 125, 250 mg. Dose: > 6 mo: 100 mg/kg/d PO QID, max 1 gm/d.

Pentobarbital (Nembutal) How supplied: caps: 50, 100; suppository: 30, 60, 120, 200 mg; injection: 50 mg/1 mL. Dose: sedation: 2–6 mg/kg/dose PO, max 100 mg/dose; coma: 3–5 mg/kg/dose IV initially, then 2–3.5 mg/kg/dose Q1H prn.

Phenazopyridine (Pyridium) How supplied: tabs: 100, 200 mg. Dose: children, 100 mg/dose PO TID after meals; adult, 200 mg/dose PO TID after meals.

Phenobarbital How supplied: tabs: 15, 30, 60, 100 mg; elixir: 20 mg/5 mL; injection: 65, 130 mg/1 mL. Dose: sedation: 2–3 mg/kg/dose PO or IM Q6–8H prn; seizures: 10–25 mg/kg/dose IM or IV initially, then 4–6 mg/kg/d PO Q12H (adults 150–250 mg/d).

Phenytoin (Dilantin) How supplied: tabs: 50 mg; caps: 30, 100 mg; suspension: 30, 125 mg/5 mL; injection: 50 mg/1 mL. Dose: seizures: 10–20 mg/kg/dose slow IV initially, not to exceed 1 mg/kg/min, then 4–8 mg/kg/d PO or IV QD–TID; adult, 300–600 mg/d PO or IV QD–TID.

Physostigmine Salicylate (Antrillium) How supplied: 1 mg/1 mL. Dose: 0.02 mg/kg/dose IM or IV, no more than 0.5 mg/min, repeat Q5–10 min up to max total dose of 2 mg.

Potassium Iodide How supplied: syrup: 325 mg/5 mL; solution: 1 gm/mL. Dose: children, 100–300 mg/d PO BID–TID; adult, 300–900 mg/d PO TID.

Potassium Supplement How supplied: potassium chloride: effervescent tabs: 25, 50 mEq; caps: 4, 8, 10 mEq; liquid: 5%, 10%, 20% (5% = 10 mEq/15 mL); powder: 15, 20 mEq/packet, 25 mEq/scoop; injection: 2 mEq/1 mL. Dose: maintenance: approx 1–2 mEq/kg/d PO QD–QID (40–80 mEq/d for adults); hypokalemia: 0.5–1.0 mEq/kg/dose slow IV.

Pralidoxime (Protopam) How supplied: tabs: 500 mg; injection: 1 gm/20 mL. Dose: 20–40 mg/kg/dose slow IV, as 5% solution, repeat Q1H prn; adult 1–2 gm/dose slow IV, dose may be given SC, IM, or PO if necessary.

Prazosin (Minipress) How supplied: tabs: 1, 2, 5 mg. Dose: NOT APPROVED FOR USE IN CHILDREN; adult: initial 1 mg/dose PO BID–TID, slowly increase to a total daily dose of 20 mg; usual dose 6–15 mg/d.

Prednisone How supplied: tabs: 1, 2.5, 5, 10, 20, 25, 50 mg; syrup: 5 mg/5 mL. Dose: physiologic replacement: 4–5 mg/m^2/d PO BID; asthma: 0.5–1.0 mg/kg/d PO QD–BID, max 20–40 mg/d for 3–5 days; anti-inflammatory: 0.5–2 mg/kg/d PO BID–QID.

Primidone (Mysoline) How supplied: tabs: 50, 250 mg; suspension: 250 mg/5 mL. Dose: < 8 yr, days 1–3: 50 mg/dose PO QHS; days 4–6: 50 mg/dose PO BID; days 7–9: 100 mg/dose PO BID; day 10 on: 125–250 mg/dose PO TID; usual maintenance dose 10–25 mg/kg/d PO TID; > 8 yr, days 1–3: 100–125 mg/dose PO QHS; days 4–6: 100–125 mg/dose PO BID; days 7–9: 100–125 mg/dose PO TID; day 10 on: 250 mg/dose PO TID, slowly increased to max 750–1500 mg/d TID–QID.

Probenecid (Benemid) How supplied: tabs: 500 mg. Dose: > 2 yr: 25 mg/kg/dose PO once, then 40 mg/kg/d PO QID; > 14 yr: 1–2 gm/dose PO once, then 2 gm/d PO QID.

Procainamide (Pronestyl) How supplied: tabs: 250, 375, 500 mg; sustained-release tabs: 500 mg; caps: 250, 375, 500 mg; injection: 100, 500 mg/1 mL. Dose: children, oral: 15–50 mg/kg/d PO Q3–6H, max 4 gm/d; IV: 10–15 mg/kg/dose IV over 30 min, then 20–80 μg/kg/min continuous IV infusion; adult, oral: approx 50 mg/kg/d PO Q3–6H, usually 250–500 mg/dose Q3–6H, max 4 gm/d; IV: 500–600 mg IV over 30 min, max 1 gm, then 2–6 mg/min continuous IV infusion.

Prochlorperazine (Compazine) How supplied: tabs: 5, 10, 25 mg; sustained-release caps: 10, 15, 30 mg; syrup: 5 mg/5 mL; suppository: 2.5, 25 mg; injection: 5 mg/1 mL. Dose: oral 9–13 kg: 2.5 mg/dose PO or PR QD–BID; 14–18 kg: 2.5 mg/dose PO or PR BID–TID; 19–40 kg: 2.5–5 mg/dose PO or PR BID–TID; adult: 5–10 mg/dose PO TID–QID, or 25 mg PR BID; IM: children: 0.13 mg/kg/dose; adult: 5–10 mg/dose Q3–4H (max 40 mg/d).

Promethazine (Phenergan) How supplied: tabs: 12.5, 25, 50 mg; syrup: 6.25, 25 mg/5 mL; suppository: 12.5, 25, 50 mg; injection: 25, 50 mg/1 mL. Dose: antihistamine: children,

0.1 mg/kg/dose PO TID and 0.5 mg/kg/dose PO QHS; adult, 12.5–25 mg/dose PO TID and QHS; nausea: children, 0.25–0.5 mg/kg/dose PO, PR, or IM Q4–6H prn; adult, 12.5–25 mg/dose PO, PR, or IM Q4–6H prn; sedation: children, 0.5–1 mg/kg/dose PO, PR, or IM Q6H prn; adult, 25–50 mg/dose PO, PR, or IM Q6H prn; motion sickness: children, 0.5 mg/kg/dose PO or PR BID prn; adult, 25 mg PO or PR BID prn.

Propranolol (Inderal) How supplied: tabs: 10, 20, 40, 60, 80, 90 mg; extended-release caps: 80, 120, 160 mg; injection: 1 mg/1 mL. Dose: hypertension: children: initial 0.5–1 mg/kg/d PO BID, maintenance 2–4 mg/kg/d PO BID; adult: initial 40 mg/dose PO BID, then increase slowly to maintenance dose of 120–240 mg/d PO Q8–12H (max dose 640 mg/d); arrhythmias: children: 0.01–0.1 mg/kg/dose slow IV (max 1 mg/dose), then 0.5–4 mg/kg/d adult: 1–3 mg/dose slow IV, then 10–30 mg/d PO TID–QID; tetralogy spells: 0.15–0.25 mg/kg/dose slow IV, may repeat once, max 10 mg/dose, then 1–2 mg/kg/dose PO Q6H; migraine prophylaxis: < 35 kg: 10–20 mg/dose PO TID; > 35 kg: 20–40 mg/dose PO TID; adult: 80 mg/d PO TID–QID, may increase to 160–240 mg/d.

Propylthiouracil (PTU) How supplied: tabs: 50 mg. Dose: initial 6–7 mg/kg/d PO Q8H, then maintenance usually ⅓–½ of initial dose; initial adult dose usually 300 mg/d PO Q8H.

Prostaglandin E₁ (Prostin) How supplied: injection: 500 μg/1 mL. Dose: to maintain patency of ductus arteriosus dose is 0.05–0.1 μg/kg/min as continuous IV infusion.

Protamine sulfate How supplied: injection: 5, 10 mg/1 mL. Dose: 1 mg will neutralize approx 100 U of heparin (max dose is 50 mg per 10-min period).

Pseudoephedrine (Sudafed, Novafed, others) How supplied: tabs: 30, 60 mg; syrup: 30 mg/5 mL. Dose: 4 mg/kg/d PO QID; adult 30–60 mg/dose PO Q6–8H.

Pyridostigmine (Mestinon) How supplied: tabs: 60 mg; extended-release tabs: 180 mg; syrup: 60 mg/5 mL; injection: 5 mg/1 mL. Dose: children, 7 mg/kg/d PO Q4–6H, adjust prn; adult: usual dose 600 mg/d PO prn.

Quinidine How supplied: gluconate (62% quinidine base): tabs: 324 mg (202 mg base); extended-release tabs: 324 mg (202 mg base); sulfate (83% quinidine base): tabs: 100, 200, 300 mg (88, 176, 264 mg base). Dose: (as base) children, test dose: 2 mg/kg/dose PO once; maintenance dose: 15–60 mg/kg/d PO Q6H; adult, test dose: 1 tab PO; maintenance: 100–600 mg/dose PO Q6–8H.

Ranitidine (Zantac) How supplied: tabs: 150, 300 mg; injection: 25 mg/1 mL. Dose: children, oral: 2–4 mg/kg/d PO BID; parenteral: 1–2 mg/kg/d IM or IV Q6–8H; adults, oral: 150–300 mg/d PO QD–BID; parenteral: 50 mg/dose IM or IV Q6–8H.

Scopolamine Hydrobromide (Transderm Scōp, others) How supplied: tabs: 400, 600 mg; transderm patch: releases 1.5 mg over 3 days. Dose: 0.006 mg/kg/dose PO, transderm patch 1 per 3 days.

Secobarbital (Seconal) How supplied: tabs: 50, 100 mg; caps: 50, 100 mg; elixir: 22 mg/5 mL; suppository: 30, 60, 120, 200 mg; injection: 50 mg/1 mL. Dose: 6 mg/kg/d PO or PR Q8H; adult 20–40 mg/dose PO or PR BID–TID.

Sodium Polystyrene Sulfonate (Kayexalate) How supplied: powder: 3.5 gm/tsp (exchanges approx 1 mEq K/gm). Dose: children, oral: 1 gm/kg/dose PO Q6H; rectal: 1 gm/kg/dose PR Q2–6H; adult, oral: 15 gm/dose PO QD–QID; rectal: 30–50 gm/dose PR Q6H.

Spironolactone (Aldactone) How supplied: tabs: 25, 50, 100 mg. Dose: 1–3.3 mg/kg/d PO QD–BID; adults 25–200 mg/d PO QD–BID.

Succinylcholine (Anectine) How supplied: injection: 20 mg/1 mL. Dose: infants, small children: 2 mg/kg/dose IV; adolescents and older children: 1 mg/kg/dose IV; adult: 0.3–1.1 mg/kg/dose IV; may be given IM if necessary, 3–4 mg/kg/dose IM (max 150 mg/dose).

Sucralfate (Carafate) How supplied: tabs: 1 gm. Dose: > 12 yr: 1 gm/dose PO QID.

Sulfasalazine (Azulfidine) How supplied: tabs: 500 mg; enteric-coated tabs: 500 mg; suspension: 250 mg/5 mL. Dose: > 2 yr: initial 40–100 mg/kg/d PO Q4–8H, then 30 mg/kg/d PO QID; adult: initial 3–4 gm/d PO Q4–8H, then 2 gm/d PO QID, max 6 gm/d.

Terbutaline (Brethine) How supplied: tabs: 2.5, 5 mg; inhaler: 200 μg/puff, approx 300 puffs/inhaler; injection: 1 mg/1 mL (may be used for nebulization). Dose: oral: < 12 yr: 0.05–0.1 mg/kg/dose PO TID; > 12 yr: 2.5–5 mg/dose PO TID; inhalation: 2 puffs Q4–6H prn; nebulization: (not FDA approved for this use) 0.1 mg/kg/dose Q1H prn, max 2.5 mg/dose; subcutaneous: 0.005–0.01 mg/kg/dose SC Q15–30 min × 2 (max 0.25 mg/dose).

Terfenadine (Seldane) How supplied: tabs: 60 mg. Dose: > 12 yr, 60 mg/dose PO BID.

Theophylline (many trade names) How supplied: (see also Aminophylline) tabs: 100, 200, 300 mg; syrup: 80 mg/15 mL;

sustained-release tabs: 100, 200, 300, 450 mg; sustained release caps: Slo-Bid gyrocaps: 50, 100, 200, 300 mg; Slo-Phyllin gyrocaps: 60, 125, 250 mg; Theo-Dur sprinkles: 50, 75, 125, 200 mg. Dose: neonatal apnea: loading dose 5 mg/kg/dose PO once; maintenance: < 36 wk: 1–2 mg/kg/d PO Q8–12H; > 36 wk: 2–4 mg/kg/day PO Q8–12H; asthma: loading dose of 1 mg/kg will raise serum level approx 2 μg/mL; 0–2 mo: 3–6 mg/kg/d PO Q6–8H; 2–6 mo: 6–15 mg/kg/d PO Q6–8H; 6–12 mo: 15–22 mg/kg/d PO Q6–8H; 1–6 yr: 22 mg/kg/d PO Q6–8H; 6–9 yr: 24 mg/kg/d PO Q6–12H; 9–12 yr: 20 mg/kg/d PO Q6–12H; 12–16 yr: 18 mg/kg/d PO Q6–12H; > 16 yr: 13 mg/kg/d PO Q6–12H (max 900 mg/d).

Thiopental (Pentothal) How supplied: injection: 250, 400, 500 mg/syringe; 500, 1000 mg/vial. Dose: PR: 10–20 mg/kg/dose PR once; IV: 2 mg/kg/dose IV for induction; adults 3–5 mg/kg/dose.

Thioridazine (Mellaril) How supplied: tabs: 10, 15, 25, 50, 100, 150, 200 mg; liquid: 30, 100 mg/1 mL; suspension: 25, 100 mg/5 mL. Dose: 2–12 yr: 0.5–3 mg/kg/d PO BID–QID; adult: initial 50–100 mg/dose PO TID, then gradually increase to 200–800 mg/day PO BID–QID.

Tolazoline (Priscoline) How supplied: injection: 25 mg/1 mL. Dose: initial 1–2 mg/kg/dose IV, then 1–2 mg/kg/hr as continuous IV infusion.

Tolmetin Sodium (Tolectin) How supplied: tabs: 200 mg; caps: 400 mg. Dose: > 2 yr: 15–30 mg/kg/d PO TID–QID; adult: 600–1800 mg/d PO TID–QID.

Trimethaphan (Arfonad) How supplied: injection: 50 mg/1 mL. Dose: children, 50–100 μg/kg/min continuous IV infusion; adult, 0.5–1 mg/min continuous IV infusion.

Trimethobenzamide (Tigan) How supplied: caps: 100, 250 mg; suppository: 100, 200 mg; injection: 100 mg/1 mL. Dose: < 15 kg: 100 mg/dose PR TID–QID; 15–40 kg: 100–200 mg/dose PO or PR TID–QID; adult: 200–250 mg/dose PO or PR TID–QID; 200 mg/dose IM TID–QID.

Valproic Acid (Depakene, Depakote) How supplied: tabs: 250 mg; enteric-coated tabs: 125, 250, 500 mg; syrup: 250 mg/5 mL. Dose: initial 15 mg/kg/d PO BID, then increments every week of 5–10 mg/kg/d, max 60 mg/kg/d.

Vasopressin (Pitressin) How supplied: nasal spray (as lypressin): 2 U/spray, 50 U/1 mL; injection: aqueous: 20 U/1 mL; in oil: 5 U/1 mL. Dose: intranasal: 1–2 squirts in each nostril Q4–6H, adjust prn; injection: aqueous: 5–10 U SC or IM BID–TID prn; in oil: 1.5–5 U IM, repeat Q1–3/d prn.

Vecuronium (Norcuron) How supplied: injection: 1, 2 mg/1 mL. Dose: 0.08–0.1 mg/kg/dose IV repeated Q30–60 min prn.

Verapamil (Calan, Isoptin) How supplied: tabs: 40, 80, 120 mg; sustained-release caplets: 240 mg; injection: 2.5 mg/1 mL. Dose: IV: children: 0.1–0.3 mg/kg/dose slow IV (max 5 mg/dose), may repeat once Q30 min; adult: 5–10 mg/ dose slow IV, may repeat once Q30 min.

Vitamin K (AquaMEPHYTON, Konakion) How supplied: (as phytonadione) tabs: 5 mg; injection: 2, 10 mg/1 mL. Dose: neonatal prophylaxis: 0.5–1 mg/dose SC, IM, or IV once, IM preferred route; anticoagulant overdose: 2.5–10 mg/ dose PO, SC, IM, or IV, may repeat once, up to 25 mg/dose; hypoprothrombinemia: 2.5–25 mg/dose PO, SC, IM, or IV, up to 50 mg/dose.

FORMULARY OF ANTI-INFECTIVES AND ANTIBIOTICS

Acyclovir (Zovirax) How supplied: ointment: 5%; caps: 200 mg; injection: 500 mg. Dose: topical: Q3H; 200 mg PO 5 times/ day; 15–30 mg/kg/d IV Q8H. Coverage: herpes simplex; varicella-zoster. Comments: Ointment is efficacious only in initial herpes genitalis. Capsules are efficacious in suppression and treatment of initial and recurrent herpes genitalis. Injections are currently used for varicella only in immuno-compromised hosts. Decrease dose in renal failure.

Amantadine (Symmetrel) How supplied: syrup: 50 mg/5 mL; caps: 100 mg. Dose: 5–9 mg/kg/d PO Q12H; max 200 mg/d. Coverage: influenza A. Comments: Must be started within 24–48 hr of onset of symptoms.

Amikacin (Amikin) How supplied: injection: 100 mg/2 mL; 500 mg/2 mL; 1 mg/4 mL. Dose: 15 mg/kg/d IV or IM Q8H; max 1.5 g/d. Coverage: gram negatives. Toxicity: renal, VIII nerve. Comments: Peak 15–30 μg/mL, trough < 5 μg/mL.

Aminosalicylic acid How supplied: tabs: 500 mg, 1 g (4 g package). Dose: 300 mg/kg/d PO Q8H–Q12H; max 12 g/d. Coverage: *mycobacterium tuberculosis*. Toxicity: renal, goitrogenic.

Amoxicillin (Amoxil, Polymox, Trimon, Wymox) How supplied: caps: 250, 500 mg; suspension: 125, 250 mg/5 mL; chewable tabs: 125, 250 mg. Dose: 40 mg/kg/d PO Q8H. Coverage: non-penicillinase producing gram-positive cocci *Listeria, E Coli, Salmonella, Shigella.*

Amoxicillin and potassium clavulanate (Augmentin) How supplied: suspension: 125 mg amox + 31.25 mg clav/5 mL, 250 mg amox + 62.5 mg clav/5 mL; chewable tabs: 125 mg amox + 31.25 mg clav, 250 mg amox + 62.5 mg clav/5 mL; tabs: 250 mg amox + 125 mg clav, 500 mg amox + 125 mg clav. Dose: same as amoxicillin. Coverage: β-lactamase-producing gram negatives and gram positives.

Amphotericin B (Fungizone) How supplied: injection: 50 mg. Dose: 0.25–1 mg/kg/d IV over 2–6 h Q24H. Coverage: *Aspergillus; Candida; Cryptococcus; Blastomyces; Sporotrichum; Coccidioides; Histoplasma; mucormycoses.* Toxicity: renal.

Ampicillin (Omnipen, Polycillin, Principen) How supplied: suspension: 125, 250, 500 mg/5 mL; chewable tabs: 125 mg; drops: 100 mg/mL; caps: 240, 500 mg; injection: 0.125, 0.25, 0.5, 1, 2, 43 g. Dose: 50 mg/kg/d PO Q6H; 100–400 mg/kg/d IV or IM Q4–Q6H. Coverage: same as Amoxicillin.

Aztreonam (Azactam) How supplied: injection: 0.5, 1, 2 g. Dose: 90–120 mg/kg/d IV or IM Q6–Q8H. Coverage: gram negatives including *Pseudomonas aeruginosa.*

Carbenicillin (Geocillin, Geopen) How supplied: tabs: 382 mg; injection: 2, 5 g. Dose: 30–50 mg/kg/d PO Q6H; 400–600 mg/kg/d IV Q4–Q6H. Coverage: gram negatives except *Klebsiella.* Toxicity: platelet dysfunction. Comments: Some *Serratia and Pseudomonas* are resistant.

Cefaclor (Ceclor) How supplied: suspension: 125, 250 mg/5 mL; caps: 250, 500 mg. Dose: 40 mg/kg/d PO Q8–Q12H. Coverage: streptococci; some *H influenzae;* some *S aureus.*

Cefamandole (Mandol) How supplied: injection: 0.5, 1, 2 g. Dose: 100–150 mg/kg/d IV or IM Q4–Q6H. Coverage: same as cefaclor; some *Klebsiella* and *Proteus;* anaerobes.

Cefazolin (Ancef, Kefzol) How supplied: injection: 0.25, 0.5, 1 g. Dose: 500–100 mg/kg/d IM or IV Q6–Q8H. Coverage: gram–positive cocci; some gram negatives.

Cefixime (Suprax) How supplied: suspension: 100 mg/5 mL; tabs: 400 mg. Dose: 8 mg/kg/d PO Q24H. Coverage: gram negatives including *H influenzae;* gram positives except staphylococci and enterococci. Comments: Only oral third-generation cephalosporin.

Cefoperazone (Cefobid) How supplied: injection: 1, 2 g. Dose: NOT APPROVED FOR USE IN CHILDREN; 100–150 mg/kg/d IM or IV Q8–Q12H. Coverage: same as Cefixime.

Cefotaxime (Claforan) How supplied: injection: 1, 2 g. Dose: 100–200 mg/kg/d IM or IV Q8–Q12H; meningitis, 200 mg/kg/d IM or IV Q6H. Coverage: same as Cefixime; does not cover *Listeria.*

Cefoxitin (Mefoxin) How supplied: injection: 1, 2 g. Dose: 80–160 mg/kg/d IM or IV Q4–Q6H. Coverage: same as Cefazolin.

Ceftazidime (Fortax, Tazicef, Tazidime) How supplied: injection: 0.5, 1, 2 g. Dose: 100–150 mg/kg/d IM or IV Q8H; meningitis, 150 mg/kg/d IM or IV Q8H. Coverage: same as Cefotaxime; most *Pseudomonas*.

Ceftriaxone (Rocephin) How supplied: injection: 1.25, 0.5, 1, 2 g. Dose: 50–100 mg/kg/d IM or IV Q12–Q24H; meningitis, 100 mg/kg/d IM or IV Q12H. Coverage: same as Cefotaxime.

Cefuroxime (Ceftin, Kefurox, Zinacef) How supplied: injection: 0.75, 1.5 g. Dose: 100–150 mg/kg/d IM or IV Q8H. Coverage: streptococci; some staphylococci. Comments: May result in delayed CSF sterilization.

Cephalexin (Keflet, Keflex, Keftab) How supplied: drops: 100 mg/mL; suspension: 125, 250 mg/5 mL; tabs/caps: 0.25, 0.5, 1 g. Dose: 25–50 mg/kg/d PO Q6H. Coverage: gram-positive cocci.

Cephapirin (Cefadyl) How supplied: injection: 0.5, 1, 2, 4 g. Dose: 40–80 mg/kg/d IM or IV Q6H. Coverage: gram-positive cocci.

Cephradine (Anspor, Velosef) How supplied: suspension: 125, 250 mg/5 mL; caps: 250, 500 mg; injection: 0.25, 0.5, 1 g. Dose: 25–50 mg/kg/d PO Q6H; 50–100 mg/kg/d IM or IV Q6H. Coverage: same as Cephalexin.

Chloramphenicol (Chloromycetin) How supplied: suspension: 150 mg/5 mL; caps: 250 mg; injection: 1 g. Dose: 50–75 mg/kg/d PO or IV Q6H; meningitis, 75–100 mg/kg/d. Coverage: gram positives and gram negatives; *Rickettsiae; Chlamydiae*. Comments: Peak 10–25 μg/mL, trough 5–10 μg/mL.

Chloroquine (Aralen PO₄, Plaquenil, Aralen HC1) How supplied: tabs: 500 mg (300 mg base); tabs: 200 mg (155 mg base); injection: 250 mg (200 mg base). Dose: suppression: 5 mg/kg base QWK; acute treatment: 10 mg/kg base; 6 hr later, 5 mg/kg base; 18 hr later, 5 mg/kg base; 24 hr later, 5 mg/kg base. Coverage: *Plasmodium* sp (some *P falciparum* resistant); *Entameoba histolytica* (extraintestinal). Toxicity: retinal. Comments: Suppressive therapy should begin 2 weeks prior to potential exposure.

Ciprofloxacin (Cipro) How supplied: tabs: 250, 500, 750 mg. Dose: NOT APPROVED FOR USE IN CHILDREN; 20–30 mg/kg/d PO Q12H. Coverage: gram negatives including *Pseudomonas*.

Clindamycin (Cleocin) How supplied: solution: 75 mg/5 mL;

caps: 75, 100 mg; injection: 150, 300, 600 mg. Dose: 20–30 mg/kg/d PO Q6H; 25–40 mg/kg/d IM or IV Q6–Q8H. Coverage: anaerobes and some gram-positive cocci.

Cloxacillin (Tegopen) How supplied: solution: 125 mg/5 mL; caps: 250, 500 mg. Dose: 50–100 mg/kg/d PO Q6H. Coverage: penicillinase-producing staphylococci.

Colistin (Coly-Mycin) How supplied: suspension: 125 mg/5 mL. Dose: 5–15 mg/kg/d PO Q8H. Coverage: enteropathogenic *E coli; Shigella.*

Dicloxacillin (Dycill, Dynapen, Pathocil) How supplied: suspension: 62.5 mg/5 mL; caps: 125, 250, 500 mg. Dose: 12–25 mg/kg/d PO Q6H. Coverage: same as cloxacillin.

Doxycycline (Doryx, Vibramycin, Vibra-Tabs) How supplied: suspension: 25 mg/mL; syrup: 50 mg/mL; caps: 50, 100 mg; injection: 100, 200 mg. Dose: > 7 yr: 4 mg/kg/d PO Q12H for 24 hr then 2 mg/kg/d PO Q24H; 2–4 mg/kg/d IV over 2 hr Q24H. Coverage: gram positives; *Rickettsiae; Chlamydiae; Mycoplasma; Brucella; Bacteroides.* Toxicity: permanent tooth discoloration when given during tooth development.

Erythromycin (E.E.S, E-mycin, EryPed, Ery-Tab, Ethril, others) How supplied: drops: 100 mg/mL, 100 mg/2.5 mL; suspension: 125, 200, 250, 400 mg/5 mL; chewable tabs: 125, 200, 250 mg; tabs: 250, 330, 400, 500 mg; caps: 125, 250 mg; topical solution: 2%; ophthalmic solution: 0.5%; amps: 0.25, 0.5, 1 g; injection: 1.5, 1 g. Dose: 20–40 mg/kg/d PO Q6–Q8H; 20–50 mg/kg/d IV Q6H; acne: topical; eye: topical. Coverage: same as Doxycycline; *Legionella; Bordetella pertussis; Corynebacterium diphtheriae; Clostridia.*

Erythromycin and sulfisoxazole (Pediazole) How supplied: suspension: 200 mg ery + 600 mg sulf/5 mL. Dose: 40 mg/kg of ery PO Q6–Q8H. Coverage: same as erythromycin; *H influenzae.*

Ethambutol (Myambutol) How supplied: tabs: 100, 400 mg. Dose: 15 mg/kg/d PO Q24H. Coverage: *M tuberculosis.* Toxicity: optic neuritis.

Flucytosine (Ancobon) How supplied: caps: 250, 500 mg. Dose: 50–150 mg/kg/d PO Q6H. Coverage: *Candida; Cryptococcus.* Toxicity: Bone marrow suppression. Comments: Check sensitivities; many candida species are resistant.

Furazolidine (Furoxone) How supplied: suspension: 50 mg/15 mL; tabs: 100 mg. Dose: 5–8 mg/kg/d PO Q6H. Coverage: *Vibrio cholerae; Giardia.* Comments: Turns urine brownish color.

Gentamicin (Garamycin) How supplied: injection: 20, 60, 80 mg; ophthalmic solution; ophthalmic ointment. Dose: 6–7.5 mg/

kg/d IM or IV; eye: topical solution, Q4H; ointment, Q6H. Coverage: same as Amikacin. Toxicity: same as Amikacin. Comments: Peak 8–10 μg/mL, trough < 2 μg/mL.

Griseofulvin (Fulvicin P/G, Fulvicin U/F, Grifulvin, others) How supplied: suspension: 125 mg/5 mL; tabs: 125, 165, 250, 330, 500 mg; caps: 125, 250, 500 mg. Dose: 10–15 mg/kg/d PO Q24H. Coverage: *Trichophyton* sp; *Microsporum* sp; *Epidermophyton floccosum*. Comments: Contraindicated in patients with porphyria or hepatocellular failure.

Imipenem-Cilastatin (Primaxin) How supplied: injection: 250, 500 mg. Dose: NOT APPROVED FOR USE IN CHILDREN; up to 50 mg/kg/d IM or IV; max 4 g/d. Coverage: gram negatives and positives including *Pseudomonas; Serratia; Enterobacter; Proteus*.

Iodoquinol (Yodoxin) How supplied: tabs: 210, 650 mg. Dose: 40 mg/kg/d PO Q8H. Coverage: *Entamoeba histolytica* (intestinal).

Isoniazid (INH, Laniazid) How supplied: syrup: 50 mg/5 mL; tabs: 50, 100, 300 mg. Dose: 10–20 mg/kg/d PO Q24H. Coverage: *M tuberculosis*. Toxicity: hepatic; neuro due to pyridoxine deficiency. Comments: Supplement with pyridoxine; use < 10 mg/kg/d when given with rifampin.

Kanamycin (Kantrex) How supplied: injection: 75, 500 mg, 1 g; caps: 500 mg. Dose: 15 mg/kg/d IM or IV Q8–12H; 50–100 mg/kg/d PO Q6H. Coverage: same as Amikacin; *Vibrio, Salmonella, Shigella*. Toxicity: same as Amikacin. Comments: Oral dosing not absorbed–used for bowel sterilization. Peak 15–30 μg/mL, trough < 10 μg/mL.

Ketoconazole (Nizoral) How supplied: cream: 2% in 15, 30, 60 g tubes; tabs: 200 mg. Dose: topical: to affected area Q24H; 4–7 mg/kg/d PO Q24H. Coverage: some dermatophytes; *Candida; Blastomyces, Coccidioides; Histplasma*. Toxicity: hepatic.

Mebendazole (Vermox) How supplied: chewable tabs: 100 mg. Dose: 100 mg PO; pinworms: one dose; other nematodes: Q12H for 3 days. Coverage: *Trichuris; Enterobius; Ascaris; Ancylostoma; Necator*.

Methicillin (Staphcillin) How supplied: injection: 1, 4, 6 g. Dose: 150–200 mg/kg/d IM or IV Q6H. Coverage: same as Cloxacillin.

Metronidazole (Flagyl, Metric-21, Protostat) How supplied: tabs: 250, 500 mg; injection: 500 mg. Dose: 15–50 mg/kg/d PO Q8H; 30 mg/kg/d IV Q6H. Coverage: anaerobes; *Giardia; Entamoeba histolytica;* trichomoniases.

Mezlocillin (Mezlin) How supplied: injection: 1, 2, 3, 4, g. Dose: 200–300 mg/kg/d IV Q4–6H. Coverage: gram negatives.

Miconazole (Monistat) How supplied: cream, lotion: 2%; vaginal cream: 2%; vaginal suppository: 100, 200 mg; injection: 200 mg. Dose: topical: to affected area Q12H; vaginal: 1 applicator QHS; vaginal: 100–200 mg QHS; 20–40 mg/kg/d IV Q8H. Coverage: some dermatophytes; *Candida; Cryptococcus; Coccidioides.* Comments: May also be administered intrathecally.

Mupirocin (Bactroban) How supplied: ointment: 2% in 15 g tube. Dose: topical Q8H. Coverage: Impetigo due to *S aureus,* B-hemolytip strep, *S pyogenes.*

Nafcillin (Nafcil, Unipen) How supplied: solution: 250 mg/5 mL; caps: 250 mg; tabs: 500 mg; injection: 0.5, 1, 2 g. Dose: 50–100 mg/kg/d PO Q6H; 150 mg/kg/d IM or IV Q6H. Coverage: same as Cloxacillin.

Niclosomide (Niclocide) How supplied: tabs: 500 mg. Dose: 11–34 kg; 1 g PO single dose; 34–59 kg: 1.5 g PO single dose; > 59 kg: 2 g PO single dose; for *H nana,* as above, then: 11–34 kg; 0.5 g PO Q24H; 34–59 kg: 1 g PO Q24H; > 59 kg: 2 g PO Q24H. Coverage: *Taenia saginata; Diphyllobothrium latum; Hymenolepis nana.*

Nitrofurantoin (Furadantin, Macrodantin) How supplied: suspension: 25 mg/5 mL; caps: 25, 50, 100 mg; tabs: 50, 100 mg. Dose: 5–7 mg/kg/d PO Q6H. Coverage: gram negatives. Toxicity: primaquine-sensitive hemolytic anemia. Comments: Used only for UTI.

Nystatin (Mycostatin, Milstat, Nystex) How supplied: cream, ointment, powder: 100,000 U/g; suspension: 100,000 U/mL; tabs: 500,000 U. Dose: topical: to affected area Q12H; infants: 2 mL/dose Q6H; children: 4–6 mL/dose or 1 tab/dose Q6H. Coverage: *Candida.* Comments: Also comes in vaginal preparations.

Oxacillin (Bactocill, Prostaphlin) How supplied: suspension: 250 mg/5 mL; caps: 250, 500 mg; injection: 0.25, 0.5, 1, 2, 4 g. Dose: 50–100 mg/kg/d PO Q6H; 150–200 mg/kg/d IM or IV Q6H. Coverage: same as Cloxacillin.

Oxytetracycline (Terramycin) How supplied: caps: 250 mg; injection: 50, 100, 250 mg. Dose: > 7 yr: 20–50 mg/kg/d PO Q6H; 15–25 mg/kg/d IM Q12H. Coverage: same as Doxycycline. Toxicity: same as Doxycycline.

Penicillin G (Pentids, Prizerpen G) How supplied: suspension: 125, 250, 500 mg/5 mL; tabs: 125, 150, 250, 500 mg; injection: 1, 2, 5, 10, 20 million U. Dose: 25–50 mg/kg/d PO Q6–Q8H; 0.1–0.25 million U/kg/d IM or IV. Coverage: some gram-positive cocci; some gram-negative cocci; oral anaerobes.

Penicillin G, benzathine (Bicillin) How supplied: injection: 0.6, 0.9, 1.2, 3 million U. Dose: 50,000 U/kg IM single dose. Coverage: Streptococci groups A, C, G, H, L, M.

Penicillin G, procaine (Wycillin) How supplied: injection: 0.3, 0.6, 1.2, 2.4 million U. Dose: 25,000–50,000 U/kg/d IM. Coverage: same as penicillin G; spirochetes.

Penicillin V (Betapen-VK, Ledercillin VK, Pen Vee VK, Veetids) How supplied: solution: 125, 250 mg/5 mL; tabs: 125, 250, 500 mg. Dose: 25–50 mg/kg/d PO. Coverage: streptococci groups A, C, G, H, L, M; oral anaerobes.

Pentamidine (Pentam 300) How supplied: injection: 300 mg. Dose: 4 mg/kg/d IM or IV. Coverage: *Pneumocystis carinii*. Toxicity: hypotension.

Piperacillin (Pipracil) How supplied: injection: 2, 3, 4, g. Dose: NOT APPROVED FOR USE IN CHILDREN; 200–300 mg/kg/d IV. Coverage: gram negatives; anaerobes.

Praziquantel (Biltricide) How supplied: tabs: 600 mg. Dose: 60 mg/kg/d PO Q8H for 3 doses. Coverage: *Schistosoma* sp.

Pyrantel (Antiminth) How supplied: suspension: 250 mg/5 mL. Dose: 11 mg/kg PO as single dose. Coverage: *Enterobius*; *Ascaris*.

Pyrimethamine (Daraprim) How supplied: tabs: 25 mg. Dose: For prophylaxis: < 4 yr: ¼ tab PO QWK; 4–10 yr: ½ tab PO QWK; > 10 yr: 1 tab PO QWK. For *T gondii:* 1 mg/kg/d PO Q12H with a sulfa. Coverage: *Plasmodium* sp; *Toxoplasma gondii*.

Quinacrine (Atabrine) How supplied: tabs: 100 mg. Dose: 6 mg/kg/d PO Q8H. Coverage: *Giardia*. Toxicity: hepatic; hemolysis in G6PD deficiency. Comments: Turns skin yellow.

Ribavirin (Virazole) How supplied: vial: 6 g. Dose: 6 g aerosolized over 12–18 hr Q24H. Coverage: Respiratory syncytial virus. Comments: Must be started within the first 3 days of RSV lower respiratory tract infection.

Rifampin (Rifadin, Rimactane) How supplied: caps: 150, 300 mg. Dose: 10–20 mg/kg/d PO Q12–24H, max 600 mg/dose. For *H influenzae* prophylaxis: 20 mg/kg/d Q24H for 4 doses. For *N meningitidis* prophylaxis: 20 mg/kg/d Q24H for 4 doses. Coverage: *Mycobacterium; Neisseria; H influenzae*. Toxicity: hepatic. Comments: All body secretions may be colored red-orange.

Spectinomycin (Trobicin) How supplied: injection: 2, 4 g. Dose: 40 mg/kg IM single dose; max 2 g IM. Coverage: *N gonorrhoeae*.

Streptomycin How supplied: injection: 1, 5 g. Dose: 20–30 mg/

kg/d IM Q12H. Coverage: *M tuberculosis;* some gram negatives. Toxicity: vestibular.

Sulfadoxine and pyrimethamine (Fansidar) How supplied: tabs: 500 mg SDX/25 mg PMA. Dose: For prophylaxis: < 4 yr: ½ tab PO Q2WK; 4–8 yr: 1 tab PO Q2WK; 9–14 yr: 1½ tab PO Q2WK; > 14 yr: t tab PO Q2WK; *or* half the above doses QWK. Same quantity may be used as a single dose for an acute attack. Coverage: *Plasmodium* sp including chloroquine-resistant *P falciparum.* Toxicity: hemolysis in G6PD deficiency; Stevens-Johnson syndrome. Comments: Fansidar-resistant *P falciparum* now exist.

Sulfamethizole (Thiosulfil) How supplied: tabs: 500 mg. Dose: CONTRAINDICATED IN INFANTS < 2 MO; 30–45 mg/kg/d PO Q6H. Coverage: *E coli; Klebsiella; Enterobacter; S aureus; Proteus; H influenzae.* Comments: Used only for UTI.

Sulfamethoxazole (Gantanol) How supplied: suspension: 500 mg/5 mL; tabs: 500 mg. Dose: CONTRAINDICATED IN INFANTS < 2 MO; 50–60 mg/kg/g PO Q12H. Coverage: same as sulfamethizole; malaria. Comments: Primarily used for UTI.

Sulfisoxazole (Gantrisin) How supplied: suspension: 500 mg/5 mL; tabs: 500 mg. Dose: CONTRAINDICATED IN INFANTS < 2 MO; 150 mg/kg/d PO Q6H; max 6 g/d. Coverage: same as sulfamethizole. Comments: Use in half daily dose for prophylaxis of otitis media.

Tetracycline (Achromycin, Sumycin) How supplied: syrup: 125 mg/5 mL; suspension: 125 mg/5 mL; caps: 250, 500 mg; tabs: 250, 500 mg; injection: 100, 250, 500 mg. Dose: > 7 yr: 25–50 mg/kg/d PO Q6H; 15–25 mg/kg/d IM Q8–Q12H; 10–20 mg/kg/d IV Q8–Q12H. Coverage: same as Doxycycline. Toxicity: same as Doxycycline.

Thiabendazole (Mintezol) How supplied: suspension: 500 mg/5 mL; chewable tabs: 500 mg. Dose: 50 mg/kg/d PO Q12H; max 3 g/d. Coverage: strongyloidiasis; cutaneous larva migrans; visceral larva migrans; trichinosis.

Ticarcillin (Ticar) How supplied: injection: 1, 3, 6 g. Dose: 200–300 mg/kg/d IV Q4–Q6H. Coverage: same as Carbenicillin. Toxicity: Platelet dysfunction.

Ticarcillin and clavulanate (Timentin) How supplied: injection: 3/0.1, 3/0.2 g. Dose: NOT APPROVED FOR USE IN CHILDREN; same as Ticarcillin. Coverage: same as Ticarcillin; *Klebsiella, S aureus, H influenzae.*

Tobramycin (Nebcin) How supplied: injection: 20, 80 mg, 1.2 g. Dose: 3–5 mg/kg/d IM or IV Q8H. Coverage: gram negatives including *Pseudomonas*. Toxicity: same as Amikacin. Comments: May need higher doses in patients with cystic fibrosis; peak 8–10 μg/mL, trough < 2 μg/mL.

Trifluridine (Viroptic) How supplied: ophthalmic solution: 1%. Dose: 1 drop Q2H to affected eye. Coverage: herpes simplex.

Trimethoprim (Proloprim, Trimpex) How supplied: tabs: 100, 200 mg. Dose: 4 mg/kg/d PO Q12H. Coverage: *E coli, Proteus mirabilis, Klebsiella pneumoniae, Enterobacter,* coagulase-negative staphylococci.

Trimethoprim-sulfamethoxazole (Bactrim, Septra) How supplied: suspension: 40 mg TMP/200 mg SMX/5 mL; tabs: 80 mg TMP/400 mg SMX, 160 mg TMP/800 mg SMX; injection: 400 mg TMP/2000 mg SMX. Dose: CONTRAINDICATED IN INFANTS < 2 MO; 6–12 mg TMP/kg/d PO Q12H; 20 mg TMP/kg/d IV Q6H. Coverage: gram positives and gram negatives; *Salmonella; Shigella, P carinii.*

Vancomycin (Vancocin, Vancoled, Vancor) How supplied: pulvules: 125, 250 mg; bottle: 1, 10 g; injection: 0.5, 1 g. Dose: 20–40 mg/kg/d PO Q6H; max 2 g/d; 40 mg/kg/d IV Q6H. Coverage: *Clostridium difficile;* gram-positive cocci including methicillin-resistant. Toxicity: rash, hypotension, renal, 8th cranial nerve.

Vidarabine (Vira-A) How supplied: ophthalmic ointment: 3%; injection: 1 g. Dose: topical: 1/2 in. to affected eye 5 times/day; 10–15 mg/kg/d IV over 12–24 hr Q24H. Coverage: herpes simplex.

Zidovudine (AZT) (Retrovir) How supplied: solution: 150 mg/5 mL; caps: 100 mg. Dose: 720 mg/m^2/d Q6H. Coverage: HIV. Toxicity: granulocytopenia; anemia.

9 | Immunization Procedures, Vaccines, Antisera, & Skin Tests

Mark A. Colloton, MS, PA-C, & John W. Ogle, M.D.

Active immunity to infectious diseases occurs following inoculation of bacterial, viral, and parasitic antigens, either in a live attenuated form, as inactivated whole organisms, or as portions or products of organisms. New vaccines are being developed and tested and are introduced periodically. In addition, vaccine composition, recommended schedules, and contraindications continue to change. Readers are advised to consult the recommendations of the Advisory Committee for Immunization Practices (ACIP) and the *Report of the Committee on Infectious Diseases* of the American Academy of Pediatrics (the *Red Book*) to supplement the information given in this chapter.

Passive immunity, administered in the form of intravenous gamma globulin (IVIG) or as one of several specific immune globulins or animal serum, provides temporary protection against infection or disease. Only a limited number of infectious agents are susceptible to passive antibody; in general, it is preferable to use a vaccine for a disease (if available) to provide active immunity than to provide passive protection.

PROCEDURES FOR ACTIVE IMMUNIZATION

General Principles

A. Sources of Information: *Always* consult authoritative sources before using any of the vaccines, sera, or immune globulins. Among these sources are (1) the CDC's *Morbidity and Mortality Weekly Report* (MMWR), (2) the American Academy of Pediatrics' periodic updates of the *Report of the Committee on Infectious Diseases* (the *Red Book*), (3) the manufacturer's package insert that accompanies each biologic product, and (4) the CDC's *Health Information for International Travel*. The package inserts are reasonably complete, but the recommendations may contain conflicting information (usually occasioned by legal considerations), in which case it is best to follow the advice of the CDC or the American Academy of Pediatrics.

B. Informed Consent: Prior to immunization, the parents or guardians must be provided information about the risks and benefits of each biologic product and the potential risks of the diseases to be prevented, and must provide signed informed consent. Convenient forms prepared by the CDC are available from local health departments; they can also be found in copies of the *Red Book* published before 1988.

C. Storage and Administration of Vaccines: Scrupulous attention should be paid to proper handling of vaccines and other biologic products. Consult the package insert for specifications for each product, as instructions vary for different types of products and manufacturers.

Aseptic technique should be used in removing vaccine from a vial, preparing the injection site, and administering the vaccine. Intramuscular injections are best given to children in either the lateral thigh or, in older children, the deltoid muscle. Administration in the gluteal region can cause injury to the sciatic nerve and should therefore be avoided. The tissue at the injection site should be compressed and the needle should be inserted in the upper lateral quadrant of the thigh with the syringe directed inferiorly at a 45-degree angle to the long axis of the leg and posteriorly at a 45-degree angle to a line parallel to the table top. Before injecting the vaccine, the syringe plunger should be pulled back; if blood appears, the needle should be withdrawn, new vaccine drawn up into a new syringe, and injected into a different site. To decrease the likelihood of local reactions to vaccines, a needle long enough to enter the muscle—2.5 cm or 1 inch—is recommended for intramuscular injections in children of all ages. When injecting an irritating material, the injection site should be rotated at subsequent inoculations and the injection site noted in the chart. Two vaccines should never be injected into the same site, and separate vaccines should never be mixed in one syringe.

D. Monitoring and Reporting Adverse Reactions: Parents should be informed of any possible adverse reactions and given specific instructions for reporting such reactions. Severe reactions require a physical assessment of the child and appropriate therapeutic intervention. The parents should be given an immunization record, which should be updated each time a vaccine is given. The National Childhood Vaccine Injury Act, which went into effect on March 21, 1988, requires health care providers to record certain information and events. The health care provider who administers the vaccine should enter into the permanent medical record the following information: date of vaccine administration; vaccine manufacturer; vaccine lot number; and name, address, and title of the person administering the vaccine. Certain reportable adverse events after vaccination are listed in Table 9–1. Procedures for reporting such events are given in Table 9–2. Adverse events due to vaccines purchased with public funds should be reported to the CDC through local, county, or state health departments using the Adverse Events Following Immunization form (CDC form 71.19). With privately purchased vaccines, adverse events should be reported to the Food and Drug Administration (FDA) with the Adverse Reaction Form (FDA form 1639), which is available from the FDA at HFN-730, Rockville, MD 20857. The forms are also available in the *Physicians' Desk Reference, USP Drug Information for Health Care Providers,* and *AMA Drug Evaluations.*

E. General Precautions and Contraindications: The physician should be aware of the recommended precautions and contraindications for each vaccine. The following are general guidelines: (1) Avoid giving live vaccines to women during pregnancy. (2) Do not administer a live vaccine to any person suspected or proved to be immunodeficient (eg, a patient with a known or suspected congenital defect, a patient with an acquired immunodeficiency disease, or a patient receiving immunosuppressive therapy or corticosteroids). (3) Vaccines are generally given only to healthy children; however, minor illness, whether there is fever or not, is not a contraindication to live viral vaccine administration. DPT should not be given to children who have a febrile illness because the symptoms may be attributed to the vaccine. However, if a child has a nonfebrile upper respiratory tract infection, DPT vaccine can be administered as scheduled, to prevent multiple visits or a delay in completing the immunization schedule.

PRIMARY IMMUNIZATION OF CHILDREN IN THE FIRST YEAR OF LIFE

The recommended schedule of immunizations is listed in Table 9–3. Adequate protection against diphtheria, pertussis, tetanus, and poliomyelitis should be initiated early in infancy and carried through with the recommended ''booster'' doses of vaccine. A combination product containing measles, mumps, and rubella vaccines (MMR) is administered once at 15 months of age. *Haemophilus influenzae* b conjugate vaccine (PRP-D) is recommended for use in children 18 months of age or older. By the time of school entry, the healthy child should have received all vaccines in the primary series and thereafter need only be given booster doses of the adult preparation of diphtheria-tetanus toxoid (Td) at 10-year intervals. Pertussis vaccine should not be given after 7 years of age, and no additional doses of poliovirus vaccine are required.

The following guidelines pertain to variations from the schedule shown in Table 9–3:

(1) If a child misses any of the DTP doses, ignore the interval and proceed with completion of the schedule.

(2) If pertussis vaccine is contraindicated in a child under 7 years of age, the pediatric preparation of diphtheria–tetanus toxoid (DT) should be substituted for DTP.

IMMUNIZATION OF CHILDREN NOT IMMUNIZED IN INFANCY

The schedule for immunization of persons not immunized in infancy is shown in Table 9–4. The following guidelines should be observed:

(1) Pediatric DT is used only for children 7 years of age. Adult Td is used for primary immunization of older children and adults (Table 9–5).

(2) Live oral poliovirus vaccine (OPV) should not be given to persons over 18 years of age. Inactivated (killed, Salk) poliovirus vaccine (IVP) should be used instead. Follow the manufacturer's instructions for dosage and booster intervals.

(3) MMR can be administered to persons of any age.

(4) *Haemophilus influenzae* b conjugate vaccine should be given to all children between the ages of 18 months and 5 years. Only those children at high risk (eg, splenectomized children, children with sickle cell disease or immunodeficiency) should receive the vaccine after the fifth birthday if they have never received it before.

IMMUNIZATION OF INSTITUTIONALIZED CHILDREN

Children who are residents of institutions, particularly institutions for the mentally retarded, may be at high risk of acquiring contagious diseases. Each resident should be immunized either before admission to the institution or at entry. The vaccines and

Table 9–1. Reportable events following vaccination.*

Vaccine/Toxoid	Event	Interval from Vaccination
DTP,P, DTP/polio combined	A. Anaphylaxis or anaphylactic shock	24 hours
	B. Encephalopathy (or encephalitis)†	7 days
	C. Shock-collapse or hypotonic-hyporesponsive collapse†	7 days
	D. Residual seizure disorder†	(See Aids to Interpretation}
	E. Any acute complication or sequela (including death) of above events	No limit
	F. Events in vaccinees described in manufacturer's package insert as contraindications to additional doses of vaccine† (such as convulsions)	(See package insert)
MMR, DT, Td, tetanus toxoid	A. Anaphylaxis or anaphylactic shock	24 hours
	B. Encephalopathy (or encephalitis)†	15 days for MMR vaccines; 7 days for DT, Td, and T toxoids
	C. Residual seizure disorder†	(See Aids to Interpretation}
	D. Any acute complication or sequela (including death) of above events	No limit
	E. Events in vaccinees described in manufacturer's package insert as contraindications to additional doses of vaccine†	(See package insert)
Oral polio vaccine	A. Paralytic poliomyelitis:	
	in a nonimmunodeficient recipient	30 days
	in an immunodeficient recipient	6 months
	in a vaccine-associated community case	No limit

	B. Any acute complication or sequela (including death) of above events	No limit
	C. Events in vaccinees described in manufacturer's package insert as contraindications to additional doses of vaccine†	(See package insert)
Inactivated polio vaccine	A. Anaphylaxis or anaphylactic shock	24 hours
	B. Any acute complication or sequela (including death) of above event	No limit
	C. Events in vaccinees described in manufacturer's package insert as contraindications to additional doses of vaccine†	(See package insert)

† **Aids to interpretation:** Shock-collapse or hypotonic-hyporesponsive collapse may be evidenced by signs or symptoms such as decrease in or loss of muscle tone, paralysis (partial or complete), hemiparesis, hemiparesis, loss of color or turning pale white or blue, unresponsiveness to environmental stimuli, depression of or loss of consciousness, prolonged sleeping with difficulty arousing, or cardiovascular or respiratory arrest.

Residual seizure disorder may be considered to have occurred if no other seizure or convulsion unaccompanied by fever or accompanied by a fever of less than 102°F occurred before the first seizure or convulsion after the administration of the vaccine involved, *and*, if in the case of measles-, mumps-, or rubella-containing vaccines, the first seizure or convulsion occurred within 15 days after vaccination or in the case of any other vaccine, the first seizure or convulsion occurred within 3 days after vaccination, *and*, if 2 or more seizures or convulsions unaccompanied by fever or accompanied by a fever of less than 102°F occurred within 1 year after vaccination.

The terms *seizure* and *convulsion* include grand mal, petit mal, absence, myoclonic, tonic–clonic, and focal motor seizures and signs. *Encephalopathy* means any significant acquired abnormality of, injury to, or impairment of function of the brain. Among the frequent manifestations of encephalopathy are focal and diffuse neurologic signs, increased intracranial pressure, or changes in level of consciousness lasting at least 6 hours, with or without convulsions. The neurologic signs and symptoms of encephalopathy may be temporary with complete recovery, or they may result in various degrees of permanent impairment. Signs and symptoms, such as high-pitched and unusual screaming, persistent unconsolable crying, and bulging fontanel are compatible with an encephalopathy, but in and of themselves are not conclusive evidence of encephalopathy. Encephalopathy usually can be documented by slow wave activity on an electroencephalogram.

The health-care provider must refer to the CONTRAINDICATION section of the manufacturer's package insert for each vaccine.

* Reprinted with permission from MMWR 1988;37:197–200.

239

Table 9–2. Reporting of events occurring after vaccination.*

	Vaccine Purchased with Public Money	VaccinePurchased with Private Money
Who Reports	Health-care provider who administered the vaccine	Health-care provider who administered the vaccine
What Products to Report	DTP, P, measles, mumps, rubella, DT, Td, T, OPV, IPV, and DTP/polio combined	DTP, P, measles, mumps, rubella, DT, Td, T, OPV, IPV, and DTP/polio combined
What Reactions to Report	Events lised in Table 9–1 including contraindicating reactions specified in manufacturer's package inserts	Events listd in Table 9–1 including contraindicating reactions specified in manufacturer's package inserts
How to Report	Initial report taken by local, county, or state health department. State health department completes CDC form 71.19	Health-care provider completes Adverse Reaction Report-FDA form 1639 (include interval from vaccination, manufacturer, and lot number on form)
Where to Report	State health departments send CDC form 71.19 to: MSAEFI/IM (E05) Centers for Disease Control Atlanta, GA 30333	Completed FDA form 1639 is sent to: Food and Drug Administration (HFN-730) Rockville, MD 20857
Where to Obtain Forms	State health departments	FDA and publications such as *FDA Drug Bulletin*

* Reprinted with permission from MMWR 1988;**37:**197–200.

schedule to be used will depend on the age of the resident (see Tables 9–3, 9–4, and 9–5).

All residents should be protected against measles, mumps, and rubella. Previous immunization documented by a physician is the only acceptable reason for not administering MMR on or shortly before admission.

Influenza vaccine should be given annually as recommended.

Poliovirus immunization should be up-to-date or should be initiated at entry if none has been given previously. For residents 18 years or older, only the inactivated vaccine (IPV) should be used.

If the child is between 18 months old and 5, *Haemophilus influenzae* type b PRP-D vaccine should be administered.

Because hepatitis may pose special risks to institutionalized children, it is recommended that immune globulin be given to all

Table 9–3. Recommended schedule for active immunization of normal infants and children.[1]

Recommended Age[2]	Vaccine(s)[3]	Comments
2 mos	DTP#1[4], OPV#1[5]	OPV and DTP can be given earlier in areas of high endemicity
4 mos	DTP#2, OPV#2	6-wk to 2-mo interval desired between OPV doses
6 mos	DTP#3,	An additional dose of OPV at this time is optional in areas with a high risk of poliovirus exposure
15 mos[6]	MMR#1[7], DTP#4, OPV#3	Completion of primary series of DTP and OPV
18 mos	PRP-D[8]	Conjugate preferred over polysaccharide vaccine[9]
4–6 yrs	DTP#5[10], OPV#4	At or before school entry
5–12 yrs	MMR#2[11]	
14–16	Td[12]	Repeat every 10 years throughout life

[1] Reprinted with permission from MMWR 1989;**38**:205–227.

[2] These recommended ages should not be construed as absolute, eg, 2 months can be 6–10 weeks. However, MMR should not be given to children less than 12 months of age. If exposure to measles disease is considered likely, then children 6 through 11 months old may be immunized with single-antigen measles vaccine. These children should be reimmunized with MMR when they are approximately 15 months of age.

[3] For all products used, consult the manufacturers' package enclosures for instructions regarding storage, handling, dosage, and administration. Immunobiologics prepared by different manufacturers can vary, and those of the same manufacturer can change from time to time. The package inserts are useful references for specific products, but they may not always be consistent with current ACIP and American Academy of Pediatrics immunization schedules.

[4] DTP = diphtheria and tetanus toxoids and pertussis vaccine, adsorbed. DTP may be used up to the seventh birthday. The first dose can be given at 6 weeks of age and the second and third doses given 4–8 weeks after the preceding dose.

[5] OPV = poliovirus vaccine live oral, trivalent: contains poliovirus types 1, 2, and 3.

[6] Provided at least 6 months have elapsed since DTP#3 or, if fewer than 3 doses of DTP have been received, at least 6 weeks since the last previous dose of DTP or OPV. MMR vaccine should not be delayed to allow simultaneous administration with DTP and OPV. Administering MMR at 15 months and DTP# 4 and OPV# 3 at 18 months continues to be an acceptable alternative.

(continued)

Table 9–3. (Continued)

[7] MMR = measles, mumps, and rubella virus vaccine, live. Counties that report fewer than 5 cases of measles among preschool children during each of the last 5 years should implement a routine 2-dose measles vaccination schedule for preschoolers. The first dose should be administered at 9 months or the first health care contact thereafter. Infants vaccinated before their first birthday should receive a second dose at about 15 months of age. Single-antigen measles vaccine should be used for children less than 1 year and MMR for children vaccinated on or after their first birthday. If resources do not allow a routine 2-dose schedule, an acceptable alternative is to lower the routine age for MMR vaccination to 12 months.

[8] PRP-D = vaccine composed of *Haemophilus influenzae* type b polysaccharide antigen conjugated to a protein carrier. Children less than 5 years of age previously vaccinated with polysaccharide vaccine between the ages of 18 and 23 months should be revaccinated with a single dose of conjugate vaccine if at least 2 months have elapsed since the receipt of the polysaccharide vaccine.

[9] If PRP-D is not available, an acceptable alternative is to give *Haemophilus influenzae* type b polysaccharide vaccine (PRP) at age over 24 months. Children at high risk for *Haemophilus influenzae* type b disease where conjugate vaccine is not available may be vaccinated with PRP at 18 months of age and revaccinated at 24 months.

[10] Up to the seventh birthday.

[11] The Red Book Committee recommends MMR#2 at 12 years of age. The ACIP recommends MMR# 2 upon entrance to kindergarten. Consult local or state health dept for recommendations on administering MMR#2.

[12] Td = tetanus and diphtheria toxoids, adsorbed (for use in persons greater than 7 years of age): contains the same amount of tetanus toxoid as DTP or DT but a reduced dose of diphtheria toxoid.

residents and staff if an outbreak of hepatitis A occurs. Hepatitis B vaccine should be administered in the prescribed regimen to all individuals who enter custodial institutions.

IMMUNIZATIONS FOR ALL CHILDREN

Diphtheria

Immunization against diphtheria is effected by administration of toxoid to stimulate antitoxin production. Levels of antitoxin are related to immunity against disease, but they do not protect against the carrier state.

A. Diphtheria-Tetanus-Pertussis (DTP): This vaccine is used routinely in infants and children. It combines diphtheria and tetanus toxoids with a suspension of killed *Bordetella pertussis* organisms. Three doses of 0.5 mL each are given intramuscularly

Table 9–4. Recommended immunization schedule for infants and children up to the seventh birthday not immunized at the recommended time in early infancy.[1, 2]

Timing	Vaccine(s)	Comments
First visit	DTP#1[3], OPV#1[4], MMR#1[5], if child is aged ≥ 15 mos and PRP-D[6] if child is aged ≥ 18 mos	DTP, OPV, and MMR should be administered simultaneously to children aged ≥ 15 mos, if appropriate. DTP, OPV, MMR, and PRP-D may be given simultaneously to children aged 18 mos–5 yrs
2 mos after DTP#1, OPV#1	DTP#2[7], OPV#2	
2 mos after DTP#2	DTP#3[7]	An additional dose of OPV at this time is optional in areas with a high risk of poliovirus exposure
6–12 mos after DTP#3	DTP#4, OPV#3	
Preschool[8] (4–6 yrs)	DTP#5, OPV#4	Preferably at or before school entry
5–12 yrs	MMR#2[9]	
14–16 yrs	Td[10]	Repeat every 10 years throughout life

[1] Reprinted with permission from MMWR 1989;**38**:205–227.
[2] If initiated in the first year of life, give DTP#1, 2, and 3 and OPV#1 and 2 according to this schedule; give MMR#1 when the child becomes 15 months old.
[3] DTP = diphtheria and tetanus toxoids and pertussis vaccine, adsorbed. DTP can be used up to the seventh birthday.
[4] OPV = poliovirus vaccine live oral, trivalent: contains poliovirus types 1, 2, and 3.
[5] MMR = measles, mumps, and rubella virus vaccine, live (see text for discussion of single vaccines versus combination).
[6] PRP-D = vaccine composed of *Haemophilus influenzae* type b polysaccharide antigen conjugated to a protein carrier. If PRP-D is not available, an acceptable alternative is to give *Haemophilus influenzae* type b polysaccharide vaccine (PRP) at age over 24 months. If PRP-D is unavailable and if the child is high risk for *Haemophilus influenzae* type b disease, PRP may be given at 18 months of age with a second dose at 24 months. Children less than 5 years who were previously vaccinated with PRP between 18 and 23 months of age should be revaccinated with a single dose of PRP-D at least 2 months after the initial dose of PRP.

(continued)

Either PRP-D or PRP can be administered up to the fifth birthday. However, they are not generally recommended for persons over 5 years of age.

[7] The second and third doses of DTP can be given 4–8 weeks after the preceding dose.

[8] The preschool doses are not necessary if the fourth dose of DTP and third dose of OPV are administered after the fourth birthday.

[9] MMR#2 may be administered upon entrance to kindergarten or during the time between kindergarten and middle or junior high school.

[10] Td = tetanus and diphtheria toxoids, adsorbed (for use in persons over 7 years): contains the same dose of tetanus toxoid as DTP or DT and a reduced dose of diphtheria toxoid.

at 2-month intervals; the first dose is usually given when the infant is 2 months of age (see Table 9–3). Booster doses may be given 6–12 months after the third DPT dose, at the 15-month examination along with MMR and OPV, if compliance is a concern, or at the 18-month visit along with PRP-D and OPV. The fifth dose of DPT is given between 4 and 6 years of age. Thereafter, the pertussis component of the vaccine is eliminated. DTP and live virus vaccines can be given at the same time. If pertussis is prevalent in the community, immunization may be started as early as 2 weeks of age and doses may be given 4 weeks apart. Reduced or split doses of vaccine may not be efficacious and are not recommended. Premature infants should be appropriately immunized according to the schedule given in Table 9–3. Altered dosages or schedules should not be used with the exception that administration of OPV should be delayed, in hospitalized newborns, until hospital discharge.

B. Diphtheria-Tetanus (DT) (Pediatric): This preparation contains full amounts of diphtheria and tetanus toxoids and is used in children for whom pertussis vaccine is contraindicated. Three doses of 0.5 mL each are given intramuscularly at 4–8 week intervals, with a booster injection 6–12 months later. DT toxoid should not be given to anyone older than 7 years.

C. Diphtheria-Tetanus (Td) (Adult): This preparation contains less diphtheria toxoid than does the DT preparation and rarely produces reactions in older children and adults. The dose is 0.5 mL intramuscularly, given at the intervals shown in Table 9–5.

D. Diphtheria (D): This toxoid is used only when combined preparations are contraindicated.

Table 9–5. Recommended immunization schedule for persons over 7 years of age not immunized at the recommended time in early infancy[1]

Timing	Vaccine(s)	Comments
First visit	Td#1[2], OPV#1[3], and MMR#1[4]	OPV not routinely recommended for persons aged ≥ 18 years
2 mos after Td#1, OPV#1	Td#2, OPV#2	OPV may be given as soon as 6 weeks after OPV#2
6–12 mos after Td#2, OPV#2	Td#3, OPV#3	OPV#3 may be given as soon as 6 wks after OPV#2
Age 12	MMR#2[5]	
10 yrs after Td#3	Td	Repeat every 10 years throughout life

[1] Reprinted with permission from MMWR 1989;38:205–227.

[2] Td = tetanus and diphtheria toxoids, adsorbed (for adult use) (for use after the seventh birthday). The DTP doses given to children less than 7 years who remain incompletely immunized at age greater than 7 years should be counted as prior exposure to tetanus and diphtheria toxoids (eg, a child who previously received 2 doses of DTP needs only 1 dose of Td to complete a primary series for tetanus and diphtheria).

[3] OPV = poliovirus vaccine live oral, trivalent: contains poliovirus types 1, 2, and 3. When polio vaccine is to be given to persons over 18 years, poliovirus vaccine inactivated (IPV) is preferred. See ACIP statement on polio vaccine for immunization schedule for IPV (2).

[4] MMR = measles, mumps, and rubella virus vaccine, live. Persons born before 1957 can generally be considered immune to measles and mumps and need not be immunized. Since medical personnel are at higher risk for acquiring measles than the general population, medical facilities may wish to consider requiring proof of measles immunity for employees born before 1957. Rubella vaccine can be given to persons of any age, particularly to nonpregnant women of childbearing age. MMR can be used since administration of vaccine to persons already immune is not deleterious (see text for discussion of single vaccines versus combination).

[5] MMR#2 may be given no less than one month after MMR#1. It is acceptable to administer M-M-R II prior to entrance into middle or junior high school.

Pertussis

Immunization with suspensions of phase I *Bordetella pertussis* prepared as vaccine can effectively reduce the risk of clinical pertussis. Infants are immunized with diphtheria-tetanus-pertussis (DTP); children over 7 years of age do not receive the pertussis component. Common adverse effects to pertussis vaccine include redness, pain or swelling at vaccination site, fever, drowsiness, fretfulness, anorexia, and vomiting. These reactions occur shortly after the vaccine and subside within 24–48 hours; however, the tendency of these reactions to occur increases with subsequent doses of the vaccine. Children who experience these reactions should receive other doses of the vaccine as scheduled; the administration of acetaminophen (15 mg/kg per dose) given at the time of vaccination and every 4 hours for 3 doses may decrease side effects to the pertussis vaccine.

More serious adverse reactions, including encephalopathy, have been reported after pertussis vaccine, but experts disagree whether the vaccine causes the reactions. None of the reported reactions are unique to pertussis vaccine; all the reactions also occur in young children who have not received pertussis vaccine. Nonetheless, future administration of pertussis vaccine is contraindicated in children who have any of the following reactions: encephalopathy within 7 days; convulsion, with or without seizure, within 3 days; persistent unconsolable screaming or crying for 3 or more hours; a high-pitched cry within 48 hours; collapse or shock-like state within 48 hours; unexplained temperature of 40.5°C (104.9°F) or higher within 48 hours; and an immediate severe or anaphylactic allergic reaction. Future administration of pertussis vaccine is contraindicated in children who have any of these more serious reactions.

Children with a neurologic disorder who have a progressive developmental delay or changing neurologic findings have an increased risk of seizures after receiving pertussis vaccine. Therefore, it may be prudent to defer pertussis vaccine because the risk of seizures after pertussis vaccine in these children may be greater than the risk of contracting pertussis itself. The decision to defer pertussis immunization should be reassessed at each visit based on the risk of postvaccine seizure compared with the risk of complications due to pertussis disease. Infants and children with well-controlled seizures may be vaccinated with pertussis because, in these children, the risk of complications owing to pertussis disease may be increased. The risk of contracting pertussis is increased in children who may travel to areas where pertussis is endemic and in children in daycare centers, special clinics, or residential care institutions. Children with neurologic conditions that predispose to seizures should not receive pertussis vaccine. These conditions include tuberous sclerosis and metabolic or degenerative disease. Such children should be observed for a time to determine the course of their neurologic involvement, an the decision whether to vaccinate should be re-evaluated at each visit. Children whose disease is controlled, resolved, or corrected may be vaccinated. A family history of seizures, SIDS, or severe reaction to pertussis vaccine by a family member is not a contraindication to pertussis immunization. All families should be informed of the risks and benefits of pertussis vaccine and given advice about appropriate medical care in the event of a seizure.

Tetanus

Tetanus toxoid is an excellent immunizing agent. Every child should receive adsorbed tetanus toxoid during infancy, usually administered in the form of DTP vaccine (see under Diphtheria, above, and Table 9–3). Older children and adults receive Td or booster injections of purified tetanus toxoid (T) every 7–10 years unless wound management dictates otherwise. More frequent boosters may be accompanied by local hypersensitivity reactions.

Poliomyelitis

Live, trivalent oral poliovirus vaccine (OPV) provides effective immunity and is the choice for immunization of infants in most countries. Some countries (eg, Sweden) utilize repeated injections of inactivated poliovirus vaccines (IPV).

A. Live Polio Vaccine (Sabin): Attenuated strains of virus types I, II, and III are grown in cell culture. Standardized suspensions of virus are stored frozen until they are administered orally. OPV is commonly administered to infants 2–3 times at 2-month intervals. This schedule usually ensures development of antibodies and immunity to all 3 types of viruses. Boosters are frequently given at 15–19 months and at 4–6 years of age; they may be given later in life under special circumstances (eg, travel to endemic regions, an outbreak of poliomyelitis).

Live monovalent vaccines are not commercially available in the USA but can be obtained from the CDC and public health departments for use in epidemic situations.

OPV is contraindicated in children with immunodeficiency diseases, including HIV infection (Table 9–6). Children who have household contacts with immunodeficiency diseases, or who are immunosuppressed because of pharmacologic or radiation therapy should receive IPV because of the possible risk of acquiring paralytic disease from virus shedding. Vaccine-associated paralysis in vaccinees or contacts have been reported to occur at a rate of one in 7.8 million. Parents and vaccinees should be informed of this rare adverse reaction.

Table 9–6. Recommendations for routine immunization of HIV-infected children—United States, 1988.[1]

Vaccine	HIV Infection	
	Known Asymptomatic	Symptomatic
DTP[2]	Yes	Yes
OPV[3]	No	No
IPV[4]	Yes	Yes
MMR[5]	Yes	Yes[6]
PRP-D[7]	Yes	Yes
Pneumococcal	No	Yes
Influenza	No	Yes

[1] Reprinted with permission from MMWR 1988;**37**:181–183.
[2] DTP = diphtheria and tetanus toxoids and pertussis vaccine.
[3] OPV = oral, attenuated poliovirus vaccine; contains poliovirus types 1, 2, and 3.
[4] IPV = inactivated poliovirus vaccine; contains poliovirus types 1, 2, and 3.
[5] MMR = live measles, mumps, and rubella viruses in a combined vaccine.
[6] Should be considered.
[7] PRP-D = *Haemophilus influenzae* type b conjugate vaccine.

B. Inactivated Polio Vaccine (Salk): Mixtures of all 3 types of viruses grown in cell culture and inactivated by formaldehyde (IPV) are available. IPV is the preparation of choice for immunization of immunodeficient children, for primary vaccination of persons over 18 years of age, and for immunocompromised adults. The new enhanced-potency IPV is the current recommended form of vaccine; the dosage schedule is 2 doses 4–8 weeks apart with the final dose given 6–12 months later. This schedule coincides with the first 2 and the fourth DPT doses given in infancy. Children who have received the earlier form of IPV should receive a dose of enhanced-potency IPV before entering school. The requirement for 5-year boosters of enhanced-potency IPV has not been established. There have been no reported serious adverse reactions to IPV.

Measles

Live attenuated measles virus vaccine is grown in cell culture. MMR is given subcutaneously according to the manufacturer's instructions. Care must be taken to ensure the potency of the MMR vaccine. MMR may be inactivated by heat and light, so the vaccine must be kept at 35.6–46.5°F or colder and must be protected from light.

The number of reported cases of measles in the United

States reached a nadir of 1497 in 1983, but rose to 6282 cases in 1986. Reported cases of measles declined in 1987 and 1988 but rose again to 14,000 cases in 1989. Measles cases occur most frequently in unvaccinated preschool-aged children and previously vaccinated school-aged children. Both children in junior high school and college students have been infected during measles outbreaks in schools.

The increase in measles cases in school-aged children prompted the ACIP and American Academy of Pediatrics to recommend a 2-dose schedule for administration of MMR vaccine. The new 2-dose schedule attempts to protect the estimated 5% of children who do not respond to the initial dose of MMR.

The first dose of MMR is usually given at 15 months of age but can be given at any age thereafter. If vaccine is given earlier than 15 months, a significant number of individuals will fail to become immune, presumably as a result of persistent transplacental antibody. The ACIP recommends a second dose of MMR upon entrance to kindergarten (4–6 years of age). This recommendation was made to fit into the pre-existing immunization schedule for children. In contrast, the Red Book Committee recommends the second dose of MMR at the time of entry to middle or junior high school (11–12 years of age).

State or local health departments may require the second dose of MMR at school entry. Practitioners should be familiar with current local requirements.

Colleges, technical schools, and post–high school educational programs should require students who were born after 1957 to provide documentation of 2 doses of measles-containing vaccine, documentation of physician-diagnosed measles disease, or laboratory evidence of measles immunity. Students who have no documentation of measles immunity should receive 1 dose of MMR at the time of school entry and a second dose of MMR no less than 1 month after the first dose. Similar recommendations apply to medical personnel.

During local measles outbreaks or in areas with recurrent measles transmission among preschool-aged children (a county with 5 cases of measles among preschool children during each of the previous 5 years, a county with a recent outbreak among unvaccinated preschool-aged children, and cities with large unvaccinated populations), monovalent measles vaccine may be given as early as 6 months of age or the first visit thereafter. Children vaccinated with MMR before 12 months of age should have a repeat vaccination at 15 months of age and a third dose at the time of entry to junior high or middle school.

During school outbreaks of measles, all children and their

siblings born after January 1, 1957, who have not received 2 doses of measles-containing vaccine after 12 months of age should be revaccinated.

The "further attenuated" measles virus vaccine (Moraten strain) is the only type of vaccine currently available in the USA. In 5% of children, the live MMR vaccine may produce a transient rash 6–14 days after vaccination. Five to 15% of children develop a fever of 39.4°C (103°F) or higher beginning 6–14 days postvaccination and lasting 1–2 days. Children with febrile seizures may be given antipyretic prophylaxis realizing that the treatment should begin before the expected onset of fever and continued for 1 week. Postvaccine encephalitis has been reported in one per 3 million doses of MMR.

Contraindications to measles vaccine include pregnancy, immunodeficiency, immunosuppression, recent administration of immune globulin, and known anaphylactic reaction to materials in the vaccine (ie, eggs, neomycin).

Although immunodeficiency is a contraindication to the administration of live virus vaccines, children with pediatric HIV should be considered for receipt of MMR (see Table 9–6). Measles is a severe disease with frequent mortality in children with HIV infection. The seemingly small risk of adverse reactions to MMR vaccine in children with symptomatic HIV infection needs to be weighed against the likelihood of acquiring measles. In most children with HIV infection, whether symptomatic or not, MMR is probably indicated.

Mumps

Mumps is usually benign but can be accompanied by aseptic meningitis, pancreatitis, orchitis, or oophoritis. Live vaccine confers immunity.

Live attenuated mumps vaccine is a chick embryo–adapted virus. It is dispensed as a freeze-dried powder that must be reconstituted before subcutaneous administration. (Follow manufacturer's directions for reconstitution). Mumps vaccine is usually combined with live measles and rubella vaccines (MMR vaccine) for administration to infants.

Contraindications to mumps vaccine are listed in the manufacturer's package insert and include immunodeficiency, hypersensitivity to eggs, and all contraindications to measles vaccine (listed above).

Rubella

Rubella is a benign disease in children, but infection in pregnant women and the resulting fetal infection can have catastrophic consequences. Maternal antibodies can fully protect the fetus.

It is urged that all infants be given live attenuated rubella vaccine (strain RA 27/3, grown in diploid cells), usually in combination with live measles and mumps vaccines (see above). The manufacturer's directions should be followed. Follow the same precautions as with measles and mumps vaccines.

Rubella vaccine may be given to prepubertal girls and to nonpregnant, susceptible women (ie, those with negative serologic test results). Such persons should be advised not to become pregnant for at least 3 months after receiving vaccine. The vaccine strain occasionally has been isolated from placental tissues of women inadvertently vaccinated during pregnancy, but no fetal abnormalities have been definitely associated with such an occurrence. Inadvertent administration of rubella vaccine to more than 250 pregnant women has not resulted in congenital rubella syndrome. Efforts should be made to ensure that other groups, such as college students, military recruits, and postpubertal males and females, are immunized. Prenatal and antepartum screening for rubella is recommended and the vaccine should be administered to susceptible women in the immediate postpartum period prior to discharge. Protection of daycare workers, school employees, and health care workers, both male and female, should be ensured either with a history of immunization or actual disease.

Adverse reactions, which may occur 5–12 days after immunization, include fever, rash, and lymphadenopathy in a small number of children. Postpubertal females may have pain in small peripheral joints 7–21 days postvaccine, but arthritis is uncommon.

Persons with sensitivities to egg may have systemic anaphylactic (hypotension, urticaria, shock, wheezing, laryngospasm, or swelling of the mouth or throat) or urticarial reactions to measles, mumps, and influenza vaccines that contain trace amounts of egg antigens. Persons with a history of egg sensitivity should not receive egg-derived vaccines until they have been skin tested using the vaccine in question. Since skin testing may result in an anaphylactic reaction, only trained personnel who are familiar with the treatment of acute anaphylaxis should perform antigen skin testing.

Haemophilus influenzae Type b Conjugate Vaccine (PRP-D)

Haemophilus influenzae type b vaccine (PRP-D) is a concentrated, purified preparation of the polyribitol antigen of the organism covalently linked to diphtheria toxoid. Conjugate vac-

cine has shown greater immunogenicity than previous polysaccharide vaccine (PRP). Children should receive 0.5 mL of the
vaccine intramuscularly at 18 months of age. Children who received polysaccharide vaccine between 18–24 months of age
should be revaccinated with PRP-D. There is no need to revac-
cinate children who received polysaccharide vaccine at 24
months or older. Children at high risk (splenectomized children,
children with functional asplenia or congenital asplenia, attendees at daycare centers, and children with malignancies associated with immunosuppression) should receive the vaccine.
Children with invasive *Haemophilus* disease before 24 months of
age should be immunized with PRP-D. The vaccine may be given
along with the DPT vaccine, although at a different site.

IMMUNIZATIONS FOR CHILDREN
WITH SPECIAL INDICATIONS

Hepatitis B Vaccine

Recombinant DNA hepatitis B vaccine became available in
July, 1986. Plasma-derived hepatitis B vaccine was available
prior to that time. The immunogenicity of the two vaccines is
comparable. Table 9–7 lists recommendations for use of the
hepatitis B vaccine. The vaccine is given in a series of 3 doses at
0, 1, and 6 months. For adults and children over 10 years of age,

Table 9–7. Persons for whom hepatitis B vaccine is recommended or
should be considered.*

Preexposure
Persons for whom vaccine is recommended:
   Health care workers having blood or needle-stick exposures
   Clients and staff of institutions for the developmentally disabled
   Hemodialysis patients
   Homosexually active men
   Users of illicit injectable drugs
   Recipients of certain blood products
   Household members and sexual contacts of HBV carriers
   Special high-risk populations
Persons for whom vaccine should be considered:
   Inmates of long-term correctional facilities
   Heterosexually active persons with multiple sexual partners
   International travelers to HBV-endemic areas
Postexposure
   Infants born to HBV positive mothers
   Health-care workers having needle-stick exposures to human blood

* Reprinted with permission from MMWR 1987;**36**:353–360.

the recommended dose is 1 mL per dose given in the deltoid muscle. Children less than 10 years old should receive 0.5 mL by the same schedule and technique. Children born to mothers who are HBsAg carriers should receive the vaccine at birth along with a single dose of HBIG, 0.5 mL, given intramuscularly into the anterolateral thigh at a different site from the hepatitis B vaccine. These children should receive the second and third doses of vaccine at 1 and 6 months of age. Adverse reactions from the vaccine are limited to soreness at the injection site.

Cholera

For children traveling to or residing in areas where cholera is endemic (or for travel to countries that require a certificate of cholera vaccination), suspensions of killed *Vibrio cholerae* vaccine give only partial protection from disease and must be repeated at 6-month intervals. The vaccination is used primarily to satisfy the requirements of several countries for vaccination prior to travel. Newer subunit or recombinant live vaccines appear safer and more efficacious in several trials and will probably replace currently available killed vaccines. Control of sanitation and use of chemoprophylaxis are also necessary. The vaccine is not recommended in the control of cholera outbreaks nor for infants less than 6 months of age.

Influenza

Epidemic influenza A or B may cause serious respiratory disease in infants or children with cardiac, pulmonary, metabolic, renal, or neurologic disease, including those with immunodeficiency and immunosuppression. Institutionalized children or those in child-care centers are at special risk. For these individuals, influenza vaccines may reduce the risk of serious illness or complications. Routine immunization is recommended *only* for children at increased risk—not for normal healthy infants and children.

The subtypes of influenza A and B to be incorporated into vaccines are selected every year, based on the strains expected to circulate during the next season. Viruses are grown in embryonated chicken eggs, purified, chemically inactivated, and made into "split" virus products. To avoid severe febrile reactions, *only* the split virus form of vaccine should be given to children less than 12 years old. More than one injection, given 4 or more weeks apart, is usually required for primary immunization. For children previously vaccinated, boosters are indicated every year. Each year, the CDC issues recommendations for influenza vaccine usage in children. Hypersensitivity to eggs is a contraindication. (See skin testing protocol above.)

Meningococcal Meningitis

Polysaccharide preparations derived from meningococcus groups A, C, Y, and W-135 are available. The type A polysaccharide is immunogenic in children 3 months of age and older, but the other types are poorly immunogenic in infants less than 2 years of age. Meningococcal vaccine is indicated during meningococcal outbreaks, if an individual plans to visit or reside in a country with endemic meningococcal disease, for children with asplenia, and for individuals with increased susceptibility to disease owing to absence of the terminal components of the complement cascade. The manufacturer's directions for dosage regimens should be followed. The vaccine is well tolerated.

Plague

Killed *Yersinia pestis* vaccine may be used in children traveling in or residing in areas where plague is highly endemic, but is not recommended for routine use in plague enzootic areas of the country. The vaccine should be given in doses recommended by the manufacturer. Control of exposure to vectors and use of chemoprophylaxis are necessary.

Pneumococcal Vaccine

A mixture of capsular polysaccharides from 23 types of pneumococci, including those that account for about 80% of bacteremic infections, is available. This preparation is not recommended for routine immunization. It should be considered for use in children at high risk of death from pneumococcal infection and in children over 2 years of age who suffer from sickle cell disease, asplenia, nephrosis, and B cell immunodeficiencies. Vaccination of children with recurrent otitis media is controversial, but the vaccine may be beneficial. The vaccine is well tolerated in children, but some children 2 years of age or older fail to develop adequate antibody responses. Children in high-risk groups must receive penicillin prophylaxis against life-threatening pneumococcal infections. The manufacturer's directions for dosage regimen, limitations, and side effects should be followed.

Rabies

Rabies develops following bites by rabid animals. It is almost always fatal. Because the disease is so feared, many persons receive rabies treatment after contact with an animal even when the chance may be very small that the animal was rabid.

Rabies Vaccine Adsorbed was licensed on March 18, 1988. This is a new cell culture–derived rabies vaccine for use in humans for both preexposure and postexposure use. The Biologic Products Program of the Michigan Department of Health developed and now produces and distributes the vaccine. The vaccine currently is available only to residents of Michigan but may soon be available outside that state. RVA differs from other human diploid cell rabies vaccines (HDCV) in the manufacturing process but the preexposure and postexposure immunization schedule is the same. Preexposure immunization requires three 1 mL doses of vaccine given intramuscularly on days 0, 7, and 28. Postexposure vaccination in previously unimmunized individuals consists of five 1-mL intramuscular doses on days 0, 3, 7, 14, and 28. The vaccine should not be given in the buttock; the deltoid muscle is the preferred site in adults, and the anterolateral thigh should be used in children. For postexposure vaccination, 20 IU/kg of rabies immune globulin (RIG) is recommended. One half the dose is infiltrated around the wound and the remainder is given intramuscularly at a site separate from the vaccine. Persons with previous vaccination need only 1 mL of RVA given intramuscularly on days 0 and 3. Adverse reactions to RVA are similar to those to HDCV and include pain, redness, and swelling at injection site in 85–90% of vaccinees, and fever, nausea, and arthralgia in 10%. Approximately 6% of persons vaccinated wiht HDCV developed a serum sickness–like allergic reaction.

Smallpox

Live vaccinia virus was long used and was highly effective for the prevention of smallpox. It was a major factor in the eradication of that disease from the world in 1980. At present, no indication exists for the use of this vaccine in civilians. However, since military personnel are still being immunized with the vaccine, it is important to be aware of complications of vaccinia. The vaccine should never be given to persons with eczema, other forms of dermatitis, or impaired cell-mediated immunity, because it may produce eczema vaccinatum, vaccinia necrosum, or postvaccinial encephalitis.

Tuberculosis

Bacille Calmette-Guérin (BCG) is an attenuated strain of *Mycobacterium bovis;* different substrains of the organism are produced as vaccine in different countries. These substrains exhibit marked differences in invasiveness and immunogenicity. Studies of the effectiveness of BCG vary significantly, and therefore use of BCG is controversial. Administration of BCG is limited to individuals who have negative results in the tuberculin skin test and who are at very high risk of infection because of (1) intimate and prolonged contact with persons untreated or ineffectively treated for pulmonary tuberculosis, or (2) exposure to persons with isoniazid- or rifampin-resistant tuberculosis and who cannot be removed from the source of exposure. BCG is also recommended for infants and children who live in areas where the rate of new infections exceeds 1% per year and where usual treatment programs have failed. The manufacturer's recommendations must be followed. BCG is not recommended for health care workers. These workers should be monitored by periodic tuberculin skin testing and isoniazid therapy for skin test–positive workers. Use of BCG varies widely in different countries, depending on socioeconomic conditions and on available measures for medical and public health control of active tuberculosis. Any form of immune deficiency is an absolute contraindication to the administration of BCG because of the possibility of disseminated and fatal BCG infection. The tuberculin skin test in a child injected with BCG will yield positive results, at least temporarily. The PPD should be repeated 2–3 months after immunization; immunization should be repeated if the child remains PPD negative. Immunization with BCG should not supplant isoniazid prophylaxis, which is of proved efficacy.

Typhoid

Children traveling to areas where exposure to typhoid is likely, or children who have intimate exposure to a documented typhoid carrier, may be given inactivated *Salmonella typhi* vaccine as recommended by the manufacturer. The vaccine causes fever, swelling, and pain at the injection site in the majority of recipients and provides only partial protection against infection. To maintain resistance, booster injections are required at intervals.

Varicella-Zoster

A vaccine of live attenuated varicella-zoster, OKA strain, has been used extensively in normal children in Japan; in this country, similar vaccines have been tested extensively in susceptible immunosuppressed children receiving chemotherapy for neoplasia. This vaccine appears to be protective and safe, but is not currently licensed.

Yellow Fever

For children 9 months of age or older living in or visiting areas where yellow fever is endemic, a single injection of live attenuated vaccine (consisting of the 17D strain of yellow fever virus) is indicated. The vaccine is administered only by certain public health officials and may be repeated 6–8 years later. A valid certificate for yellow fever vaccination is required for travel to some countries.

MATERIALS USED FOR PASSIVE IMMUNIZATION

IMMUNE GLOBULINS

Standard immune globulin (IG) is prepared from pooled plasma and contains sufficient antibodies against measles, hepatitis, and other pathogens to be used as follows:

(1) For **measles prophylaxis** in unimmunized individuals exposed to the disease, give 0.25 mL/kg intramuscularly as a single dose; the maximum dose is 15 mL. For immunocompromised susceptible individuals, the dose is 0.5 mL/kg.

(2) For **hepatitis A prophylaxis** in individuals exposed to hepatitis A virus, give 0.02 mL/kg intramuscularly. Susceptible individuals include family contacts of the index case and daycare workers and children in the same classroom as the index case. If the daycare setting involves children who are not yet toilet trained and HAV infection is identified in an employee or child, or if household contacts of 2 children in a daycare setting contract HAV, all employees and enrolled children should receive IG. If the exposure is continuous, such as occurs in endemic areas of the world, this dose should be repeated in 5 months.

Recent studies have shown that intravenous immunoglobulin is more effective than intramuscular immune globulin. Several preparations of IVIG are now available for use in a number of conditions, yet its use in other conditions remains controversial. There is good evidence that IVIG is efficacious in the following conditions: primary hypogammaglobulinemia, neonates predisposed to group B streptococcal infections, selected cases of idiopathic thrombocytopenic purpura, Kawasaki disease, bone marrow and renal transplant recipients at risk for cytomegalovirus infections, and patients with lymphocytic leukemia.

Several special immune globulins are available: tetanus (TIG), rabies (RIG), varicella-zoster (VZIG), and hepatitis B (HBIG). Consult the product brochure, and follow the advice of the CDC and the Infectious Diseases Committee of the American Academy of Pediatrics for their use in specific situations.

SKIN TESTS

Coccidioidin Skin Test

A. Test Materials: A 1:100 dilution of the filtrate obtained from a culture of *Coccidioides immitis* grown in a synthetic medium. Spherulin (derived from spherules of *Coccidioides* in culture) is more sensitive but less specific than coccidioidin as a skin testing material.

B. Indications: For detecting sensitivity to *C immitis*. The test does not evoke humoral antibodies.

C. Dosage and Administration: The 1:100 material is injected intradermally and read at 24 and 48 hours. Patients with coccidioidal erythema nodosum are likely to be very sensitive; therefore, an initial testing with 1:10,000 dilution is advisable. If this test is negative, 1:100 can be used.

D. Results and Interpretation: Induration over 4 mm in diameter at either 24 or 48 hours is considered positive. Positive reactions may be obtained 2–3 weeks after infection and remain positive for many years.

Histoplasmin Skin Test

A. Test Material: Culture filtrate of *Histoplasma capsulatum*.

B. Indications: For epidemiologic studies. The histoplasmin skin test stimulates a rise in antibodies and is therefore rarely used in diagnosis. There are probably cross-reactions with other fungi. Serologic tests have taken the place of the histoplasmin skin test.

C. Dosage and Administration: 0.1 mL of a 1:100 dilution is injected intradermally and read at 48 and 72 hours.

D. Results and Interpretation: The reaction is positive if at either reading the area of induration is more than 5 mm in diameter.

Tuberculin Skin Test (Mantoux Test)

A. Test Material: Purified protein derivative of tuberculin (PPD). PPD is a highly purified protein fraction isolated from culture filtrates of human-type strains of *Mycobacterium tuberculosis*.

B. Indications: For determination of tuberculin sensitivity. Annual testing should be completed on high-risk groups such as American Indians and Eskimos or children from neighborhoods with a tuberculosis case rate higher than the national average. Low-risk children should be screened at 12–15 months of age, before school entry, and at 14–16 years of age. Tuberculosis testing is indicated for contacts of persons with known tuberculous disease.

C. Dosage and Administration: A 0.1 mL injectin of 5 TU-PPD should be made intradermally on the flexor surface of the forearm so as to raise a small bleb. PPD should be stored in a cool dark place and should be injected as soon as it is drawn up into a syringe.

D. Results and Interpretation: The Mantoux test should be read at 48–72 hours. Reactions of 10 mm or more are considered positive. If the child has a reaction of 5 mm or more, a complete history, physical examination, and chest roentgenogram should be taken. The Mantoux test should be repeated at 4–6 weeks in those with a reaction < 10 mm. Once a child has exhibited a positive result to the tuberculin skin test, the test should not be repeated.

· Tuberculosis skin testing may be done on same day as administration of the MMR, but PPD should not be given within 4–6 weeks of the MMR vaccine because of possible suppression of reactivity. Negative results in the Mantoux test occur in patients with measles and other viral illnesses, persons who have received live virus vaccines, and patients who are immunosuppressed or immunocompromised. False-positive results in the Mantoux test (often indurations of small diameter) occur in patients with infections due to nontuberculous mycobacteria.

Tuberculin Skin Test (Tine Test)

A. Test Material: Dried purified protein derivative of tuberculin (PPD) or old tuberculin (OT) on disposable metal tines.

B. Indications: For screening apparently healthy groups. This test should not be used for diagnosis of tuberculosis. It is less sensitive and less specific than the intradermal Mantoux test with PPD.

C. Dosage and Administration: The volar surface of the mid forearm is cleansed, and the tines are firmly but briefly pressed into the skin. The metal tines deliver an approximate dose of intermediate strength when pressed into the skin. The results are read in 48 hours.

D. Results and Interpretation: Size of induration is compared with the pattern provided by the manufacturer. If significant induration is found in a healthy child, results should be confirmed by Intradermal Mantoux test before chemoprophylaxis is considered.

10 | The Newborn Infant: Assessment & General Care

David W. Boyle, MD, &
Gerald B. Merenstein, MD, FAAP

Assessment and care of the newborn infant can be divided into 3 distinct phases: antenatal evaluation, delivery room management, and postnatal care.

ANTENATAL EVALUATION

The antenatal evaluation begins with a thorough history that includes the medical history of the mother and father (including relevant genetic history), the previous obstetric history of the mother, and the history of the current pregnancy. Particular attention should be paid to chronic illnesses in the mother; use by the mother of medications, drugs, alcohol, or cigarettes; and acute problems in the mother such as bleeding, pregnancy-induced hypertension, or gestational diabetes (Table 10–1).

Anticipation of the delivery of an infant at high risk has allowed for a steady decline in neonatal mortality (Fig 10–1a,b). The risk of neonatal mortality and morbidity is increased in pregnancies associated with a variety of maternal, labor and delivery, and fetal conditions (Table 10–2). High-risk pregnancies should be identified early and monitored carefully for evidence of fetal distress. Whenever possible, arrangements should be made to deliver mothers with high-risk pregnancies at perinatal centers, to avoid transport of the infant after delivery.

DELIVERY ROOM MANAGEMENT

Transition from Fetus to Newborn

Successful resuscitation of the neonate begins with an understanding of the normal physiologic events that occur during the transition from fetal to newborn life. In the fetus the placenta

Table 10–1. Maternal drugs and effects in the fetus and newborn.

Drug	Effect
Progestins, testosterone, and other hormones	Virilization and advanced bone age of female fetus
Thalidomide	Phocomelia
Nitrofurantoin	Hemolysis
Sulfonamides, novobiocin, oxacillin, cephalothin, sodium benzoate, and salicylates	Competitive binding with albumin in serum with resultant hyperbilirubinemia due to displacement of bilirubin
Chloramphenicol	Cardiovascular collapse and the "gray baby syndrome"
Aminopterin, methorexate, and chlorambucil	Anomalies and abortions
Dicumarol	Hemorrhage and fetal death
Heroin, morphine, and other narcotics	Tremors, neonatal death, and neonatal withdrawal symptoms in maternal addiction
Smoking	Intrauterine growth retardation
Streptomycin	Deafness
Cancer chemotherapeutic agents and phenothiazines	Parkinsonism-like syndrome
Mepiracaine and lidocaine	Central nervous system depression or seizures and irritability
Thiazides	Electrolyte imbalance, thrombocytopenia, and leukopenia
Inorganic mercury	Brain damage with cerebral palsy
Reserpine	Nasal congestion, bradycardia, hypothermia, and drowsiness
Tetracyclines	Retarded bone growth and mottled and stained teeth
Magnesium sulfate	Depression or convulsions (rare)
General anesthetics	Respiratory distress
Spinal anesthetics	Maternal hypotension with fetal distress
Paracervical block	Fetal bradycardia
Oxytocin induction	Water intoxication in the mother and hyponatremia, hypotension, and hypotonia in the infant
Vitamin K_3	Hyperbilirubinemia
Salicylates	Coagulation defects with neonatal bleeding
Quinine	Thrombocytopenia and deafness
Ganglionic blocking agents	Paralytic ileus
Phenobarbitol	Increase the rate of neonatal drug metabolism; a large dose may depress the infant; barbiturate withdrawl; neonatal

(continued)

Table 10–1. (Continued)

Drug	Effect
	hemorrhage due to depletion of vitamin K–dependent factors
Hexamethonium	Ileus
Atropine	Tachycardia
Prochlorperazine	Depression
Chloroquine	Retinal damage
Corticosteriods	Adrenal insufficiency
Oral hypoglycemic agents	Hypoglycemia
Radioiodine	Fetal thyroid destruction
Thiouracil derivative, potassium iodide, and potassium perchlorate	Congential goiter
Phenytoin	Congenital anomalies (fetal hydantoin syndrome); neonatal hemorrhage due to depletion of vitamin K–dependent factors

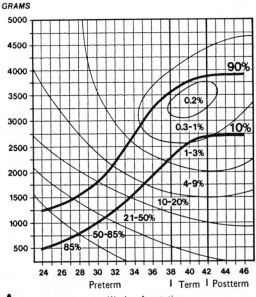

A

Figure 10–1a. Neonatal mortality risk by birth weight and gestational age, 1958–1969, based on 14,436 live births at the University of Colorado Health Sciences Center. (Reproduced, with permission, from Koops BL, Morgan LJ, Battaglia FC: Neonatal mortality risk in relation to birth weight and gestational age: An update. *J Pediatr* 1982;**101**:969.)

is the organ of gas exchange. The fetal circulation represents 2 circuits in parallel (Fig 10–2). Oxygenated blood from the placenta is carried by the umbilical vein (P_{O_2} approximately 35 torr) through the ductus venosus to the inferior vena cava (P_{O_2} approximately 28 torr). Inferior vena cava blood flows preferentially through the right atrium to the left atrium via the foramen ovale, where it mixes with pulmonary venous return, and then into the left ventricle (P_{O_2} approximately 26 torr). The left ventricular output supplies the myocardium, brain, and upper body via the ascending aorta and returns to the right atrium via the superior vena cava (P_{O_2} approximately 12 torr). Superior vena cava blood flows preferentially through the right atrium to the right ventricle (P_{O_2} approximately 16 torr) and out through the main pulmonary artery. Since pulmonary vascular resistance is high owing to constriction of the pulmonary arterioles, and systemic vascular

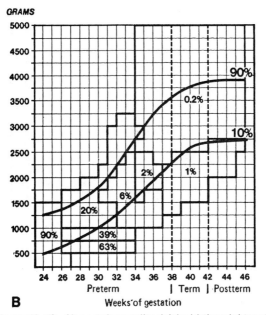

GRAMS

B

Weeks of gestation

Figure 10–1b. Neonatal mortality risk by birth weight and gestational age, 1974–1980, based on 14,413 live births at the University of Colorado Health Sciences Center. (Reproduced, with permission, from Koops BL, Morgan LJ, Battaglia FC: Neonatal mortality risk in relation to birth weight and gestational age: An update. *J. Pediatr* 1982;**101**:969.)

Table 10–2. Factors that increase neonatal morbidity and mortality.

Maternal Conditions	Labor and Delivery Conditions	Fetal Conditions
Previous neonatal death	Premature/prolonged rupture of membranes	Multiple gestation
Previous congenital anomalies	Prolapsed umbilical cord/cord compression	Premature delivery
Incompetent cervix	Abnormal presentation (face, brow, breech, transverse, lie, dystocia)	Fetal distress (abnormal heart rate or rhythm; passage of meconium; acidosis, fetal scalp capillary pH < 7.20)
Antepartum hemorrhage (placenta previa, abruptio placenta)	Prolonged labor	Oligo/polyhydramnios
Blood type or group isoimmunization	Mid or high forceps delivery	Intrauterine growth retardation
Maternal infection (rubella, cytomegalovirus, human immunodeficiency virus, hepatitis B virus, varicella-zoster, chlamydia, herpes simplex virus, gonorrhea, group B streptococcus, listeria, syphilis, tuberculosis, toxoplasmosis, etc)	Cesarean section	Macrosomia
Chronic maternal illness (hyertension, diabetes [including gestational], renal disease, thyroid disease, cardiovascular disease, anemia, collagen or vascular disease, convulsive disorders, etc)	Complications of analgesia or anesthesia	Fetal malformations
Maternal age <16 or >35 years	Maternal hypotension	Evidence of immaturity of pulmonary surfactant system (low lecithin: sphingomyelin ratio/absence of phosphatidylglycerol in amniotic fluid)
No prenatal care	Chorioamnionitis	
Ethanol or other substance abuse		
Smoking		

264

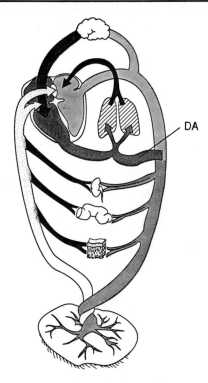

Figure 10–2. A schematic representation of the fetal circulation. Highest oxygenated blood is without stippling; lowest oxygenated blood is with heaviest stippling. DA = ductus arteriosus. (Reproduced, with permission, from Avery GB: *Neonatology: Pathophysiology and Management of the Newborn.* Philadelphia, J.B. Lippincott Company, 1987.)

resistance is low owing to the placenta, most of the right ventricular output is shunted across the ductus arteriosus mixing with blood from the ascending aorta to supply the lower body via the descending aorta (P_{o2} approximately 20 torr). Blood returns to the placenta via the umbilical arteries.

With delivery of the infant and the onset of respiration, the lungs become the organ of gas exchange. The neonate must convert from fetal to adult circulation (Fig 10–3). With lung expansion, pulmonary vascular resistance falls and pulmonary blood flow increases owing to uncoiling of pulmonary vessels and

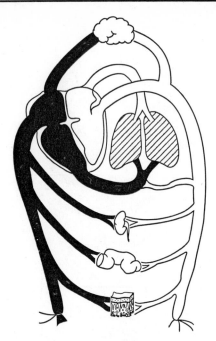

Figure 10–3. A schematic representation of the circulation in the normal newborn. Oxygenated blood is light; deoxygenated blood is dark. (Reproduced, with permission, from Avery GB: *Neonatology: Pathophysiology and Management of the Newborn.* Philadelphia, J.B. Lippincott Company, 1987.)

vasodilatation as a result of increasing P_{O_2}. Pressures fall in the pulmonary artery, right ventricle, and right atrium, while left atrial pressure rises because of an increase in pulmonary venous return and an increase in systemic vascular resistance owing to the removal of the placenta from the circulation. Left atrial pressure exceeds right atrial pressure, thus closing the foramen ovale. Systemic pressure exceeds pulmonary pressure and shunting through the ductus arteriosus is reversed. Increasing arterial oxygen tension leads to constriction of the ductus arteriosus. Failure of the normal circulatory adaptations leads to persistent pulmonary hypertension.

Successful transition also requires that the neonate remove the liquid present in the lung prior to birth and establish the neonatal lung volume. As much as 30 mL of fetal lung fluid is removed during passage through the birth canal as a result of the "physiologic squeeze." Active removal of fluid via absorption by alveolar epithelial cells as well as increases in pulmonary blood and lymphatic flows allows for clearance of fetal lung liquid in the first few hours after normal vaginal delivery. Retention of fetal lung fluid, as occurs in preterm infants, infants of diabetic mothers, and infants born by cesarean section, results in transient tachypnea of the newborn.

Many factors are responsible for the onset of postnatal breathing: sensory stimuli such as cold, light, noise, gravity, and pain; chemical stimuli such as hypoxemia, hypercapnia, and acidosis; and mechanical gasp reflexes caused by the elastic recoil of the thorax after delivery. The initial lung inflation may require pressure of 30–40 cm H_2O, but pressures as great as 60–70 cm H_2O are not uncommon. Subsequent breaths in the normal newborn require 15–20 cm H_2O pressure.

Blood gases and pH in the neonate normalize shortly after birth. The pH of fetal blood is only slightly lower (0.05 pH unit) than the adult value. During labor the pH falls slightly but is generally normal (blood pH approximately 7.4) within 1–3 hours after birth. Fetal P_{co2} is slightly higher than maternal P_{co2}. Following recovery from birth, the normal neonate has a lower P_{co2} (approximately 32 torr) than does the adult. As noted above, fetal P_{o2} is much lower than the adult value. During the first 24 hours of life, the Pa_{o2} increases from about 55 torr shortly after birth to about 90 torr.

Physiology of Asphyxia

Failure of the organ of gas exchange prenatally, intrapartum, or postnatally will lead to hypoxemia and respiratory acidosis. If this condition persists, tissue hypoxia and metabolic acidosis will develop, with subsequent end organ injury. The physiology of asphyxia is illustrated in Figure 10–4. The initial response to hypoxia is an increase in the frequency of respiration and a rise in heart rate and blood pressure. Respirations then cease (primary apnea) as heart rate and blood pressure begin to fall. At this point tactile stimulation and free-flow oxygen are adequate to induce respirations (see Neonatal Resuscitation, below). However, if asphyxia continues, the infant develops gasping respirations followed by secondary or terminal apnea, while heart rate and blood pressure continue to fall. Positive-pressure ventilation is then required for resuscitation. A feature of the defense against hypoxia is that cardiac output is redistributed such that perfusion of the vital organs (brain and heart) is maintained at the expense of peripheral tissues (skin, muscle,

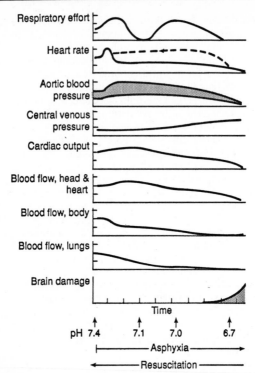

Respiratory effort

Heart rate

Aortic blood
pressure

Central venous
pressure

Cardiac output

Blood flow, head &
heart

Blood flow, body

Blood flow, lungs

Brain damage

Time

pH 7.4   7.1   7.0   6.7

├── Asphyxia ──→

←── Resuscitation ──

Figure 10–4. Schematic sequence of cardiopulmonary changes with asphyxia and resuscitation. (Adapted from Dawes G: *Foetal and Neonatal Physiology.* Chicago, Year Book Publishers, 1968.) (Reproduced, with permission, from Avery GB: *Neonatology: Pathophysiology and Management of the Newborn.* Philadelphia, J.B. Lippincott Company, 1987.)

and gastrointestinal tract). The above sequence of changes can occur in utero; therefore, one must assume that an infant who is apneic at birth is in secondary apnea and resuscitative efforts should proceed quickly. The physiologic response to resuscitation is the reverse of that of asphyxia.

Neonatal Resuscitation

Preparation and anticipation are the keys to successful neonatal resuscitation. The supplies and equipment necessary are listed in Table 10–3. At least one person skilled in initiating

Table 10–3. Equipment for neonatal resuscitation.*

Suction Equipment
  Bulb syringe
  DeLee mucus trap with #10 French catheter and mechanical suction
  Suction catheters #5 or #6, #8, #10 French
  #8 French feeding tube and 20-mL syringe
Ventilation Equipment
  Infant resuscitation bag connected to a pressure manometer or with
    a pressure-release valve; bag should be capable of delivering
    90–100% oxygen
  Soft-rimmed face masks—newborn and premature sizes
  Oral airways—newborn and premature sizes
  Oxygen with flowmeter and tubing
Intubation Equipment
  Neonatal laryngoscope with #0 and #1 straight blades
  Endotracheal tubes—sizes 2.5, 3.0, 3.5, 4.0 mm OD
  Stylet
Administration of Medications
  Sterile umbilical catheterization tray
  Umbilical catheters—#3.5 and #5.0 French
  Sterile syringes and needles
  Medications (as listed in text)
  Betadine and alcohol sponges
Miscellaneous
  Clock with sweep second hand
  Radiant warmer
  Gloves, gown, mask, goggles (universal precautions)
  Stethoscope
  Adhesive tape (1/2- or 3/4-inch width) and benzoin
  Scissors

* Modified and reproduced, with permission, from American Heart Association, American Academy of Pediatrics: *Textbook of Neonatal Resuscitation.* Dallas, AHA, 1987.

resuscitation should be present at every delivery. Intrapartum steps to support the infant include maintenance of maternal blood pressure, maternal oxygen therapy, and positioning of the mother to improve placental perfusion. Specific measures regarding management of the delivery of an infant through meconium-stained amniotic fluid will be addressed below.

The steps to be taken in neonatal resuscitation are as follows (Fig 10–5):

(1) Prevent heat loss.

(a) Transfer infant to a preheated radiant warmer.

(b) Dry infant thoroughly with warmed towel; remove wet towel.

(2) Open airway.

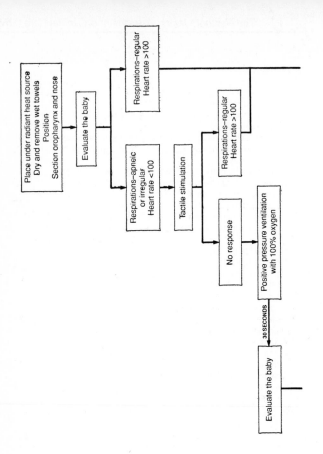

270

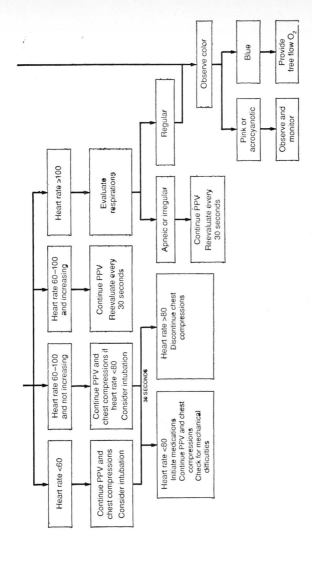

Figure 10–5. Delivery room management of the newborn. (Modified and reproduced, with permission, from American Heart Association and American Academy of Pediatrics: *Textbook of Neonatal Resuscitation.* Dallas, AHA, 1987.)

(a) Position infant on back or side in a slight Trendelenburg position with neck slightly extended.

(b) Gently suction the oropharynx and nose with a bulb syringe or #10 French suction catheter attached to wall suction.

(3) Evaluate the infant.

(a) Respirations.

(b) Heart rate.

(c) Color.

(4) If the infant's respirations are regular and the heart rate is greater than 100 beats per minute (bpm), observe color and provide free-flow oxygen at 5 liters per minute if there is evidence of central cyanosis. Slowly withdraw oxygen if infant remains pink.

(5) If the infant is apneic or has irregular respirations, or has a heart rate below 100 bpm, provide tactile stimulation by flicking the bottom of the foot or by rubbing the back, and provide free-flow oxygen at 5 liters per minute. Do not provide tactile stimulation for more than 10–15 seconds as the infant may be in secondary apnea and be unresponsive to these measures.

(6) If there is no response to tactile stimulation, proceed to positive-pressure ventilation with 100% oxygen using a resuscitation bag and a soft-rimmed mask. For the initial inflation, pressures of 30 to 40 cm H_2O may be necessary to overcome surface-active forces within the lung and expand the chest. In premature infants pressures of 40 to 60 cm H_2O may be needed. For subsequent breaths, pressures of 15 to 20 cm H_2O are often adequate to expand the chest unless pulmonary disease with decreased lung compliance is present. In the latter situation pressures of 20 to 40 cm H_2O may be needed. Ventilation of the infant should be performed at a rate of 40 to 60 per minute.

(7) Continue positive-pressure ventilation for 30 seconds and reevaluate the infant.

(a) If the heart rate is less than 60 bpm, continue positive-pressure ventilation and initiate chest compressions at a rate of 120 per minute to a depth of 1/2 to 3/4 inch.

(b) If the heart rate is between 60 and 100 bpm and increasing, continue positive-pressure ventilation. If the heart rate is between 60 and 100 bpm and not increasing, continue positive-pressure ventilation; initiate chest compressions if the heart rate is less than 80 bpm.

(c) If the heart rate is above 100 bpm, check for spontaneous respirations; if present, discontinue positive-pressure ventilation and provide free-flow oxygen for central cyanosis.

(8) Reevaluate the infant every 30 seconds. Discontinue chest compressions when the heart rate is greater than 80 bpm. If

the heart rate remains below 80 after 30 seconds of positive-pressure ventilation with 100% oxygen and chest compressions, medications are indicated. The drug of choice is epinephrine at a dose of 0.01 mg/kg (0.1 mL/kg of 1:10,000 epinephrine) given rapidly intravenously or per endotracheal tube. Epinephrine may be readministered every 5 minutes if required. Epinephrine is also indicated for a heart rate of 0.

(9) Most neonates will respond to positive-pressure ventilation with 100% oxygen. Rarely should a neonate require cardiac massage or drugs. In the event that an infant is not responding to resuscitative measures, mechanical difficulties should be ruled out or corrected (Table 10–4).

(10) Other medications to consider include:

(a) Volume expanders (whole blood, 5% albumin/saline solution, plasmanate, normal saline, Ringer's lactate). Give 10 mL/kg via umbilical venous line over 5–10 minutes if there is evidence of acute bleeding or signs of hypovolemia. May be repeated if necessary. Be careful not to induce fluid overload in the severely asphyxiated infant.

(b) Sodium bicarbonate. Give 1–2 meq/kg of 0.5 meq/mL (4.2% solution) intravenously over at least 2 minutes only after effective ventilation has been established. Should be given for *documented* metabolic acidosis.

(c) Naloxone hydrochloride. Give 0.1 mg/kg of Narcan (0.4 mg/mL or 1 mg/mL) rapidly intravenously, intramuscularly, subcutaneously, or intratracheally when there is *persistent* respiratory depression after resuscitation and a history of maternal narcotic administration within 4 hours of delivery. Naloxone

Table 10–4. Mechanical causes of failed resuscitation.*

Cause	Examples
Equipment failure	Malfunctioning bag, oxygen not connected or running
Endotracheal tube malposition	Esophagus, right main stem bronchus
Occluded endotracheal tube	
Insufficient inflation pressure to expand lungs	
Space-occupying lesions in the thorax	Pneumothorax, pleural effusions, diaphragmatic hernia
Pulmonary hypoplasia	Extreme prematurity, oligohydramnios

* Reproduced, with permission, from Rosenberg AA, Battaglia FC: The newborn infant. Chapter 4 in: *Current Pediatric Diagnosis and Treatment*, 10th ed. Hathaway WE et al (editors). Lange, 1990.

should not be given to an infant of a suspected drug-addicted mother as it might precipitate acute, severe withdrawal in the infant. Infants who receive naloxone should be closely observed for recurrence of respiratory depression as the duration of action of the narcotic may exceed that of naloxone.

(11) Apgar scores (Table 10–5) should be assigned at 1 and 5 minutes and every 5 minutes thereafter until 20 minutes have passed or until 2 consecutive scores of 7 or higher are obtained.

Before removing the infant from the delivery room, a brief screening examination, should be performed checking for gross abnormalities, adequate chest expansion and air exchange, heart tones, abdominal masses, torsion of testes, evidence of birth trauma, and color and perfusion of the skin. The umbilical cord should be checked for the number of vessels, and the placenta examined for size, identification of membranes and vessels, and evidence of infarcts and hemorrhage. Finally, the infant must be identified with a hospital bracelet. The pediatrician should encourage parental contact in the delivery room if the infant's condition permits.

Owing to the potential of infection with bloodborne pathogens such as human immunodeficiency virus and hepatitis B virus, the Centers for Disease Control recommends that all persons assisting in deliveries wear gloves, gowns, surgical masks,

Table 10–5. Apgar score of newborn infant.*

Sign	Score		
	0	1	2
A Appearance (color)	Blue; pale	Body pink; extremities blue	Completely pink
P Pulse (heart rate)	Absent	<100	>100
G Grimace (reflex irritability in response to stimulation of sole of foot)	No response	Grimace	Cry
A Activity (muscle tone)	Limp	Some flexion of extremities	Active motion
R Respiration (respiratory effort)	Absent	Slow;irregular	Good strong cry

* Practical epigram of Apgar Score. (Reproduced, with permission, from Butterfield J, Covey M: JAMA 1962;181:353. Copyright American Medical Association.)

and goggles; ie, practice universal precautions. Gloves should be worn when handling the placenta or infant until blood and amniotic fluid have been removed from the infant's skin. After the gloves are removed, hands and other skin surfaces contaminated with blood should be washed thoroughly with soap and water.

Special Considerations in Neonatal Resuscitation

A. Intubation: Endotracheal intubation should be considered in the following situations:

1. When the amniotic fluid is stained with meconium (see below).

2. In the preterm infant, especially those below 1000 grams.

3. When a diaphragmatic hernia is suspected.

4. When bag-and-mask ventilation is ineffective (eg, anatomic upper airway obstruction).

5. For prolonged positive-pressure ventilation.

6. In skilled hands, when there is a need for chest compressions.

To minimize hypoxia during intubation provide free-flow oxygen at 5 liters per minute near the baby's mouth and limit intubation attempts to 20 seconds.

B. Management of Infants with Meconium-Stained Amniotic Fluid:

1. Careful obstetric monitoring of fetal well-being is required.

2. As soon as the baby's head is delivered, pass a DeLee catheter or #10 French suction catheter attached to wall suction through the nares to the level of the nasopharynx and aspirate any meconium. Suction the mouth and hypopharynx.

3. If the meconium is thin or watery, complete delivery in the usual manner and provide routine resuscitation of the infant.

4. If the meconium is thick or particulate, immediately hand the baby to the pediatrician with minimal stimulation. Position the baby appropriately on the warmer and dry his/her face lightly. Suction out any residual meconium in the oropharynx using a #10 French catheter attached to wall suction.

5. If obstetric suctioning has been good and the baby already has vigorous respiratory efforts, no further intervention is indicated.

6. If obstetric suction has not been done (eg, precipitous delivery) or if the infant has not had respiratory efforts, perform direct laryngoscopy and endotracheal suctioning via an endotracheal tube and wall suction. When the airway is cleared of meconium, complete resuscitation in the usual manner.

Tracheobronchial saline lavage is not recommended and may lead to increased morbidity. Wall suction pressure should not exceed 100 mm Hg. Infants who have had meconium recovered from their trachea and who have been depressed should be watched closely for respiratory symptoms and arterial hypoxia. Oxygen should be used liberally to keep Pa_{O_2} greater than 80 mm Hg or Sa_{O_2} greater than 95%.

POSTNATAL CARE

Immediate Care of the Newborn

Place the infant in a heated crib or under a radiant warmer and maintain a stable axillary temperature between 36.3°C and 36.9°C. Avoid heat loss by drying the baby thoroughly and postponing the initial bath until the infant has stabilized and the temperature is normal. Cooling may interfere with the normal cardiovascular adjustments previously described and lead to persistent pulmonary hypertension. Assess gestational age based on the maternal menstrual history, obstetric milestones and gestational age assessment (eg, early ultrasound examination), and physical examination of the neonate (Figure 10–6). Weigh and measure length and head circumference and plot growth parameters versus gestational age to determine if the infant is appropriate size-for-gestational-age (AGA), small-for-gestational-age (SGA), or large-for-gestational-age (LGA) (Figure 10–7). This determination will assist in the identification of infants at increased risk for illness. Administer vitamin K_1 oxide (phytonadione) in a single parenteral dose of 0.5–1.0 mg within 1 hour of birth to prevent hemorrhagic disease of the newborn. Instill 1% silver nitrate, 0.5% erythromycin, or 1% tetracycline into the eyes for prophylaxis against gonococcal ophthalmia. In areas where chlamydial infection is low, silver nitrate is recommended, especially if penicillinase-producing *Neisseria gonorrhoeae* are present. However, in areas where chlamydial conjunctivitis is common, topical erythromycin or tetracycline may be preferable. Instillation may be delayed up to 1 hour following birth. A mild conjunctivitis may result.

The stabilization period takes from 2 to 12 hours depending on the circumstances surrounding labor and delivery. The physiologic changes that occur during this time are illustrated in Figure 10–8. During the stabilization period, temperature, heart rate, rate and quality of respirations, blood pressure, color, adequacy of perfusion, level of consciousness, muscle tone, and activity should be recorded at least once per hour until the neonate's condition has remained stable for 2 hours. Neonates at risk for hypoglycemia should have their blood sugar screened. Infants who have abnormal bleeding during labor, perinatal asphyxia, respiratory distress or an oxygen requirement, pallor, plethora, or hypoglycemia, as well as infants of multiple gestations and infants at increased risk for polycythemia (SGA, LGA/ infants of diabetic mothers) should have their hematocrits determined at 3–6 hours of age.

If the baby is clinically well, the above nursing may be done in the mother's room. Infants who are at increased risk of becoming ill should be transferred to a special-care nursery. Transportation of ill or high-risk infants to a referral nursery should be done swiftly, with a nurse or physician accompanying the infant if possible. Portable incubators with adequate means for temperature and oxygen support are essential.

Physical Examination

All infants should have a complete physical examination within 12 hours of birth. Sick babies should have a thorough examination as soon as they are stable. A term newborn has the following characteristics at birth and shortly thereafter.

A. Resting Posture: Extremities are flexed and somewhat hypertonic (determined to some extent by intrauterine position [eg, following frank breech presentation, the neonate's thighs may be flexed onto the abdomen]). Fists are clenched. Asymmetries of skull, face, jaw, or extremities may result from intrauterine pressures.

B. Skin: Skin is usually ruddy and often mottled. Localized cyanosis of hands and feet (acrocyanosis) normally disappears after several days except when the infant is cool. Subcutaneous tissues may feel full and slightly edematous in the term newborn; skin may appear dry and peeling in the postterm newborn. Check for bruising, meconium staining, and jaundice.

1. Lanugo (fine downy growth of hair) may be present over the shoulders and back.

2. Vernix caseosa (whitish or clay-colored, cheesy, greasy material) may cover the body but is usually on the back and scalp and in the creases of the term infant.

3. Milia of the face (distended sebaceous glands producing tiny whitish papules) are especially prominent over the nose, chin, or cheeks.

4. Mongolian spots (benign bluish pigmentation over the lower back, buttocks, or extensor surfaces) may be found in infants of dark-skinned races.

NEUROMUSCULAR MATURITY

	0	1	2	3	4	5
Posture						
Square window (wrist)	90°	60°	45°	30°	0°	
Arm recall	180°		100°–180°	90°–100°	<90°	
Popliteal angle	180°	160°	130°	110°	90°	<90°
Scarf sign						
Heel to ear						

Apgar _____ 1 min _____ 5 min _____ (hr)
Age at exam _____
Race _____ Sex _____
B.D. _____
LMP _____
EDC _____
Gestational age by dates _____ (wk)
Gestational age by exam _____ (wk)
Birth weight _____ (g) _____ percentile
Length _____ (cm) _____ percentile
Head circum. _____ (cm) _____ percentile
Clin. dist. _____ None _____ Mild _____ Mod. _____ Severe

	0	1	2	3	4	5
Skin	gelatinous red, transparent	smooth pink, visible veins	superficial peeling and/or rash, few veins	cracking pale areas, rare veins	parchment, deep cracking, no vessels	leathery, cracked, wrinkled
Lanugo	none	abundant	thinning	bald areas	mostly bald	
Plantar creases	no creases	faint red marks	anterior transverse crease only	creases anterior two-thirds	creases cover entire sole	
Breast	barely perceptible	flat areola, no bud	stippled areola, 1–2 mm bud	raised areola, 3–4 mm bud	full areola, 5–10 mm bud	
Ear	pinna flat, stays folded	Slightly curved pinna, soft with slow recoil	well-curved pinna, soft but ready recoil	formed and firm with instant recoil	thick cartilage, ear stiff	
Genitals ♂	scrotum empty, no rugae	testes descending, few rugae	testes down, good rugae	testes pendulous, deep rugae	
Genitals ♀	prominent clitoris and labia minora	majora and minora equally prominent	majora large, minora small	clitoris and minora completely covered	

MATURITY RATING

Score	Weeks
5	26
10	28
15	30
20	32
25	34
30	36
35	38
40	40
45	42
50	44

PHYSICAL MATURITY

Figure 10–6. Assessment of neonatal maturity. (Reproduced, with permission, from American Academy of Pediatrics and American College of Obstetricians and Gynecologists: *Guidelines for Perinatal Care,* 2nd ed. Evanston, Ill., AAP and ACOG, 1988.)

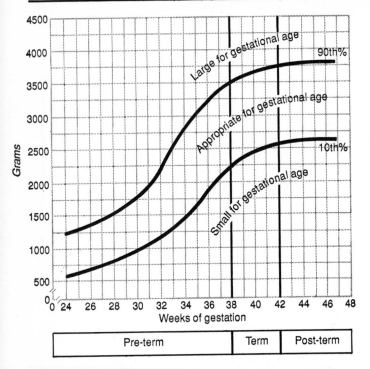

Figure 10–7. University of Colorado Medical Center classification of newborns by birth weight and gestational age. (Adapted from Battaglia FC, Lubchenco LO: *J Pediatr* 1967;**71**:159. (Reproduced, with permission, from Avery GB: *Neonatology: Pathophysiology and Management of the Newborn.* Philadelphia, J.B. Lippincott Company, 1987.)

5. Capillary hemangiomas ("flame nevi") are common on the eyelids, forehead, and neck.

6. Petechiae are sometimes present over the head, neck, and back, especially in association with nuchal cord; if generalized, thrombocytopenia should be suspected.

7. Miliaria, caused by blocked sweat gland ducts, are pustules without a red base.

8. Newborns of 32 weeks' or more gestational age may perspire when too warm. The forehead is usually the first site noted.

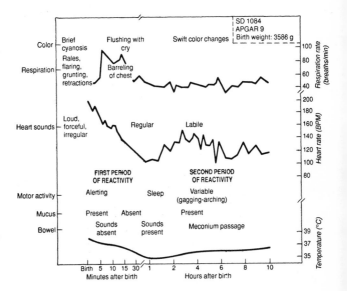

Figure 10–8. Physiologic changes in an infant with a high Apgar score delivered under spinal anesthesia without prior medication. (Adapted from Desmond MM, Rudolph AJ, Phitaksphraiwan P: *Pediatr Clin North Am* 1966;**13**:651.) (Reproduced, with permission, form Avery GB: *Neonatology: Pathophysiology and Management of the Newborn.* Philadelphia, J.B. Lippincott Company, 1987.)

9. Erythema toxicum is characterized by erythematous raised areas with a pustule filled with eosinophils.

10. Pustular melanosis is a pustular rash that has pigment when the pustule ruptures. The pustules are noninfectious but may contain neutrophils.

C. Head: The head is large in relation to the rest of the body; it may exhibit considerable molding with overriding of the cranial bones.

1. Caput succedaneum (localized or fairly extensive ill-defined soft tissue swelling) may be present over the scalp or other presenting parts. It usually extends over a suture line.

2. Cephalhematoma (see Chapter 11).

3. Anterior and posterior fontanelles may measure 0.6–3.6 cm in any direction and are soft. They may be small initially. A third fontanelle between these 2 is present in approximately 6% of infants and is more likely to occur in children with various abnormalities.

4. Transillumination normally produces a circle of light no greater than 1.5 cm beyond the light source in term infants.

5. Craniotabes (slight indentation and recoil of parietal bones elicited by lightly pressing with the thumb) is normal in newborns.

D. Face: Unusual facies occur with syndromes. Check face for bruising or forceps marks and facial nerve palsy.

1. Eyes–The irises are slate-gray except in dark-skinned races. Tears may or may not be present. Most term infants look toward a light source and transiently focus on a face. Subconjunctival, scleral, and retinal hemorrhages occur with birth trauma. The pupillary light reflex is present. Lens opacities are abnormal. A red reflex can be seen on ophthalmoscopic examination. The infant will turn to follow a face more than other stimuli.

2. Ears–Eardrums may be difficult to visualize but have a characteristic opaque appearance and decreased mobility. Severe malformation of the pinnas may be associated with abnormalities of the genitourinary tract. Normal newborns respond to sounds with a startle, blink, head turning, or cry.

3. Nose–The newborn, a preferential nose-breather, experiences respiratory distress in bilateral choanal atresia. Patency should be confirmed by passage of a nasogastric tube if obstruction is suspected.

4. Mouth–Small, pearllike retention cysts at the gum margins and in the midline of the palate (Bohn's and Epstein's pearls) are common and insignificant. Natal teeth should be removed. Rule out clefts of the lip and of the hard and soft palate. Examine the size of the tongue and mandible. The tonsils are quite small. Excessive drooling occurs with esophageal atresia.

5. Cheeks–The cheeks are full because of sucking pads.

E. Neck: Check for webbing, sinus tracts, and masses.

F. Chest: Check for fractured clavicles.

1. Breasts–Breasts are palpable in most mature males and females; size is determined by gestational age and adequacy of nutrition.

2. Lungs–Breathing is abdominal and may be shallow and irregular; rate is usually 40–60 breaths per minute, with a range of 30–100 breaths per minute. Breath sounds are harsh and bronchial. Faint rales may be heard immediately following birth and normally clear in several hours. Check for equal air entry bilaterally and position of the mediastinum.

3. Heart–Rate averages 130 beats per minute, but rates from 90 to 180 may be present for brief periods in normal infants. Sinus dysrhythmia may be present. The apex of the heart is usually lateral to the midclavicular line in the third or fourth interspace. Transient murmurs are common. Check brachial and femoral pulses to rule out aortic stenosis. Blood pressure is a function of birth weight (Figure 10–9).

6. Abdomen–The abdomen is normally flat at birth but soon becomes more protuberant; a markedly scaphoid abdomen suggests diaphragmatic hernia. Two arteries and one vein are usually present in the umbilical cord. The liver is palpable; the tip of the spleen can be felt in 10% of newborns. Both kidneys can and should be palpated. Bowel sounds are audible shortly after birth. Between 5 and 25 mL of cloudy white gastric fluid can be aspirated from the stomach.

H. Genitalia: Appearance in both sexes is dependent on gestational age (see Figure 10–6). Edema is common, particularly after breech delivery. Rule out ambiguous genitalia. In

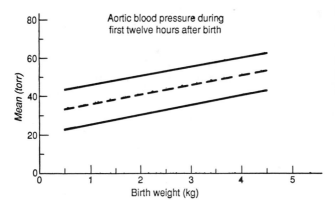

Figure 10–9. Mean aortic blood pressure versus birth weight. The solid lines are the 95% confidence limits. (Adapted from Versmold HT, Kitterman JA, Phibbs RH et al: *Pediatrics* 1981; **67**:607, copyright American Academy of Pediatrics, 1981.) (Reproduced, with permission, from Avery GB: *Neonatology: Pathophysiology and Management of the Newborn.* Philadelphia, J.B. Lippincott Company, 1987.

females an imperforate hymen may be visible. Females may develop a whitish with or without bloody discharge. In males the prepuce is adherent to the glans of the penis. White epithelial pearls 1–2 mm in diameter may be present at the tip of the prepuce.

I. Anus: Patency should be checked. An anteriorly displaced anus may be associated with stenosis.

J. Skeleton: Check for bony abnormalities (eg, absence of a bone, clubfoot, syndactyly, polydactyly). Examine for hip dislocation by attempting to dislocate the femur posteriorly and then abducting the legs to relocate the femur. Examine for extremity fractures, palsies, and arthrogryposis (limited joint movement). Rule out myelomeningoceles and other spinal deformities (eg, scoliosis).

K. Neurologic Examination:

1. Neurologic development is dependent on gestational age.

2. Assess muscle tone and strength.

3. Assess character of cry.

4. Most reflexes, including the Moro, tonic neck, grasp, sucking, rooting, stepping, Babinski, deep tendon, abdominal, cremasteric, and Chvostek reflexes, are normally present at birth.

Routine Care of the Term Infant

A. Observation:

1. Following stabilization observations should be made and recorded every 8 hours. The infant should be observed for signs of illness: temperature instability, change in activity, refusal to feed, pallor, cyanosis, jaundice, abnormal heart or respiratory rate or rhythm, delayed (beyond 24 hours) or abnormal stooling or voiding, and bilious vomiting.

2. The normal full-term neonate passes meconium in the first 24 hours of life and voids within the first 12 hours. Delays beyond 48 and 24 hours, respectively, may indicate obstruction.

3. Infants should be weighed at least daily. Term infants lose 5–10% of their body weight by the third to fifth day (more than 12% may be excessive) and regain their birth weight by the second week of life. Healthy term neonates subsequently gain about 30 grams per day.

4. One-third of healthy term infants develop clinically apparent "physiologic jaundice" during the first week of life. Clinical jaundice is not manifest until the second or third day of life, with peak bilirubin levels on days 5–7. Term infants rarely exceed indirect bilirubin levels of 12 mg/dL. Jaundice present in the first 24 hours of life should be considered abnormal.

B. Feeding: Feeding can be started as early as 2–6 hours after birth in vigorous term infants. Breast-feeding can be initiated in the delivery room. Babies are ready to feed when they are alert and vigorous; have a soft, nondistended abdomen; and have good bowel sounds, a strong rhythmic suck, and a normal hunger cry. Feedings should be delayed in infants who have had difficulties during labor and delivery. These infants should be screened for hypoglycemia and be started on an intravenous infusion of 10% dextrose. Feedings may be initiated with breast milk or 20 kcal/oz formula. Sterile water may be used for the first feeding in bottle-fed infants. The normal term infant should be allowed to feed every 2–5 hours on demand. The volume of feeds will increase from ½ to 1 ounce per feed to 1½ to 2 ounces per feed on day 3. Breast-fed infants will feed every 2–3 hours, increasing from 5 to 10 minutes on each side. Maternal medications should be screened for their safety during breast-feeding.

Bottle-fed babies receiving a standard iron-containing formula need no further supplementation except fluoride (0.25 mg/d) if they do not live in an area with a fluoridated water supply. Breast-fed infants should be supplemented with vitamin D (400 IU/d) if their mothers have a low vitamin D intake or little exposure to sunlight. In addition, breast-fed infants should receive supplemental fluoride and should be given supplemental elemental iron (2–3 mg/kg/d) when they reach 4–6 months of age.

C. Skin and Umbilical Cord Care: After the infant has stabilized, bathe the infant with water and a mild, nonmedicated soap. Techniques that minimize exposure to water may reduce the neonate's heat loss. Heat loss can also be reduced with the use of a radiant warmer. Bathing with a solution of 1% hexachlorophene followed by thorough rinsing should be reserved for infants with a significantly increased risk of skin infections. Hexachlorophene may be absorbed through intact skin and is potentially neurotoxic for neonates. After the initial bath the diaper area may be cleansed with water and cotton, with a mild soap as needed.

Cord care with triple dye (brilliant green, proflavin, and crystal violet) or bacitracin ointment can reduce colonization with staphylococci. The skin absorption and toxicity of the triple-dye agents in newborns have not been carefully studied. Alcohol hastens the drying of the cord but is probably not effective in preventing cord colonization.

In addition to techniques for bathing infants, nurseries should have policies regarding hand washing and dress codes for personnel in the nursery. Most diseases in neonates are transmitted from patient to patient on the hands of health care providers. Before entering the nursery, personnel should wash their hands and forearms up to the elbow with an antiseptic soap. Antiseptic soap should also be used before and after caring for infected neonates. Routine washing with soap and water between handlings of normal infants is adequate.

D. Laboratory Screening:

1. Cord blood–Cord blood is used for blood typing, Rh determination, and Coombs' antibody testing. These tests should be done routinely at the time of delivery if the mother has type O or Rh negative blood. Serologic tests for syphilis should be done on cord blood or on blood drawn from the neonate before discharge if the mother was not previously tested. Cord blood can also be used for electrolytes, glucose, blood culture, total protein, toxicology screen, pH, base deficit, and lactate concentration.

2. Neonatal screening–Most states have mandatory screening programs for inborn errors of metabolism (eg, phenylketonuria, maple syrup urine disease, homocystinuria, galactosemia, etc) and for congenital hypothyroidism. In addition, newborn screening can be done for other disorders, such as cystic fibrosis and hemoglobinopathies. Samples of blood for screening tests should be taken only after the infant has had adequate intake of milk for 24 hours. Infants screened before 24 hours of age should be rescreened for certain inborn errors of metabolism at one week of age.

E. Circumcision: The decision to circumcise an infant should be an individual decision by parents after consultation with the pediatrican. A possible increased risk of urinary tract infection has been suggested in uncircumcised infants. If performed, circumcision should be delayed until the infant is at least 12 hours of age.

F. Length of Hospitalization: Neonates and their mothers are routinely being discharged after 24–48 hours. Nurseries should provide good parental education on both routine newborn care and signs and symptoms of concern to watch for (eg, jaundice, lethargy, poor feeding, vomiting, and fever). Outpatient follow-up visits need to be arranged accordingly (eg, repeat blood screening at one week of age for infants discharged at or before 24 hours of age).

Care of the Preterm Infant

A. Characteristics of the Preterm Newborn: The premature infant is comparatively inactive, with a feeble cry and irregular respirations (periodic breathing). The infant has a relatively large head, prominent eyes, and a protruding abdomen. The skin is relatively translucent and is often wrinkled, red, and deficient in subcutaneous fat. The nails are soft, lanugo is prominent, and vernix is thick. The musculature is poorly developed, the thorax less rigid, and breast engorgement usually absent. Testes may be undescended.

In general, preterm infants weigh less than 2500 grams and have a crown–heel length less than 47 cm, a head circumference less than 33 cm, and a thoracic circumference less than 30 cm.

B. Observations: The preterm infant has physiologic handicaps owing to the functional and anatomic immaturity of various organs.

1. Thermoregulation–Body temperature is more difficult to maintain owing to decreased insulation by subcutaneous fat and large surface area:body weight ratio. Consequently, body temperature falls unless the environment is thermally supported. Prematurely born neonates should be cared for in isolettes designed to keep them warm and to allow them to be carefully observed with minimal handling. Infants may be placed in a neutral thermal environment servocontrolled to maintain a skin temperature of 36°C to 36.5°C. Relative humidity is maintained at about 50%. Preterm infants who weigh 1800–2000 grams or more can often maintain their body temperature out of an isolette.

2. Monitoring–Respiratory difficulties are common because of weak gag and cough reflexes (increased risk of aspiration); pliable thorax and weak respiratory musculature (which result in less efficient ventilation); deficiency of surfactant (allowing alveoli to collapse on exhalation and contributing to the respiratory distress syndrome); and defects in central nervous system control (apnea).

Infants of less than 36 weeks' gestational age have an increased risk of apnea and bradycardia. All babies less than 34 weeks' gestational age should be monitored for at least 7–10 days for apnea and bradycardia. Heart rate monitors may be used; however, these devices may not identify infants with periodic breathing who are at risk for apnea.

Apnea is a nonspecific sign of many disease processes in premature infants (eg, sepsis, necrotizing enterocolitis, seizures, intraventricular hemorrhage, meningitis, respiratory distress syndrome, pneumonia, patent ductus arteriosus metabolic abnormalities, and others). Apnea occurring in the first 24 hours of life and new onset of apnea after the first day of life warrants a physical examination and possibly laboratory screening to rule out these organic etiologies.

3. Hyperbilirubinemia–About one-half of preterm neonates develop clinically apparent "physiologic jaundice" in the first week of life because of impaired conjugation and excretion of bilirubin. Peak bilirubin levels may reach 15 mg/dL on days 5–6. The period of hyperbilirubinemia is more prolonged in preterm infants.

4. Renal function–Because of immature renal function, iatrogenic disturbances of water or electrolyte balance may occur. Large solute or water loads may not be adequately excreted.

5. Resistance to infection–The premature infant's ability to combat infection is decreased owing to inadequate placental transmission of 19S immunoglobulins; relative inability to produce antibodies; and impaired phagocytosis, leukocyte bactericidal capacity, and inflammatory response. Epidermal and mucosal barriers in preterm infants are not as effective as those in term infants.

Immunization schedules for preterm infants should be based on their chronologic age. Infants who remain in the hospital for more than 2 months should be given diphtheria, tetanus, and pertussis vaccine in the hospital. Due to the risk of cross-infection with oral polio vaccine (OPV), the OPV series of vaccination should be delayed until the time of discharge.

6. Hematologic disturbances–Hemorrhagic diathesis is more common owing to clotting factor deficiencies. Deficient antenatal accumulation of iron and vitamin E and rapid body growth and blood volume expansion as well as iatrogenic blood loss contribute to a more pronounced anemia in the first months of life. Hematocrits should be checked at least weekly in preterm infants and more frequently in the ill premature infant.

C. Feeding: Preterm newborns weighing less than 1700 grams should be given 10% dextrose solutions intravenously to supplement the inadequate oral intake that occurs during the first few days after birth. If glycosuria occurs in a markedly preterm infant, the concentration of dextrose should be reduced. Intravenous supplementation should be continued until the infant is receiving a combined intravenous and oral intake of at least 100 mL/kg/d.

Infants of less than 34–36 weeks' postconceptual age usually do not suck and swallow well enough to take nipple feedings. These infants can be gavage-fed via intermittent (or in some cases continuous) nasogastric polyethylene feeding tubes, beginning with 2–5 mL of sterile water. Subsequent feedings with full-strength formula may be increased 1–5 mL in volume every 2–3 hours. Residual gastric contents should be aspirated before each feeding to assess delayed gastric emptying and the infant's ability to tolerate an increased volume of formula. Residual gastric contents greater than 10% of the feeding should lead to caution during further feeding advancements.

When gavage-fed infants are 34–36 weeks old postconceptually and demonstrate good sucking ability, nipple feedings may be tried. In premature infants in whom conventional feedings have been poorly tolerated, nasogastric or nasojejunal feedings may be of value.

Disturbances of nutrition may be a consequence of the faulty absorption of fat, fat-soluble vitamins, and certain minerals as well as reduced stores of calcium, phosphorus, proteins, ascorbic acid, and vitamin A. The current commercially available premature infant formulas and fortified breast milk provide adequate intake of protein, fat, carbohydrate, minerals, and all vitamins, with the exception of vitamin E. Thus, vitamin E supplementation at a dose of 25 IU per day should be initiated when full enteral feedings are being tolerated. The American Academy of Pediatrics recommends that preterm infants be supplemented with elemental iron (2 mg/kg/d) beginning no later than 2 months of age.

Peripheral intravenous hyperalimentation with amino acid, glucose, and lipid solutions can been used in very premature infants and other sick neonates when oral alimentation is impossible or difficult to achieve. Neutral nitrogen balance can be achieved with intravenous alimentation containing amino acids, 2 g/kg per day, and 60 kcal/kg per day.

Preterm infants experience a greater relative weight loss than term neonates owing to decreased intake and thus may take longer to regain their birth weight.

D. Oxygen Therapy: Preterm infants should not routinely be placed in oxygen-supplemented environments. Hypoxemia is the only indication for augmented oxygen therapy. Infants who are cyanotic may be placed temporarily in an oxygen-rich environment sufficient to relieve cyanosis, but it is essential to determine arterial P_{o2} for management of more prolonged oxygen exposure. Therapy should be aimed at maintaining the arterial P_{o2} between 50 and 80 mm Hg (higher in the case of infants with persistent pulmonary hypertension) to avoid retinopathy of prematurity. Monitoring devices such as transcutaneous oxygen monitors and pulse oximeters may be used as an adjunct in managing oxygen therapy; however, physicians using these devices must be aware of the limitations of the particular instrument being used and be capable of correctly interpreting the data it provides.

E. Laboratory Screening: Premature infants need careful monitoring of their blood sugar, especially when receiving intravenous fluids. Attempts should be made to maintain blood sugar between 60 and 100 mg/dL. Hematocrit should be monitored as indicated previously. Newborn screening for inborn errors of metabolism and hypothyroidism should be done at 7 days of age.

Care of the Small-for-Gestational Age (SGA) Infant

All infants whose birth weight is ≤2500 grams are referred to as low birth weight. Regardless of gestational age, the SGA infant's weight is less than the tenth percentile for that age (see Figure 10–7). The infant often appears malnourished. With increasingly severe growth retardation, the infant's length and head circumference are compromised. It is important to distinguish between symmetric growth retardation (weight, length, and head circumference ≤10%) and asymmetric growth retardation (sparing of growth in length and head circumference). Asymmetric growth retardation implies a problem late in pregnancy (placental insufficiency of any etiology), whereas symmetric growth retardation implies an early pregnancy event (chromosomal abnormality, drug or alcohol use, congenital viral infection).

SGA infants have higher morbidity and mortality rates than do AGA infants (see Figure 10–1b). SGA infants may present with severe asphyxia in the delivery room. SGA infants should be carefully examined for congenital anomalies and evaluated for intrauterine infections. Approximately two-thirds of preterm SGA infants and one-third of term SGA infants develop neonatal hypoglycemia (blood glucose <30 mg/dL). These infants are optimally managed by the prophylactic administration of intravenous dextrose solutions; blood glucose should be determined frequently during the first few days of life. SGA infants are also more likely to develop polycythemia/hyperviscosity and feeding difficulties. SGA infants often have problems with thermal regulation; however, they may not require as warm an isolette as do preterm AGA infants of the same weight.

Care of the Large-for-Gestational Age (LGA) Infant

An LGA neonate is one whose birth weight is greater than the 90th percentile for gestational age (see Figure 10–7). Only a portion of LGA neonates are infants of diabetic mothers. Birth injuries (brachial plexus injuries, fractures of the clavicle, intracranial hemorrhage) and hypoglycemia are more common in LGA infants. Transient tachypnea (not progressing to respiratory distress syndrome) is also more common in LGA infants delivered by cesarean section.

Infants of diabetic mothers have a characteristic macrosomic appearance. They are obese and plethoric and have round, full faces. In addition to the above problems, they also have an increased incidence of renal vein thrombosis (manifested by flank mass and hematuria), congenital anomalies (especially skeletal and frequently below the waist), and cardiomyopathy, as well as an increased incidence of respiratory distress syndrome, polycythemia/hyperviscosity, hypocalcemia, and hyperbilirubinemia.

While term LGA infants have the same mortality rate as AGA infants (see Figure 10–1b), particular attention must be given to LGA newborns. Their large size may fail to stimulate an adequate level of concern in those caring for them even though they actually have a much higher risk of morbidity for a given gestational age than do AGA infants. LGA infants should be observed carefully for the development of the complications outlined above.

Multiple Births

Twins may be monozygotic (identical) or dizygotic (fraternal). The intrauterine growth of each twin parallels that of a singleton until about 34 weeks of gestation. Thereafter, the fetal growth rate is less than that for a singleton. As a consequence, many twins (and triplets) are small for gestational age.

The two main complications of multiple pregnancies are intrauterine growth retardation and prematurity. Gestation length tends to be inversely related to the number of fetuses carried. It is the prematurity that tends to increase the mortality or morbidity of twin pregnancies. In addition to the development of intrauterine growth retardation, monozygotic twins may become discordant (birth weights of the twins discrepant by 10% or more) if there is an arterial venous shunt from one twin circulation to the other. This situation results in a small, anemic donor twin and a large, plethoric recipient twin. It is the larger of the twins who is more likely to develop morbidity due to hypervolemia leading to congestive heart failure and polycythemia/hyperviscosity.

Prognosis

Factors that affect mortality rate include the following: (1) gestational age, (2) birth weight, (3) high-risk obstetric history, (4) low Apgar score at 5 minutes, (5) difficult or prolonged resuscitation, (6) severe birth injury, and (7) abnormal physical findings at birth. Neonatal morbidity risk is increased by all the factors that raise the mortality risk.

11 | The Newborn Infant: Diseases & Disorders

Steven B. Spedale, MD, &
Adam A. Rosenberg, MD

DISEASES OF THE RESPIRATORY SYSTEM

APNEA

Clinical Findings

An apneic episode is defined as a respiratory pause longer than 20 seconds that is accompanied by cyanosis and bradycardia; such episodes occur mainly in preterm infants. Apnea must be differentiated from periodic breathing, which is regularly occurring ventilatory cycles interrupted by short pauses not associated with bradycardia or color changes. Various causes of apnea are listed in Table 11–1.

Prematurity is the most common cause of apnea owing to the immaturity of central respiratory regulation centers and of protective mechanisms that aid in maintaining airway patency. The onset is in the first 2 weeks of life, with a gradual increase in frequency of apnea spells over time. Apnea due to other causes can be suspected in an infant with sudden onset of frequent or severe spells.

Treatment

Therapy should be guided toward the underlying cause. If apnea is due to prematurity, prophylactic cutaneous stimulation may relieve mild symptoms. If apnea is frequent or severe, intubation and ventilation or pharmacologic therapy with theophylline (loading dose 5 mg/kg; maintenance dose 1–2 mg/kg every 6–12 h) or caffeine (loading dose 10 mg/kg-base or 20 mg/kg-citrate; maintenance dose 2.5–5.0 mg/kg every 24 h) are helpful. Drug levels must be followed (normal, 5–10 μg/mL).

Table 11–1. Causes of apnea in premature infants.

1. Temperature instability—cold or heat stress
2. Response to passage of a feeding tube
3. Gastroesophageal reflux
4. Hypoxemia: pulmonary parenchymal disease, patent ductus arteriosus, possible anemia
5. Infection: sepsis (viral or bacterial) necrotizing enterocolitis
6. Metabolic: hypoglycemia, hyponatremia
7. Intracranial hemorrhage
8. Posthemorrhagic hydrocephalus
9. Seizures
10. Drugs (eg, morphine)
11. Apnea of prematurity

Prognosis

In the majority of premature infants, apnea and bradycardia cease by 34–36 weeks' postconception. If they persist at time of discharge, home monitoring should be considered as well as continued use of methylxanthines.

RESPIRATORY DISTRESS IN THE NEWBORN

Clinical Findings

Respiratory distress is one of the most common problems seen in the newborn. It can have both noncardiopulmonary and cardiopulmonary causes (Table 11–2).

In general, the most important clinical features include respiratory rate greater than 60 per minute, with or without associated cyanosis; nasal flaring; intercostal and sternal retractions; and expiratory grunting. Most noncardiopulmonary causes of respiratory distress can be ruled out by the history, physical examination, and a few simple laboratory tests (eg, glucose chemstrip, blood gas, hematocrit). The evaluation of cardiovascular disorders will be discussed in the next section of this chapter.

The differential diagnosis of common causes of respiratory distress in term infants is presented in Table 11–3.

HYALINE MEMBRANE DISEASE

Clinical Findings

Premature infants, by virtue of their overall immaturity, represent a significant portion of infants with respiratory dis-

Table 11–2. Causes of respiratory distress in the newborn.

Noncardiopulmonary
  Hypo- or hyperthermia
  Hypoglycemia
  Polycythemia
  Metabolic acidosis
  Drug intoxications, drug withdrawal
  CNS insult
    Asphyxia
    Hemorrhage
  Neuromuscular disease
  Phrenic nerve injury
  Skeletal abnormalities
    Asphyxiating thoracic dystrophy
Cardiovascular
  Left-sided outflow tract obstruction
    Hypoplastic left heart
    Aortic stenosis
    Coarctation of the aorta
  Cyanotic lesions
    Transposition of the great vessels
    Total anomalous pulmonary venous return
    Tricuspid atresia
  Right-sided outflow tract obstruction
Pulmonary
  Upper airway obstruction
    Choanal atresia
    Vocal cord paralysis
    Lingual thyroid
  Meconium aspiration
  Clear fluid aspiration
  Transient tachypnea
  Pneumonia
  Pulmonary hypoplasia
  Hyaline membrane disease
  Pneumothorax, pleural effusions
  Mass lesions
    Lobar emphysema
    Cystic adenomatoid malformation

tress. The most common cause is hyaline membrane disease (HMD), or deficiency of surfactant. Surfactant deficiency results in poor lung compliance and atelectasis. The diagnosis is based on the gestational age of the infant, clinical presentation, and chest x-ray findings. Incidence is 5% at 35–36 weeks' gestation and rises to 65% at 29–30 weeks. Physical examination features include tachypnea, retractions, expiratory grunting, and poor air entry. On chest x-ray, the lung fields classically have a "ground glass" appearance with normal to small lung volumes and evidence of atelectasis as shown by the appearance of air bronchograms.

Table 11-3. Common causes of respiratory distress in the term infant.

Condition	Presentation	Diagnosis	Course
Delayed absorption of amniotic fluid (TTN)*	Slightly preterm infant or term infant delivered by C-section. Tachypnea, cyanosis, grunting, retractions soon after birth	CXR-hyperexpansion, perihilar infiltrates, fluid in fissures	Usually require <40% FIO$_2$; resolves in 12–24 h
Amniotic fluid aspiration	Tachypnea, cyanosis, grunting, retractions soon after birth	CXR-hyperexpansion; patchy infiltrates	Protracted course of 4–7 d; may require FIO$_2$ 30–60%
Meconium aspiration	As for clear fluid aspiration; barrel chest, fetal distress	CXR-hyperexpansion, coarse irregular infiltrates	Resolves in 4–7 d, may require high FIO$_2$. At risk for PPHN† and air leaks. 25% mortality
Pneumonia	Onset of respiratory symptoms within 6–12 h of birth, history of prolonged rupture of membranes, +/− chorioamnionitis, associated shock, absolute neutropenia on CBC	CXR-variable; can mimic TTN, aspiration syndromes, HMD‡	Variable; 10–15% mortality rate
Pneumothorax	Tachypnea, shifted heart sounds, cyanosis	CXR; transillumination	Resolves in 24–48 h. Rarely requires drainage. FIO$_2$ requirement usually <40%

* TTN: transient tachypnea of newborn.
† PPHN: persistent pulmonary hypertension of the newborn.
‡ HMD: hyaline membrane disease.

Treatment

The goal of therapy is to maintain a Pa_{O2} of 60–70 mm Hg and oxygen saturations of 92–95%. Hypo- and hyperoxia should be avoided, as these increase the risk of persistent pulmonary hypertension of the newborn (PPHN) and retinopathy of prematurity (ROP), respectively. Initial therapy includes supportive care of the preterm infant (glucose, fluids, colloid infusions for hypotension, antibiotics, etc). Respiratory assessment includes arterial blood gas sampling and noninvasive oxygen monitoring with pulse oximetry or transcutaneous P_{O2} monitoring. Arterial access through either a peripheral or umbilical artery catheter should be obtained if the infant requires an FIO_2 greater than 0.40. The need for intubation is present if the infant is unable to maintain a Pa_{O2} greater than 60 and a Pa_{CO2} less than 50 mm Hg in FIO_2 greater than 0.60. Infants greater than 30 weeks' gestation may benefit from a trial of continuous positive airway pressure (CPAP) alone. Initial ventilator settings should include peak inspiratory pressure (PIP) sufficient for adequate chest expansion (usually 18–24 cm H_2O), positive end-expiratory pressure (PEEP) 4–6 cm H_2O, and a rate of 20–50 per minute.

Currently, clinical trials are being undertaken to evaluate the benefits of artificial surfactant. It may be administered in the delivery room or in rescue fashion. Early benefits have shown decreased ventilator settings and FIO_2 over the first 3 days of life, but findings are still inconclusive regarding mortality and the incidence of chronic lung disease.

Prognosis

Mortality from HMD is less than 10% for infants over 28 weeks' gestation. The major long-term sequela is the development of chronic lung disease in 20% of the survivors.

DISEASES OF THE CARDIOVASCULAR SYSTEM

Neonates with cardiovascular causes of respiratory distress can be divided into two major groups—those with structural heart disease (presenting with cyanosis or congestive heart failure) and those with shunting through fetal pathways and a structurally normal heart.

STRUCTURAL HEART DISEASE

Clinical Findings

Examples of cyanotic lesions are transposition of the great vessels, total anomalous pulmonary venous return, tricuspid atresia, certain types of truncus arteriosus, and right heart obstruction (pulmonary/tricuspid atresia). Cyanosis presents early and may not be associated with any respiratory distress. However, over time many infants will develop respiratory symptoms due to increased pulmonary blood flow or secondary to metabolic acidosis from hypoxia. Diagnostic aids include failure of an infant's Pa_{O_2} to increase significantly when placed in 100% oxygen (all lesions), decreased pulmonary lung markings on chest x-ray (right heart obstruction), and left-sided forces predominating on ECG (tricuspid atresia). Diagnosis can be confirmed with echocardiography.

Infants presenting with congestive heart failure in the newborn period usually have some form of left outflow obstruction (aortic stenosis, aortic atresia, coarctation). Lesions involving left-to-right shunting (VSD) do well until the pulmonary vascular resistance drops (3–4 weeks) and shunting becomes significant, leading to heart failure. Infants with obstructive lesions present when the patent ductus arteriosus, which previously had provided for most or all of the systemic flow, closes (1–2 days). At this time heart failure and metabolic acidosis develop. Diagnostic aids include abnormal pulses (either poor throughout or differential pulses) on physical examination. Chest x-ray shows a large heart with pulmonary edema. Arterial blood gases are remarkable for profound metabolic acidosis.

SHUNTING THROUGH FETAL PATHWAYS

Clinical Findings

A. Persistent Pulmonary Hypertension of the Newborn (PPHN): This occurs in full or postterm infants who have experienced perinatal asphyxia. It represents a failure of the postnatal decrease in pulmonary vascular resistance normally seen. It is also associated with hypothermia, meconium aspiration, hyaline membrane disease, polycythemia, sepsis, chronic intrauterine hypoxia, and pulmonary hypoplasia. The clinical syndrome is characterized by (1) onset on the first day, usually from birth; (2) respiratory distress; (3) poor response of Pa_{O_2} in 100% O_2; (4) possible myocardial depression with hypotension; and (5) right-to-left shunting at the level of patent ductus arteriosus (PDA) or foramen ovale.

B. Patent Ductus Arteriosus: This is the most frequent cardiovascular disorder seen in the preterm infant. Presentation may occur on day 1 or 2 in small prematures, but most often becomes clinically significant on days 3–7 as the infant is recovering from HMD. Clinical findings include a hyperdynamic precordium, increased peripheral pulses, widened pulse pressure, and possible systolic murmur. Respiratory support may need to be increased. Echocardiogram may be confirmatory.

Treatment

Each infant with the various structural lesions may require basic stabilization. Specific therapy includes infusion of prostaglandin E_1, 0.1 μg/kg/min, to maintain ductal patency. In some cyanotic lesions, this will improve pulmonary blood flow and Pa_{o2} by allowing shunting through the ductus to the pulmonary artery. In left-sided outflow tract obstructions, systemic blood flow is ductal-dependent, so prostaglandin E_1 will improve systemic perfusion and resolve the baby's acidosis. Further specific therapies are given in Chapter 19.

Therapy of PPHN involves supportive therapy for related postasphyxial problems (eg, anticonvulsants for seizures, careful fluid and electrolyte management for renal failure). Specific therapy is designed to raise systemic pressure higher than pulmonary pressure in order to reverse the right-to-left shunting through fetal pathways. Therapy includes (1) O_2 and ventilation, which lowers the pulmonary vascular resistance; (2) colloid infusions (10–30/mL/kg) to improve systemic pressure; (3) systemic pressors to aid compromised cardiac function (dopamine 5–20 μg/kg/min and/or dobutamine 5–20 μg/kg/min); (4) alkalosis to raise pH to 7.55–7.65 (done by hyperventilation with systemic bicarbonate administration if necessary); and (5) pulmonary vasodilators (isuprel 0.1–1.0 μg/kg/min, tolazoline, 1–2 mg/kg IV push followed by an infusion of 0.2–1.0 mg/kg/h). Caution should be exercised with the use of vasodilators as they may cause severe systemic hypotension. Infants who fail to respond to this therapy may benefit from extracorporeal membrane oxygenation (ECMO).

Management of PDA is both medical and, if needed, surgical. Indomethacin (0.2 mg/kg IV) in a schedule dependent on the infant's age may close the ductus in about two-thirds of cases. If the ductus reopens, a second trial may be undertaken. If this fails, surgical ligation is indicated. A major side effect of indomethacin is a transient oliguria, which can be treated by fluid restriction until urine output improves. Indomethacin does not increase the incidence and severity of intracranial hemorrhage. The drug should not be used if the infant is hyperkalemic, the creatinine is greater than 2.0 mg/dL, or the platelet count is less than 50,000/mm^3.

Prognosis

The prognosis for structural heart lesions is dependent on the type of lesion and is reviewed in Chapter 19. PPHN carries a mortality rate of approximately 10–15%, with long-term neurologic morbidity approximately 10%. The other major long-term problem is chronic lung disease secondary to the extensive ventilator support required by many of these infants.

BIRTH INJURIES

Birth injuries occur during both labor and delivery. Predisposing factors include macrosomia, cephalopelvic disproportion, prematurity, dystocia, prolonged labor, and abnormal presentation.

Soft tissue injury consisting of petechiae, erythema, and ecchymosis is common. It usually involves the presenting part of the infant and most often requires no treatment. It should be noted that petechiae away from the presenting part may represent an underlying hemorrhagic disorder.

Cephalhematoma is present in 0.4–2.5% of live births and represents a subperiosteal collection of blood caused by localized trauma. Cephalhematoma presents as a lump on day 1 that does not cross suture lines. Most commonly, the lumps are over the parietal bone. Rarely there can be enough bleeding to cause shock or anemia. Subgaleal bleeds occur beneath the scalp and are not restricted by sutures. This type of injury is rare, but can result in significant blood loss. Subdural and subarachnoid bleeds can also be seen as the result of a traumatic delivery.

The most common fracture resulting from birth trauma is to the clavicle. It may be clinically palpable or may be suspected in an infant who does not move an upper extremity. Therapy is usually not necessary; healing occurs with good callus formation in 7–10 days. The most common long-bone fracture is to the humerus.

Nerve injuries most often involve the brachial plexus or facial nerves. Three types of brachial plexus injuries are described: (1) Duchenne-Erb, an upper arm paralysis resulting from damage to the fifth and sixth cervical nerve; (2) Klumpke's (lower arm), damage to the eight cervical and first thoracic nerves; and (3) entire arm. Treatment involves physical therapy to prevent contractures. Most infants will recover good arm function, although 15% will suffer significant handicap. Phrenic nerve injuries, like brachial plexus injuries, occur during deliveries where the neck is severely stretched. Eighty to ninety percent of phrenic injuries are associated with brachial plexus damage. The clinical presentation of a phrenic nerve injury is tachypnea and cyanosis. Facial nerve injuries occur at the point where the nerve emerges from the stylomastoid foramen. Unilateral facial muscle weakness will be seen with complete resolution over several days in most cases.

NEONATAL HYPERBILIRUBINEMIA

BILIRUBIN METABOLISM

The two sources of bilirubin in the neonate are from breakdown of circulating RBCs (75%) and from ineffective erythropoiesis and tissue heme proteins (25%). Heme is converted to unconjugated (lipid soluble) bilirubin in the reticuloendothelial system and is transported bound to albumin to the liver. In the liver it is conjugated with glucuronic acid in a reaction catalyzed by glucuronyl transferase. The conjugated bilirubin (water soluble) is secreted into the biliary tree for excretion via the GI tract. The enzyme B-glucuronidase is present in the small bowel and hydrolyzes some of the conjugated bilirubin. This unconjugated bilirubin can then be reabsorbed into the circulation, adding to the total load of unconjugated bilirubin (enterohepatic circulation).

PHYSIOLOGIC HYPERBILIRUBINEMIA
(Physiologic Jaundice)

This is a transient hyperbilirubinemia occurring in the first week of life; it is seen in most newborns (average, 5–7 mg/dL). It occurs secondary to low levels of glucuronyl transferase and increased bilirubin load from an increased RBC volume with decreased survival, increased ineffective erythropoiesis, and enterohepatic circulation. Clinically, physiologic jaundice (1) should not present on day 1; (2) total bilirubin should rise by less than 5 mg/dL/d, peaking at less than 12.9 mg/dL on days 3–4 (term infant) and 15 mg/dL on days 5–7 (preterm infant); (3) conjugated fraction should be less than 2 mg/dL; and (4) jaundice should persist no longer than 1 week in the term infant and 2 weeks in the preterm infant.

NONPHYSIOLOGIC HYPERBILIRUBINEMIA

If criteria are not met for a diagnosis of physiologic jaundice, the cause of the jaundice must be investigated. Appropriate laboratory tests at this time include CBC, platelets, reticulocyte count, Coombs' test, and peripheral blood smear. The various etiologies are as follows:

A. Overproduction of bilirubin
  1. Increased rate of hemolysis (increased unconjugated bilirubin and reticulocyte count)
    a. Positive Coombs'—Rh incompatibility, ABO incompatibility, other blood group sensitization
    b. Negative Coombs'—RBC membrane defects (spherocytosis, elliptocytosis, pyknocytosis, stomatocytosis)
    c. RBC enzyme defects (glucose-6-phosphate deficiency, pyruvate kinase deficiency, hexokinase deficiency)
  2. Nonhemolytic causes (increased unconjugated bilirubin, normal reticulocyte count)
    a. Extravascular hematoma—cephalhematoma, bruising, CNS hemorrhage
    b. Polycythemia
    c. Exaggerated enterohepatic circulation—GI obstruction, ileus
B. Decreased rate of conjugation (increased unconjugated bilirubin, normal reticulocyte count)
  1. Physiologic jaundice
  2. Criggler-Najjar (type I glucuronyltransferase deficiency, autosomal recessive)
  3. Type II glucuronyltransferase deficiency, autosomal dominant
  4. Breast milk jaundice
C. Excretion or reabsorption abnormalities (increased conjugated and unconjugated bilirubin, Coombs' negative, normal reticulocyte count)
  1. Hepatitis (viral, bacterial, parasitic, toxic)

2. Metabolic (galactosemia, glycogen storage disease, cystic fibrosis, hypothyroidism)
3. Biliary atresia
4. Choledochal cyst
5. Obstruction of the ampulla of Vater
6. Sepsis

BILIRUBIN TOXICITY

The importance of monitoring serum bilirubin is to prevent kernicterus (staining of basal ganglia and hippocampus). It occurs when unconjugated bilirubin enters nerve cells and produces cell death. Mortality is high. Clinical symptoms include lethargy, refusal to feed, high-pitched cry, hypertonicity, opisthotonos, seizures, and apnea. Sequelae include athetoid cerebral palsy, high-frequency hearing loss, paralysis of upward gaze, and dental dysplasia. The risk of kernicterus in a given infant is not well defined. The only group in which a specific bilirubin level (20 mg/dL) has been associated with an increased risk of kernicterus is infants with Rh hemolytic disease. This observation has been extended to the management of other neonates with hemolytic disease, although no definitive data exist for these infants. The risk is likely negligible for term infants without hemolytic disease, even at levels greater than 20 mg/dL. Premature infants of 32 to 38 weeks' gestation are probably safe up to levels of 20 mg/dL, while meaningful data for infants less than 32 weeks' gestation are not available.

Treatment

Two modalities are in use today for treatment of hyperbilirubinemia. In phototherapy, unconjugated bilirubin in the skin is converted to a water-soluble photoisomer and excreted in the bile and urine. The infant's eyes should be shielded and fluid administration should be increased to compensate for evaporative losses. Side effects are loose stools, skin rashes, and problems with thermoregulation. In term and near-term infants, phototherapy is started at levels 4–5 mg/dL below exchange transfusion levels. In babies with hemolytic disease, phototherapy can be instituted earlier (eg, level of 10 mg/dL on day 1 and 13 mg/dL on day 2). In very immature babies, many centers institute "prophylactic" phototherapy.

Double-volume exchange transfusions are used when the bilirubin level approaches toxic ranges to rapidly decrease serum bilirubin (Table 11–4). In addition, exchange transfusions are

Table 11–4. Serum bilirubin for exchange transfusion.*,†

Birth Weight	Normal Infants‡	Abnormal Infants(g)§
<1000	10.0	10.0 ‖
1001–1250	13.0	10.0 ‖
1251–1500	15.0	13.0
1501–2000	17.0	15.0
2001–2500	18.0	17.0
>2500	20.0	18.0

* Reproduced, with permission, from American Academy of Pediatrics: Page 95 in *Standards and Recommendations for Hospital Care of Newborn Infants*, 6th ed. American Academy of Pediatrics, 1977. Copyright American Academy of Pediatrics, 1977.

† These guidelines have not been validated.

‡ Normal infants are defined for this purpose as having none of the problems listed below.

§ Abnormal infants have one or more of the following problems: perinatal asphyxia, prolonged hypoxemia, acidemia, persistent hypothermia, hypoalbuminemia, hemolysis, sepsis, hyperglycemia, elevated free fatty acids or presence of drugs that compete for bilirubin binding, signs of central nervous system deterioration.

‖ There have been case reports of basal ganglion staining at levels considerably lower than 10 mg.

also used in the care of erythroblastic infants. A partial isovolemic exchange done with packed red cells (35 mL/kg) corrects the anemia and adjusts blood volume. An early double-volume exchange with whole blood will remove the sensitized cells, hopefully decreasing the number of subsequent exchange transfusions to remove bilirubin. Indications for early double-volume exchange are cord hematocrit less than 40% and/or bilirubin greater than 6.0 mg/dL.

SPECIFIC CAUSES OF HYPERBILIRUBINEMIA

Breast Milk Jaundice

Breast milk jaundice is an unconjugated hyperbilirubinemia that peaks late (usually by days 6–14). The infant is well, and bilirubin levels are approximately 12–20 mg/dL. It can be distinguished from other causes by a prompt reduction in bilirubin upon substituting formula feeds for 1–2 days. This entity is to be distinguished from jaundice in the breast-fed infant during the first week of life. Breast-fed infants, when compared with formula-fed infants, have higher bilirubin levels owing to decreased intake over the first several days of life. The treatment is not to stop breast-feeding, but rather to increase the frequency of feedings.

ABO Incompatibility

ABO incompatibility is an indirect hyperbilirubinemia secondary to destruction of neonatal RBCs by maternal IgG that crosses the placenta into the fetal circulation (mother O, infant A or B). The infants may have anemia with or without jaundice, jaundice with or without anemia, or neither. Since the amount of circulating IgG antibody varies, it is not possible from one pregnancy to another to predict the severity of the process. Guidelines for phototherapy for term infants are day 1 bilirubin levels > 10, day 2 levels > 13, day 3 and later levels > 15 mg/dL. Exchange transfusion should be performed when bilirubin levels are greater than 20 mg/dL.

Erythroblastosis

Erythroblastosis is caused by isoimmunization to Rh (D, C, E, d, c, or e), Kell, Duffy, Lutheran, or Kidd antigens. Most commonly, D antigen is involved. Fetal blood may enter the maternal circulation as the initiating event. The problem worsens with subsequent pregnancies. Clinically, some infants are more affected than others. The more severely affected will have hydrops (pleural effusions, ascites) secondary to intrauterine high-output failure from anemia and hypoproteinemia. Less severe cases are characterized by hepatosplenomegaly, anemia, and jaundice.

Extravascular Hemorrhage

Extravascular hemorrhage within the body (eg, cephalhematoma, bruising, CNS hemorrhage) may result in an unconjugated hyperbilirubinemia secondary to an extra bilirubin load for the liver. The jaundice tends to peak at 3–4 days of age.

Gastrointestinal Tract Obstruction

Gastrointestinal tract obstruction (functional or structural) can result in unconjugated hyperbilirubinemia owing to enhanced enterohepatic circulation of bilirubin.

INFECTION OF THE NEWBORN

Clinical Findings

There are 3 major routes of perinatal infection: (1) bloodborne transplacental infection of the fetus (eg, CMV, rubella, syphilis); (2) ascending infection with disruption of the barrier provided by the amniotic membranes (eg, bacterial infection after ruptured membranes); and (3) infection upon passage through an infected birth canal or exposure to infected blood at delivery (eg, herpes simplex, hepatitis B infections).

Early onset bacterial infections are related to perinatal risk factors and usually present on the first day of life. Symptoms include respiratory distress (most common), poor perfusion, and hypotension. Late onset disease is more subtle and may present with poor feeding, lethargy, hypotonia, temperature instability, altered perfusion, new or increased oxygen requirement, and apnea. Laboratory findings may include an abnormal CBC (decreased total count, neutropenia, increased immature/mature neutrophil ratio, thrombocytopenia), hyperglycemia, and an unexplained metabolic acidosis. Counterimmune electrophoresis on a urine sample may be helpful in the diagnosis of Group B streptococcus. Definitive diagnosis is made from positive blood and CSF cultures. Signs suggestive of congenital viral infection include small size for gestational age, petechiae, jaundice, and hepatosplenomegaly. A review of specific neonatal infections is presented in Table 11–5.

Treatment

Guidelines for evaluation and management of term infants are listed in Table 11–6. It must be remembered that respiratory distress in a preterm infant might also be evidence of infection. Preterm infants have a fivefold risk for infection compared with term infants; each premature infant with respiratory distress should have blood cultures obtained. Empiric antibiotics should be given for 48–72 hours, until cultures are negative. Infants with strong clinical signs of sepsis should have their CSF examined. Intravenous gamma globulin (500 mg/kg) may be given to infants with known or clinically suspect infections.

Prognosis

The prognosis for neonatal infection is dependent upon the specific agent and type of infection.

DISORDERS OF THE GASTROINTESTINAL SYSTEM

TRACHEOESOPHAGEAL FISTULA/ ESOPHAGEAL ATRESIA

Clinical Findings

Tracheoesophageal fistula (TEF) and esophageal atresia consist of a blind esophageal pouch and fistulous connection

Table 11–5. Characteristics of specific neonatal infections.

Infection	Etiologies	Clinical Tips	Treatment
Bacterial sepsis	GBS[1], gram-negative enteric (E coli), S aureus, L monocytogenes, Enterococcus, S epidermidis	Early onset—shock, pneumonia; late onset—meningitis, local infection. Maternal diarrhea may be associated with listeria. S epidermidis is increased with indwelling lines.	Ampicillin plus aminoglycoside or third-generation cephalosporin. Vancomycin for S epidermidis. Duration of therapy 10–14 d. Intrapartum penicillin/ampicillin has had some success against early GBS.
Fungal sepsis	C albicans	High-risk group: VLBW infants with indwelling lines.	Amphotericin B.
Meningitis	GBS, gram-negative enterics, viral (enterovirus)	Infants with bacterial sepsis at risk. CSF: protein >250 mg/dL, glucose <20mg/dL, WBC >25/μL, positive gram stain.	Appropriate antibiotics for 21 days.
Pneumonia	Bacterial, viral (CMV[2], RSV[3], adenovirus, influenza, parainfluenza), Ureaplasma, Mycoplasma, Chlamydia	Can be infected in utero or upon passage through birth canal. Older neonates: look for new-onset respiratory distress or an increase in FIO$_2$ or ventilator settings in infants receiving respiratory support.	Specific therapy when known. Ventilatory support as needed.
Urinary tract infection	Gram-negative enterics	Uncommon early onset infection; usually associated with GU anomalies. Obtain urine culture by aspiration or catheterization.	Treat for 10–14 days. Evaluate for GU anomalies.

306

Osteomyelitis	GBS, *S aureus*	See Chapter 15.
Otitis media	Usual bacterial agents, gram negatives	Uncommon in neonates. Usually late onset disease. Appropriate antibiotics.
Omphalitis	Group A strep, *S aureus*, gram negatives	Seen with increased incidence in infants with prolonged endotracheal intubation. Some degree of purulent material at the base of cord is common. Diagnosis of omphalitis requires erythema, edema of surrounding soft tissues. Infection more common with cords manipulated for venous or arterial access. Broad-spectrum antibiotics.
Congenital viral infection	CMV[2]	Most common virus transmitted in utero. Clinical disease: SGA, hepatosplenomegaly, petechiae, thrombocytopenia, increased conjugated bilirubin. Mortality 20% with symptomatic CMV, sequelae in 90% of survivors. Sequelae: hearing loss, mental retardation, delayed motor development, chorioretinitis, optic atrophy, seizures, language delay, learning disabilities. Rate of sequelae is 5–15% in asymptomatic infants; most frequently hearing loss. Frequency of viral transmission to	No known therapy.

(continued)

Table 11-5. (Continued).

Infection	Etiologies	Clinical Tips	Treatment
		the fetus and symptomatic neonatal infection is highest with primary infection in the mother. Transmission of secondary infection occurs in 0–1% of cases. Postnatal infection can occur (acquired from transfusions). Can see hepatitis, pneumonia, and neurological illness in compromised seronegative prematures. Diagnosed by culture of virus (blood, CSF, urine, throat, placenta, amniotic fluid).	
	Rubella	Infant affected secondary to maternal infection during pregnancy. 80% of fetal infection during first trimester. Clinical syndrome: adenopathy, bone radiolucencies, encephalitis, cardiac defects, cataracts, retinopathy, SGA, hepatosplenomegaly, thrombocytopenia, purpura. Sequelae: mental retardation, hearing loss. Diagnosis: Compare	No therapy. Prevention: Maternal immunization.

	Varicella	infant and maternal IgG; specific IgM in infant. Cultures of pharyngeal secretions. Congenital varicella (first/second trimester) rare. Findings: limb hypoplasia, cutaneous scars, microcephaly, cortical atrophy, cataracts, chorioretinitis. Perinatal exposure (5 days before–2 days after delivery) causes severe fatal disseminated varicella. Diagnosis: Rise in maternal IgG, IgM in infant. Culture vesicles.	Prevention: VZIG[4] to baby in perinatal period. Can treat illness with acyclovir.
Congenital parasitic	Toxoplasmosis (*Toxoplasma gondii*)	Infection during pregnancy (2–6 mos). 40% children infected (15% severe clinical damage). Exposure to cat feces, raw meat. Sequelae: SGA, chorioretinitis, seizures, jaundice, hydrocephalus, microcephaly, hepato-splenomegaly, adenopathy, cataracts, thrombocytopenia, pneumonia. Diagnosis: maternal IgG serologies, IgM in infants.	Can potentially treat known cases transplacentally by treating mother.
Perinatal acquired viral infections	Herpes simplex	Usually acquired upon passage through birth canal. May be primary or reactivated disease. Risk likely low to infant with	Acyclovir prevents progression of local disease. Decreases mortality with disseminated and CNS disease.

(continued)

309

Table 11–5. (Continued).

Infection	Etiologies	Clinical Tips	Treatment
		reactivated disease. Primary disease carries higher risk to infant, but is usually asymptomatic in the mother. Local/disseminated disease (onset 5–14 days): up to 70% of infants present initially with local skin or oral vesicles. Progression of disease occurs in a significant number of cases. Disseminated disease: pneumonia, shock, hepatitis. CNS (onset 14–18 days): lethargy, instability, seizures. Diagnosis: Viral cultures usually grow in 48–72 hours.	
Hepatitis B		Screen high-risk mothers with HBsAg[5] (IV drug abuser, far eastern origin). Clinical illness rare at birth. Exposed infants at risk to be chronic carriers.	HBsAg in mother. If positive give HBIG[6] immediately followed by vaccination. If unavailable, give HBIG at birth and await results before giving vaccine.
Enterovirus		Late summer/fall: maternal illness (fever, diarrhea, rash) in week prior to delivery. Infant: fever, rash, diarrhea, lethargy. May be more severe with meningoencephalitis, myocarditis, hepatitis, pneumonia, shock, DIC. Diagnosis: Viral cultures—rectal, CSF, blood.	No therapy. Prognosis good except for disseminated disease.

Human immunodeficiency disease (HIV)	Clinical features: SGA, microcephaly, prominent forehead, flattened nasal bridge, prominence of eyes, blue sclera, hypertelorism, long philtrum, patulous lips. Transmission may be transplacental or perinatal. Majority of infected infants present before 2 years.	See Chapter 14.
T pallidum	Transplacental infection. Symptoms: mucocutaneous lesions, lymphadenopathy, hepatitis, bony changes, hydrops. Usually asymptomatic at birth. Diagnosis: darkfield identification of organism. Presumptive—rising serologies (VDRL); FTA-IgM. CSF exam indicated looking for CNS infection.	IV/IM penicillin.
Neisseria gonorrhea	Onset 3–7 days. Gram-negative intracellular diplococci on gram stain.	Systemic penicillin.
Conjunctivitis		
Chlamydia	Onset 5 days–several weeks. Congestion, edema, and discharge.	Oral erythromycin.

1 Group B streptococcus.
2 Cytomegalovirus.
3 Respiratory syncytial virus.
4 Varicella zoster immune globulin.
5 Hepatitis B surface antigen.
6 Hepatitis B immune globulin.

Table 11–6. Management of bacterial infection in the term infant.

Risk Factor	Clinical Signs*	Evaluation and Treatment
24-h rupture of membranes	None	Observation
>24-h rupture of membranes; chorioamnionitis	None	CBC, blood cultures, 48–72 h broad-spectrum antibiotics
>24-h rupture of membranes, chorioamnionitis, maternal antibiotics	None	CBC, blood cultures, urine CIE, 48–72 h broad spectrum antibiotics
None or any of the above	Present	CBC, blood, CSF cultures, ± urine culture, broad-spectrum antibiotics†

* In any infant without signs consistent with infection, it is reasonable to observe without treatment, provided close observation is possible.
† Any infant, irrespective of age of presentation, who appears infected by clinical criteria should have a CSF examination. Urine culture is indicated in the evaluation of infants who are initially well and develop symptoms after 2–3 days in the nursery.

between either the proximal or distal esophagus and airway. There is often a maternal history of polyhydramnios; significant clinical findings include copious secretions, choking, cyanosis, and respiratory distress. Chest x-ray following placement of a nasogastric tube will show the tube in the blind pouch. If a TEF is present to the distal esophagus, gas will be present in the abdomen.

Treatment

Surgery provides the definitive therapy. It may be staged if initial reanastomosis of the esophageal ends is not possible. A gastrostomy may also be performed until reanastomosis heals. Prior to surgery, the goal is to minimize aspiration of gastric fluid through the fistula into the lungs. Infant should be supported with IV fluids and glucose; the head of the crib should be elevated; and a nasogastric tube in the proximal pouch should be attached to continuous suction.

Prognosis

Prognosis is determined primarily by the presence or absence of associated anomalies (vertebral, cardiac, limb, or anal).

OBSTRUCTIVE LESIONS

Clinical Findings

Obstructive lesions are classified as high or low based on their location with respect to the ligament of Treitz. Clinical findings suggestive of high obstruction include a maternal history of polyhydramnios, and early onset of emesis, often bilious (Table 11–7).

Distal obstructions present with increasing intolerance of feedings, abdominal distention, and decreased or absent stooling. Imperforate anus should be sought out early as it is often missed on a cursory examination. Other causes include meconium ileus, Hirschsprung's disease, meconium plug, small left colon, and ileal and colonic atresia. Plain films will show gaseous distention with air through a considerable portion of the bowel and air-fluid levels. Meconium ileus or plug and small left colon are diagnosed by contrast enema. Contrast enema and rectal biopsy are used to diagnose Hirschsprung's disease.

Treatment

Definitive treatment is surgical, with the exception of meconium plug and small left colon. Prior to surgery, infants should have nasogastric suction and administration of IV fluids.

Prognosis

Most lesions carry a good prognosis. Ten percent of infants with meconium plug will have cystic fibrosis, while all infants with meconium ileus will have cystic fibrosis. Imperforate anus is

Table 11–7. High intestinal obstruction in the neonate.

Lesion	Clinical Tips
Duodenal atresia	Nonbilious emesis. Abdominal x-ray will show double bubble (stomach/dilated duodenum). May be associated with trisomy 21.
Malrotation with volvulus	Bilious emesis. Abdominal x-ray often needs to be supplemented with contrast studies for diagnosis (contrast enema looking for location of caecum or upper GI study). *Prompt* surgical repair necessary to prevent ischemic damage from torsion of intestine and superior mesenteric artery.
High jejunal atresia	Bilious emesis. Diagnosis confirmed with upper GI exam.

associated with other anomalies (vertebral, renal, cardiac, limb), and duodenal atresia is associated with trisomy 21. Otherwise, after surgical repair, most of these infants do well.

ABDOMINAL WALL DEFECTS

Omphaloceles are formed by incomplete closure of the anterior abdominal wall after the return of the mid gut to the abdominal cavity. The defect is usually covered by a sac, with the umbilical cord inserted into the center of the defect. The size of the defect varies but may contain intestine, stomach, liver, and spleen. There is a high incidence of associated anomalies including cardiac, other gastrointestinal, and chromosomal anomalies. Acute therapy includes covering the defect with sterile warm saline to prevent fluid loss, nasogastric decompression, and administration of IV fluids and glucose. Definitive therapy is surgery.

Gastroschisis is a defect in the anterior abdominal wall lateral to the umbilicus. There is no covering sac, and herniated viscera is limited to the intestine. The underlying etiology may be an infarct to the abdominal wall. Other than intestinal atresia, associated anomalies are uncommon. Acute therapy is as for omphalocele, and definitive therapy is surgical.

DIAPHRAGMATIC HERNIA

Diaphragmatic hernia is a herniation of abdominal organs into the hemithorax, usually the left, and is caused by a defect in the posterior lateral diaphragm. Infants present in the delivery room with respiratory distress, cyanosis, decreased breath sounds on the side of the hernia, and shift of the mediastinum to the opposite side of the hernia. Definitive repair is surgical but infants often require extensive resuscitation including intubation and nasogastric decompression. Postoperative course is often complicated by PPHN.

ACQUIRED CONDITIONS

Necrotizing enterocolitis (NEC) is the most commonly seen acquired GI emergency in the newborn period, usually affecting premature infants. The pathogenesis is multifactorial and is related to previous ischemic episodes, bacterial or viral infection, and immunologic immaturity of the GI tract.

Clinical Findings

The primary presenting sign is abdominal distension with or without associated vomiting, increased gastric residual, heme-positive stool, abdominal tenderness, temperature instability, increased apnea and bradycardia, decreased urine output, and poor perfusion. CBC may show increased WBCs with bandemia and decreased platelets. Diagnosis is confirmed by the presence of pneumatosis intestinalis (air in bowel wall on x-ray).

Treatment

Surgery is required if evidence of necrotic bowel (perforation with free air on x-ray, fixed dilated loop on serial films, abdominal wall cellulitis, progressive deterioration) is present. Otherwise, medical management consisting of nasogastric decompression, IV fluids, withholding feedings, and antibiotics is usually sufficient. Infants should not be refed until disease is resolved, examination of the abdomen is normal, and x-ray reveals resolution of pneumatosis. This usually takes 10–14 days.

Prognosis

Mortality rate is 10%. Surgery is needed in fewer than 25% of cases. Long-term prognosis depends on the amount of intestine lost.

DISEASES OF THE BLOOD/HEMATOPOIETIC SYSTEM

BLEEDING DISORDERS

Clinical Findings

Bleeding in newborns may result from either inherited clotting disorders or acquired disorders, including deficiency of vitamin K–dependent clotting factors, hemorrhagic disease of the newborn (HDN), disseminated intravascular coagulation (DIC), liver failure, and thrombocytopenia. Clinical features of coagulation disorders are presented in Table 11–8 and the differential diagnosis of thrombocytopenia (platelet count < 150,000) in Table 11–9.

Treatment

Treatment for coagulation disorders is presented in Table 11–8. Thrombocytopenia is treated with 10 mL/kg of platelets. Indication for transfusion in the term infant is clinical bleeding or a total count less than $10,000–20,000/mm^3$. In the preterm infant

Table 11–8. Features of infants bleeding from HDN, DIC, or liver failure.

	HDN	DIC	Liver Failure
Clinical	Well infant, no prophylactic vitamin K	Sick infant, hypoxia, sepsis, etc	Sick infant— hepatitis, inborn errors of metabolism, shock
Bleeding	GI tract, umbilical cord, circumcision, nose	Generalized	Generalized
Onset	2–3 d	Anytime	Anytime
Platelet count	Normal	Decreased	Normal or decreased
PT	Prolonged	Prolonged	Prolonged
PTT	Prolonged	Prolonged	Prolonged
Fibrinogen	Normal	Decreased	Decreased
Factor V	Normal	Decreased	Decreased
Treatment	Vitamin K, 1 mg	Address underlying condition. Replace factors.	Similar to DIC

Table 11–9. Differential diagnosis of neonatal thrombocytopenia.

Disorder	Clinical Tips
Immune	
Passively acquired antibody (ITP, SLE, drug induced)	Proper history, maternal thrombocytopenia
Isoimmune sensitization to PLA-1 antigen	Positive antiplatelet antibodies in baby's serum, sustained rise in platelets by transfusion of mother's platelets
Infections	
Bacterial	Sick infants with other signs
Congenital viral infections	consistent with infection
Syndromes	
Absent radii	
Fanconi's anemia	Congenital anomalies, associated pancytopenia
DIC	Sick infants, abnormalities of clotting factors
Giant hemangioma	
Thrombosis	Hyperviscous infants, vascular catheters
High-risk infant with RDS, pulmonary hypertension, etc.	Isolated decrease in platelets is not uncommon in sick infants even in the absence of DIC

at risk for intraventricular hemorrhage, transfusion is indicated for counts less than 40,000–50,000/mm³. Isoimmune thrombocytopenia requires transfusion of maternal platelets. In some cases infants born to mothers with ITP respond to corticosteroids.

ANEMIA

Clinical Findings

Anemia can be caused by hemorrhage, hemolysis, or failure of RBC production. Evaluation of anemia includes (1) clinical assessment for signs of acute blood loss; (2) laboratory evaluation consisting of CBC, peripheral smear, reticulocyte count, and direct and indirect Coombs' test. Anemia in the first 24–48 hours of life is due to hemorrhage or hemolysis. The Kleihauer–Betke test on maternal blood should be performed when a fetomaternal bleed is suspected.

Hemorrhage can occur in utero (fetoplacental, fetomaternal, twin–twin), perinatally (cord rupture, placental previa, placental incision at cesarean section), or internally (intracranial, rupture of liver or spleen). Infants with chronic blood loss (eg, fetomaternal) will be pale at birth but will compensate without signs of volume loss. Initial hematocrit will be low. Acute bleeding will present with hypovolemia (tachycardia, poor perfusion, hypotension) and a normal or low initial hematocrit. Hemolysis is caused by blood group incompatibility, enzyme/membrane abnormalities, infection, and DIC.

Treatment

Acute treatment is provision of volume (10–20 mL/kg) as 5% albumin or with whole blood to restore normovolemia. Later treatment with packed red cells is indicated for symptomatic anemia.

ANEMIA IN THE PREMATURE NEONATE

Anemia of prematurity is due to decreased erythropoietin production in response to a low red-cell mass. Symptoms include poor feeding, lethargy, tachycardia, poor weight gain, and apnea. Transfusion may be indicated if the infant is symptomatic (usually occurs with a hematocrit < 25%).

Premature infants are also at risk for vitamin E deficiency, which presents at 4–6 weeks with a hemoglobin of 6–10 mg/dL, increased reticulocytes, thrombocytosis, and edema. Prevention is possible with 25 IU vitamin E given daily.

Supplemental iron should be started in premature infants at 2–4 months of age to prevent iron-deficiency anemia.

POLYCYTHEMIA

Clinical Findings

Polycythemia occurs in 2–5% of live births. Etiologies include twin–twin transfusion, maternal–fetal transfusion, intrapartum transfusion from the placenta associated with fetal distress, and chronic intrauterine hypoxia. The consequence is hyperviscosity, which decreases effective perfusion of capillary beds in the microcirculation. Clinical consequences can relate to any organ system and are presented in Table 11–10. Venous hematocrit greater than 70% at less than 12 hours of age and greater than 65% after 12 hours should be considered indicative of hyperviscosity.

Treatment

Treatment with partial exchange transfusion is recommended for symptomatic infants. Whether or not to treat asymptomatic infants based only on hematocrit is controversial. Albumin (5%) is transfused over a constant rate through a peripheral IV while blood is removed through an umbilical venous line. The amount to exchange is as follows:

$$\frac{\text{Peripheral venous Hct} - \text{desired Hct}}{\text{Peripheral venous Hct}} \times \text{blood volume/kg} \times \text{Body wt}$$

Desired hematocrit is 50–55%; blood volume 80 mL/kg.

Table 11–10. Organ-related symptoms of hyperviscosity

Central nervous system	Irritability, jitteriness, seizures, lethargy
Cardiopulmonary	Respiratory distress secondary to congestive heart failure or persistent pulmonary hypertension
Gastrointestinal	Vomiting, heme-positive stools, distension, NEC
Renal	Decreased urine output, renal vein thrombosis
Metabolic	Hypoglycemia
Hematologic	Hyperbilirubinemia, thrombocytopenia

Prognosis

Follow-up studies at 1–2 years have revealed that infants with hyperviscosity have more motor problems, more abnormal neurologic examinations, and delayed speech development. At 7 years of age, some subtle findings persist. Whether or not this outcome can be improved by treatment is unclear.

METABOLIC DISORDERS

HYPOGLYCEMIA

Hypoglycemia is defined as a blood glucose level less than 40 mg/dL. Although glucose concentration normally decreases in all infants during the postpartum period, most term babies have stable glucose (50–80 mg/dL) by 3 hours of age. Two high-risk groups for hypoglycemia are infants of diabetic mothers and infants with intrauterine growth retardation.

In infants of diabetic mothers (IDM), hypoglycemia develops because of an imbalance in insulin-glucagon secretion due to hyperinsulinemia from islet-cell hyperplasia. Infants are macrosomic because other sites grow abnormally in utero secondary to an increased flow of nutrients. They may also have asymmetric septal cardiac hypertrophy, small left colon, hypercoagulability, and polycythemia. As these infants are immature for gestational age, there is an increased risk for HMD, hypocalcemia, and hyperbilirubinemia. IDMs are also at increased risk for congenital anomalies, likely related to first-trimester glucose control.

Intrauterine growth retarded infants have appropriate endocrine control but low carbohydrate stores in the form of glycogen.

Other causes of hypoglycemia include other disorders with islet-cell hyperplasia (Beckwith-Wiedemann, nesidioblastosis, erythroblastosis fetalis), inborn errors (leucine sensitivity, glycogen storage diseases, galactosemia), and endocrine disorders (panhypopituitarism). Hypoglycemia may also be associated with birth asphyxia and sepsis.

Clinical Findings

Symptoms can be nonspecific and include lethargy, irritability, poor feeding, and regurgitation. More severe symptoms include cardiorespiratory distress, apnea, and seizures.

Catecholamine-related symptoms may be present and include pallor, sweating, cold extremities, and increased heart rate. Hypoglycemia may be detected by commercially available test strips, but these may be unreliable with glucose levels below 40 mg/dL. All low glucose levels should be verified by direct measurement with a glucose analyzer.

Treatment

A treatment regimen is present in Table 11–11.

Prognosis

Prompt therapy improves prognosis. CNS sequelae occur with hypoglycemic seizures.

HYPOCALCEMIA

Hypocalcemia is defined as a total serum concentration less than 7–8 mg/dL (equivalent to calcium activity of 3–3.5 meq/L). Early onset on day 1–2 is seen in IDM, sepsis, asphyxia, prematurity, and maternal hyperparathyroidism; late onset (1–2 weeks of age) is seen in infants receiving modified cow's milk with high phosphorus content.

Clinical Findings

Clinical signs include a high-pitched cry, jitteriness, tremulousness, and seizures. ECG may show a prolonged QT interval.

Table 11–11. Hypoglycemia: suggested therapeutic regimens.

Screening Test	Symptoms	Action
Test strip 20–40 mg/dL	None	Confirm with blood glucose; if infant is alert and vigorous, feed; follow with frequent test strips. If the baby continues after 1 or 2 feeds to have test strips <40 mg/dL, provide intravenous glucose at 6 mg/kg/min.
Test strip <40 mg/dL	Present	Confirm with blood glucose; provide bolus (2 mL/kg) of D10W followed by an infusion of 6 mg/kg/min.
Test strip <20 mg/dL	±	Confirm with blood glucose; provide bolus (2 mL/kg) of D10W followed by an infusion of 6 mg/kg/min. If IV access cannot be obtained immediately, an umbilical venous line should be utilized.

Treatment

Calcium gluconate (0.5–1 g/kg/d) may be given orally (45–90 mg/kg elemental calcium). It is administered IV for frank tetany or seizures. Cautious IV use is necessary to prevent the right-atrial calcium concentration rising too quickly, which can cause bradycardia. Close observation for tissue infiltrates is important. The dosage is 10% calcium gluconate as a 2 mL/kg bolus over 10–20 minutes. Do not add calcium salts to IV solutions with sodium bicarbonate as they will precipitate.

Prognosis

Prognosis is excellent.

INFANTS OF MOTHERS WITH DRUG ABUSE

Drug abuse is an increasing problem in all parts of the country. Maternal history of abuse is often difficult to obtain but must be pursued. Withdrawal symptoms are common with many drugs, narcotics and alcohol being most prominent (Table 11–12).

RENAL DISORDERS

Renal function is dependent on postconceptional age. Normal renal function and tests are presented in Table 11–13. Normal urine output is 1–3 mg/kg/min.

The most common renal disorders seen in newborns are renal failure, renal vein thrombosis (RVT), and congenital anomalies.

RENAL FAILURE

Clinical Findings

Renal failure is often seen following an asphyxial episode, hypovolemia, or sepsis. Two phases are present: (1) anuria/oliguria (first 2–3 days) associated with hematuria, proteinuria, and increased creatinine, and (2) polyuria with increased urine losses of sodium and bicarbonate.

Table 11–12. Drugs commonly abused during pregnancy.

Drug	Clinical Tips	Treatment and Prognosis
Narcotics (heroin, methadone, propoxyphene, codeine)	Heroin/methadone withdrawal similar, with methadone having longer duration. Early onset 1–2 d, although methadone withdrawal may be delayed. Symptoms: irritability, hyperactivity, tremors, high-pitched cry, excessive hunger, salivation, sweating, sneezing, yawning, nasal stuffiness, tachypnea, diarrhea, and seizures.	Supportive care (quiet environment, swaddling) usually sufficient. Medical control: phenobarbital (loading dose 15–20 mg/kg; maintenance dose 5 mg/kg divided BID), valium, paregoric. Prognosis good but mortality can occur in severe cases. Increased incidence of sudden infant death syndrome.
Ethanol	Fetal/newborn effects proportional to abuse amount. Effects— SGA, dysmorphic features (short palpebral fissures, microcephaly), cardiac and joint anomalies; withdrawal similar to narcotics.	Treat as in narcotic withdrawal. Postnatal growth may be slow, mental retardation, hyperactivity in severe cases.
Tobacco	SGA	Maternal education regarding prevention important.
Cocaine	May see abruptio placenta and CNS infarct of infant secondary to vasoconstrictive properties of drug. Genitourinery anomalies also reported.	Screen infant for metabolites with suspected maternal history. Close observation, no specific therapy.

Treatment

The initial step is fluid resuscitation, if necessary, followed by fluid restriction equal to insensible water losses (40–60 mL/kg/d) plus urine losses. Hyperkalemia must be observed for in the presence of oliguria/anuria. During the polyuric phases, the

Table 11–13. Summary of neonatal renal function.

Function	Premature	Full-term	2 wk	8 wk	1 Yr
Glomerular filtration (mL/min/1.73 m)	13–58	15–60	50	63–80	120
Concentrating ability (mosm/L)	480	800	900	1200	1400
Tests		**Gestational age**			
Creatinine (mg/dL)	<28 wk	29–32 wk	33–36 wk	36–42 wk	
0–2 d	1.2	1.1	1.1	0.8	
28 d	0.7	0.6	0.45	0.3	

infant should be allowed to diurese if fluid overloaded, with careful attention paid to water, salt, and acid–base balance.

RENAL VEIN THROMBOSIS

RVT is seen most frequently in IDMs and infants with dehydration and polycythemia. Clinically, one might suspect RVT on basis of a new renal mass (usually unilateral), hematuria, and proteinuria. Anuria may be present if RVT is bilateral. Diagnosis can be confirmed with renal ultrasound. Treatment involves correcting the predisposing condition and heparinization. Systemic hypertension has been noted in some infants.

CONGENITAL ANOMALIES

Abdominal masses in the newborn are most frequently due to renal enlargement—multicystic/dysplastic kidney and hydronephrosis. Anomalies might also be suspected on the basis of a maternal history of oligohydramnios, which can be associated with renal agenesis or posterior urethral valves. Diagnosis in most cases is aided by renal ultrasound.

NEUROLOGIC DISORDERS

HYPOXIC ISCHEMIC ENCEPHALOPATHY

Hypoxic ischemic encephalopathy (HIE) occurs in both preterm and term infants. In the preterm infant it is often associated with intraventricular hemorrhage.

Clinical Findings

Infants with evidence of fetal distress before and during labor are at risk. Clinical features include (1) birth to 12 hours: decreased level of consciousness, hypotonia, decreased spontaneous movement, periodic breathing or apnea, possible seizures; (2) 12–24 hours: seizures, apnea, jitteriness, weakness; (3) over 24 hours: decreased level of consciousness, progressive apnea, onset of brainstem dysfunction, hypotonia, poor feeding.

The severity of clinical signs and the length of time the signs persist correlate with the severity of insult. Other helpful diagnostic tools include EEG, CT scan, evoked potentials, and technetium scan.

Treatment

The mainstay of therapy is to provide adequate oxygen to the injured brain and to maintain normal Pa_{O2} and blood pressure. Fluids may be modestly restricted, glucose normalized, and anticonvulsants given for seizures.

Prognosis

The best predictor of outcome is the severity of clinical encephalopathy (severe symptoms are correlated with a 75% chance of death and 100% rate of neurologic sequelae). Major sequelae in survivors are cerebral palsy and mental retardation.

INTRACRANIAL BLEEDING

A. Subdural Hemorrhage: Subdural bleeding is usually related to birth trauma and occurs in 3 locations (tentorial laceration, falx laceration, and rupture of superficial cerebral veins). Major complications of the first 2 types is extension of bleeding infratentorially, causing brainstem compression that requires immediate surgical drainage. Bleeds in the third location are the most common and may be asymptomatic or may cause seizures on days 2–3. Diagnosis can be confirmed with CT scan. The prognosis is poor for bleeding in the first 2 locations; 75% of infants with bleeding of the third type have normal follow-up.

B. Subarachnoid Hemorrhage: Subarachnoid bleeding is the most common type of hemorrhage. In prematures it is associated with germinal matrix bleed and in term infants with birth trauma. The most common presentation is with seizures and irritability on day 2 of life. Diagnosis is aided by CT scan and lumbar puncture. Prognosis is good.

C. Periventricular/Intraventricular Hemorrhage: Intraventricular hemorrhage is seen almost exclusively in premature infants. The incidence is 25–35% in infants less than 31 weeks' gestation and 1500 grams. Other risk factors include birth asphyxia, severe respiratory distress, and pneumothorax. Bleeding is most commonly seen in the subependymal germinal matrix but may extend into the ventricular cavity. Primary parenchymal hemorrhages can be seen as well. Fifty percent of bleeds occur by 24 hours of age, and the vast majority by 4 days. Clinically, these bleeds range from asymptomatic to rapidly catastrophic presentations (coma, hypoventilation, acidosis, shock, drop in hematocrit). Diagnosis is by real time ultrasound. The grading system is as follows: Grade I, germinal matrix bleed only (60% of bleeds); Grade II, intraventricular bleed without enlargement of the ventricles; Grade III, intraventricular bleed with enlargement of the ventricles; Grade IV, any of the above plus intracerebral hemorrhage.

Routine screening is performed at 4–7 days in infants less than 31 weeks' gestation or any "sick" infant at 31–35 weeks. Follow-up for Grade I/II is at 2 weeks of age; Grade III/IV within 1 week of initial screen. Further follow-ups are dictated by progression of ventricular enlargement. One should also seek evidence of periventricular leukomalacia (cystic changes in periventricular white matter), which is usually evident by 17–21 days of age.

Treatment

Initial treatment should be based on the infant's status; the more severely affected may require volume resuscitation, transfusion, and increased ventilatory support. If progressive posthemorrhagic hydrocephalus develops, it can be controlled by decreasing CSF production (Lasix 1 mg/kg/d plus Diamox, increasing doses from 25–100 mg/kg/d) or by removal of CSF with daily lumbar puncture.

Prognosis

There is no mortality with Grade I/II bleeds, while Grade III/IV carry a 10–20% mortality risk. Ventriculomegaly is rare with Grade I, but is found in 54–87% of Grade II–IV bleeds. Long-term neurologic risk in Grade I/II is no different from premature infants who experience no bleeding; with grade III/IV, sequelae severe occur in 20–25%, mild in 35%, and absent in 40%. The major severe long-term sequelae include hydrocephalus, cerebral palsy, and mental retardation.

SEIZURES

Organized tonic-clonic seizures in infants are rare owing to incomplete cortical organization and a preponderance of inhibitory synapses. The most common type of seizure is characterized by a constellation of findings including horizontal deviation of eyes with or without jerking, eyelid blinking, or fluttering; sucking, smacking, drooling; swimming, rowing, or paddling movements; and apneic spells. One can also see strictly tonic or

Table 11–14. Differential diagnosis of neonatal seizures.

Diagnosis	Comment
Hypoxic-ischemic encephalopathy	Most common cause (60%); onset within first 24 hours
Intracranial hemorrhage	Up to 15% of cases: PVH/IVH, subdural or subarachnoid bleeds
Infection	12% of cases
Hypoglycemia	SGA, IDM
Hypocalcemia, hypomagnesemia	Low-birth-weight infant, IDMs
Hyponatremia	Rare, seen with SIADH (syndrome of inappropriate secretion of antidiuretic hormone)
Disorders of amino and organic acid metabolism, hyperammonemia	Associated acidosis, altered level of consciousness
Pyridoxine dependency	Seizures refractory to routine therapy; cessation of seizures after administration of pyridoxine
Developmental defects	other anomalies, chromosomal syndromes
Drug withdrawal	
No cause found	10% of cases

multifocal clonic episodes. The differential diagnosis of neonatal seizures is given in Table 11–14.

Treatment

Supportive therapy to ensure adequate ventilation and perfusion should be provided. Hypoglycemia should be promptly treated; other therapy is directed toward the specific underlying cause. Phenobarbital (20 mg/kg loading with supplemental doses of 5 mg/kg/d up to 40 mg/kg) can be utilized. If seizures persist, therapy with dilantin, sodium valproate, lorazepam, and paraldehyde may be tried. A trial of pyridoxine for refractory seizures is indicated.

Prognosis

Prognosis is related to the cause of the seizure—the more difficult they are to control, the worse the prognosis. Seizures due to hypoglycemia and CNS infection, some inborn errors of metabolism, and developmental defects also have a high rate of poor outcome.

12 | Emotional Problems

Ruth S. Kempe, MD

Very early in life, the infant's behavior—limited as it is by genetic endowment, temperament, and medical history—reflects the success with which bodily needs are recognized, interpreted, and satisfied, chiefly by the mother. Knowledge about and mastery of the infant's own body and physical environment develop simultaneously, and the interplay between development in the physical and emotional environments may be harmonious or conflictual. Serious conflict in either area is apt to affect performance in the other—eg, the motor development of emotionally deprived infants is slow. With time, experience becomes integrated and internalized, and the infant becomes a complex person capable of reacting in a highly individualized way to new experiences.

For the very young child, emotional life grows from many additive emotional interchanges in the relationship with the parents, especially the mother. As the child grows, the emotional environment expands to include siblings, extended family, babysitters, and peers. By 2 or 3 years of age, as contacts with outsiders increase, the child will already have developed many attitudes and learned ways of reacting to others. As relationships develop, conflict is unavoidable and must be dealt with; how the conflict is resolved can contribute to the child's maturity and self-esteem or can create further difficulty.

For the parent, too, the child's development can present opportunities for emotional gratification or sometimes create problems. Parents often have difficulty dealing with problems in their children that they themselves have resolved poorly or that caused difficulty when they were children. It is an indication of maturity in parents if they are able to help a child develop freely without seizing on a "second chance" to gratify their own unfulfilled wishes.

ROLE OF THE PHYSICIAN

Pediatricians have a unique opportunity as physicians to promote emotional health as well as physical health and to practice preventive psychiatry. No other health professionals are in a position to be so knowledgeable about the interplay of genetic, physical, social, cultural, and interpersonal influences on the developing child. Yet it is likely that only about one-half of the mental health problems present in a pediatric practice are ordinarily detected by the pediatrician.

The first chance to assess the relationship between parents and child is immediately after birth, while mother and child are still in the hospital. If there are doubts about whether normal bonding between parents and infant will occur, the physician should stand ready to help the parents adjust to their new roles and be prepared to intervene promptly if necessary. In many cases, the pediatrician is the only contact the infant may have with the outside world. Many parent–child problems can be prevented if the pediatrician schedules early and frequent office visits, encourages inquiries by telephone, and makes provision for extra visits by public health nurses or family aides in cases in which the child is considered to be at special risk.

At each regular check-up, the pediatrician should inquire about the child's social and emotional adjustment. A useful question about a very young child might be, ''What kind of baby is Johnny?'' or ''What kind of personality does Susie have?'' Routinely checking the child's emotional adjustment during regular medical care alerts parents to its importance, makes it easier to give the parents appropriate information about variations in normal development, reassures parents about common problems, and recognizes serious parenting difficulties or emotional problems in the child.

Families often ask for advice, and the pediatrician has the opportunity to further the child's healthy development by anticipating and encouraging appropriate recognition of developmental needs, providing reassurance when parental anxiety becomes restrictive, and helping delineate parental limit-setting when the child's impulses are unacceptable.

In times of family crisis, the pediatrician must be available to and supportive of the child by recognizing the child's probable needs, providing advocacy in school or hospital, and providing support when parents are overwhelmed.

The pediatrician is often the first person the parents turn to for help with the emotional problems of their children. An interested physician can be very helpful; one who is uncomfortable in the role of psychologic counselor should be wary of giving casual advice and should find another professional for consultation or referral. Many common problems that arise in families do not need the attention of a specialist in child psychiatry. Pediatricians capably practice much more psychologic medicine than is commonly recognized.

One of the pediatrician's first concerns will be to assess the severity of the problem and decide whether to refer the patient to a specialist for further care. The pediatrician should be thoroughly familiar with normal development in children and the wide variations compatible with it. Since many children have transitory behavior difficulties during times of personal stress, the physician may wish to follow the patient for a time to see whether the problem resolves spontaneously, but must avoid giving a blanket assurance that "He'll grow out of it."

Severe emotional illness is usually easy to recognize, and the physician's goal in such cases will be to make a successful referral to a psychiatrist. Less obvious problems can be considerably more difficult to evaluate, and detailed examination is worthwhile.

If a detailed evaluation in the physician's office does not clarify possible treatment objectives, consultation with a psychiatrist or a behavioral pediatrician may help. Some pediatricians meet regularly with a child psychiatrist or have developed an informal consultation relationship that can be educational for both and allows some patients to be treated in the setting of a pediatric practice. If little progress is observed after several interviews, referral can be discussed with the parents.

The role of the physician should also be considered from a more personal viewpoint. Physicians' attitudes undoubtedly influence their reactions to their patients' problems. Like parents, physicians sometimes have difficulty helping children with problems they themselves have not been able to overcome. Thus, physicians must be conscious of the part their personal attitudes play in their professional thinking. This does not mean, of course, that people with personal difficulties cannot help others; it does mean that we must understand how our personal concerns might influence our professional attitudes so we can minimize that influence.

SPECIAL PROBLEMS OF PARENTING

Although everyone finds parenting tiring, stressful, and unrewarding at times, some parents seldom find it rewarding and some are unable to care adequately for a child. It is important to identify such parents as early as possible, to keep track of their performance as parents, primarily in order to offer extra support, and to intervene promptly if abuse or neglect occurs.

Some parents have great difficulty in bonding with one of their children but can love and respond well to the others. Even if physical abuse or gross neglect does not occur, the "unwanted" child may have developmental or behavioral difficulties brought on by unconscious or overt parenting difficulties. By discussing that child's development, encouraging daycare or preschool placement, and offering early referral for psychiatric help, the pediatrician can be of help to a child whose parents offer no direct opportunities for intervention involving them.

Hints that a parent (or guardian or step-parent) may be at risk for poor parenting can be listed as follows:

(1) A history of abuse, neglect, or deprivation as a child.

(2) A suspected or explicit history of abuse or neglect of another child.

(3) Low self-esteem, depression, or social isolation.

(4) Signs of social stress, eg, marital discord, recent loss of an important personal relationship, frequent moves, layoffs or other financial difficulties.

(5) Unrealistic expectations of the child's performance and a lack of understanding of normal development in children.

(6) A belief that the child is willfully difficult or provocative and that physical punishment is "good for children."

(7) Difficulty in forming a bond with the child; a rejecting attitude.

(8) A history of mental illness, alcohol or drug abuse, or criminal activity.

(9) Violent outbursts of temper.

Child Abuse and Neglect

Physical abuse, neglect, emotional deprivation, and sexual abuse occur in families at all educational and economic levels. In the USA, physicians and nurses (and other specified classes of child-care professionals) are legally required to report known or reasonably suspected cases of child abuse or neglect.

Cardinal signs of abuse are physical injuries inadequately explained by the history, injuries (including poisoning) that are implausible or discrepant with the child's developmental age, and delay in seeking medical care. In the USA, reports of possible abuse are filed for about 2 million children each year. Over 50% of these cases involve neglect, while the remainder involve physical abuse (> 25%), sexual abuse (> 15%), and emotional abuse (> 10%). Each year, 2000 to 5000 physically abused children die, and there are indications that the number of deaths from neglect may be higher than that from physical abuse. Any combination of abuses may occur in a given family.

Signs of physical abuse include pathognomonic bruises left by lashing, grabbing, slapping, tying, choking, and pinching. Forcible feeding of a crying infant may produce bruises of the frontal dental ridge. The pediatrician should recognize burns inflicted by cigarettes, heating grates, and dunking of the lower body in very hot water. Over half of subdural hematomas in infants occur without fractures or signs of scalp trauma and are the result of violent shaking. Retinal hemorrhages can usually be seen on ophthalmoscopic examination and their duration accurately estimated. Unexplained abdominal injuries such as ruptured spleen, ruptured bowel, intramural hematoma of the duodenum, or pseudocyst of the pancreas are usually inflicted injuries. A skeletal survey will often confirm the diagnosis by disclosing multiple bone changes due to fractures at different stages of healing that were caused by violent wrenching or pulling of the extremities. These findings may include metaphyseal chip fracture, subperiosteal calcification, epiphyseal displacement ("nursemaid's elbow"), and cortical thickening.

Signs of neglect include poor physical care, with inadequate nutrition, health care, and personal hygiene. Occipital baldness in an infant may be a sign that the infant is being left unattended in a crib for long periods. There may be failure to recognize and satisfy developmental and emotional needs and lack of supervision, exposing the child to a risk of accidental injury. These acts of omission may lead to growth retardation; frequent illnesses or accidents; and retarded motor, cognitive, or social development. Emotional deprivation may lead to severe delays and distortions of personality development.

Growth failure due to insufficient caloric intake (*nonorganic failure to thrive*) is common in infants during the first 2 years of life. It is seen as retardation or cessation of growth (especially of weight gain) in the absence of a discernible physical cause such as neurologic or heart disease. Unless the parent is cooperative and there is rapid response to initial outpatient treatment, the infant should be hospitalized for a basic physical evaluation, observation of the parent–infant interaction (especially in feeding and play), and evaluation of the infant's response to adequate feeding. Some mothers have difficulties with breast-feeding and need advice and support. Others—through negligence or ignorance—have not obtained, understood, or followed instructions for good formula-feeding techniques. A few infants are difficult to feed because of delay in development of motor (sucking) skills, chalasia, and so on, and need special feeding techniques.

A higher percentage of admissions for growth failure are due to **reactive attachment disorder of infancy,** in which the deprivation of social interaction and love—which in these cases accompanies the inadequate feeding—causes severe delays in development. In addition to malnutrition, the infants show poor emotional development, with lack of early eye contact, smiling, affection, and the ability to be comforted. Such infants are socially unresponsive, often also to the mother, and may ignore or look away from social contacts. They are apathetic and may show little or no interest in playing with toys. Physical development suffers and is characterized by weakness, poor muscle tone, and delayed gross and fine motor development.

This syndrome is a result of both inadequate feeding and inadequate parenting, as can be demonstrated by placing the infant with an adequate substitute mother. Rapid recovery occurs when the infant's physical, emotional, and social needs are met. If the infant remains with the mother and parenting is only partially improved (eg, the infant is adequately fed but there is no improvement in the emotional relationship between parent and infant), delays in development and emotional difficulties persist, making the infant vulnerable to stress. Long-term medical and psychiatric follow-up are needed.

Sexual abuse is the involvement of a dependent, developmentally immature person in sexual activities. A child or adolescent may be sexually abused by an adult or by an older child or adolescent. In some studies 20–40% of adults admit to an episode of sexual abuse before adulthood. Sexual abuse includes exhibitionism (indecent exposure); molestation (pedophilia); seduction with oral, anal, or genital intercourse; forcible rape; incest; child prostitution; and child pornography. Most sexual abuse (> 90% of cases) involves an offender known to the child, and over half of cases of repeated abuse involve a member of the family.

Physical signs of sexual abuse (eg, vaginal or anal lesions) may be present in about one-third of cases. However, symptoms may be primarily emotional, including sexualized or seductive behavior, anxiety, fear, depression, poor self-esteem, preoccupation, poor school performance, or symptoms of posttraumatic stress disorder. Depression, running away, promiscuity, prostitution, and substance abuse (eg, drugs, alcohol) in adolescents are often linked to sexual abuse. Masked sexual abuse presents as vague physical symptoms such as eating and sleeping problems, abdominal or joint pains, and depression. Boys who are victims of sexual abuse usually complain to no one. The pediatrician is often the only person with an opportunity to make the diagnosis of sexual abuse (including incest), which should be considered in children with poorly defined complaints. Reporting of sexual abuse is mandatory and treatment of victims and perpetrators of child sexual abuse is necessary.

Emotional abuse is recognized not only as an integral part of physical and sexual abuse but often as a devastating problem in itself. It can be difficult to demonstrate, and the physician often must use the treatment of other symptoms as a means of aiding or arranging help for the child. Denigration, rejection, ignoring, corruption, and exploitation are common forms of emotional abuse.

Intentional causing of illness or poisoning of a child by the mother ("Munchausen-by-proxy" syndrome) is rare but less so than supposed. It may continue during visiting hours while the child is in the hospital for diagnosis. Medications may be given to produce vomiting, diarrhea, cardiac symptoms, etc. False evidence of bleeding or infection may be produced. Barbiturates, tranquilizers, alcohol, and heroin are among the substances implicated; salt feeding may also take place. Guarding the child and setting up a drug screen can assist in the diagnosis. Seeking treatment for false or manufactured symptoms in the child serves unconscious needs of the parent, putting the child at grave risk. Protection, placement, and a trial of therapy for the parent are indicated.

ASSESSMENT OF THE CHILD

It is often helpful to schedule two closely spaced interviews when evaluating a difficult emotional problem. The interval allows time to arrange for additional testing if needed and gives the parents an opportunity to ponder questions raised during the first interview, recall additional pertinent information, and perhaps view the child with greater insight, which may be revealing.

The history of an emotional problem is best taken in an unhurried, informal manner. For this reason, it is often wise to allow for a lengthy interview. The physician's ability to listen calmly, attentively, and with understanding is an important factor in determining the source of the problem. Parents should be encouraged to speak freely and to stress areas of greatest concern. Noting the parents' modes of "body language" and other nonverbal communication can open unexpected channels of information. Nonverbal communications include facial expressions, hesitancy, restlessness, defensiveness, sudden angry tones of voice, tearfulness, and evidence of anxiety.

The pediatrician needs to formulate an impression of the parents as individuals and an impression of the problems they face apart from those they have as parents. Care must be taken not to assume that only the parents are at fault; this is rarely true and can foredoom to failure any attempt at therapeutic intervention. Understanding the parents' own needs, even when they are in conflict with the child's needs, and recognizing their abilities as parents can do much to support and improve the quality of the parent–child relationship. Most people genuinely wish to be good parents. The anxiety and frustration aroused in parents by a child's difficult behavior need to be alleviated through supportive discussion and management. The physician also needs to recognize any emotional problems in the parents; their need for psychiatric therapy may be as urgent as the child's need for help.

The relationship between the child's presenting problem and coincident family events may be a clue to diagnosis. Thus, a brief family history should be taken to place the child's problem in a historic setting.

The child should be present for part of the evaluation to let the physician see how the child and parents interact in talking about the difficulty. This is also a time when the physician may wish to assure the child that his or her feelings of unhappiness or helplessness are recognized and to offer the parents an opportunity to recognize the child's point of view.

Evaluation of Emotional Problems in Children (Sample Outline)

A. Presenting Symptoms: Description of symptoms; duration and severity; time of onset and accompanying circumstances (possible precipitating cause); history of previous attempts to deal with the problem and attitudes toward it.

B. Other Symptoms: Description of past and present symptoms.

C. Adjustment of the Child: Description of overall and present adjustment; interactions in family, school, peer situations; description of personality traits, abilities, activities.

D. Developmental History: History of the pregnancy;

mother's attitude toward pregnancy; initial reaction to infant; evidences of bonding. Child's psychomotor development; feeding, toilet-training, sleep, or disciplinary problems; curiosity about sex and other topics.

E. Family History: Major events such as births of siblings, moves, illnesses, accidents, deaths, separations, parental discord.

F. Parent–Child Relationships: Past difficulties; parents' areas of special concern about the child; differences of opinion between parents about the child. Is child's symptom a reaction to serious problems in a parent?

G. Observations of the Patient:

1. Observations of child with parents together and their joint discussion of the problem helps delineate their relationship and views on the difficulty.

2. Play interview with the child:

a. Usually the easiest format to put child at ease as doctor discusses problem with him/her.

b. Crayons and paper, a doll family, and/or play dough are usually most helpful toys, allowing expression of feelings roused by the conversation.

c. Confidentiality (as far as it can be guaranteed) should be offered the child.

d. Expression of the physician's desire to help and the importance of the child's point of view.

e. Allowing the child opportunity to ask questions.

f. Offering the child further opportunity to talk if desired (for older children the doctor may give the child his or her phone number).

3. Mental status of the child:

a. Will include observations of how child relates socially.

b. Child's emotional state, especially as related to specific topics.

c. Thought content with worries, unusual thought content, fantasies, dreams.

d. Language with developmental level and ability to communicate.

e. Motor activity, attention span.

f. Cognitive.

H. Behavior Questionnaires: A behavior questionnaire filled out by the parents either before the assessment or during the child interview will help ensure good coverage of potential problem behaviors. The Achenbach Child Behavior Checklist is probably the most used and very complete. The Pediatric Symptoms Checklist is much shorter but is effective and can be used as a screening tool with parents.

I. Special Examinations: Screening examinations for developmental problems, tests of vision or hearing, or referral for psychologic testing.

J. Outside Opinions: Advisability of soliciting opinions from teachers, psychologists, or others after obtaining a written release from the parents.

Diagnostic Considerations & Treatment Planning

(1) Transitory or recent symptoms are usually more easily treated than those that have remained unchanged for months or years; they may even disappear spontaneously. If symptoms arise in response to a particular crisis and can be understood as an appropriate response to the crisis, supportive counseling may lead to resolution and increasing maturity. When no precipitating causes are apparent, intrapsychic stress is more likely and a review of the history may show previous episodes of maladjustment.

(2) Generalized adjustment difficulties—with several symptoms that affect performance in school, at home, and with peers—indicate a more pervasive pathologic process.

(3) Two of the most common responses to assess in young children are the cessation of developmental progress and the partial reversal of developmental progress (regression). They occur with physical as well as with emotional illness and may be the only signs of problems in infants.

(4) The parents' special concern about the child may not be shared by the child. If the symptom (eg, obesity or a phobia) produces little discomfort in the child or provides an effective mechanism for avoiding the child's underlying anxiety, the child may not want help until changes in lifestyle make the symptom less acceptable. If the symptom is disturbing only to the parents, a decision must be made about whether the parents' expectations are too high or the parents are reacting to personal intrapsychic distress, or whether therapy is indicated because of the nature of the symptom.

Review of the Evaluation

As an understanding of the child's emotional difficulties develops during an evaluation, a further course of action may become self-evident. The evaluation itself can help parents and child to express their feelings openly, often for the first time, and to communicate them to one another, with the reassuring support of the physician. Exploration of the family's history and current situation can lead to better understanding, particularly when the physician helps interpret the relationship between events and the child's behavior. In such cases, interpretation would not center on unconscious dynamics but on educating the family about the usual limitations or capacities of children to respond to stress. With continued support from the physician, the parents and child may try new ways of coping with the problem, and the physician may be able, through suggestion, to urge them in the direction of healthier behavior. Continued interest, follow-up, and support may lead to resolution of the problem. If not, psychiatric consultation can be recommended.

DEVELOPMENTAL DISORDERS

MENTAL RETARDATION

The physician has a major role in helping the family with a mentally handicapped child.

Diagnosis
(1) Usually suspects and confirms the diagnosis.
(2) Usually informs the parents of diagnosis. Counsels family concerning realistic educational and social expectations for child. Helps family to mourn loss of perfect child and cope with feelings of responsibility, guilt, and resentment. Arranges genetic counseling.

Treatment
(1) Specific treatment for type of retardation when available.
(2) Advocacy at school for special tutoring and program needs, which may be government-mandated.
(3) Advocacy in community for sports and social programs—often available through referral to Aid for Retarded Children or other parent groups.
(4) Counseling to family regarding child's diminished capacity for adaptation and increased likelihood of emotional disturbance.
(5) Development of social judgment and interpersonal coping skills are major goals.

MILD MENTAL HANDICAP

Children with IQs from 70 to 90 are not diagnosed as retarded but are handicapped, a problem that often is not recognized early. Such children often are considered lazy or un-cooperative, and may feel inadequate. A less demanding academic program allows for success. Appropriate vocational skill training uses child's personal strengths. Help in development of interpersonal skills and special abilities such as music or sports promote success and self-esteem.

EDUCATIONAL UNDERACHIEVEMENT WITH NORMAL OR SUPERIOR INTELLIGENCE

Etiology

(1) Specific developmental disorders and attention deficit disorder should be diagnosed and treated, if present.

(2) Early environmental deprivation or distorted parental expectations may have resulted in poor problem-solving techniques, lack of motivation, and avoidance of potential failure.

(3) Emotional disturbance with depression or high levels of anxiety or anger may cause child to be too preoccupied to perceive and integrate new knowledge or to retrieve what has been learned.

(4) Sudden change in academic performance may signal a traumatic experience.

Diagnosis

(1) Family history, with particular attention to parental expectations and child's early coping responses.

(2) Physical, neurologic, and psychologic evaluations are needed.

(3) Current symptoms of emotional disturbance.

Treatment

(1) Any specific etiology needs specific treatment.

(2) Educational consultation and perhaps tutoring in learning strategies for "catch-up."

(3) Referral for psychotherapy, when indicated.

SPECIFIC DEVELOPMENTAL DISORDERS OF READING, ARITHMETIC, OR SPEECH

These disorders are due to delays in development of the respective capacities. They are not due to inadequate intelligence or a known specific cause, and may sometimes persist into adulthood. They may appear together or in association with attention deficit disorder or, if diagnosed late, in conjunction with school and social behavioral symptoms. Not infrequently, parents or other family members have had similar difficulty.

Diagnosis

(1) Physical and neurologic examination (including soft signs); careful visual, hearing, and perhaps speech evaluations.

(2) Complete psychologic testing of intelligence and of academic achievement in relevant areas.

(3) Careful educational history, plus family and adjustment history to ascertain contributory or secondary symptoms.

Treatment

(1) Tutoring by skilled personnel in specific educational area.

(2) Treatment of any contributory condition such as attention deficit disorder.

(3) Counseling of family regarding nature of disorder, appropriate expectations, and supportive attitudes.

(4) Counseling or psychotherapy of child, depending on degree to which child adjusts realistically or has developed a maladaptive emotional response.

AUTISTIC DISORDER (INFANTILE AUTISM)

Clinical Findings

A severe distortion in development.

(1) Lacking the ability to relate emotionally to other persons.

(2) Lacking the ability to communicate both verbally and nonverbally.

(3) Causing restriction of interests and a lack of capacity to adapt to environmental changes, even in a minor degree, without severe anxiety.

(4) Associated with a wide range of intelligence, although more often it is in the retarded range.

Symptoms vary in severity from the child who remains nonverbal with an IQ under 50 who requires lifelong institutionalization to perhaps 30% of patients who are able to live semi-independent to independent lives, with residual social awkwardness and restricted interests but evidence of good intelligence.

Etiology

Presumed to be related to faulty brain development, but in a manner not yet known. Seizure activity occurs in about 25% of patients after childhood, usually in the more severely handicapped patients.

Diagnosis

Onset by age 30 months. The lack of awareness of other's feelings or interest in relationships is accompanied by distortions in communication; the preoccupation with inanimate objects and narrowness of interests are present in a degree commensurate with the intellectual capacity. Thus, autistic disorder presents particular developmental distortions that remain fairly consistent in quality over a spectrum of intellectual capacity.

Treatment

(1) Psychiatric management.

(2) Children often require hospitalization initially. Institutionalization may be necessary later for the most handicapped.

(3) Special education (usually in the public school system) and later sheltered workshops allow many to earn a partial living and live in a protected setting. A small number make a comparatively good work adjustment with highly circumscribed but effective skills and an independent lifestyle.

(4) Behavioral modification is often the most effective tool if adapted to the education needs of the given autistic child to improve social interaction and effective use of language.

(5) A large amount of research has evaluated the efficacy of many drugs in autistic disorder, without any remarkable benefit. Haloperidol and phenothiazines make some children more available to educational measures but do not change the basic characteristics of the disorder.

CHILDHOOD-ONSET PERVASIVE DEVELOPMENTAL DISORDER

Appears after age 30 months; may be milder but similar in symptomatology to autistic disorder.

COMMON DEVELOPMENTAL PROBLEMS

These problems do not constitute a psychiatric disorder but may cause parents considerable worry and lead to requests for advice. They include variations in response to normal developmental steps and difficult responses to environmental crises.

BEHAVIORAL DISORDERS

ATTENTION DEFICIT HYPERACTIVITY DISORDER

Clinical Findings
Before the age of 7, the child shows problems of inattention and impulse control, usually with hyperactivity. Symptoms include the following:

(1) restless, squirming behavior,
(2) difficulty remaining seated,
(3) easily distracted by extraneous stimuli,
(4) difficulty awaiting turn,
(5) difficulty following instructions,
(6) difficulty sustaining attention,
(7) works without planning,
(8) shifts activity frequently,
(9) requires supervision for task completion,
(10) talks excessively, and,
(11) always "on the go" (sometimes even in sleep).

Etiology
The cause is not known. It was called minimal brain dysfunction in the past but neurologic status is not clear. There is a slightly increased familial incidence. The diagnosis is based on the child's behavior. Other causes of hyperactivity (brief and age-appropriate) or poor attention span due to anxiety or to a chaotic environment should be ruled out.

Treatment
(1) Highly structured and mildly restricted routine.
(2) Provision of an environment with few distractions.
(3) Additional one-to-one supervision.
(4) Remedial tutoring if academic work has suffered.
(5) Methylphenidate (Ritalin) or dextroamphetamine is often remarkably effective. However, because these drugs have side effects, their use must be monitored and discontinued occasionally for evaluation of their continued need.

CONDUCT DISORDER
(Including Delinquency)

Types
(1) Group type—usually occurs in a peer group, often as a gang, which serves to provide emotional warmth and approval to

gang members and a set of group rules that alleviate individual guilt.

(2) Solitary aggressive type—often have a history of no satisfactory relationships, have no guilt or empathy for victims, and often go on to become antisocial personalities in late adolescence or adulthood.

Etiology

(1) Neurologic abnormalities are not infrequent; central nervous system injuries or dysfunction is sometimes evident. Frequent history of injuries.

(2) A high percentage of these children come from disturbed homes with parents who are drug or alcohol addicted, sociopathic in behavior, or psychiatrically disturbed.

(3) Emotional deprivation and/or physical or sexual abuse are frequently present.

(4) Some apparently well-adjusted, successful parents may appear strict and law-abiding but reveal in their own behavior conflicts about antisocial behavior.

(5) Educational handicaps are common on the basis of environmental deprivation, specific developmental disorders, or emotional difficulty.

Diagnosis

Persistent behavior that violates societal rules in a major way. It may represent a spectrum of disorders.

(1) Rule-breaking behavior, which may involve property damage (but does not include violence to persons) such as stealing, lying, running away, fire setting, truancy, housebreaking, car theft, or destruction of property.

(2) Some of the above, plus cruelty to animals, frequent fighting, forcible sexual activity, using a weapon in a fight, robbery with violence, and physical cruelty.

Treatment

Treatment must be multidimensional, based on a good diagnostic assessment and flexible in its goals according to the specific needs of the child. For some children, a single episode of delinquent behavior if it meets with prompt parental concern and therapeutic intervention may lead to better adjustment.

(1) Medical or neurologic handicaps need to be treated when possible.

(2) Educational deficits require remedial help and appropriate educational placement.

(3) Placement at home, group home, hospital, or institution.

(4) Milieu therapy, individual or group psychotherapy, behavior modification management as they can be used by each child.

(5) Pharmacotherapy for neurologic symptoms, attention deficit disorder, anxiety, or depression.

(6) An ongoing support system to oversee all treatment and provide for future needs.

OPPOSITIONAL DEFIANT DISORDER

A disorder in which the child frequently loses temper, argues, defies rules, deliberately annoys, and blames others; is resentful and vindictive; and uses unacceptable language.

Treatment includes evaluation followed by behavior modification, individual play therapy, or family therapy as appropriate to history.

ILLNESS AND PHYSICAL HANDICAPS

HOSPITALIZATION

Effects depend upon the age of the child, but fear and regression are frequent.

(1) Infants and young children suffer acute separation anxiety with loss of primary attachment figure. Every effort should be made to make the mother or other family member available to child as much as is compatible with ward functioning and home responsibilities. Painful procedures are frightening and difficult to understand. Hospitalization may be interpreted as punishment.

(2) Older children also fear separation, mutilation and pain. They may fear dependence and loss of bodily control, especially in procedures or anesthesia. (See section on posttraumatic stress.)

Treatment preparation, when possible, includes familiarization to hospital and personnel. Family should be educated to accept regressed, anxious, or withdrawn behavior of child following illness.

CHRONIC ILLNESS AND PHYSICAL HANDICAPS

Child may have to adapt to pain, visible signs of illness, loss of function or activity, and social limitations. Lack of understanding increases feelings of inferiority or of being punished. Restrictions may cause resentment with feelings of rebellion against parents, doctors, and treatment regimen. Parents also may feel depressed, responsible, somehow guilty, or angry. They may be ashamed of a visibly handicapped child and resent the child or the burden the child represents. Parents may make unrealistic demands of child to overcome the handicap, be overprotective, or be overindulgent. They may neglect siblings.

Treatment

(1) Good treatment of the illness or physical handicap.

(2) Programs of physical or occupational therapy that allow as much normal activity as possible.

(3) Counseling of parents and child separately and together as a family. Recognition of underlying feelings, fantasies, and fears, and encouragement of innovative ways to improve social capabilities and motivation for compliance.

FATAL ILLNESS

Diagnosis of a fatal illness taxes the physician's capacity to remain helpful to the child and family. Once diagnosis is certain, the parents must be told and helped to deal with their shock, grief, anger, and possible guilt. The physician needs to remain available, to listen, provide information, and support. The decision whether to tell the child directly or indirectly of the prognosis will depend on the age of the child and the child's understanding of the seriousness of the illness, expressed concerns, parents' readiness to cope with open discussion, and the apparent capacity of the family to share this information in some form. Sometimes a child is ready to face the issue before the parents are or the parents may withdraw somewhat from the relationship because they cannot cope for a time. It is the physician who can then be available to the child (as well as the family) to provide support. The physician also may appropriately need help in maintaining his or her capacity to remain available to the patient.

ADJUSTMENT DISORDERS

These include maladaptive responses to stress that persist and cause difficulty in school or social relationships. They may be described as associated with anxiety, depression, conduct disturbance, or a combination of these.

Treatment may consist of recognition of the stress and its removal. More often, there may be residual symptoms or the stressful situation persists (as with parental divorce or the onset of a serious chronic illness). Then individual, or sometimes group, psychotherapy is helpful, usually with the support and involvement, as needed, of the parents.

FEEDING & EATING DISORDERS

Feeding difficulties of a minor nature are common in infants during the early months, especially infants with inexperienced mothers. The feeding process is often a good indicator of how the mother and infant are handling the early tasks of development, ie, mutual regulation of the infant's physiologic states; of feeding and sleep periods and ways to deal with crying; of adaptation of mother and child to some kind of schedule; and of development of social interactive behavior. An early effort by the pediatrician to make the feeding experience a success often enhances the whole mother–infant interaction.

A major feeding difficulty in infants between 6 and 15 months of age may involve the issue of autonomy. A mother who insists in putting food in the infant's mouth without allowing any awkward and messy self-feeding can deprive her infant of the opportunity to learn a satisfying skill. Cooperative feeding, in which both the mother and the infant participate, can provide mutual pleasure.

A normal decrease in the infant's appetite accompanies the slower growth that occurs during the second year of life. This decrease may arouse anxiety in the parent. Urging the child to eat produces resistance, which further decreases appetite. The physician can help by explaining this cycle to the parent, reassuring the parent about nutritional needs, and watching the infant's weight and growth curves (and perhaps prescribing vitamins). In severe feeding problems, the mother's anxiety about feeding is based on unconscious conflicts concerning nurturing, and psychiatric help may be required.

Pica is the continued eating of nonnutritive substances, often unpleasant or dangerous, usually during the second or third year of life. Retardation, neglect, and iron or zinc deficiency may be implicated. Prevention of poisoning or bezoar formation and provision of additional attention for the child may be important.

OBESITY

Genetics may determine the number of fat cells each child has, but caloric intake balanced by energy expenditure and influence of metabolic rate determines the amount of fat stored in those cells.

Predisposing Factors
(1) Food habits of the obese family.
(2) Parental anxiety or conflict about nurturing expressed as overfeeding.
(3) Food used by child to assuage feelings of deprivation, inadequacy, or being unloved.
(4) Inactivity and sedentary habits.

Treatment
(1) Enlisting help of family and addressing family diet.
(2) Education of parents and child about healthy weight parameters and the importance of exercise and social activity.
(3) Encouragement of physical-skill developments in sports and other activities.
(4) Referral to group therapy for overweight children.
(5) Individual psychotherapy, also involving parents, if emotional factors seem to be primary.

ANOREXIA NERVOSA

Refer to Chapter 13.

BULIMIA

Refer to Chapter 13.

PSYCHOSOCIAL DWARFISM

An uncommon disorder with onset at age 18–24 months, with failure of linear growth and, to some extent, of weight gain. Bizarre eating habits are common and children show behaviors consistent with their emotionally deprived and often abusive family environment.

Etiology

Not yet clear. A concomitant sleep disorder in stage III–IV sleep has been described with possible disturbance in the release of growth hormone at this time. The emotional environment seems to be the major factor.

Treatment

(1) Hospitalization may be necessary to promote growth.

(2) Parents are usually uncooperative in therapy.

(3) There is usually a history of inadequate parenting with development of a hostile mother–child relationship not readily amenable to change.

(4) At present, removal to a nurturing, emotionally supportive environment seems to be necessary, often with termination of parental rights.

(5) Individual psychotherapy for child and parents.

SLEEP DISORDERS

Sleep disturbances are most marked in children between 2 and 6 years of age, but they may also occur during the first year of life if the parents are very uncertain or permissive about developing regularity in the family schedule. The young child who refuses to sleep alone may reflect normal fears concerning object constancy and separation. The physician may help by offering reassurances to the parents and child and by recommending sensible restrictions on the sleeping arrangements and night feedings.

Nightmares are common in children after 3 years of age. They accompany rapid eye movement (REM) sleep, usually in the latter part of the sleep period, and can often be traced to some exciting or frightening event of the preceding day or to a recent trauma. Night terrors sometimes are called dreams but occur earlier in the sleep period and are associated with non-REM

(NREM) sleep. They are accompanied by difficult arousal and signs of intense anxiety, agitation, and confusion; the child is usually amnesic for the episode. Sleepwalking occurs also in NREM sleep and is accompanied by difficult arousal, poor coordination, and amnesia. Night terrors and sleepwalking have no reported associations with emotional disturbances in children.

Treatment involves soothing the child with a bedtime ritual and use of a transitional object when sleep is interrupted. Encouraging the child to discuss nightmares may help. For sleepwalking, safety precautions to prevent accidents are important. However much the anxious child may want to sleep in the parents' bed, this is not the long-term answer to sleeping problems, for it can delay resolution of separation anxiety, encourage unconscious sexual fantasies, and eventually increase the child's anxiety.

Children who sleep excessively during infancy may be reacting to deprivation (reactive attachment disorder of infancy).

BLADDER CONTROL

Toilet-training methods are in large part culturally determined; only recently have bladder function and children's physiologic and cognitive capacities for control been studied in any depth. Although some children can become continent before 2 years of age, many are not ready for toilet training before 3 years of age. They must first acquire bladder control (ie, the ability to retain a fairly large amount of urine and to be aware of the need to urinate). If they are able to understand the purpose of toilet training and are not in an oppositional phase, they are then presumably ready for training. If the child is spontaneously interested in body functions and self-control, this would be an optimal time for training. Toilet training, whatever method is used, must be noncoercive; modeling and praise are very helpful. Displeasure must be exhibited with caution, and angry shaming is contraindicated.

ENURESIS

Enuresis is involuntary urination, usually at night, in children over 5 years of age; it is about twice as common in boys as in

girls. If day-time "dribbling" is not due to organic factors, its use
as a deliberate negativistic symptom must be suspected.

Etiology

A. Maturational Delay: Longitudinal experience and sleep
studies involving many children emphasize that the development
of bladder musculature plays an important role in the ability of
the bladder to withstand increased intravesical pressure without
involuntary voiding. Particularly in children who have never
achieved bladder control for prolonged periods, a delay in this
process of development should be considered.

B. Toilet Training: Toilet training may have been absent
or, more often, too early or too coercive. If the only form of
training was vague verbal instruction, the child may not know
what is required. A child who was expected to perform before
being physiologically ready may be confused or disheartened. If
training was coercive, with shaming and punishment for accidents (which are often the nearly successful attempts to void that
occur just before or after the child is placed on the toilet seat), the
child may be confused, resentful, and resistant to further efforts.
Retraining with positive, gentle encouragement is needed.

C. Emotional Disturbances:

1. Enuresis may be a temporary symptom of regression, and
attention to the source of upset will usually result in improvement.

2. Enuresis sometimes seems to be a passive-aggressive
response to parents who are thought to be too controlling, intru-
sive, or critical.

3. Enuresis may be associated with symptoms that indicate
more difficult problems of adjustment, such as educational disability or an anxiety disorder. The evaluation of total adjustment
is then indicated. Psychiatric evaluation is required when enuresis is associated with predelinquent behavior, fire setting, and
problems of impulse control; the child's history is often one of
emotional deprivation and longstanding family difficulty.

D. Physical Disease: Although physical disease is not common, this should be ruled out.

1. Spina bifida or other lower spinal cord lesions, if significant, are usually accompanied by neurologic sensory changes
that may be noted on physical examination.

2. Congenital anomalies of the genitourinary tract, especially the urethral valve, may be present. The test for residual
urine is diagnostic. Urethral dilation is psychologically very traumatic as a treatment procedure and should be avoided.

3. Cystitis (a common cause) or other infections of the uri-

nary tract usually produce dribbling during the day as well as at night.

4. Enuresis may be an early symptom of diabetes.

5. Nocturnal epilepsy may rarely be accompanied by enuresis.

Treatment

(1) Clarify motivational and developmental capacity of child, evaluate appropriateness of past toilet training.

(2) For some young children under age 6, support, prevention of punitive parental responses, and encouragement of patience with developmental delay may be enough.

(3) Recognition of recent stress when present in the case of sudden secondary enuresis, with supportive counseling.

(4) Behavioral modification techniques.

(a) The use for 5–12 weeks of a bell-alarm pad that awakens the child when urination occurs is most effective. If relapse occurs, another period of treatment may be successful.

(b) The dry bed technique is intensive behavior training, usually not well accepted by parents.

(5) Use of medication—imipramine—is often rapidly effective but has a high relapse rate and also may have undesirable side effects.

(6) Psychotherapy for the child, combined with counseling of the parents, is the treatment of choice when an emotional etiology is recognized. A brief course of medication may also be used in older children at the onset of psychotherapy.

BOWEL CONTROL

Permanent bowel control is usually more easily achieved than bladder control, probably in part because of individual differences in neurologic maturation. If movements are regular, training for bowel control may be begun after age 18 months, somewhat earlier than for bladder control. Many children, however, are not ready to start bowel training until after age 2 years.

Constipation occurs frequently in children between ages 2 and 3 years and seems to be part of the "negative phase" of this period. Withholding bowel movements seems to represent an attempt to exercise some autonomy against demanding, controlling parents. Treatment is aimed at diverting parental interest from the gastrointestinal tract; usually the child's interest will gradually decline as well. Physical causes for chronic constipation should be ruled out.

ENCOPRESIS

Encopresis is voluntary or involuntary passage of feces in an inappropriate place (eg, in the clothing) by a child over 4 years of age. The condition is called primary encopresis if bowel control has never been established and secondary encopresis if bowel control was established and incontinence recurred.

Etiology
(1) The difficulty may be traced to lack of toilet training or training that is inadequate, too early, or too coercive. These problems in training may cause a child who is physiologically, emotionally, or cognitively incapable of complying to be blamed by the parents for being uncooperative. Family, peers, and school contacts may react to encopresis with disgust and disapproval; the child may make great efforts to prevent discovery of the problem but nevertheless may have lost awareness of the need to defecate or of the smell after defecation has occurred.

(2) Encopresis may involve painful retention of hard fecal material in the colon, with the passage of softer stool, usually involuntarily around the impacted feces. Diagnosis of this situation should be confirmed by x-ray.

(3) Encopresis may be a response to stress or the physiologic expression of emotional conflict of some duration, usually accompanied by other symptoms of emotional distress.

Treatment
(1) Supportive counseling of the parents and child together, to reduce anxiety, disapproval, and stress concerning the encopresis, accompanied by a regular toileting routine.

(2) There is sometimes disagreement among psychiatrists and pediatricians about how vigorously to treat the symptoms when retention is present. Pediatricians sometimes recommend bowel evacuation followed by diet, use of stool softeners, reinstitution of a toilet-training routine with the child advised by the pediatrician, and promoting support and cessation of criticism by the parents.

(3) Psychotherapy (play therapy) for the child is indicated

whenever the course of action in method (1) above has not been sufficient or the child shows evidence of emotional disorder. Again, concomitant involvement of the parents would be necessary, in order to provide understanding of the problems and support for the child.

PSYCHOSEXUAL DEVELOPMENT

Recognition of the genitalia as pleasure-producing may occur in infancy. In the prepubertal child, masturbation is usually a transient habit, and parents should treat it with understanding. Reasonable restrictions (eg, emphasizing privacy) can be placed on the activity for social reasons. Continued or excessive masturbation may have limited sexual significance; in some cases, it can be viewed as a symptom of anxiety indicative of other emotional conflicts. Excessive masturbation or sexually provocative behavior in young children, however, may also be a clue to sexual abuse, especially repeated abuse (see Child Abuse and Neglect, above).

In the postpubertal child, masturbation would undoubtedly be universal if adult prohibitions were not so strong. Here the conflict is more severe because of genital maturing and accounts for much of the "nonspecific" guilt found in adolescents. Emphasis should be focused on the child's emotional needs, not on the act itself.

Young children are aware of sex differences just as they are aware of social differences between the sexes in dress, games, and mannerisms. Parental anxiety about manifestations of sexuality in children is based on the assumption that these are equivalent to adult sexuality and are abnormal. Television viewing should be controlled and sexual abuse ruled out (see above); premature sexual experience can be anxiety producing.

Sexual concerns such as gender identity issues during childhood or early adolescence may be brought to the physician's attention by the parent or child if a good relationship exists, and the concerns should be taken seriously. Gender confusion and fears of being homosexual, for example, should not be dismissed but should be discussed confidentially with the pediatrician or with a mutually agreed upon consultant.

TICS AND OTHER STEREOTYPED MOVEMENTS

Atypical stereotyped movements include head banging, rocking, or other movements and are usually seen in children during infancy and preschool years. They are voluntary and repetitive; they seem to provide release of tension; and they are probably related to insufficient fondling, cuddling, and other expressions of affection. Head banging can have a self-punitive quality and in toddlers is sometimes a sign of frustration or anger.

Tics appear during childhood and are recurrent, involuntary, rapid movements, usually of facial or other small muscle groups. They can be voluntarily controlled for short periods and may disappear during periods of intense concentration or distraction; they are never present during sleep. Tics are made worse by stress, and although they may originate from some kind of physical irritation, they usually represent a response to emotional stress and tension. For example, an only child reared in a family in which aggression is rigidly controlled and conformity is expected in all areas of behavior may find no outlet for feelings of anger and worry. The facial tic allows some limited and distorted expression of tension but does not provide permanent relief. Treatment should be directed toward recognition and relief of tension.

Gilles de la Tourette's syndrome is a familial disorder that originates in childhood and continues in a course of fluctuating severity. It is characterized by hyperactivity, extensive involuntary movements, and vocal tics, which may include grunts, shouts, and compulsive uttering of obscenities (coprolalia). Recently, an association with attention deficit disorder (with or without hyperactivity) has been described. Obsessive compulsive behavior is common. Although the tics can often be controlled voluntarily for minutes to hours, they are often worse during times of stress and may be disabling in social situations, at school, or at work. Considerable relief is experienced with the use of haloperidol or clonidine, although these drugs have the side effects common to neuroleptic drugs. Because of the necessity for titrating a minimum effective dose of medication with maximum symptom reduction, referral to an expert may be advisable. Supportive therapy for the patient and family members and contact with the Tourette Syndrome Association may help with adjustment to the disorder.

ANXIETY DISORDERS

Etiology

There may be a biologic vulnerability or genetic component to anxiety but these have not yet been clarified and there is little doubt that fears (and anxiety) are to some extent learned within the family. In addition, separation anxiety presumably has roots in the early parent–child experience in the separation–individuation phase or in later neurotic conflict or stress. Both parents and child play a part in these disorders.

Diagnosis:

Disorders in which anxiety is the main symptom either in generalized form or in relation to specific situations.

A. Overanxious Disorder: Worry is excessive about future, past, or current events, especially competence. Somatic complaints (headaches and stomachaches), tension, self-consciousness, and need for reassurance may all be present.

B. Separation Anxiety Disorder: There is excessive anxiety concerning separation from key attachment figures with fears of harm to them or to the child, with avoidance of separation by school attendance, going to sleep alone, or remaining alone in the house. Nightmares about separation, physical complaints, and excessive distress at any separation are frequent symptoms.

School refusal is more often due to separation anxiety but may also be related to fear of school attendance because of problems in school. Treatment must distinguish between these etiologies in order to be effective.

C. Avoidant Disorder: The child is pathologically shy, avoiding social activities and unfamiliar people; clings to familiar persons and activities to detriment of social development.

Treatment

Treatment is usually individual and/or family psychotherapy, often using some behavioral modification techniques when appropriate. The use of medication, especially imipramine, has been found very helpful in maintaining attendance in the early treatment stages of school refusal although the potential toxic effects of imipramine must be considered; psychotherapy is the long-term treatment of choice.

POSTTRAUMATIC STRESS DISORDER

Etiology
A well-defined traumatic experience.

Clinical Findings
(1) Re-experiencing of the event through recollection, repetitive thematic play, recurrent nightmares, and distress at reminder experiences.
(2) Avoidance of associations to traumatic event by amnesia, dissociation, regression, avoidance of associated activities, withdrawal, preoccupation, or daydreaming.
(3) Symptoms of hypervigilance such as difficulty concentrating, startle responses, irritability, or temper outbursts.

Treatment
(1) Psychotherapy.
(2) Help in recalling the traumatic event in a supportive therapeutic relationship.
(3) Resolution of the issues of helplessness and being overwhelmed.

PSYCHONEUROTIC DISORDERS

1. SOMATOFORM DISORDERS
(Hysterical Neurosis, Conversion Type)

Etiology
Symptoms of conversion disorder represent a neurotic use of physical complaints (pain, anesthesia, paralysis, blindness, etc) as a substitute for expression of unconscious impulses. It is important to rule out physical illness promptly in order to emphasize the role of psychiatric treatment.

Diagnosis
The close relationship between the emotions and physiologic functions is established during early infancy and persists throughout life. It is necessary to recognize the physical components of emotional states, ranging from mild physiologic deviations such as urinary frequency accompanying apprehension over an approaching examination to such life-threatening conditions as anorexia nervosa. A comfortable working relationship between psychiatrist and pediatrician can contribute to the suc-

cessful treatment of patients with underlying emotional conflicts and physical symptoms.

Conversion disorder is characterized by physical complaints with no apparent bodily change noted on physical examination. Complaints involve pain or disturbance of function. The symptom often has a significant relation to the patient's history but it may never become explicit.

Treatment

(1) Prompt diagnosis of no physical disease.

(2) Help to the patient in removal of symptoms by reassurance, suggestions, or benign procedures.

(3) Focus in therapy on support, problem-solving, and, when intensive, on the nature of the psychopathology superficially expressed by the symptom.

(4) Primary case follow-up, in order to pick up new symptoms, especially when recommendation for continued treatment is not accepted.

2. HYSTERICAL NEUROSIS, DISSOCIATIVE TYPE
(Psychogenic Fugue, Psychogenic Amnesia, and Multiple Personality Disorders)

Dissociative phenomena do occur in childhood but are rarely diagnosed. Multiple personality disorder is said to have its origin in early childhood, usually with a history of severe, sadistic, physical and sexual abuse; however, although the history of dissociation begins in childhood the diagnosis is rarely made until later adolescence.

DRUG AND SUBSTANCE ABUSE
(See also Chapter 13)

In recent years, children have increasingly abused alcohol, cigarettes, marijuana, sedatives, cocaine and its derivative "crack," heroin, hallucinogens, nitrous oxide, and paint and glue solvent vapors. Suspecting that the problem exists is often the clue to diagnosis. Sometimes use begins during the latency or prepubertal years, usually as experimentation or at the instigation of an older child, but most drug and substance abuse begins during adolescence and may rapidly progress to severe abuse.

Many of these children fail in school and become truant, and they may become alienated from family and friends. Drug abuse may be part of the regular behavior of a child's peer group, or it may be an individual activity that severely isolates a child. Marked personality change comes with continued intoxication, and activities are often focused on how to obtain the drug even at the expense of important relationships or work progress, Theft, prostitution, and other forms of delinquency may be the means of paying for drugs.

Although the drug problem may be limited to episodic use, the decision on how to help the child involves a complete evaluation. Supportive treatment is rarely adequate and psychotherapy or most often hospitalization in a specific drug abuse program is usually necessary. Long-term monitoring is needed, for recidivism is frequent.

One important issue is drug monitoring of teenage pregnant mothers. Infants born following exposure to drugs during pregnancy, especially cocaine, are at risk of premature birth, delayed withdrawal symptoms, and possible permanent central nervous system damage.

DEPRESSION
(See also Chapter 13)

Depression may occur in children at any age, from infancy through adolescence. It is often unrecognized, because the depressed child may not complain of feeling sad and may attempt to avoid behavior that reflects unhappy feelings.

DEPRESSION IN INFANTS AND YOUNG CHILDREN

In infants, depression is usually the result of object loss (eg, loss of the mother, caretaker, or sibling), lack of attention, or depreciation and rejection by the parents. A good mother substitute may reverse the mood, which is expressed as apathy and lack of interest in surroundings.

Depression takes three forms in children:

Reactive depression is an acute reaction, often caused by sudden object loss (especially of a parent or sibling), in a child who previously appeared to be fairly well adjusted. Sadness may be evident but is often not sustained, leading to the false as-

sumption of quick recovery. Young children may need help to
mourn.

Chronic depression is sometimes expressed in sadness,
crying, withdrawal, poor self-image, and apathy. Often disinterest, lack of developmental progress, and distrust of the future are
the major signs. The life history of children with chronic depression often reveals why they are depressed.

Masked depression often takes the form of aggressive or
difficult behavior, which may be a mechanism to avoid feelings of
hopelessness and helplessness or may be an expression of some
of the child's angry feelings that led to depression; the behavior
does not relieve the feeling of sadness or promote love and
acceptance. During early childhood, depressive feelings may be
channeled into fantasy and play as a way of masking sadness.
During acute and chronic depression, children often do not express unhappiness in tearfulness or sad rumination; they may
show apathy, psychomotor retardation, poor appetite, or sleep
disturbances.

Depression is common in adolescents, partly because of the
stress of biologic maturation, dependence–independence conflicts with parents (who may be critical or rejecting), and anxiety-
provoking school and social demands. The discrepancy between
an adolescent's self-image and ideal (changeable as the latter
may be) results in feelings of anxiety, inadequacy, and helplessness. The reality of the inability to change oneself quickly or to
alter circumstances may lead an adolescent to feel hopeless and
depressed, especially when the environment presents difficult
stresses. Symptoms may include vague psychosomatic complaints, withdrawal, boredom, anorexia or overeating, and insomnia or excessive sleeping. Preoccupation with the self and
excessive guilt or depressive rumination may lead to school
failure by a child with a record of being a good student. Acting-
out behavior may take the form of alcohol or drug abuse, running
away from home, or delinquency; in these cases, the adolescent
often denies the depression.

Some children will show cyclothymic variations in affect
before adolescence, bringing up the possibility of future bipolar
disease. Genetic predisposition and possible biochemical indicators are currently the objects of research.

Treatment

(1) Antidepressant drugs are not ordinarily used before 6
years of age and should be used with caution and very careful
monitoring during latency.

(2) Psychotherapy with child and parents is probably still

the best mode of dealing with childhood depression, with special attention to the entire history of the parent–child relationship, emotional unavailability of parents though present, losses without the opportunity to mourn, and on-going stress that is not being recognized by the family.

BIPOLAR AFFECTIVE ILLNESS

By adolescence, a few children will show clear signs of bipolar illness, sometimes with a manic episode being the first indication. Manic episodes present as elevated or expansive mood, marked increase in activity with little need for sleep, increased talkativeness with flight of ideas, inflated self-esteem, distractibility, and poor judgment. Swings from manic to depressive episodes may be rapid and require hospitalization with careful monitoring.

Treatment

(1) Careful diagnostic assessment.

(2) Hospitalization during acute episodes.

(3) Medications, usually lithium (must be carefully monitored for effective blood levels and possible toxicity).

(4) Psychotherapy when patient is available after effective medication.

(5) Long-term treatment planning.

(6) Educational planning as part of the long-term plan.

(7) Family evaluation and treatment of family members as indicated.

SUICIDE
(See also Chapter 13)

Suicide does occur in children during the latency period, although the incidence increases dramatically during adolescence, when it becomes the second most frequent cause of death.

Suicidal ideation occurs in young children, mostly in terms of retaliation against people who have made them unhappy. ("How sorry they'll be when I'm dead!") Some children who feel unloved and unwanted assume it is their fault and thus have a poor self-image. Some attention-getting suicide attempts may be accidentally successful. The angry, impulsive suicidal gesture of the adolescent usually indicates a need for help from others or a need for environmental change. Gestures are more common in girls; successful suicides are more common in boys, perhaps because of the methods used. Suicidal gestures may be impulsive but may be successful. All suicidal threats or ideation should be taken seriously, especially when they occur after a major bereavement, following the suicide of a friend, or in an adolescent with a major depressive illness. Protection, psychotherapy, the use of an antidepressant medication, and hospitalization are often needed. It is also important to evaluate the family's response and to prevent family members from giving the child the unconscious message, "We don't really want you."

PSYCHOSIS

Psychosis is rare in prepubertal children. The very early psychoses of infantile autism and symbiotic psychosis are categorized as pervasive developmental disorders, an appropriate description of their natural history (see above). The possibility of schizophrenia-like illness occurring in early and mid childhood is not well defined.

When a child presents with apparent psychosis, it is important to rule out organic disease; this includes certain metabolic diseases, neurologic disease, brain tumor, and chronic poisoning. A psychiatric evaluation alone is not necessarily sufficient to make the diagnosis, for symptoms of emotional disorder and a pathogenic environment can co-exist with organic disease.

Schizophreniform psychosis occurs during prepubertal childhood and later; it tends to be shorter in duration than the later schizophrenias. Symptoms include delusions, auditory hallucinations, thought disorder, inappropriate affect, and isolation and withdrawal. Severe "neurotic" symptoms such as phobias or compulsions may occur. Bizarre behavior may also take place and includes unusual motor activity, such as twirling, and destructive behavior directed outward or at the self. There is clear deterioration from the child's previous level of behavior.

Treatment

(1) Psychiatric evaluation, with medical evaluation to rule out organic illness.

(2) Psychiatric hospitalization.

Table 12-1. Overview of childhood psychopharmacology.*

Drug Class	Drug (Trade) Name	Daily Dose Range	Clinical Indications	Side Effects
Psychostimulants	Methylphenidate (Ritalin)	.2–5 mg/kg/dose (5–20 mg/dose) at AM, noon, ± 4 PM	ADHD	Trouble falling asleep, diminished appetite, increase in pulse and BP, growth retardation, dysphoria & tearfulness, headache and stomachache, lethargy, emergence of tics, interdose rebound
	Dextroamphetamine (Dexedrine)	2.5 mg–10 mg/dose at AM, noon, ± 4 PM		
	Magnesium pemoline (Cylert)	37.5–112.5 mg/d in single AM dose		
Antidepressants	Imipramine (Tofranil)	1–3 mg/kg/d (higher doses with EKG monitoring)	Major depression	Sedation, dry mouth, stuffy nose, orthostatic hypotension, tachycardia & mild hypertension, risk of
	Desipramine (Norpramin)		ADHD	
			Enuresis	

	Nortriptyline (Aventyl)	1/3 the daily dose of imipramine and desipramine (except for enuresis, daily dosage divided B-TID)	Panic anxiety	cardiac conduction abnormalities in doses greater than 3.0 mg/kg/d, irritability
Neuroleptics	Haloperidol (Haldol)	.5–4.0 mg/d	Autistic disorder, Childhood schizophrenia Tourette's syndrome	Sedation, weight gain, photosensitivity, dry mouth, stuffy nose, orthostatic hypotension, acute dystonias, akathisia, parkinsonian tremor, tardive dyskinesias
	Thioridazine (Mellaril)	20–200 mg/d (daily dosage frequently divided B-TID)	Psychotic disorders, Temporary control of agitation	
Mood stabilizer	Lithium carbonate	Serum lithium 0.6–1.2 meq/L	Bipolar disorder	Gastrointestinal upset, tremor, polyuria & polydipsia, acne, goiter, possible renal damage

*Reproduced, with permission, from Hathaway WE et al (eds): *Current Pediatric Diagnosis and Treatment.* Lange, 1990.

(3) Antipsychotic medication.

(4) Long-term follow-up.

PSYCHOSES IN OLDER CHILDREN AND ADOLESCENTS

Acute confusional state is usually a fairly brief psychotic episode characterized by anxiety, depression, confusion, and feelings of depersonalization and diffusion of identity. Hospitalization, with a delay in the use of antipsychotic drugs (which may exacerbate confusion and feelings of helplessness), usually helps; the psychotic episode is generally followed by a need for intensive psychotherapy to aid in the support and re-establishment of identity.

Schizophrenia of the type found in adults may have its early onset in postpubertal children. Occasionally, only one psychotic episode occurs. The illness may have all the characteristics of adult schizophrenia and is often gradual in onset. Characteristics include thought disorder, delusions, and hallucinations, followed by disorganized behavior, combativeness, withdrawal, or depression. Hospitalization, use of neuroleptic drugs, and supportive psychotherapy help bring about some integration. A long period of regression then follows, accompanied by on-going reintegration and requiring long-term therapy. Even after the acute symptoms have improved, the adolescent is still vulnerable, and long-term support, continued medications as needed, and psychotherapy are recommended.

Treatment

(1) Psychiatric evaluation, with medical evaluation to rule out organic illness.

(2) Psychiatric hospitalization with milieu therapy.

(3) Antipsychotic (neuroleptic) medication following diagnosis.

(4) Psychotherapy to support integration.

(5) A period (often shorter than in adults) of regression accompanied by re-integration requires psychotherapy.

(6) Long-term follow-up, often with psychotherapy and continued medication.

USE OF PSYCHOTROPIC DRUGS IN CHILDREN

The response to drugs given to modify behavior may be different and less satisfactory in children than in adults. The best long-term results are obtained by using drugs very conservatively and helping the parents to use behavior modification techniques in specific repetitive situations and to improve interpersonal relationships. The drugs listed in Table 12–1 have been shown to be helpful.

For sedation or treatment of anxiety in acute situations, the benzodiazepines (chlordiazepoxide and diazepam) in small doses are probably the safest and best-known drugs. These agents should not be used for long periods; symptoms are better controlled by diagnosis and treatment of the underlying cause. The use of tranquilizers such as thioridazine for treatment of sleep disorders in young children is not justifiable.

In children who have attention deficit disorder with hyperactivity, methylphenidate or dextroamphetamine, in morning and noontime doses, can be effective in reducing hyperactivity and allowing the child to attend better to classroom activity.

Haloperidol or clonidine is effective in suppressing the more severe symptoms of Gilles de la Tourette's syndrome. In patients with enuresis, imipramine is useful for short periods when rapid achievement of continence is an important first step in treatment. Imipramine has also been used effectively in children with school phobia but must be monitored.

Major depression is best treated with an antidepressant, usually a tricyclic such as imipramine.

The major antipsychotic tranquilizers such as haloperidol are of benefit for the treatment of patients with psychosis during late childhood and adolescence. They are also used extensively in the management of aggressive behavior in institutionalized children who are retarded or who have antisocial conduct disorder, but lithium may be more effective due to its apparent antiaggressive qualities. There is evidence that better management techniques can help by allowing lower drug doses and, therefore, less sedation or side effects. Children with antisocial conduct disorder who have symptoms of major depression—and perhaps also those with attention deficit disorder—may benefit from antidepressant drugs such as imipramine.

Because most of these drugs can have serious, and occasionally dangerous, side effects, their use should be closely monitored for toxicity. Pediatric doses should always be calculated carefully.

13 | Adolescence

David W. Kaplan, MD, MPH,
& Kathleen A. Mammel, MD

Adolescence is a unique period of rapid physical, emotional, cognitive, and social growth and development bridging childhood and adulthood. Generally, adolescence "begins" at age 11–12 years and ends between ages 18 and 21. Although most teenagers complete puberty by ages 16–18 years, in Western society, for educational and cultural reasons, the adolescent period is prolonged to allow for further psychosocial development before adult responsibilities are assumed.

The developmental passage from childhood to adulthood encompasses:

(1) Completing puberty and somatic growth.

(2) Developing socially, emotionally, and cognitively— moving from concrete to abstract thinking.

(3) Establishing an independent identity and separating from the family.

(4) Preparing for a career or vocation.

DEMOGRAPHY

In the United States in 1986, 18.6 million adolescents were between the ages of 15 and 19 years and 20.4 million were 20–24 years of age. The adolescent/young adult population—15–24 years—comprises 16% of the US population.

MORTALITY

The 3 leading causes of mortality in the adolescent population ages 15–19 years in 1986 were unintentional injuries 55.4% (78% of all unintentional injuries were caused by motor vehicle crashes), suicides 11.7%, and homicides 11.5%. During the past 20 years, mortality due to motor vehicle crashes, suicide, and homicide have increased between 300 and 400%. The major threats of death for the adolescent population are due to cultural and environmental, rather than organic, factors.

MORBIDITY

The major morbidity during adolescence is primarily psychosocial: unintended pregnancy, sexually transmitted disease, substance abuse, smoking, dropping out of school, depression, running away from home, physical violence, and juvenile delinquency. Early identification of the teenager at risk for these problems is important not only to prevent the immediate complications but also to prevent any future associated problems. High-risk behavior in one area is often associated with or may lead to problems in another area (Figure 13–1).

Some of the early indicators of an adolescent at high risk include:

(1) Decline in school performance.

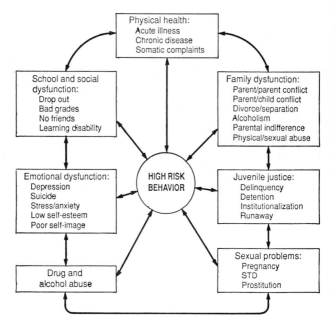

Figure 13–1. Interrelationship of high-risk adolescent behavior.

(2) Excessive school absences or cutting class.

(3) Frequent or persistent psychosomatic complaints.

(4) Changes in sleeping or eating habits.

(5) Difficulty concentrating or persistent boredom.

(6) Signs or symptoms of depression, extreme stress, or anxiety.

(7) Withdrawal from friends or family, or change to a new group of friends.

(8) Unusually severe violent or rebellious behavior, and/or radical personality change.

(9) Parent–adolescent conflict.

(10) Sexual acting out.

(11) Conflict with the law.

(12) Expressing suicidal thoughts or preoccupation with themes of death.

(13) Drug and alcohol abuse.

(14) Running away from home.

DELIVERY OF HEALTH SERVICES

How, where, why, and when adolescents seek health care depends on a number of different factors: ability to pay for care, distance, transportation, accessibility of services, time out of school, and privacy. Teenagers having concerns about pregnancy or contraception, symptoms of a sexually transmitted disease or depression, or problems with substance abuse are often reluctant to confide in their parents for fear of disappointing them and being punished. For the physician, establishing a trusting and confidential relationship is basic to meeting an adolescent patient's health-care needs. If the patient senses the physician is going to tell parents about a confidential problem, the patient may lie or not disclose information essential for proper diagnosis and treatment.

RELATING TO THE ADOLESCENT PATIENT

The manner in which the physician initially approaches the adolescent may determine the success or failure of the visit. The physician should act in a simple and honest fashion, without an authoritarian or excessively "professional" aura. Because many young adolescents have a fragile self-esteem, the physician must be careful not to overpower and intimidate the patient. In communicating with an adolescent, the physician needs to be especially sensitive to developmental level, recognizing that physical appearance and chronological age may be misleading as a measure of cognitive development.

CONFIDENTIALITY

It is helpful at the beginning of the visit to talk with the adolescent and his or her parents as to what to expect. Confidentiality should be addressed, telling the parents you want to meet with the teenager alone, and then with them. Adequate time must be spent with both the patient and parent or important relevant information may be missed. At the beginning of the interview with the patient, it is useful to say something like "I am likely to ask you some personal questions. This is not because I am trying to snoop into your private life, but it may be important to your health. I want to assure you that what we talk about is confidential, just between the two of us. If there is something I feel we should discuss with your parents, I will ask your permission first, unless I feel it is life-threatening."

THE INTERVIEW

How the interview is conducted in the first few minutes of the visit may determine whether a trusting relationship can be established. Spending a few minutes getting to know the patient is time well spent.

The history should include an assessment of progress with psychodevelopmental tasks as well as those health behaviors that are potentially detrimental to the patient's health. The review of systems should include questions about:

(1) Nutrition: Number and balance of meals, calcium, iron, cholesterol intake.

(2) Sleep: Number of hours, problems with insomnia or frequent wakening.

(3) Seatbelt: Regularity of use.

(4) Self care: Knowledge of testicular or breast self examination, dental hygiene, and exercise.

(5) Family relationships: Parents, siblings, relatives.

(6) Peers: Best friend, involvement in group activities, boy/girl friend.

(7) School: Attendance, grades, activities.

(8) Educational and vocational interests: College, career, short- and long-term vocational plans.

(9) Tobacco: Use of cigarettes, snuff, chewing tobacco.

(10) Substance abuse: Frequency, extent and history of alcohol and drug use.

(11) Sexuality: Sexual activity, contraceptive use, pregnancies, history of sexually transmitted disease, number of sexual partners, risk for AIDS.

(12) Emotional health: Signs of depression or excessive stress.

The physician's personal attention and interest is likely to be a new experience for the teenager who has probably only experienced medical care through his or her mother. The teenager should leave the visit with a sense of having his or her "own physician."

THE PHYSICAL EXAMINATION

During early adolescence many teenagers may be quite shy and modest, especially if examined by a physician of the opposite sex. The examiner should address this concern directly as it can usually be allayed by verbally acknowledging the uneasiness, explaining the purpose of the examination, and commenting on the findings during the examination. A pictorial chart of sexual development (Figure 13–2) is extremely useful to show the patient current development and the changes to expect in the future.

GROWTH AND DEVELOPMENT

PHYSICAL GROWTH

Pubertal growth and physical development are a result of activation in late childhood of the hypothalamic–pituitary–gonadal axis. Before the onset of puberty, pituitary and gonadal hormones remain at very low levels. With the onset of puberty, the inhibition of gonadotropin-releasing hormone (GnRH) in the hypothalamus is removed, thus allowing pulsatile production and release of the gonadotropins, luteinizing hormone (LH) and follicle-stimulating hormone (FSH). In early to middle adolescence, there is an increase in pulse frequency and amplitude of LH and FSH secretion, which stimulates the gonads to produce sex steroids (estrogen or testosterone). In the female, FSH stimulates ovarian maturation, granulosa cell function, and estradiol secretion. LH is important in ovulation of the mature ovum and is also involved in corpus luteum formation and progesterone secretion. Initially, estradiol has an inhibitory effect on the release of LH and FSH. Eventually, estradiol becomes stimulatory and the secretions of LH and FSH become cyclic. There is a progressive increase in estradiol that results in maturation of the female genital tract and development of the breasts.

In the male, LH stimulates the interstitial cells of the testes, which produce testosterone. FSH stimulates the production of spermatocytes in the presence of testosterone. The testes also produce inhibin, which is a Sertoli-cell protein that inhibits the secretion of FSH. During puberty circulating testosterone increases more than 20-fold. Levels of testosterone correlate with the physical stages of puberty and the degree of skeletal maturation.

Tanner's scale of sexual maturation is useful clinically to categorize genital development. Tanner staging includes age ranges of normal development and specific descriptions for each stage of pubic hair growth, penis and testes development in boys, and breast maturation in girls. Figures 13–2 A and B graphically represent the chronologic development of this process with reference to each Tanner stage.

The pubertal growth spurt usually takes 2–4 years. It begins nearly 2 years earlier in girls than in boys, but lasts longer in boys. Girls reach their peak height velocity (PHV) between 11.5 and 12 years of age and boys at ages 13.5–14 years. Linear growth at peak velocity is 9.5 ± 1.5 cm per year for boys and 8.3 ± 1.2 cm per year for girls. During adolescence, a teenager's weight doubles, and height increases by 15–20%. In the US, the average age of menarche is 12¾ years. However, menarche may be delayed until age 16 or begin as early as age 10. The first conspicuous sign of puberty in girls is development of breast buds between the ages of 8 and 11 years. The first sign of puberty in the male, usually between the ages of 10 and 12, is thinning of the scrotum and testicular growth.

PSYCHOSOCIAL DEVELOPMENT

Adolescents are struggling to find out who they are, what they want to do in the future, and what their personal strengths

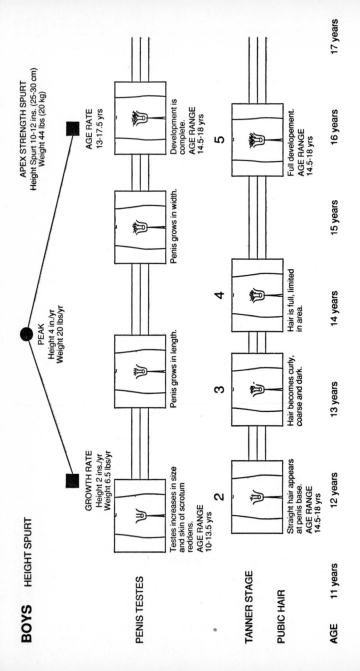

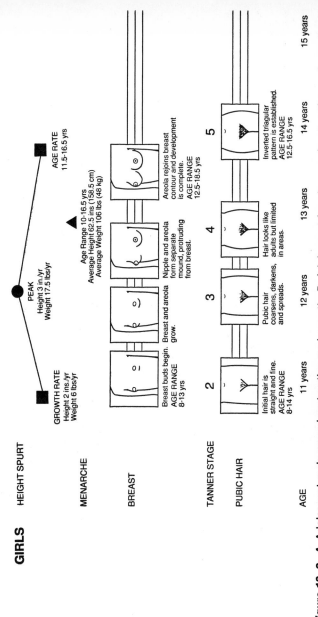

Figure 13–2. *A.* Adolescent male sexual maturation and growth. *B.* Adolescent female sexual maturation and growth. (Adapted from Tanner JM: *Growth at Adolescence.* Blackwell, 1962.)

373

and weaknesses are to accomplish that end. These questions arise primarily because teenagers are in the process of establishing their own identity. Adolescence is a period of progressive individuation and separation from the family. Because of the rapid physical, emotional, cognitive, and social growth that occur during adolescence, it is useful to divide the period into 3 sequential phases of development. Early adolescence occurs roughly between ages 10 and 13, middle adolescence between ages 14 and 16, and late adolescence at age 17 and older.

Early Adolescence

Early adolescence (ages 10–13) is characterized by rapid growth and development of secondary sex characteristics. Young adolescents are often preoccupied with the physical changes taking place in their bodies. Because of the rapid physical changes, body image, self-concept, and self-esteem fluctuate dramatically. Worries about how their growth and development deviates from their friends may be of great concern, especially issues of short stature in boys and delayed breast development or delayed menarche in girls. As the young teenager begins to become more independent, and family ties loosen, allegiance shifts from parents to peers, who become much more important. Young teenagers still think concretely and cannot easily conceptualize about the future. They may have vague and unrealistic professional goals such as becoming a lead singer in a rock group or a famous movie star.

Middle Adolescence

During middle adolescence (14–16 years), with the rapid pubertal growth of early adolescence decreasing, teenagers begin to adjust and become more comfortable with their "new" bodies. Intense emotions and wide mood swings are typical. Cognitively, as teenagers move from concrete thinking to formal operations, they develop the ability to think abstractly. With this new mental power comes a sense of omnipotence and a belief that the world can be changed merely by thinking about it. Sexually active teenagers may believe they don't need to worry about using contraception because they "can't get pregnant—it won't happen to me." In an effort to establish their own identity, relationships with other people, including peers, are primarily narcissistic, and experimenting with different images is quite common. Peers determine the standards for identification, behavior, activities, and fashion, and provide emotional support, intimacy, empathy, and the sharing of guilt and anxiety, during the struggle for autonomy.

Late Adolescence

Late adolescents (17 years and older) are less self-centered and begin caring much more about others. Social relationships shift from the peer group to the individual. Dating becomes much more intimate. The older adolescent becomes more independent from the family. The ability to think abstractly allows older adolescents to think more realistically in terms of future plans, actions, and careers. Morally, older adolescents have very rigid concepts of right and wrong. Late adolescence is a period of idealism.

BEHAVIORAL AND PSYCHOLOGIC HEALTH

Adolescents with emotional disorders often present with somatic symptoms that do not appear to have biologic cause, eg, abdominal pain, headaches, dizziness/syncope, fatigue, sleep problems, and chest pain. The emotional basis of such a complaint may be varied: somatoform disorder, depression, or stress and anxiety.

PSYCHOPHYSIOLOGIC SYMPTOMS AND CONVERSION REACTIONS

The most common somatoform disorders during adolescence are conversion reactions. A **conversion reaction** is a psychophysiologic process in which unpleasant feelings, especially anxiety, depression and guilt, are communicated through the use of a physical symptom. The symptom may appear at times of stress such as parental conflict, serious illness in a parent or grandparent, or a change in school. Psychophysiologic symptoms result when anxiety activates the autonomic nervous system, resulting in tachycardia, hyperventilation, and vasoconstriction. The degree to which the conversion symptom lessens anxiety, depression, or the unpleasant feeling is referred to as "primary gain." Conversion symptoms not only diminish unpleasant feelings, but also benefit the adolescent by removing him or her from conflict or an uncomfortable situation. This is referred to as "secondary gain." Specific symptoms may be based on existing or previous illness such as pseudoseizures in adolescents with epilepsy. Adolescents with conversion symptoms tend to have overprotective parents and to become increasingly dependent on their parents as the symptom becomes the major focus of both the parent's and adolescent's life.

Diagnosis and Treatment

In cases of suspected conversion reaction, history and physical findings are usually inconsistent with anatomic and physiologic concepts. It is critical that from the onset the physician emphasize to the patient and the family that both physical and emotional etiologies for the symptom need to be considered. The relationship between physical causes of emotional pain and emotional causes of physical pain needs to be described. The patient should be encouraged to understand that the symptom may persist, and that at least a short-term goal is to help the patient continue normal daily activities in school and with friends. Medication is rarely helpful in relieving or resolving the symptom. Discussion of the symptom itself should be minimized; however, the physician should be supportive and never suggest that the pain is not real. As the parents gain further insight into the etiology of the symptom, they will become less indulgent of the complaints, facilitating the resumption of normal activities. If management is successful, the adolescent will acquire increased coping skills and become more independent, with decreasing secondary gain.

If the symptom persists in interfering with daily activities, school attendance, participation in extracurricular activities, and involvement with peers, and the patient and parents feel that no progress is being made, psychologic referral is definitely indicated.

DEPRESSION

Presentation

Serious depression during adolescence may present in a variety of ways. It may be similar to the presentation in adults, with vegetative signs such as depressed mood nearly every day, crying spells or inability to cry, discouragement, irritability, sense of emptiness and meaninglessness, negative expectations of self and the environment, low self-esteem, isolation, helplessness, markedly diminished interest or pleasure in most activities, significant weight loss or weight gain, insomnia or hypersomnia, fatigue or loss of energy, and diminished ability to think or concentrate. However, it is not unusual for a serious depression to be "masked" because the teenager cannot tolerate the severe feelings of sadness. The teenager may present with recurrent or persistent psychosomatic complaints, such as abdominal pain, chest pain, headache, lethargy, weight loss, dizziness and syncope, or other nonspecific symptoms. Other behavioral manifestations of a masked depression may include school truancy, running away from home, defiance of authorities, self-destructive behavior, drug and alcohol abuse, sexual acting out, and delinquent acts.

Diagnosis

A complete history and physical examination should be performed, including a careful review of the patient's past medical and psychosocial history. The family history should be explored for psychiatric problems.

The teenager should be questioned directly about any specific symptoms of depression (as noted above), expression of suicidal thoughts, or preoccupation with themes of death. The history should include an assessment of the patient's school performance, change in work or other outside activities, changes in the family, or death of a close relative. The teenager may have withdrawn from friends or family, or changed to a new group of friends. Is there a history of drug and alcohol abuse, conflict with law, sexual acting out, running away from home, unusual severe violent or rebellious behavior, or radical personality change?

Because a number of physical disorders can mimic, cause, or exacerbate major depression, adolescents presenting with significant symptoms of depression deserve a thorough medical evaluation to rule out any contributing or underlying medical illness. Commonly prescribed medications in this age group, such as birth control pills and anticonvulsants, may be responsible for depressive symptoms, as may illicit drugs such as marijuana, phencyclidine, and amphetamine and cocaine.

The majority of physical disorders presenting with symptoms of depression are usually evident by history of present illness, past medical history, and physical examination. However, some routine laboratory studies are indicated, including CBC, sedimentation rate, urinalysis, electrolytes, BUN, calcium, T_4 and TSH, serology, and liver enzymes.

The risk of depression appears to be greatest in families with a history of depression of early onset and chronicity of depressive symptoms.

Treatment

The primary care physician may be able to counsel adolescents and parents if an underlying depression is mild or seems to be the result of an acute identifiable personal loss or frustration, and if the patient is not contemplating suicide or at risk for other life-threatening behaviors. If there is evidence of a longstanding depressive disorder, suicidal thoughts, or psychotic thinking, or if the physician does not feel competent or have the interest in counseling the patient, a psychologic referral should be made.

ADOLESCENT SUICIDE

In 1986 there were over 5000 suicides in persons aged 15 through 24. In the 15–19-year-old age group, males had a rate 400% higher than females, and white males had the highest rate. The estimated ratio of attempted suicides to actual suicides is estimated to be 50:1 to 100:1, and is 3 times higher in females than in males. Among actual suicides, deaths due to firearms are the number one cause for both males and females, accounting for over 60% of the suicide deaths.

Acute depressive reactions (transient grief responses) to the loss of a close family member or friend, due to death or separation, may result in depression lasting for weeks or even months. If an adolescent is unable to work through the grief and becomes increasingly depressed, is unable to function at school or socially, has sleep and appetite disturbances, and feelings of hopelessness and helplessness, the magnitude of the depression fulfills the criteria of a major depression and the teenager should be considered to be at increased risk for suicide. As discussed in the section on depression, symptoms of depression during adolescence may be "masked."

Another group of suicidal adolescents is composed of angry teenagers attempting to affect their environment. They may be only mildly depressed, and may not have a longstanding wish to die. Teenagers in this group—usually females—may "attempt" or "gesture" suicide as a way of getting back at someone, or gaining attention by scaring another person.

The last group of adolescents at risk for suicide is made up of teenagers with a serious psychiatric problem such as acute schizophrenia or a true psychotic depressive disorder.

Diagnosis

The physician must determine the extent of the teenager's depression and the risk of the adolescent trying to self-inflict harm. The evaluation should include interviews with both the teenager and the family. The history should include the medical, social, emotional, and academic background, as described above. When seeing depressed patients, the physician should always inquire about thoughts of suicide: "Are things ever so bad that life doesn't seem worth living?" "Have you thought of taking your life?" If the patient has thoughts of suicide, the immediacy of risk can be assessed by determining if there is a concrete, feasible plan. Although the patients who are at greatest risk have a concrete plan that can be carried out in the near future, especially if they have rehearsed the plan, the physician should not dismiss the potential risk of suicide in the adolescent who does not describe a specific plan. The physician should pay attention to "gut feelings." There may be subtle nonverbal signs that the patient is at greater risk than is apparent on the surface.

Management

The primary care physician is often in a unique position to identify an adolescent at risk for suicide, because many teenagers who attempt suicide seek medical attention within weeks preceding the attempt. These visits are often for vague somatic complaints or subtle signs of depression. If there is evidence of depression, the physician must assess the severity of the depression and suicidal risk. The physician should always get emergency psychologic consultation for any teenager who is severely depressed, psychotic, or acutely suicidal. It is the psychologist's or psychiatrist's responsibility to assess the seriousness of suicidal ideation and decide whether hospitalization or outpatient treatment is most appropriate.

SUBSTANCE ABUSE

Substance abuse is a growing problem in our society of quick fixes for complex problems. In 1986, a national survey of high-school seniors reported that 65.3% had used alcohol, 27.1% smoked marijuana, and 13.9% used hallucinogens, cocaine, stimulants, or sedatives, in the past 30 days; 16.9% reported they had tried cocaine.

Risk Factors

The causes of substance abuse are multifactorial, including personality characteristics, genetic influences, peer pressure, and parental and cultural influences.

Children whose parents give clear messages against drugs and provide consistent authoritative discipline involving warmth and discussion, those whose peers do not use drugs, those with knowledge of the consequences of substance abuse, and those possessing personal values placing importance on health and achievement tend to be protected from substance abuse.

Stages of Substance Abuse

Chemical dependency is the result of a gradual process. Donald Macdonald, MD, has suggested five stages of substance abuse, 0–4, which are outlined in Table 13–1. Progression through these stages may occur at a variable rate, and not every user will progress to stage 4. However, the younger the user, the greater the risk for development of chemical dependency.

Substances Abused

While tobacco and alcohol are considered "gateway" drugs, marijuana is also commonly used during adolescence. See Table 13–2 for a list of drugs commonly abused and their effects.

Diagnosis

History is the key to diagnosis of substance abuse, and a history obtained in a nonjudgmental manner may be highly enlightening. In later stages of involvement, however, denial may cause the adolescent to minimize use. Clues to diagnosis include episodes of acute drug abuse (such as overdose or suicide gestures), deteriorating school performance, personality changes (mood swings, lack of motivation), worsening family relationships, change of peer groups, trouble with the law, or persistent regular drug use despite parental or physician discussion with the teenager. When substance abuse is suspected or established in an adolescent, an assessment of the adolescent's involvement with the drug (age at onset, drugs used, duration of use, frequency of use, attitude toward use), involvement with a drug-using peer group, family relationship, and psychologic profile (any preexisting psychiatric, developmental, or educational difficulties) will assist in decisions on appropriate management. Information should also be obtained from the parents, who may suspect substance abuse or may be enabling the adolescent and therefore deny its significance.

Physical examination will provide few clues. Laboratory tests are generally helpful only with acute intoxication, when a blood alcohol and urine toxin screen should be obtained. When it is known that one chemical has been used at the time of acute intoxication, a drug screen should be obtained to look for other substances due to the possibility of multiple drug abuse or adulteration or misrepresentation of material. Drug testing outside of an episode of acute intoxication or a drug-free maintenance program is generally of little help and may endanger the patient–physician relationship.

Management

Prevention and early intervention during experimental use is most effective. Management will depend on the stage of involvement (see Table 13–1).

EATING DISORDERS

It is estimated that 5–10% of adolescent girls and young women have an eating disorder. The typical patient is a middle or upper-middle class female, but this trend is changing. The causes of eating disorders remain unclear. There are contributing psychosocial and cultural factors, with the emphasis in today's society on thinness and the "superwoman" image.

Presentation and Diagnosis

Often the patient presents with abdominal pain, nausea, fainting spells, hair loss, or amenorrhea, and it is the clinician who discovers the true diagnosis. In some instances, a school nurse, coach, or parent may become suspicious after observing weight loss, overconcern with weight, or unusual eating and exercise behaviors. Bulimics, however, may present on their own and may feel relieved to share their burden with someone.

The diagnosis of anorexia nervosa or bulimia nervosa is largely based on history and meeting specific diagnostic criteria (Table 13–3). The history needs to include the presenting symptoms; weight history, including desired weight; dietary intake, unusual eating behaviors, or avoided foods; history of any purging behaviors such as vomiting, excessive exercise, or use of diet pills, diuretics, emetics, or laxatives; and menstrual history for irregular cycles, secondary amenorrhea, or delay in menarche. Social history may provide clues to a perfectionistic drive in anorexics or impulsiveness in bulimics (eg, substance abuse or sexual promiscuity), or family dysfunction. Review of systems should focus on symptoms of possible complications of the above behaviors and on symptoms of other diseases in the differential diagnosis.

Physical Findings

The physical examination is most often normal, but this does not rule out the diagnosis of an eating disorder. The anorexic's weight will quantitate the actual loss; however, bulimics are usually of normal weight or within 10 pounds (under or over) of normal weight. The vital signs of the anorexic may show hypothermia, bradycardia, or hypotension. Other findings in anorexia include dry skin, presence of fine, downy lanugo hair on the body

Table 13–1. Stages of substance abuse.*

Stage	Drugs	Sources	Frequency	Feelings	Behavior	Treatment
Stage 0 Curiosity	None	Available— but not used	—	Curious	Risk-taking Desire for acceptance	Optimum time. Anticipatory guidance to develop good coping skills and strong self-esteem. Clear family guidelines on drug and alcohol use. Drug education.
Stage 1 Experimentation	Tobacco Alcohol Marijuana	House supply Friends Siblings	Weekend use for recreational purposes	Excitement Pleasure Few consequences Learns how easy it is to feel good	Lying Little change	Drug education. Attention to societal messages. reduce supply. Strict, loving rules at home. Drug-free alternative activities established.
Stage 2 Regular use	As above, plus hashish or hash oil, tranquilizers, sedatives, amphetamines	Buying	Progresses to mid-week use. Purpose is to get high.	Excitement followed by guilt	Mood swings Faltering school performance Truancy Changing peer groups	Drug-free self-help groups (Alcoholics or Narcotics Anonymous). Family involvement.

382

					Changing style of dress	Psychiatric counseling
						unhelpful unless family therapy and after-care provided.
Stage 3 Psychologic or chemical dependency	As above, plus stimulants, hallucinogens	Selling to support their habit. Possibly stealing or prostitution in exchange for drugs.	Daily	Euphoric highs followed by depression, shame, guilt, and perhaps suicidal thoughts	Pathologic lying School failure Family fights Involvement with the law over curfew, truancy, vandalism, shoplifting, or driving under the influence, breaking and entering, violence	Inpatient or foster-care programs that require family involvement and provide after-care.
Stage 4 Using drugs to feel "normal"	As above; any available drug, including opiates	Any way possible	All day	Euphoria rare and harder to achieve Chronic depression.	Drifters with repeated failures and psychologic symptoms of paranoia and agression Overdosing, blackouts, amnesia occur regularly Chronic cough, fatigue, malnutrition	Inpatient or foster-care programs that require family involvement and provide after-care.

*Reproduced, with permission, from Macdonald DI: *Drugs, Drinking, and Adolescents.* Year Book, 1984. © 1984 Year Book Medical Publishers, Inc.

Table 13–2. Subjective, objective, and adverse effects of commonly abused drugs.

Drug	Street Names	Subjective Effects	Objective Effects	Adverse/Overdose Reactions
Cannabis Marijuana Hashish Hash oil THC	Pot Grass Weed Maryjane Hash Tea Reefer Joint	Sedation Tranquilization Mild hallucination or pleasurable change in perception	Tachycardia Conjunctival irritation Impaired abstract thinking, reading comprehension, verbal ability, short-term memory, counting, color discrimination Impaired driving ability	Acute anxiety Serious reaction uncommon unless adulterated with hallucinogens
Alcohol	Booze	Stimulation as blood level rises Subsequent sedation, release of inhibitions	Slurred speech Ataxia Impaired driving performance	Poor judgment Impaired cognitive and motor abilities Emotional changes Respiratory depression Decrease in temperature Coma, shock, death
CNS Stimulants Cocaine Amphetamines	Cocaine Coke Snow Dust Amphetamines Uppers Speed Meth Bennies Dexies	Euphoric effects: exhilaration, calmness, sense of power; omnipotence and unlimited energy in high doses Perception of decrease in appetite, thirst, fatigue Dysphoria or "wired" irritability after euphoric phase	Local anesthetic Sympathomimetic: mydriasis, hypertension, tachycardia, tachypnea, temperature elevation, tremor, agitation	Anxiety Elevated temperature Seizures Respiratory arrest Arrhythmia Death Hallucinations and paranoia

CNS Depressants Group I Sedatives Tranquilizers	Downers Quaaludes, Ludes Blues, Bluebirds Reds, Red devils Yellows, Yellow jackets	Relaxation Facilitation of social behavior With higher doses, loss of inhibitions, sedation, drowsiness	Nystagmus on lateral gaze Slurred speech, ataxia Impulsiveness	Coma Death
CNS Depressants Group II Nitrous oxide Toluene Trichlorethylene Methanol Acetone Gasoline Fluorinated hydrocarbons		Sedation Heightened visual imagery Hallucination Euphoria	Drowsiness Rhinitis, bronchitis Odor of inhalant on breath Metabolic abnormalities	Coma is rare Idiosyncratic reaction to fluorinated hydrocarbons resulting in sudden death by cardiac arrhythmia
Nitrites Amyl nitrite Isobutyl nitrite	Rush Lockerroom Poppers Bolt	Sudden, transient, pleasurable tingling Headache Pounding heart	Tachycardia Hypotension	Exacerbation of preexisting cardiac disease, syncope Elevated intraocular pressure Coma, rarely sudden death Methemoglobinemia
Hallucinogens Group I Lysergic acid diethylamide Mescaline Psilocybin	Acid LSD Peyote Button Mesc Mushrooms	Vivid sensory stimulation and distortion Introspection Awareness of drug-induced state	Dizziness, nausea Paresthesias Sympathomimetic effects Varying mental status as changes from hallucinating to coherent recountings	Idiosyncratic "bad trips" or panic reactions with terrifying hallucinations that may last from hours to more than a day

385

Table 13–2. *(Continued)*

Drug	Street Names	Subjective Effects	Objective Effects	Adverse/Overdose Reactions
Hallucinogens Group II Phencyclidine	PCP Angel dust	Low doses (1–5 mg) produce floating euphoria or numbness Doses of 5–15 mg cause confusion, agitation, impairment of communication, and distorted body perception Higher doses may cause psychotic reactions lasting from days to months	Sympathomimetic effects Drooling Rotatory nystagmus Decreased response to pain Combative and aggressive or silent and withdrawn	Muscle rigidity, opisthotonus, seizures, coma Toxic psychosis (rotatory nystagmus and fever may be the only signs to differentiate from nontoxic psychosis) Hypertensive crises with CNS hemorrhage and death
Opiates Heroin Morphine Meperidine Propoxyphene Methadone Codeine	Dope H Horse Smack Meth	With IV use a sudden "rush" and sensation similar to orgasm With other routes, euphoria, drowsiness, decreased appetite and libido Nausea, vomiting, and dizziness may occur in novices	Oriented but indifferent Slurred speech, unsteady gait Slowed heart and respiratory rates Pinpoint pupils Needle tracks in IV users	CNS and respiratory depression responsive to naloxone (Narcan) Pulmonary edema 24–36 hours after use, not responsive to naloxone Death

Table 13–3. Diagnostic criteria for eating disorders.*

Anorexia Nervosa:

A. Weight loss or failure to gain weight during growth such that weight is 15% below that expected for age and height.

B. Fear of weight gain or fatness despite being underweight.

C. Distorted body image—feels all or part of the body is fat even when severely underweight.

D. Interruption of menstrual cycles for at least 3 months (secondary amenorrhea) or failure to menstruate when expected (primary amenorrhea).

Bulimia Nervosa

A. Repeated binge eating (large number of calories in short period of time) with a frequency of at least twice a week for 3 or more months.

B. Perception by patient that eating behavior is out of control.

C. Recurrent purging behavior to prevent weight gain–self-induced emesis; use of laxatives, diuretics, or emetics; excessive exercise; or severely restricted intake.

D. Overly focused on body image.

* Modified and reproduced, with permission, from *Diagnostic and Statistical Manual of Mental Disorders,* Third edition-Revised. American Psychiatric Association, 1987.

or more pigmented body hair, limpness and loss of shine to the scalp hair, excoriation over the sacral spine from excessive sit-ups, prominent ribs, atrophied breasts, scaphoid abdomen, palpable hard stool in the rectal vault, cold extremities, squaring off of the convergence of the thighs, or edema of the extremities. In patients with self-induced emesis there may be loss of tooth enamel, particularly on the posterior aspect of the front teeth, or callouses on the dorsum of the fingers.

Laboratory Findings

The goal of laboratory tests is to exclude other diagnoses and to assess the patient's status. Most laboratory studies will not change until late in the disease. A CBC is useful to assess nutritional status and a sedimentation rate to help exclude other disorders such as inflammatory bowel disease or collagen vascular disease. Electrolytes may detect the presence of hypochloremic alkalosis and hypokalemia from vomiting or the metabolic acidosis of laxative abuse. Serum total protein and albumin are usually normal until late; low serum phosphorus and magnesium levels are an ominous sign. Other laboratory studies, such as thyroid function tests, x-rays, upper gastrointestinal series, or CT scan of the head need only be done as indicated by the presentation.

Differential Diagnosis

The list of causes of weight loss is legend. Etiologies such as malignancy, collagen vascular disease, diabetes mellitus, hyperthyroidism, malabsorptive syndromes, inflammatory bowel disease, or chronic renal, pulmonary, or cardiac disease warrant consideration in the suspected anorexic. However, with these disorders there may be weight loss but there is no associated disturbance of body image or fear of obesity. One must also remember that a number of psychiatric disturbances, including depression, may be associated with loss of appetite and weight loss. Some unusual central nervous system disorders may present like bulimia, but again there is no distorted body image or overconcern with body shape or weight.

Complications

Eating disorders can result in severe consequences to nearly every system of the body including electrolyte and acid–base disturbances; depressed gonadotropins; altered thyroid tests; disturbed menstruation; dysrhythmias; congestive heart failure; osteoporosis; disturbed thermoregulation; constipation; gastric dilatation, delayed emptying, and rupture; and bone marrow suppression.

Management

The patient needs to know that the clinician appreciates her struggle, aims to restore her to health, won't let her become fat, and will help her to regain control. The parents need to understand that eating disorders are symptoms of underlying issues, often a family problem; that the family is very important to the solution; and that treatment requires the intervention of the mental health disciplines.

Restoration of the nutritional and physiologic state is an early goal. An individualized contract can be drawn up and signed by the patient that addresses such issues as long-term weight goal, rate of weight gain, amount of exercise, frequency of visits and of labwork, minimal weight signalling need for hospitalization, and consequences of failed weight goals.

Most often, the patient can eat adequately to replace nutrient deficits and to gain weight. In extremely malnourished and noncompliant hospitalized patients, nasogastric tube feedings or hyperalimentation may initially be necessary. Hospitalization may become necessary for medical or psychiatric reasons (Table 13–4).

Table 13–4. Criteria for hospitalization of eating-disorder patients.

Medical
Weight loss greater than 30% of body weight over 3 months
Severe metabolic disturbance
  HR < 40
  T < 36°C
  SBP < 70
  Serum K^+ < 2.5 despite oral K^+ replacement
  Severe dehydration
Severe binging and purging

Psychiatric
Severe depression or risk of suicide
Psychosis
Family crisis
Failure to comply with a therapeutic contract, or inadequate response
  to outpatient treatment

Prognosis

It appears that 40–60% of significantly ill anorexics make a good physical and psychosocial recovery and that 75% improve weight. The mortality rate ranges from 0 to 19%, and is at least 5% in those receiving therapy. As few as 40–50% of treated bulimics are felt to be "cured," and there is a greater likelihood of serious medical complications, risk of suicide, and death than for anorexics without bulimic behavior.

EXOGENOUS OBESITY

Background

If a child enters adolescence obese, the odds are 4:1 against later achievement of normal weight; but if a child leaves adolescence obese, the odds are 28:1 against later normal weight. The associated medical risks of obesity include pediatric and adult hypertension, elevated triglyceride levels, cerebrovascular accidents, diabetes mellitus, gallbladder disease, slipped capital-femoral epiphyses, degenerative arthritis, and pregnancy complications. The psychosocial hazards of obesity tend to be the greatest consequence for adolescents, who may experience alienation, distorted peer relations, poor self-esteem, guilt, depression, or distorted body image.

Diagnosis

History should include onset of obesity, eating and exercise habits, amount of time spent in sedentary activities such as television watching, problem foods, previous successful and unsuccessful attempts at weight loss, and family history of obesity. In addition, one needs to assess the patient's readiness to lose weight. A complete physical examination should be performed. Height, weight, and weight index should be plotted; an index greater than 1.2 is considered diagnostic of obesity. Triceps skinfold (TSF) thickness is the most practical way to measure obesity in children and teenagers, but reproducibility is inconsistent. A TSF more than one standard deviation above the mean (85th percentile) defines obesity; one at the 95th percentile indicates superobesity. Laboratory evaluation should include CBC, urinalysis, and cholesterol level. Endocrine causes such as hypothyroidism or Cushing's disease can generally be excluded on the basis of history and physical examination, but in individual cases exclusion of these may require additional studies.

Management

An age-appropriate behavior modification program incorporating good dietary counseling and exercise is optimal (Table 13–5).

SCHOOL FAILURE

When children graduate from grade school to middle school or junior high school, the course work content, amount, and complexity increases significantly. Academic failure presenting at adolescence has a broad differential diagnosis: 1) limited intellectual abilities, 2) specific learning disability, 3) depression or emotional problems, 4) physical causes such as visual or hearing problems, 5) excessive school absenteeism secondary to chronic disease such as asthma or neurologic dysfunction, 6) lack of ability to concentrate, 7) attention deficit disorder, 8) lack of motivation, or 9) drug and alcohol problems. Each of these possible etiologies must be explored in depth.

Diagnosis

A thorough history, physical examination, appropriate laboratory studies, and educational and psychologic testing should be performed. A detailed medical history looking for the presence of chronic disease or any sensory deficits should be evaluated. The amount of school missed secondary to absences and the response

Table 13–5. Program components for weight-control interventions.*

Component	Specific Aspects
Physical activity Cardiovascular fitness High calorie equivalent	a. Frequency: 3–4 ×/week b. Intensity: 50–60% maximal ability (55–65% max heart rate) c. Duration: 15 min at start, building to 30–40 min d. Mode: use of large muscle activity such as walk/jog, swim, or cycle e. Interest: encourage a wide variety of recreational activities f. Enjoyment: focus on the fun of movement and the enjoyment of being physically active
Nutrition education	a. Teach critical aspects of quality nutrition, ie, food groups, serving requirements, and variety b. Develop understanding for calorie balance: calories in vs calories out c. Alert children to pressures of media advertising d. Instruct on role of snacks and ideas for "good" snacking e. Assist children on balancing fast-food eating and calorie intake f. Teach children to reduce intake of high-calorie, low-nutrition treats
Behavior modification Change eating habits Increase habitual physical activity	a. Identify those cues that affect eating, eg, location of meals, size of plates, food in easy-to-see places b. Identify behavior that negatively affects weight control: speed of eating, chronic second portions, high calorie food choices, "pickiness" c. Contract for increased levels of activity using record cards or activity contracts d. Develop strategies for more functional activity, such as walking to school, taking stairs, sitting rather than lying e. Develop interest in a variety of recreational areas: tennis, dance, skating, etc f. Identify cues that lead to inactivity: frequent TV watching, lying down after school or meals, friends who do not like active play

*Reproduced, with permission, from Ward DS, Bar-Or O: Role of the physician and physical education teacher in the treatment of obesity at school. *Pediatrician* 1986;**13**:44.

of the parents, eg, "too sick to go to school," overlaps with school avoidance. A history of attention deficit disorder or stimulant medication use in the past may be an indication of ongoing problems with concentration. Educational records including previous educational and intelligence testing is important background information to obtain. The emotional history may reveal past episodes of counseling for depression or other significant psychiatric problems. The presence of conflict in the family, such as divorce or alcoholism, may have an important role, distracting the adolescent from academic responsibilities. There may be a family history of school problems in other siblings or family members.

Treatment

Management must be individualized to address specific needs, foster strengths, and implement a feasible program. With specific learning disabilities an individual prescription for regular and special educational courses, teachers, and extracurricular activities is important. Counseling is helpful to work on coping skills, self-esteem, and socialization. If there is a history of hyperactivity or attention deficit disorder, with poor concentrating ability, a trial of stimulant medication may be useful. If the teenager appears to be depressed, or other serious emotional problems are uncovered, further psychologic evaluation should be recommended.

BREAST DISORDERS

The breast examination should become part of the routine physical exam in females as soon as breast budding occurs. The breast examination begins with inspection of the breasts for symmetry and Tanner stage. Asymmetry is usually a normal variation but may be due to unilateral breast hypoplasia or amastia, absence of the pectoralis major muscle, or virginal hypertrophy.

BREAST MASSES

Most breast masses in adolescents are benign; however, approximately 150 cases of adenocarcinoma are reported each year in the US in women under 25 years of age. Fibroadenomas account for 90% of breast lumps in teenagers seen in referral clinics, with the remainder being cysts. In practice, cysts may account for as many as 50% of breast masses in adolescents, but they are readily diagnosed and many spontaneously resolve. Suspicious lesions should be immediately referred to a surgeon (Table 13–6).

GALACTORRHEA

In teenagers, **galactorrhea,** or inappropriate nipple discharge, is most often benign, although a careful history and work-up are necessary. Numerous prescribed and illicit drugs are associated with galactorrhea (Table 13–7), as are a number of CNS, endocrine, or chest-wall disorders (Table 13–8).

Evaluation
If there is no history of pregnancy or drug use, TSH and prolactin levels should be obtained. An elevated TSH confirms the diagnosis of hypothyroidism. An elevated prolactin and normal TSH, often accompanied by amenorrhea, suggests a hypothalamic or pituitary tumor, and CT scan is indicated. When the prolactin level is normal, uncommon causes such as adrenal, renal, or ovarian tumors should be considered. For those with a negative work-up and persistent galactorrhea, careful follow-up is required. In many cases symptoms resolve spontaneously without a diagnosis.

Treatment
Treatment of galactorrhea depends upon the underlying cause. Prolactinomas may be surgically removed or suppressed with bromocriptine. Bromocriptine may also be beneficial to some amenorrheic females with normal prolactin levels.

GYNECOMASTIA

Gynecomastia is a common concern of male adolescents, the majority of whom (60–70%) develop transient subareolar breast tissue during Tanner stage II–III development. Proposed etiologies include testosterone-estrogen imbalance, increased prolactin level, or abnormal serum binding protein levels.

Table 13-6. Breast lesions.

Type	Clinical Findings	Progression	Treatment
Fibroadenoma	Rubbery, well-demarcated, nontender mass, usually in upper outer quadrant. Most < 5 cm; 25% will be multiple or recurrent.	Slow growing, quiescent after teen years.	Follow for 2–3 menstrual cycles. If no change, ultrasound differentiates solid tumor from cyst. Solid tumors should be referred for excisional biopsy.
Cysts	Tender, spongy masses, often multiple. Increased symptoms premenstrually.	About half of cysts spontaneously regress over 2–3 menstrual cycles.	Persistent cysts may be drained by needle aspiration. Refer suspicious lesions to breast surgeon.
Fibrocystic breasts	Cyclical tenderness and nodularity bilaterally, most common in third and fourth decades, but seen in adolescence.	Increase and diminish under cyclical influence of estrogen–progesterone balance.	Reassurance. Oral contraceptives reduce the risk of fibrocystic breasts. Some women report decreased symptoms after vitamin E treatment or when methylxanthines are limited in the diet, but recent studies have not proven this.
Breast abscess	Unilateral breast pain with overlying inflammatory changes, breast mass palpable late in course. Often due to *Staphylococcus aureus*.	Infection may extend deeper than suspected on exam.	Surgical incision and drainage when fluctuant. Oral antibiotics (dicloxacillin or cephalosporin) for 2–4 weeks.

Adenocarcinoma	Hard, nonmobile, well-circumscribed, painless mass.	Generally indolent course. Refer for surgical treatment.
Cystosarcoma phylloides	Firm, rubbery, tender, warm, cystic; associated with skin necrosis.	May suddenly enlarge. Most often benign; rarely metastasizes. Surgical removal is indicated.
Giant juvenile fibroadenoma	Remarkably large fibroadenoma with overlying dilated superficial veins.	Benign. Requires excision to prevent breast atrophy for cosmetic reasons.
Intraductal papilloma	Cylindrical tumor arising from epithelium duct; often subareolar but may be in periphery in adolescents; associated nipple discharge.	Most are benign. Requires excision for cytologic diagnosis.
Fat necrosis	Localized inflammatory process in one breast; follows trauma in half of cases.	Subsequent scarring may be confused with malignancy. Biopsy if suspicious in scarring stage.
Virginal or juvenile hypertrophy	Massive enlargement of both, or less often one, breasts, attributed to end-organ hypersensitivity to normal hormone levels around menarche.	Benign. May cause embarrassment. Cosmetic reduction may be done at a later date.

395

Table 13–7. Drugs associated with breast symptoms (galactorrhea, gynecomastia, pain, mass).*

**Street drugs
(illicit or abused)**
Marijuana
Opiates
Amphetamines
Meprobamate

Hormones or related drugs
Oral contraceptives
Estrogens
Tamoxifen
Bromocriptine withdrawal
Methyltestosterone
Human chorionic gonadotropin

Chemotherapeutic agents
Vincristine
Busulfan

Prescription medications
Antidepressants
Benzodiazepines
Butyrophenones
Cimetidine
Digoxin
Isoniazid
Methyldopa
Phenothiazines & derivatives
Reserpine
Spironolactone

*Modified and reproduced, with permission, from Beach RK: Routine breast exams: A chance to reassure, guide, and protect. *Contemp Pediatr,* 1987;**Oct:**70.

Clinical Findings

In type I idiopathic gynecomastia the adolescent presents with a unilateral (20% bilateral), tender, firm mass beneath the areola. More generalized breast enlargement is classified as type II. Pseudogynecomastia refers to excessive fat tissue or prominent pectoralis muscles.

Differential Diagnosis

Gynecomastia may be drug-induced (see Table 13–7) or related to any one of a host of disorders (Table 13–9).

Table 13–8. Causes of galactorrhea.*

1. Hypothalamic disorders
     Functional
         Postpartum
         Without pregnancy
     Pathologic
         Infiltrative
             Sarcoid
             Histiocytosis X
             Hypothalamic tumors
         Section of pituitary stalk
2. Drug therapy
     Tranquilizers
     Tricyclic antidepressants
     Methyldopa
     Rauwolfia alkaloids
     Oral contraceptives
     Estrogens
3. Neoplasms
     Pituitary tumors
         Prolactin secretion only
         Prolactin and ACTH secretion (Cushing's disease)
         Growth hormone secretion with or without prolactin secretion
             (acromegaly)
     Ectopic prolactin-secreting tumors
4. Hypothyroidism
5. Neurogenic stimulation
     Breast stimulation
     Chest-wall lesions (herpes zoster, thoracotomy)

*Reproduced, with permission, from Fraser WM, Blackard WG: Medical conditions that affect the breast and lactation. *Clin Obstet Gynecol* 1975;18:51.

Treatment

If gynecomastia is idiopathic, reassurance of the common and benign nature of the process should be given. Resolution may take several months to 2 years. Pharmacotherapeutic agents, such as dihydrotestosterone heptanoate, danazol, clomiphene, and tamoxifen, have been used with variable results. Surgery is reserved for adolescents with significant psychologic trauma or severe breast enlargement.

GYNECOLOGIC DISORDERS IN ADOLESCENCE

MENSTRUAL PHYSIOLOGY

The menstrual cycle is divided into 3 phases: follicular, ovulatory, and luteal. Hypothalamic, pituitary, and ovarian hor-

Table 13–9. Disorders associated with gynecomastia.*

Klinefelter's syndrome
Traumatic paraplegia
Male pseudohermaphroditism
Testicular feminization syndrome
Reifenstein's syndrome
17-Ketosteroid reductase deficiency
Endocrine tumors (seminoma, Leydig cell tumor, teratoma, feminizing
   adrenal tumor, hepatoma, leukemia, hemophilia, bronchogenic
   carcinoma, leprosy, etc)
Hypothyroidism
Hyperthyroidism
Cirrhosis
Herpes zoster
Friedreich's ataxia

*Reproduced, with permission, from McAnarney ER, Greydanus DE: Adolescence. In: *Current Pediatric Diagnosis and Treatment*, 9th ed. Kempe CH, Silver HK, O'Brien D, Fulginiti VA (eds). Appleton and Lange, 1987.

mones work in concert through a complex system of positive and negative feedback to bring about monthly ovulation (Figure 13–3) and, if fertilization does not occur, menstruation.

MENSTRUAL DISORDERS

Amenorrhea

Amenorrhea is the lack of menses when otherwise expected to occur. It may be the result of anatomic abnormalities, chromosomal deviations, or physiologic delay (Table 13–10).

Primary amenorrhea refers to delay in menarche such that there are no menstrual periods or secondary sex characteristics by 14 years of age, or no menses in the presence of secondary sex characteristics by 16 years of age. **Secondary amenorrhea** is defined as the absence of menses for at least 3 cycles after regular cycles have been established. In some instances evaluation should begin immediately, without waiting for the specified age or duration of lapsed periods, for example, in suspected pregnancy, short stature with the stigmata or Turner's syndrome, or an anatomic defect.

Figure 13–3. Physiology of the normal ovulatory menstrual cycle: gonadotropin secretion, ovarian hormone production, follicular maturation, and endometrial changes during one cycle. FSH = follicle-stimulating hormone; LH = luteinizing hormone.

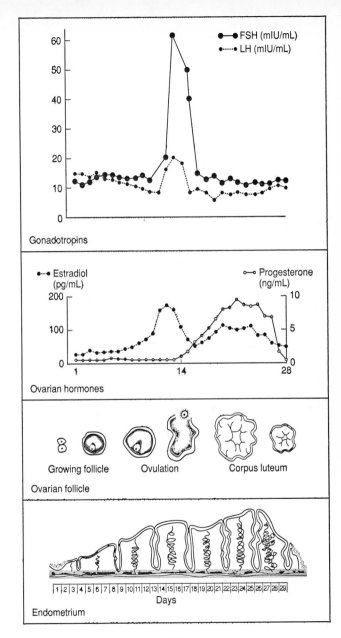

Gonadotropins

- ●—● FSH (mIU/mL)
- ●····● LH (mIU/mL)

Ovarian hormones

- ●—● Estradiol (pg/mL)
- ○—○ Progesterone (ng/mL)

Ovarian follicle

Growing follicle   Ovulation   Corpus luteum

Endometrium

| 1 | 2 | 3 | 4 | 5 | 6 | 7 | 8 | 9 | 10 | 11 | 12 | 13 | 14 | 15 | 16 | 17 | 18 | 19 | 20 | 21 | 22 | 23 | 24 | 25 | 26 | 27 | 28 | 29 |

Days

Table 13–10. Causes of amenorrhea.

Hypothalamic–Pituitary Axis
Hypothalamic repression
  Emotional stress
  Depression
  Chronic disease
  Weight loss; severe dieting
  Obesity
  Strenuous athletics
  Drugs (post-BCP, phenothiazines)
CNS lesion
  Pituitary lesion–adenoma, prolactinoma
  Craniopharyngioma and other brainstem or parasellar tumors
  Head injury with hypothalamic contusion
  Infiltrative process (sarcoidosis)
  Vascular disease (hypothalamic vasculitis)
Congenital conditions*
  Kallman's syndrome

Ovaries
Gonadal dysgenesis*
  Turner's syndrome (XO)
  Mosaic (XX/XO)
Injury to ovary
  Autoimmune disease (may include thyroid, adrenal, islet cells)
  Infection (mumps, oophoritis)
  Toxins (alkylating chemotherapeutic agents)
  Irradiation
  Trauma, torsion (rare)
Polycystic ovary syndrome (Stein-Leventhal)
  (virilization may be present)
Ovarian failure
  Premature menopause—may result from causes of ovarian injury
  above
  Resistant ovary
  Variant of gonadal dysgenesis (mosaic)

Uterovaginal Outflow Tract
Müllerian dysgenesis*
  Congenital deformity or absence of uterus, fallopian tubes, or vagina
Imperforate hymen, transverse vaginal septum, vaginal agenesis,
agenesis of the cervix*
Testicular feminization (absent uterus)*
Uterine lining defect
  Asherman's syndrome (intrauterine synechiae postcurettage or
  endometritis)
  TB, brucellosis

Defect in Hormone Synthesis/Action (virilization may be present)
Adrenal hyperplasia*
Cushing's syndrome
Adrenal tumor
Ovarian tumor (rare)
Drugs (steroids, ACTH)

*Indicates condition usually presenting as primary amenorrhea.

A. Evaluation for Primary Amenorrhea: The history should include whether puberty has commenced and the age at menarche for other female relatives. A careful physical examination should be performed, keeping in mind that estrogen is responsible for breast development; maturation of the external genitalia, vagina, and uterus; and menstruation. If pelvic examination reveals normal female external genitalia and pelvic organs, a vaginal smear for estrogen influence or a progesterone challenge may be done (Fig 13–4).

If signs of virilization are present (Fig 13–5), LH level should be obtained as the first step, to rule out polycystic ovaries. If the LH level is low in the face of virilization, an adrenal disorder is the most likely diagnosis. Endocrinologic and gynecologic consultations may assist in determining the diagnosis.

If physical examination reveals the absence of a uterus (see Fig 13–6), karyotyping should be performed to differentiate testicular feminization from Müllerian duct defect, since the managements differ.

B. Evaluation and Management of Secondary Amenorrhea: Secondary amenorrhea results when there is unopposed estrogen stimulation, maintaining the endometrium in the proliferative phase. The most common causes are pregnancy, stress, or Stein-Leventhal syndrome (polycystic ovaries) (see Table 13–11). The history should focus on issues of stress, weight change, strenuous exercise, sexual activity, and contraceptive use. Review of systems should include questions about headaches, visual changes, and galactorrhea. Physical examination should be sure to include a careful funduscopic examination, visual fields, palpation of the thyroid, measurement of blood pressure and heart rate, compression of the areola to check for galactorrhea, and a search for signs of androgen excess such as hirsutism, clitoromegaly, severe acne, or ovarian enlargement.

The first laboratory study obtained is a pregnancy test, even if the patient denies sexual activity. If the test is negative, vaginal smear for estrogen or progesterone challenge should be done to determine whether the patient has an estrogen-primed uterus that will respond with withdrawal bleeding.

Dysmenorrhea

Dysmenorrhea is the most common gynecologic complaint of adolescent girls, with an incidence of about 60%. Dysmenorrhea can be divided into primary and secondary dysmenorrhea on the basis of whether there is any underlying pelvic pathology. **Primary spasmodic dysmenorrhea** accounts for 80% of adoles-

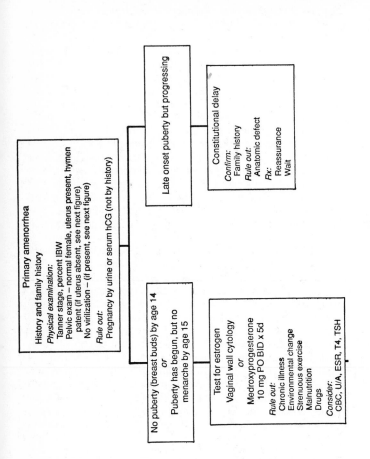

Primary amenorrhea

History and family history

Physical examination:
Tanner stage, percent IBW
Pelvic exam – normal female, uterus present, hymen
patent (if uterus absent, see next figure)
No virilization – (if present, see next figure)

Rule out:
Pregnancy by urine or serum hCG (not by history)

No puberty (breast buds) by age 14
or
Puberty has begun, but no menarche by age 15

Test for estrogen
Vaginal wall cytology
or
Medroxyprogesterone
10 mg PO BID x 5d

Rule out:
Chronic illness
Environmental change
Strenuous exercise
Malnutrition
Drugs

Consider:
CBC, U/A, ESR, T4, TSH

Late onset puberty but progressing

Constitutional delay

Confirm:
Family history
Rule out:
Anatomic defect
Rx:
Reassurance
Wait

402

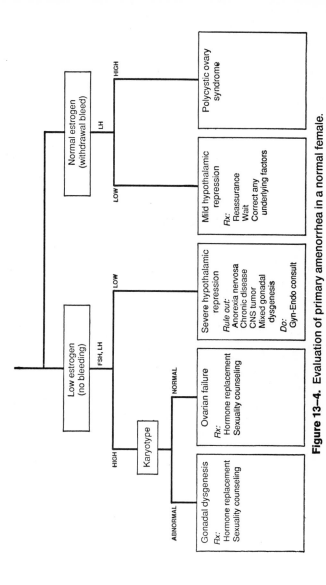

Figure 13–4. Evaluation of primary amenorrhea in a normal female.

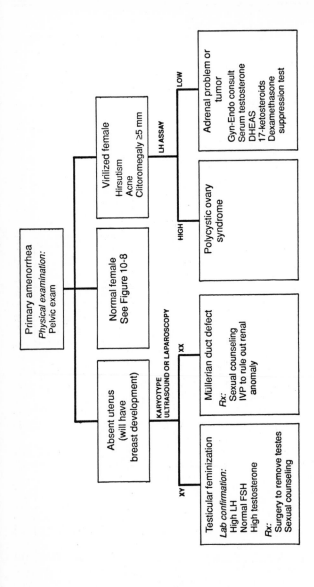

Figure 13-5. Evaluation of primary amenorrhea in a virilized female or one whose uterus is absent.

cent dysmenorrhea and most often affects women under 25 years of age. **Secondary dysmenorrhea** is most often due to sexually transmitted infection, endometriosis, congenital anomalies, or a complication of pregnancy (Table 13–12).

Dysfunctional Uterine Bleeding

Dysfunctional uterine bleeding (DUB) may be referred to as hypermenorrhea or polymenorrhea. It results when an endometrium that has proliferated under unopposed estrogen stimulation finally begins to slough, but incompletely, causing irregular, painless bleeding. The unopposed estrogen stimulation occurs during anovulatory cycles, common in younger adolescents who have not been menstruating for long, but also seen in older adolescents during times of stress or illness.

A. Findings: Typically, the adolescent will present with a history of several years of regular cycles; she then begins to have menses every 2 weeks, or complains of bleeding for 2–3 weeks after 2–3 months of amenorrhea. A past history of painless, irregular periods at intervals of less than 3 weeks may also be elicited. Bleeding for more than 10 days should be considered abnormal. Dysfunctional uterine bleeding must be considered a diagnosis of exclusion (Table 13–13).

B. Management: A pregnancy test and pelvic examination with appropriate cultures should be performed in sexually active patients. A CBC with platelets should also be obtained. Additional coagulation or hormonal studies can be based on the history and physical findings. Management depends on the severity of the problem. For mild DUB a menstrual calendar and reassurance may be sufficient. Mefenamic acid, 500 mg 3 times a day during menses, may reduce flow, and an iron supplement may be considered as anemia can contribute to dysfunctional uterine bleeding as well as result from it.

For moderate DUB in which there is mild anemia, cycles are moderately heavy and prolonged, or the interval between menses remains shortened, medroxyprogesterone, 10 mg once or twice a day for 10 days starting on day 14 of the cycle, may be used for 3–6 months. To acutely stop bleeding in progress, one cycle of Ovral may be given, followed by cycling with medroxyprogesterone for 3–6 months. An iron supplement should also be given.

Severe dysfunctional bleeding requires hospitalization if the patient presents with a low hemoglobin and orthostatic symptoms in the face of heavy vaginal bleeding with disruption of menstrual cycles. Clotting studies should be obtained. Premarin, 25 mg intravenously, may be given for its hemostatic

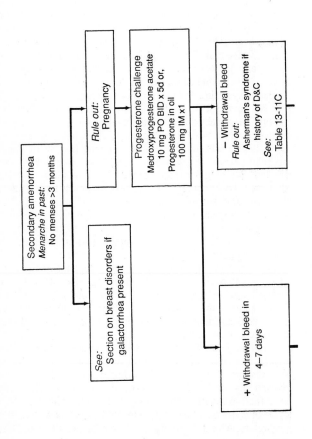

Secondary amenorrhea
Menarche in past:
No menses >3 months

See:
Section on breast disorders if galactorrhea present

Rule out:
Pregnancy

Progesterone challenge
Medroxyprogesterone acetate
10 mg PO BID x 5d or,
Progesterone in oil
100 mg IM x1

− Withdrawal bleed
Rule out:
Asherman's syndrome if history of D&C
See:
Table 13-11C

+ Withdrawal bleed in 4–7 days

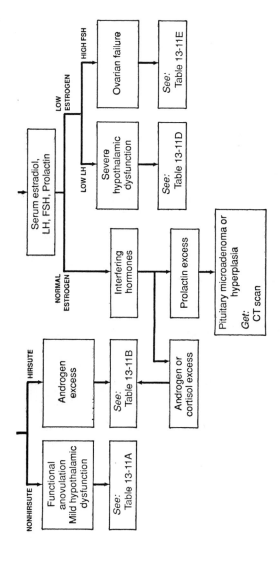

Figure 13–6. Evaluation of secondary amenorrhea.

Table 13–11. Management of secondary amenorrhea by cause.

	Cause	Lab	Management
Mild hypothalamic dysfunction	Recent pregnancy Physical illness Weight loss Obesity Emotional stress Environmental change Strenuous athletics Drugs (post birth control pills, phenothiazines)	CBC, urinalysis ESR T_4, TSH, etc (as indicated)	Reassurance; assessment of birth control needs Repeat of progesterone test every 3 months (after ruling out pregnancy) LH, FSH, prolactin if no menses for 1 year
Androgen excess	Polycystic ovary syndrome (PCO) Cushing's syndrome Adrenal hyperplasia Adrenal tumor Ovarian tumor Drugs (steroids, ACTH)	LH, FSH (high LH suggests PCO); consultation with endocrinologist to help evaluate adrenals	If PCO, birth control pills (Demulen) to control hirsutism and menses Treatment of underlying problem

Asherman's syndrome	Uterine synechiae post TAb or D&C	No bleeding after 1 cycle of combination oral contraceptive (Ovulen)	Referral to gynecologist
Severe hypothalamic dysfunction	Anorexia nervosa Severe emotional stress Chronic systemic disease CNS tumor Pituitary infarction	Low estrogen Low LH Check T_4, TSH, ESR, neurologic exam	Treatment of cause; slow hormone recovery expected
Ovarian failure	Variant of gonadal dysgenesis (mosaicism XX/XO) Postirradiation Postchemotherapy Autoimmune oophoritis Resistant ovarian syndrome Premature menopause	Chromosomes Antiovarian antibodies Laparoscopy Ovarian biopsy	Referral to gynecologist; hormone replacement therapy

Table 13–12. Dysmenorrhea in the adolescent.

Primary Dysmenorrhea—no pelvic pathology					
	Etiology	Onset and Duration	Symptoms	Pelvic Exam	Treatment
Primary spasmodic	Excessive amount of prostaglandin F2α which attaches to myometrium causing uterine contractions, hypoxia, and ischemia. Also, directly sensitizes pain receptors.	Begins with onset of flow or just prior and lasts 1–2 days. Does not start until 6–18 months after menarche, when cycles become ovulatory	Lower abdominal cramps radiating to lower back and thighs. Associated nausea, vomiting, diarrhea, and urinary frequency also due to excess prostaglandins.	Normal. May wait to examine if never sexually active and history is consistent with primary spasmodic dysmenorrhea.	Mild—heating pad, warm baths, nonprescription analgesics. Moderate–severe: prostaglandin inhibitors at onset of flow or pain. Oral contraceptives for sexually active patients
Psychogenic	May have history of sexual abuse or may have difficulty adjusting to womanhood. May have secondary gain from school or work avoidance.	Starts at menarche. Pain begins with anticipation of menses and lasts throughout flow.	Abdominal cramps.	Normal.	Educate regarding normal menstrual function. Reassure that pain does not indicate pathology. Relaxation techniques and biofeedback. Counseling to understand underlying issues.

Secondary Dysmenorrhea—underlying pathology present. (Always perform pelvic exam if secondary dysmenorrhea suspected or patient is sexually active. Gonorrhea culture, test for chlamydia, CBC, and ESR should be obtained.)

Infection	Most often due to a sexually transmitted disease such as chlamydia or gonorrhea.	Recent onset of pelvic cramps.	Pelvic cramps, excessive bleeding, intermenstrual spotting or vaginal discharge.	Mucopurulent or purulent discharge from cervical os, cervical friability, cervical motion tenderness, adnexal tenderness, positive culture for STD.	Appropriate antibiotics.
Endometriosis	Aberrant implants of endometrial tissue in pelvis or abdomen; may result from reflux.	Generally starts more than 2 years after menarche.	Pelvic pain, may occur intermenstrually.	Two thirds are tender on exam, especially during late luteal phase.	Hormonal suppression by oral contraceptives or danazol. Surgery may be necessary for extensive disease.
Complication of pregnancy	Spontaneous abortion, ectopic pregnancy.	Acute onset.	Pelvic cramps associated with a delay in menses.	Positive hCG, enlarged uterus or adnexal mass.	Immediate gynecologic consult.
Congenital anomalies	Transverse vaginal septum, septate uterus, or cervical stenosis.	Onset at menarche.	Pelvic cramps.	Underlying congenital anomaly may be apparent. May require exam under anesthesia.	Gynecologic consult for ultrasound, hysteroscopy, or laparoscopy.

(continued)

Table 13–12. (Continued)

Primary Dysmenorrhea—no pelvic pathology

Primary spasmodic	Etiology	Onset and Duration	Symptoms	Pelvic Exam	Treatment
IUD	Increased uterine contractions, or increase risk for pelvic infection.	Onset after placement of IUD or acutely if due to infection.	Pelvic cramps, heavy menstrual bleeding, may have vaginal discharge.	Normal, or see Infection above.	Prostaglandin inhibitors or mefenamic acid may be drug of choice because it also reduces flow. Appropriate antibiotics and consider removal of IUD if infection is present. Surgery.
Pelvic adhesions	Previous abdominal surgery or pelvic inflammatory disease.	Delayed onset after surgery or PID.	Abdominal pain, may or may not be associated with menstrual cycles; possible alteration in bowel pattern.	Variable.	

Table 13–13. Differential diagnosis of dysfunctional uterine bleeding in adolescents.

Pelvic inflammatory disease

Complication of pregnancy: ectopic pregnancy, threatened abortion, incomplete abortion, missed abortion

Breakthrough bleeding on oral contraceptives

Blood dyscrasias: iron deficiency, thrombocytopenia, coagulopathy, von Willebrand's disease, leukemia

Endocrine disorders: hypothyroidism, hyperthyroidism, diabetes mellitus, adrenal disease, hyperprolactinemia

Trauma

Foreign body

Uterine, vaginal, ovarian, abnormalities: carcinoma, fibroids, adenosis from DES, premature menopause

effect. Ortho-Novum or Norinyl 2 mg should be given every 4 hours until bleeding stops, then once a day for 21 days. This should be followed by cycling on Ovral or Demulen for 3–4 months and iron therapy. Gynecologic consult should be obtained, as a D&C may be necessary if there is no improvement within 24 hours.

Mittelschmerz
Mittelschmerz refers to the pain caused by spillage of fluid from the ruptured follicular cyst at the time of ovulation, irritating the peritoneum. The patient presents with a history of midcycle, unilateral dull or aching abdominal pain lasting a few minutes or as long as 8 hours. Rarely this pain mimics the acute abdominal findings of appendicitis, torsion or rupture of an ovarian cyst, or ectopic pregnancy, in which case a laparoscopy may be necessary. The patient should be reassured and treated symptomatically.

Ovarian Cysts
Functional cysts account for 20–50% of ovarian masses in adolescents and are a variation of the normal physiologic process. They may be asymptomatic, or may cause menstrual irregularity, constipation, or urinary frequency. Functional cysts, unless large, rarely cause abdominal pain. However, tor-

sion or hemorrhage of an ovarian cyst may present as an acute or subacute abdomen. **Follicular cysts** account for the majority of ovarian cysts; they are usually less than or equal to 4 cm in diameter, and resolve spontaneously. **Lutein cysts** occur less commonly, and may be 5–10 cm in diameter. The patient should be referred to a gynecologist for laparoscopy if she is premenarchal, the cyst has a solid component or is larger than 5 cm by ultrasound, there are symptoms or signs suggestive of hemorrhage or torsion, or the cyst fails to regress after 2 to 3 menstrual cycles.

CONTRACEPTION

Sexually active adolescent females wait an average of 1 year before seeking contraception. However, one half of teen pregnancies in the United States occur in the first 6 months of initiating sexual intercourse. Sexuality, contraception, and pregnancy prevention are areas with which the pediatrician has become familiar out of necessity.

Counseling Teenagers About Contraception

Adolescents may have poorly formulated skills for making decisions of any kind, and often benefit from a decision-making framework that can be applied to a variety of situations, particularly those involving peer pressure. By talking with teenagers about their alternatives to sexual intercourse and the implications of coitus (unintended pregnancy; sexually transmitted diseases; possible emotional trauma; and effects on education, career, income, and responsibilities if a pregnancy occurs) the physician can help them to make better-informed decisions before they find themselves in a dilemma.

Abstinence is the most commonly used method of birth control. However, it is prudent to encourage the adolescent to use contraception at the time they do initiate sexual intercourse. Adolescents should understand the menstrual cycle and be taught either that there is no "safe" period or that ovulation occurs 2 weeks before the next menstrual period and may be difficult to predict. Since teenagers frequently have irregular cycles and sexual intercourse is often spontaneous and unplanned, the rhythm or calendar method is not very effective for them. Adolescents also need to be educated that withdrawal is not a method of contraception (Table 13–14).

A. Beginning Birth Control Pills and Follow-up: Before beginning oral contraceptives, a careful menstrual history, medical history, and family medical history should be taken. In addition, baseline weight and blood pressure should be established, breast and pelvic examination should be performed, and specimens for urinalysis, Papanicolaou smear, gonorrhea culture, and chlamydia culture or antigen-detection test obtained.

If there are no contraindications (Table 13–15), the patient may begin her first pack of pills with her next menstrual period. A triphasic or a low-dose combined oral contraceptive is used for teenagers without contraindications to the use of estrogen. It is wise to always use 28-day packs with adolescents rather than 21-day packs, to reduce the chance of missed pills. The patient should be instructed on the use of her type of pills, as well as possible risks and side effects and their warning signs. She should use a back-up method such as condoms and foam for the first 2 weeks to assure protection. A follow-up visit in 1 month and then every 2–3 months for the first year may improve compliance, as teenagers often discontinue birth control pills for nonmedical reasons or because of minor side effects.

B. Management of Side Effects: A different type of combined oral contraceptive should be tried if the patient has a persistent minor side effect for more than the first 2 or 3 months. Adjustments should be made on the basis of hormonal effects. Changes are most often made for persistent breakthrough bleeding not related to missed pills.

PREGNANCY

There are more than 1 million teen pregnancies in the US each year. Of these, about 40% result in abortion, 13% in miscarriage, and 47% in live births. About 45% of 15–19-year-old females are sexually active and more than one third of these become pregnant within 2 years of the onset of sexual intercourse. More than 80% of these pregnancies are unintended, and about 60% of pregnancies in women less than 20 years old occur out of wedlock.

Young maternal age and associated maternal risk factors have been linked to adverse neonatal outcome, including higher rates of low-birth-weight babies (< 2500 g) and neonatal mortality. The psychosocial consequences for the teen mother and her infant are extensive.

Presentation

An adolescent may present with delayed or missed menses, or may even request a pregnancy test, but often they present with

Table 13–14. Commonly used contraceptives in the United States.

Method	Action	Effectiveness(%)	Side Effects	Benefits	Comments
Condoms	Barrier, spermicidal action of nonoxynol-9 in some	88–98	None	Protect against STD	Require no medical visit or prescription
Spermicides	Spermicidal action	79–97	Local irritation	Non-oxynol 9 is bactericidal and viricidal	
Sponges	Barriers, spermicidal	72–95	Possible risk of toxic shock syndrome		Higher failure rates in parous than nulliparous women
Combined oral contraceptives	1) Suppress ovulation 2) Thicken cervical mucus and make sperm penetration difficult 3) Atrophy of endometrium diminishes chance of implantation	96–99	Risk of thromboembolism, MI, stroke, hypertension, hepatoma, death exist but rare in teenagers	Improve dysmenorrhea and acne	May be method of choice for adolescents who have unplanned intercourse. Serious risks increase after age 30, especially in smokers. See Table 13–14 for contraindications.

Method	Mechanism	Efficacy (%)	Disadvantages		Comments
Mini pill	1) Thicken cervical mucus 2) Atrophy of endometrium 3) Ovulation suppressed in only 15–40% of cycles	97–98	Less predictable menstrual patterns		May be used in patients who should avoid exogenous estrogens
IUD	Prevent implantation through local inflammatory response and local production of prostaglandins	95–98	STDs, PID and its sequelae, heavy menstrual flow, dysmenorrhea	No temporal relationship to sexual activity	Not the most ideal method for teens who have multiple partners and their childbearing years ahead of them, given STD risk
Diaphragm	Barrier Spermicidal action of contraceptive gel used in conjunction	82–97	None		Must be comfortable inserting and checking fit

Table 13–15. Contraindications to combined birth control pills.*

Absolute contraindications
History of thrombophlebitis, thromboembolic disorder, cerebrovascular disorder, ischemic heart disease
Known or suspected carcinoma of the breast or estrogen-dependent neoplasia
Known or suspected pregnancy
History of benign or malignant liver tumor
Undiagnosed abnormal vaginal bleeding

Strong relative contraindications
Severe vascular or migraine headaches
Hypertension
Diabetes
Active gallbladder disease
Mononucleosis, acute phase
Sickle cell disease or sickle C disease
Upcoming major surgery
Long leg cast or major injury to lower leg
Known impaired liver function at present time
Completion of term pregnancy within past 10–14 days

*Modified and reproduced, with permission, from *Contraceptive Technology 1988–1989,* 14th revised ed. Breedlove B, Judy B, Martin N (eds). Irvington Publishers, Inc., 1988.

an unrelated concern (hidden agenda) or a vague somatic complaint. Clinicians need to have a low threshold for suspecting pregnancy. If there is *any* suspicion, a urine pregnancy test should be obtained.

Diagnosis

History, as above, and physical examination may assist in making the diagnosis of pregnancy. Bluish coloring and softening of the cervix may be noted on speculum examination. The uterine fundus may be palpable on abdominal examination if sufficient time has lapsed. If uterine size on bimanual examination does not correspond to dates, one must consider ectopic pregnancy, incomplete or missed abortion, twin gestation, or inaccurate dates. Laboratory tests for human chorionic gonadotropin (hCG) are simple to perform and usually make the diagnosis.

Special Issues in Management

When an adolescent presents for pregnancy testing, it is wise to find out before performing the test what she hopes the results will be and what she thinks she will do. If she wants to be pregnant and the test is negative, further counseling into the implications of teen pregnancy should be undertaken. For those who do not wish to be pregnant, this is a good time to begin contraception.

If the adolescent is pregnant, discuss her support systems and her options with her. Many teenagers need help in involving their parents. Since teenagers are often ambivalent about their plans and may have a high level of denial, it is prudent to follow-up with her in a week to be certain that a decision has been made and to assist her into prenatal care if she has chosen to maintain the pregnancy.

It has been shown that maternal age in and of itself is not responsible for low birth weight and poor fetal outcome, but that low maternal prepregnancy weight, poor weight gain, delay in prenatal care, low socioeconomic status, and black race are contributing factors. The poor nutritional status of some teenagers and their erratic diets, habits of smoking, drinking, or substance abuse, and high prevalence of sexually transmitted diseases also play a role. Teenagers are also at greater risk of toxemia of pregnancy, iron deficiency anemia, cephalopelvic disproportion, prolonged labor, premature labor, and maternal death. Early prenatal care and good nutrition can make a difference with a number of these potential complications.

Because of the high risk of a second unintended pregnancy within the next 2 years, postpartum contraceptive counseling and follow-up is imperative.

VULVOVAGINITIS

Vaginitis has two main causes: pathogens or indigenous flora after a change in milieu of the vagina. Monilia vulvovaginitis and bacterial vaginosis (formerly referred to as gardnerella, hemophilus, or nonspecific vaginitis) may be found in non–sexually active patients and are examples of indigenous flora that may cause infection. Bacterial vaginosis is more prevalent in those who are sexually active. In sexually active patients, trichomonas or cervicitis from sexually transmitted pathogens must be considered. (See section on STDs.) For this reason, sexually active patients or those suspected to be victims of sexual abuse should have appropriate specimens taken for STDs even if yeast or bacterial vaginosis is identified.

Physiologic Leukorrhea
This is the normal vaginal discharge that begins just prior to or around the time of menarche. The discharge is typically clear or whitish, nonodorous, and of varying consistency. Early ado-

lescent girls may have concerns about such a discharge and need reassurance that it is normal. If a vaginal wet prep is examined a few squamous epithelial cells may be revealed, but there should be less than 5 polymorphonuclear cells per high power field.

Monilia Vulvovaginitis

Monilial or candidal vulvovaginitis is caused by yeast. It typically occurs after a course of antibiotic therapy, which alters the normal perineal flora and allows the yeast to proliferate. Diabetics, those with compromised immunity, and those who are pregnant or on oral contraceptives are more prone to monilial infections. The patient usually complains of vulvar pruritus or dyspareunia and a cheesy vaginal discharge. Examination of the genitals reveals an erythematous mucosa, sometimes with excoriation, and a thick, white, adherent, cheesy discharge. Leukocytes may be seen on wet prep, and KOH prep may reveal budding yeast or mycelia. Often the vaginal preps will be unhelpful, in which case the patient should be treated on the basis of the clinical examination. Nystatin, clotrimazole, or terconazole vaginal creams or suppositories designed for 3 nightly or 7 nightly doses are effective in the majority of patients. Some patients require a longer course of treatment. Patients with recurrent episodes should be given prophylactic treatment whenever they are on antibiotics. It may be helpful to simultaneously treat the partners of sexually active patients with recurrent monilial infections.

Bacterial Vaginosis

Bacterial vaginosis may be caused by any of the indigenous vaginal flora, such as gardnerella, bacteroides, peptococcus, or lactobacilli. The patient generally complains of malodorous mild discharge. On examination, a thin, homogeneous, grayish-white discharge is found adherent to the vaginal wall, with diffuse vaginal erythema. A whiff test, in which a drop of potassium hydroxide is added to a smear of the discharge on a slide, results in the release of amines causing a fishy odor. Wet prep reveals an abundance of clue cells (vaginal epithelial cells stippled with adherent bacteria) and small pleomorphic rods. Treatment is with metronidazole, 500 mg orally twice a day for 7 days. Ampicillin, 500 mg orally 4 times a day for 7 days is the alternative therapy during pregnancy.

Sexually Transmitted Diseases

See next section for cervicitis. It behooves one to do appropriate cultures even if the cervix appears normal, as sexually transmitted diseases may otherwise be missed.

Foreign-body Vaginitis

Foreign bodies, most commonly retained tampons, cause extremely malodorous vaginal discharges. Treatment is by removal of the foreign body, for which ring forceps may be useful. Further treatment is generally not necessary.

Allergic or Contact Vaginitis

Bubble baths, feminine hygiene sprays, or vaginal contraceptive foams or suppositories may cause chemical irritation of the vaginal mucosa. Discontinuing use of the offending agent is indicated.

SEXUALLY TRANSMITTED DISEASES AND PELVIC INFLAMMATORY DISEASE

The 15–19 and 20–24-year-old age groups have the highest incidence of sexually transmitted diseases (STDs) because of multiple sexual partners, lack of use of barrier methods of contraception, and delay in seeking treatment.

Chlamydia trachomatis, an obligate intracellular body half the size of the gonococcus, is the most common cause of STD, with 2–3 million new cases per year in the US; peak incidence is in 15–20 year olds. One quarter to one half of those infected are asymptomatic, and one quarter to one half are coinfected with gonorrhea. Chlamydia accounts for 20–30% of the 170,000 cases of pelvic inflammatory disease (PID) per year and is responsible for more than 60% of PID cases in women under 20 years old (Table 13–16).

Neisseria gonorrhoea is the second most common cause of STD, with peak incidence in the 15–25-year-old age group. Five to 25% of cases are associated with another STD, and more than 50% of those infected are asymptomatic (see Table 13–16).

In view of the prevalence of STD in the adolescent population and the reluctance of teenagers to talk about them, the clinician needs to routinely ask adolescents about sexual activity, number of partners, and symptoms of STD when they present for routine physical examinations or sexually related symptoms (dysuria, penile or vaginal discharge, genital lesion, or abdominal pain). As females are frequently asymptomatic, obtaining wet prep, gonorrhea culture, and test for chlamydia at the time of the annual Pap smear in sexually active females is advised. Although males are usually symptomatic, a significant

Table 13–16. Urethritis, cervicitis, and pelvic inflammatory disease.

	Agents	Symptoms	Physical Findings	Laboratory Findings	Complications
Urethritis	Chlamydia Gonorrhea *Ureaplasma* *Mycoplasma* Trichomonas	Dysuria Urethral discharge May be asymptomatic	Exam may be normal. Clear, white, or purulent penile discharge. (May occur in females, often in association with cervicitis.)	U/A: Moderate WBCs without bacteriuria Gramstain: PMNs, may show gram-negative intracellular diplococci if due to gonorrhea. Gonorrhea culture: may be positive. Chlamydia culture or antigen detection test: may be positive.	Nontender penile edema Prostatitis Epididymitis Orchitis
Cervicitis	Chlamydia Gonorrhea Herpes Trichomonas	Asymptomatic Possible vaginal discharge or dysuria	Cervix may appear normal, or may have erythema, petechial irregular raised surface, friability, or ulcerations.	Wet prep: > 10 WBCs/hpf with gonorrhea or chlamydia. Gonorrhea culture: may be positive. Chlamydia culture or	Pelvic inflammatory disease Infection of Bartholin glands

PID				
Chlamydia Gonorrhea Normal vaginal aerobic and anaerobic flora may be secondary invaders	Abdominal pain may be minimal Vaginal discharge in 75% Excessive menstrual bleeding or intermenstrual spotting in 40% Fever in 40% Dysuria in 15%	Mucopurulent or purulent cervical discharge. Lower abdominal tenderness. Uterine, adnexal, or cervical motion tenderness. Abnormal cervical discharge in half.	antigen detection test: may be positive May have elevated WBC, ESR, but may be normal. Cervical culture for gonorrhea or chlamydia may be positive.	Tuboovarian abscess Fitz-Hugh-Curtis syndrome Tubal occlusion Infertility Ectopic pregnancy Chronic abdominal pain

number of those with chlamydia are asymptomatic, or symptoms of gonorrhea may resolve, and the adolescent fails to seek treatment.

When an STD is diagnosed, the adolescent and his or her partner(s) should be treated simultaneously with the appropriate antibiotic regimen (Tables 13–17, 13–18, 13–19, and 13–20). They should be followed closely because poor compliance with treatment is common in this age group. A test-of-cure culture for gonorrhea should be obtained no sooner than 4–5 days after completion of treatment to allow clearing of antibiotic from the blood. Serology will need to be followed in the case of syphilis. It is essential to emphasize abstinence until both partners complete treatment to avoid reinfection and/or spread, and to advise use of barrier methods of contraception to prevent future infections. Possible complications and the implications of recurrent infections with regard to fertility and ectopic pregnancy should also be discussed. Adolescents should also be made aware of the possibility of transmission of an STD to the fetus.

Table 13–17. Treatment of urethritis or cervicitis in adolescents.*

	Drug of Choice	**Alternatives**
Gonorrhea	Ceftriaxone 125–250 mg IM once, followed by treatment for *Chlamydia*, below	Spectinomycin 2 g IM once or ciprofloxacin† 500 mg orally once or amoxicillin‡ 3 g orally once plus probenecid 1 g orally once plus treatment for *Chlamydia*
Chlamydia trachomatis	Doxycycline§ 100 mg orally bid for 7 days or tetracycline§ 500 mg orally 4 times daily for 7 days	Erythromycin 500 mg orally 4 times daily for 7 days

*Modified and reproduced, with permission, from Treatment of sexually transmitted diseases. *Med Lett Drugs Ther* 1990;**32**:5.
†Quinolones, such as ciprofloxacin, are contraindicated during pregnancy and in children 16 years of age or younger.
‡May be used for infections proved *not* to be penicillin-resistant gonorrhea.
§Contraindicated during pregnancy.

Table 13–18. Treatment of pelvic inflammatory disease.*

	Drug of Choice	Dosage	Alternatives
Hospitalized patients	Cefoxitin or cefotetan either one plus doxycycline followed by doxycycline†	2 gr IV every 6 hours 2 gr IV every 12 hours 100 mg IV every 12 hours until improved 100 mg orally twice daily to complete 10–14 days	Clindamycin 600 mg IV every 6 hours plus gentamicin 2 mg/kg IV once followed by gentamicin 1.5 mg/kg IV every 8 hours until improved followed by doxycycline† 100 mg orally twice daily to complete 10–14 days
Outpatients	Cefoxitin plus probenecid or ceftriaxone either one followed by doxycycline†	2 gr IM once 1 gr orally once 250 mg IM once 100 mg orally twice daily for 10–14 days	

*Modified and reproduced, with permission, from Treatment of sexually transmitted diseases. *Med Lett Drugs Ther* 1990;**32**:5.
†Contraindicated during pregnancy.

URETHRITIS

Urethritis may be caused by gonorrhea, chlamydia, *Ureaplasma, Mycoplasma,* or trichomonas.

CERVICITIS

Cervicitis may be caused by chlamydia or gonorrhea. There may also be involvement of the cervix with trichomonas vaginitis, and herpes may cause characteristic cervical ulcerations.

Table 13–19. Diagnosis and treatment of genital lesions.

Lesion	Agent	Clinical Findings	Treatment
Condyloma acuminata (genital warts)	Human papilloma virus	Verrucous skin lesion most often occurring on the glans penis or corona in males and posterior introitus in females.	Apply 20–25% Podophyllin in tincture of benzoin to wart after applying petroleum jelly to normal skin. Wash off in 4 hours. Do not use on vaginal or anal mucosa, nor during pregnancy. Refer for colposcopy if HPV effects are noted on Pap smear. (Additional treatments: liquid nitrogen, laser, 5-FU, surgical excision, interferon.)
Herpes	Herpes simplex virus (HSV-2 in 80–95% and HSV-1 in remainder)	Cluster of painful papules which progress to vesicles, pustules, ulcers, and crusts. Systemic symptoms with primary episode. Prodromal tingling with recurrences.	Acyclovir 200 mg orally 5 times a day for 7–10 days (primary) or 5 days (recurrence). May shorten duration of eruptions. Institute with prodromal symptoms.
Syphilis	Treponema pallidum		
Primary		Painless, clean ulcer with an erythematous, indurated border (chancre) which is positive on darkfield exam.	Penicillin G benzathine 2.4 million units IM once OR tetracycline 500 mg orally 4 times a day for 15 days OR Erythromycin 500 mg orally 4 times a day for 15 days.
Secondary		Broad-based, flat, mucoid	

Table 13–20. Diagnosis and treatment of sexually transmitted parasites.

	Symptoms	Clinical Findings	Treatment
Trichomoniasis	Asymptomatic or pruritic vaginal discharge in females or clear penile discharge in males.	Copious frothy vaginal discharge. Motile flagellated trichomonad seen on wet prep of vaginal discharge or spun urinalysis.	Metronidazole 2 g orally once or 250 mg orally 3 times a day for 7 days. During pregnancy, use clotrimazole 100 mg intravaginally at bedtime for 7 days instead.
Pediculosis pubis (crab lice)	Pruritic rash.	Lice and opalescent nits found anchored to pubic hairs.	Lindane or pyrethrins is applied to pubic hair and surrounding skin, lathering for 4–10 minutes, and rinsed off. Nits are combed. Fomites and linens need to be washed in hot water. Treat close contacts.
Scabies	Pruritic rash of groin, thighs, or abdomen.	Scabetic burrows and erythematous, maculopapular rash with some scaliness and tendency to impetiginize.	Lindane is applied from neck down for 8 hours, or crotamiton for 24 hours, then showered off. Repeat application in 24 hours. Fomites & close contacts must be treated.

PELVIC INFLAMMATORY DISEASE

Acute PID, or salpingitis, is the most common serious infection occurring in young women (see Table 13–16). The adolescent age group has the highest rate of PID, with an annual rate of 1.5% of females 15–19 years old. Risk factors for PID include sexual activity, multiple partners (5 times greater risk than for one partner), age less than 25, presence of an IUD (2–4 times greater risk than for nonusers), nulliparous, prior history of PID (2 times greater risk), prior history of uncomplicated STD, and prior induced abortion.

The diagnosis of PID is not straightforward, hence, the following guidelines have been suggested. The 3 major criteria of lower abdominal pain and tenderness, cervical motion tenderness, and adnexal tenderness must be present. In addition one of the following minor criteria must be present: temperature greater than 38°C, leukocytosis above 10,500 WBC/mm^3, culdocentesis yielding peritoneal fluid containing WBCs and bacteria, inflammatory mass noted on pelvic examination, or ultrasound, elevated ESR, cervical Gram stain suggestive of gonorrhea or positive chlamydia antigen detection test, or more than 5 WBCs per oil-immersion field on Gram stain of endocervical discharge.

The differential diagnosis of PID includes acute appendicitis, mesenteric lymphadenitis, cholecystitis, ectopic pregnancy, intrauterine pregnancy, ovarian cyst or tumor, endometriosis, urinary tract infection, and renal calculus.

If there is the slightest suspicion of PID the patient should be treated with appropriate antibiotics while cultures are pending (see Table 13–18). The patient should be hospitalized if she exhibits significant fever or toxicity, is unable to tolerate oral medication and fluids, has not responded to outpatient therapy or is unlikely to comply with it, is a younger adolescent, or is seriously ill with an unclear diagnosis.

GENITAL LESIONS

Condyloma acuminata, or genital warts, are caused by human papilloma virus (HPV). Warts typically occur at the site of minute skin trauma, with 50% occurring on the glans penis or corona in males and 75% at the posterior introitus in females. Diagnosis is based on the clinical appearance of a verrucous skin lesion with a negative darkfield examination. HPV may, however, be present on the cervix or the penis but be indiscernible to the unaided eye. It is now accepted that HPV is the most important etiologic agent in the development of cervical intraepithelial neoplasia and invasive cervical cancers, and appears to be associated with penile cancer (see Table 13–19).

Herpes Simplex Virus

Eighty to 95% of genital herpes cases are due to herpes simplex virus type 2 (HSV-2); the remainder are due to HSV-1. Fifty percent of new cases may be asymptomatic. The primary episode is generally more symptomatic and prolonged than recurrences, and is characterized by systemic symptoms such as fever, headache, malaise, myalgias, and a cluster of painful papules that progress to vesicles, pustules, ulcers, and finally crusts (see Table 13–19).

Syphilis

The primary stage of syphilis typically presents with a painless chancre that appears as a clean ulcer with an erythematous, indurated border. Diagnosis is by immediate darkfield examination of a microscope slide that has been pressed to the base of the lesion with a drop of saline added. VDRL can be done for further investigation, but may be negative early in the course of the disease. The chancre may be self-limited, and after a latency period of 4–6 weeks the disease may resurface in the secondary stage, characterized by a diffuse, nonpruritic, maculopapular rash that includes the palms and soles, mucous patches on the mucosal surfaces, generalized lymphadenopathy, constitutional symptoms, and the presence of condylomalata (broad-based, flat, mucoid lesions) on the genitals. At this stage, diagnosis is by VDRL. The tertiary stage is divided into early latent and late benign, and may include the cardiovascular and central nervous system complications of dissection of the ascending aorta, seizures, stroke, optic atrophy and tabes dorsalis. All stages may be treated with penicillin. The VDRL should be repeated 3, 6, and 12 months after treatment.

PARASITES

Trichomonas Vaginalis

This infection causes vaginitis in females and urethritis in males. Females may be asymptomatic or may complain of a pruritic vaginal discharge. Diagnosis is by examination of a vaginal wet prep in females, or a spun urinalysis in males, for the motile trichomonad.

Arthropods

Phthirius pubis, or crab lice, causes pubic pruritus. On physical examination lice and opalescent nits (eggs) anchored to the pubic hair are found. **Scabies** also results in an intensely pruritic rash, which is located on the groin, thighs, or abdomen in the case of sexual transmission. On physical examination the scabetic burrows and erythematous, maculopapular rash with some scaliness and the tendency to impetiginize are found.

ACQUIRED IMMUNODEFICIENCY SYNDROME (AIDS)

AIDS results from infection with the human immunodeficiency virus (HIV), which is transmitted in blood and semen, and potentially other bodily fluids, through sexual and needle contact.

About 75% of cases in the US have been in homosexual or bisexual men, and 15% in intravenous substance abusers. Although to date few cases have occurred in adolescents, they are at significant potential risk due to their propensity for multiple sexual partners and their limited use of barrier contraceptives, as well as the use of drugs by some. A large number of infected young adults 20–29 years old acquired the infection as adolescents.

Preventive measures need to be taken to ensure that adolescents have the necessary knowledge to protect themselves from AIDS in current and future relationships, and to eliminate AIDS hysteria. They need to be instructed in risk factors for AIDS, modes of transmission, means of protection, and availability of confidential testing. The safer sex practices promoted as a result of AIDS can reduce the rate of all kinds of STD if heeded. Adolescence is an ideal time to promote these practices, as it is a time when intimate relationships are beginning and sexual decisions become important.

Infectious Diseases: Viral & Rickettsial | 14

Mark J. Abzug, MD

VIRAL DISEASES

ROSEOLA INFANTUM
(Exanthema Subitum)

Roseola infantum is an acute febrile disease of infants and young children characterized by fever followed by a faint rash. The incubation period is estimated to be 5–15 days. The newly discovered virus herpesvirus-6 has been implicated as the possible causative agent.

Clinical Findings

A. Symptoms and Signs: The onset is sudden, with sustained or spiking fever as high as 41.1 °C (106 °F). Fever persists for 1–5 days (average, 3 days), falls by crisis, and then may be subnormal for a few hours just before the rash appears. Rash appears when the temperature returns to normal. It is faintly erythematous, maculopapular, and principally confined to the trunk. Individual macules resemble those of rubella. Other physical findings may include mild pharyngitis, enlargement of the postoccipital nodes, and irritability.

B. Laboratory Findings: Findings include progressive leukopenia to 3000–5000 white cells, with a relative lymphocytosis as high as 90%.

Complications

Seizures are the principal complicaton (they may be the first sign of illness) and are related to the rapidly rising temperature. A parainfectious type of encephalitis has been reported (see Chapter 27).

Treatment

A. Specific Measures: None available.

B. General Measures: Antipyretics and tepid water sponge baths may be used to minimize discomfort and the risk of febrile seizures.

C. Treatment of Complications: Barbiturate anticonvulsants may prevent febrile seizures in children with convulsive tendencies (see Table 14–1).

Prognosis

The prognosis is excellent.

MEASLES
(Rubeola)

Measles is a highly communicable disease; the highest incidence is between the ages of 2 and 14 years. The incubation period is 8–14 days, with a majority of cases occurring 10 days after exposure.

Clinical Findings

A. Symptoms and Signs:

1. Prodrome–Fever is usually the first sign and persists throughout the prodrome. It ranges from 38.3 to 40 °C (101 to 104 °F), tends to be higher just before the appearance of the skin rash, and may be lower after eruption of the rash. Sore throat, nasal discharge, and dry, "barking" cough are common during the prodrome. Nonpurulent conjunctivitis appears toward the end of the prodrome and is accompanied by photophobia. Lymphadenopathy of the posterior cervical lymph nodes may occur. The causative virus is easily transmitted via nose and throat secretions during the prodromal period, which lasts 3–5 days.

Koplik's spots are fine white spots on a faint erythematous base that appear first on the buccal mucosa opposite the molar teeth and by about the third or fourth day of the prodrome may spread over the entire inside of the mouth. They usually disappear as the exanthem becomes well established.

2. Rash–Rash appears on about the fifth day of disease. The pink, blotchy, irregular, macular erythema rapidly darkens and characteristically coalesces into larger red patches of varying size and shape. The eruption fades on pressure. The rash first appears on the face and behind the ears; it then spreads to the chest and abdomen and, finally, to the extremities. It lasts 4–7

Table 14–1. Diagnostic features of some acute exanthems.

Disease	Prodromal Signs and Symptoms	Nature of Eruption	Other Diagnostic Features	Laboratory Findings
Chickenpox (varicella)	0–1 d of fever, anorexia, headache.	Rapid evolution of macules to papules, vesicles, crusts; vesicles extremely fragile; all stages simultaneously present in successive outcroppings; lesions superficial; distribution centripetal.	Lesions on scalp and mucous membranes.	Specialized complement fixation and virus neutralization in tissue culture. Fluorescent antibody test of smear of lesions.
Drug eruption	Occasionally fever.	Maculopapular rash resembling rubella, rarely papulovesicular.		Eosinophilia.
Eczema herpeticum	No prodrome.	Vesiculopustular lesions in area of eczema.		Herpes simplex virus isolated in tissue culture; complement fixation. Fluorescent antibody test of smear of lesions.
Enterovirus infection	1–2 d of fever, malaise.	Maculopapular rash resembling rubella, rarely papulovesicular or petechial.	Aseptic meningitis.	Virus isolation from stool or cerebrospinal fluid; complement fixation titer rise.

(continued)

433

Table 14–1. (Continued).

Disease	Prodromal Signs and Symptoms	Nature of Eruption	Other Diagnostic Features	Laboratory Findings
Erythema infectiosum	No prodrome. Usually in epidemics.	Red, flushed cheeks; circumoral pallor, maculopapules on extremities.	"Slapped face" appearance.	White blood count normal.
Exanthema subitum	3–4 d of high fever.	As fever falls by crisis, pink maculopapules appear on chest and trunk; fade in 1–3 d.		White blood count low.
Infectious mononucleosis	Fever, adenopathy, sore throat.	Maculopapular rash resembling rubella, rarely papulovesicular; distribution scattered, asymmetrical.	Splenomegaly, tonsillar exudate.	Atypical lymphs in blood smears; heterophil agglutination. Slide agglutination test.
Meningococcemia	Hours of fever, vomiting.	Maculopapules, petechiae, purpura.	Meningeal signs, toxicity, shock.	White blood count high. Cultures of blood and cerebrospinal fluid.
Rocky Mountain spotted fever	3–4 d of fever, chills, severe headache.	Maculopapules, petechiae; distribution centrifugal.	History of tick bite.	Agglutination (O × 19, O × 2), complement fixation.
Rubella (German measles)	Little or no prodrome.	Maculopapular, pink; begins on head and neck, spreads downward, fades in 3 d. No desquamation.	Lymphadenopathy, postauricular or occipital.	White blood count normal or low. Serologic tests for immunity and definitive diagnosis

Disease				
Rubeola (measles)	3–4 d of fever, coryza, conjunctivitis, cough.	Maculopapular, brick-red; begins on head and neck; spreads downward. In 5–6 d, rash is brownish, desquamating.	Koplik's spots on buccal mucosa.	White blood count low. Virus isolation in cell culture. Antibody tests by hemagglutination inhibition and complement fixation or neutralization.
Scarlet fever	½–2 d of malaise, sore throat, fever, vomiting.	Generalized, punctate, red; prominent on neck, in axilla, groin, skin folds; circumoral pallor; fine desquamation involves hands and feet.	Strawberry tongue, exudative tonsilitis.	Group A hemolytic streptococci cultures from throat; antistreptolysin O titer rise.
Smallpox (variola)	3 d of fever, severe headache, malaise, chills.	Slow evolution of macules to papules, vesicles, pustules, crusts; all lesions in any area in same stage; lesions deep-seated; distribution centrifugal.		Virus isolation. Serologic tests for immunity. Fluorescent antibody test of smear of lesions.
Typhus fever	3–4 d of fever, chills, severe headache.	Maculopapules, petechiae; distribution centripetal.	Endemic area, lice.	Agglutination (O × 19), complement fixation.

(hemagglutination inhibition, complement fixation).

435

days and may be accompanied by mild itching. A fine brawny desquamation, especially of the face and trunk, may follow, lasting 2 or 3 days; light brown pigmentation may then appear.

B. Laboratory Findings: Leukopenia is present during the prodrome and early stages of the rash. There is usually a sharp rise in the white cell count with the onset of any bacterial complication. In the absence of complications, the white cell count slowly rises to normal as the rash fades.

Complications

A. Bacterial Infection:

1. Otitis media–This may appear toward the end of the prodrome or during the course of the rash (see Chapter 20).

2. Tracheobronchitis–Besides the specific inflammation due to rubeola, there may be secondary bacterial involvement. This is usually accompanied by a more productive cough.

3. Bronchopneumonia–While rubeola virus itself often causes a specific pneumonitis, secondary bacterial invasion is a relatively common complication.

B. Encephalitis: Encephalitis (see Chapter 27) occurs in about 1 of 2000 cases (no relation to severity of measles). The first sign may be increasing lethargy or seizures. Lumbar puncture shows 0–200 cells, mostly lymphocytes. Subacute sclerosing panencephalitis (SSPE) is a late degenerative central nervous system complication that results from persistent infection.

C. Hemorrhagic Measles: This rare form of the disease has a high mortality rate and is characterized by generalized bleeding and purpura.

D. Tuberculosis: Active pulmonary tuberculosis may be aggravated by measles.

Treatment

A. Specific Measures: None available.

B. General Measures: Measures include isolation for 4 days from onset of rash, and supportive therapies: rest, antipyretics, mist, and antitussives.

C. Treatment of Complications: Bacterial complications should be treated with appropriate antibacterials. Prophylaxis of bacterial infection may be instituted in children with preexisting pulmonary conditions or other debilitating diseases. For treatment of patients with encephalitis, see Chapter 27.

Prophylaxis

Live measles virus vaccine should be given at 15 months of age—or at any age thereafter in susceptible persons (see Chapter

9). Newly revised recommendations now call for a second vaccination, either at the time of school entry (ie, at approximately 5 years) or at the time of middle/junior high school entry (ie, at approximately seventh grade). Standard immune globulin can prevent the disease in exposed susceptible persons if it is administered within 6 days of exposure and at a dose of 0.25 mL/kg (0.5 mL/kg in immunocompromised children).

Prognosis

In uncomplicated cases or those with bacterial complications, the prognosis is excellent. In patients with encephalitis, the prognosis is guarded; the incidence of permanent sequelae is high.

RUBELLA
(German Measles)

Rubella is a mild febrile virus infection that frequently occurs in epidemics. Transmission is probably by the droplet route. The incubation period is 12–21 days (average, 16 days).

Clinical Findings

A. Symptoms and Signs:

1. Typical rubella–The prodrome, if present, lasts only a few days and is characterized by slight malaise, occasional tender postauricular and occipital lymph nodes, and no catarrhal symptoms. Rash may be the first sign of disease and consists of faint, fine, discrete, erythematous maculopapules, appearing first on the face and spreading rapidly over the trunk and extremities, which may coalesce. The rash generally disappears by the third day. The temperature rarely exceeds 38.3 °C (101 °F) and usually lasts less than 2 days.

2. Rubella without rash–Rubella sine eruptione occurs as a febrile lymphadenopathy that may persist for a week or more. During epidemics, this syndrome may represent over 40% of cases with infection.

3. Congenital rubella–This is a syndrome generally involving infants born to mothers affected with rubella in the first trimester of pregnancy. The majority of infants show growth retardation and microcephaly, hepatosplenomegaly, and purpura, in addition to mental deficiency and congenital defects of the heart, eye, and ear. Marked thrombocytopenia and radiographic metaphysitis are common findings. Rubella virus is easily isolated from such patients, and they must be considered to be highly contagious. A late-onset congenital rubella syndrome, with minimal signs at birth and an acute onset of severe clinical disease after 3–6 months, has been reported.

B. Laboratory Findings: Transient leukopenia is generally noted.

Complications

If rubella occurs during the first month of pregnancy, there is a 50% change of fetal abnormality. By the third month of pregnancy, the risk of abnormalities decreases to less than 10%.

Encephalitis and thrombocytopenic purpura are rare. Polyarthritis occurs in 25% of cases in persons over 16 years of age.

Treatment

A. Specific Measures: None available.

B. General Measures: Isolation is required for 7 days after the onset of rash. Infants with congenital rubella may be contagious for more than 1 year. Symptomatic measures are rarely necessary.

C. Treatment of Complications: For treatment of encephalitis and purpura, see Chapters 23 and 27, respectively.

Prophylaxis

Live rubella vaccine is normally administered in combination with measles and mumps vaccine at 15 months of age (see Chapter 9). Live rubella vaccine can be administered at any age after 12 months in susceptible persons; adolescents and young adults with no history of vaccine should be identified and vaccinated. A history of disease is unreliable and should not be used to determine the need for vaccine. Females of childbearing age should avoid pregnancy for 3 months after vaccination, although surveillance data suggest that no cases of congenital rubella syndrome have occurred in the offspring of women inadvertently given live rubella vaccine shortly before or within 3 months of conception.

Standard immune globulin is not reliable in preventing infection in pregnant women exposed to rubella virus infection and is therefore not recommended. Rubella serology should be measured immediately after exposure and then, if negative (susceptible), again at 3 and 6 weeks, to document whether maternal infection has occurred. All pregnant women—regardless of their immune status—should be cautioned against exposure to any person with an illness suggestive of rubella.

Prognosis

The prognosis in patients with acquired infection is excellent. In patients with congenital disease, the prognosis is universally poor. A progressive, degenerative panencephalitis has been reported. Late manifestations of brain damage such as behavior problems, increasing mental retardation, and minimal brain dysfunction (see Chapter 12) may occur.

ERYTHEMA INFECTIOSUM
(Fifth Disease & Parvoviruses)

Erythema infectiosum is a mild, minimally febrile contagious disease usually occurring in family or institutional epidemics. The incubation period is estimated to be 4–14 days. Human parvovirus B19 has recently been demonstrated to be the causative agent.

Clinical Findings

A. Symptoms and Signs: There is usually no prodrome. The first symptom is the rash, which appears first on the cheeks and ears as very red coalescent macules that are warm and slightly raised. Circumoral pallor is marked, leading to the "slapped cheek" appearance. This eruption fades within 4 days, followed 1 day later by a lacy, reticulated maculopapular erythematous rash that appears on the extensor surfaces of the extremities and spreads, over 2–3 days, to the flexor surfaces and trunk. The rash lasts 3–7 days but may recur over 1–3 weeks in response to environmental changes. Pruritus, headache, and arthralgia are occasional additional symptoms.

B. Laboratory Findings: The white blood cell count is normal.

Complications

Human parvovirus has been implicated in arthritis syndromes, particularly in adults, and is the cause of aplastic crises in patients with chronic hemolytic disorders. Intrauterine parvovirus infection has also been described, occasionally producing fetal hydrops and fetal death.

Treatment

Treatment in uncomplicated cases is not indicated. Patients with hemolytic conditions may require transfusions. Intrauterine transfusion has been suggested for fetal infections.

Prophylaxis

Pregnant women can be advised to avoid exposure to a known outbreak of erythema infectiosum. Should exposure occur, acute serology (IgG and IgM) can be measured; if negative (susceptible), repeat IgG and IgM titers can then be checked in 3 or more weeks to document whether maternal infection has occurred. Pregnant women with known exposure may be followed with serum alpha-fetoprotein levels and frequent ultrasound examinations for the earliest detection of fetal hydrops.

Prognosis

Prognosis of uncomplicated erythema infectiosum and aplastic crises, if adequately supported by transfusion therapy, is excellent. It appears that most intrauterine infections that produce hydrops will result in fetal loss unless transfusion therapy can be implemented.

VARICELLA (Chickenpox) & HERPES ZOSTER (Shingles)

Varicella is an acute, extremely communicable disease caused by the varicella zoster virus. It is spread from person to person by droplets from a respiratory source or by direct contact with freshly infected vesicles. Varicella is communicable from 1 to 2 days before until 6 days after appearance of the rash. The incubation period is 10–21 days (average, 15 days).

With rare exceptions, immunity to varicella after attack is probably lifelong, although the individual with a history of varicella may later develop herpes zoster.

Clinical Findings

A. Symptoms and Signs:

1. Prodrome–The prodrome is usually not apparent; there may be slight malaise and fever for 24 hours.

2. Rash–Usually, the first sign is rash. Lesions tend to appear in crops (2–4 crops in 2–6 days), and all stages and sizes may be present at the same time and in the same vicinity. Lesions occur first on the scalp and mucous surfaces and then on the body. They are numerous over the chest, back, and shoulders; less numerous on the extremities; and seldom seen on the palms and soles. Successive stages include macules, papules, vesicles on erythematous bases, and pustules or scabs.

3. Pruritus–Pruritus is minimal at first but may become severe in the pustular stage.

4. Fever–Fever may occur during the first few days of rash, but constitutional reactions are usually minimal.

5. Herpes zoster–Herpes zoster (shingles) occurs in individuals who have had varicella and is rarely seen in very young children. There may be pain in the area of the rash before the vesicles erupt. Lesions resemble those of varicella but are confined to dermatomal distributions. The most common site is the chest, but lesions may also follow the distribution of the trigeminal nerve root. The vesicles have usually dried and are healing by the fourth or fifth day.

B. Laboratory Findings: Leukopenia occurs early. The white blood count may rise with extensive secondary infection of vesicles.

Complications

There may be secondary infection of vesicles. Encephalitis, nephritis, hepatitis, arthritis, glomerulonephritis, thrombocytopenia, and Reye's syndrome occur rarely. Severe disease with visceral involvement occurs in some immunocompromised individuals and in some normal adults and newborns. Congenital infection, with cicatricial skin lesions and neurologic and eye abnormalities, occasionally result from infection during the first or early second trimester of pregnancy.

Treatment

A. Specific Measures: Antivirals, such as acyclovir, are generally reserved for complicated cases, eg, immunocompromised patients or those with disseminated, visceral involvement.

B. General Measures: Pruritus may be relieved by local application of calamine lotion or mild local anesthetic ointments, or by administration of systemic antihistamines.

C. Treatment of Complications: Treat secondary infection with antibiotics directed toward group A streptococcus and *Staphylococcus aureus*. For general measures of treatment in patients with encephalitis, see Chapter 27.

Prophylaxis

Varicella zoster immune globulin (VZIG) may modify the course of progressive disease or prevent it in susceptible immunodeficient individuals exposed to the virus (see Table 14–1). For maximal benefit, it should be administered within 96 hours of exposure. Protection with VZIG is also recommended for susceptible, exposed pregnant women and other adults, for neonates whose mothers develop chickenpox between 5 days before and 2 days after delivery, and for premature neonates exposed postnatally.

Prognosis

In uncomplicated disease, the prognosis is excellent. Scarring from secondary infection of eruptions is not uncommon. Encephalitis may lead to significant neurologic sequelae in some patients. Severe illness and death may occur in immunodeficient patients or neonates with disseminated disease. Congenital disease may result in long-term extremity, neurologic, or ocular abnormalities. In patients with herpes zoster, pain along the nerve root may persist for several months.

MUMPS
(Epidemic Parotitis)

Mumps is an acute viral disease that commonly affects the salivary glands, chiefly the parotid gland (about 60% of cases), and frequently the central nervous system. It is uncommon before 3 and after 40 years of age. Mumps is spread directly from person to person and by direct contact with contaminated articles. It is communicable from 2 days before the appearance of symptoms to the disappearance of salivary gland swelling. The incubation period is usually 12–24 days (average, 16–18 days).

Clinical Findings
  A. Symptoms and Signs:
  1. Gland involvement–A prodrome of 1 or 2 days may precede the salivary gland involvement and is characterized by fever, malaise, and pain in or behind the ear on chewing or swallowing. Tender swelling and brawning edema of the parotid gland is common (submaxillary and sublingual glands may be involved also or in the absence of parotid gland involvement). Pain is referred to the ear and is aggravated by chewing, swallowing, opening the mouth, and sometimes by ingestion of sour substances. Tenderness persists for 1–3 days and swelling is present for 7–10 days. Skin over the gland is normal. Openings of ducts of the involved gland and especially the papilla of Stensen's duct (opposite the upper second molar) may be puffy and red. Fever may be absent or as high as 40 °C (104 °F). Malaise, anorexia, and headache may be present.
  2. "Inapparent" mumps infection–This infection has a short course, with fever lasting 1–5 days and without apparent salivary gland involvement.

3. Central nervous system involvement–Mumps encephalitis may precede, accompany, or follow inflammation of the salivary glands but may occur without such involvement. Asymptomatic central nervous system inflammation with pleocytosis may be found in over half of cases of mumps. The onset of meningeal irritation is usually sudden. Headache, vomiting, stiff neck and back, and lethargy are characteristic. Fever recurs or increases, up to 41.1 °C (106 °F). Symptoms seldom last more than 5 days. Transient paresis may suggest poliomyelitis.

4. Other organ involvement–Mastitis and thyroiditis may occur. Other organs may be involved, including the following:

a. Testicles and ovaries–Involvement is usually during or after adolescence, but orchitis can occur in childhood. This may occur in the absence of distinctive salivary gland involvement.

b. Pancreas–There is a sudden onset of pain in the mid or upper abdomen, with vomiting, prostration, and usually, fever.

c. Kidney–Nephritis is rare and mild, with complete recovery in most cases.

d. Ear–Deafness occasionally occurs and may be permanent.

B. Laboratory Findings: The white blood cell count usually shows leukopenia and relative lymphocytosis. Serologic tests will confirm the diagnosis. Skin testing is unreliable as an indication of immunity in exposed persons.

Complications

Paresis of the facial nerve has been reported. Serious sequelae of central nervous system involvement are rare. Testicular involvement (usually unilateral) may produce atrophy, but sterility is rare.

Treatment

A. Specific Measures: None available.

B. General Measures: Measures include bed rest, isolation of the patient until the salivary swelling is gone, local warm or cold applications to areas of salivary gland swelling, analgesics, mouth wash with fat-free broth or slightly saline solution, and avoidance of highly flavored or acidic foods and drinks.

C. Treatment of Complications:

1. Central nervous system involvement–Treatment is symptomatic for mild encephalitis. Lumbar puncture may be useful in reducing headache.

2. Orchitis–Suspension of the scrotum in a sling or suspensory, application of ice packs, and use of analgesics may be indicated. Infiltration around the spermatic cord at the external inguinal ring with 10–20 mL of 1% procaine solution may produce dramatic relief.

3. Pancreatitis and oophoritis–Treatment is symptomatic only.

Prophylaxis

Live mumps virus vaccine is usually given in combination with measles and rubella vaccine at 15 months of age. It may be administered to any preadolescent or adolescent with a negative history for vaccine (see Chapter 9). There is no effective passive protection for mumps exposure.

Prognosis

The prognosis is excellent even with extensive organ system involvement. Sterility very rarely results from orchitis in the postadolescent male.

ENTEROVIRUS INFECTION
(Coxsackieviruses, Echoviruses, & Other Nonpolio Enteroviruses)

Enterovirus is responsible for a large variety of illnesses, chiefly occurring during epidemics in the summer and fall months. They are spread by the enteric–oral route and perhaps by the respiratory route; incubation periods are usually 3–6 days.

Clinical Findings

A. "Summer Grippe": An acute, brief febrile illness lasting 1–4 days without other signs or symptoms.

B. Exanthematous Disease: A febrile illness associated with a macular or maculopapular or petechial rash on the face, trunk, and extremities. The illness may be accompanied by pharyngitis or gastrointestinal symptoms. Frequently caused by echovirus strains.

C. Herpangina: A febrile illness lasting 1–4 days associated with pharyngitis, including hyperemia of the anterior tonsillar pillars and vesicles in the posterior oropharynx. Usually associated with Coxsackie A viruses.

D. Hand–Foot–Mouth Syndrome: Also caused by Coxsackie A viruses; a papulovesicular eruption is present on the oropharynx, hand or foot, and, often, on the buttocks.

E. Aseptic Meningitis: Caused by both Coxsackie viruses and echoviruses, this self-limited febrile illness is accompanied by headache, nausea, vomiting, meningismus, and, sometimes, rash. Spinal fluid generally shows a pleocytosis, usually less than

500/mL, and usually mononuclear cells, although this finding is variable. Paralytic disease occasionally occurs with some viral strains.

F. Pleurodynia (Bornholm Disease): Fever is accompanied by dyspnea and pleuritic chest pain, and, often, abdominal pain. Usually pleurodynia is caused by Coxsackie B viruses, and tends to occur in older children and adults.

G. Myocarditis and Pericarditis: Enteroviruses, especially Coxsackie B viruses, are a major cause of viral myocarditis. They may occasionally lead to sudden cardiac death or chronic heart failure.

H. Neonatal Infection: Infected neonates may have variable combinations of sepsis, meningoencephalitis, myocarditis (especially Coxsackie B viruses), hepatitis (especially echoviruses), and pneumonia. Epidemics in newborn nurseries have been reported.

I. Conjunctivitis: Specific serotypes have been implicated in acute (epidemic) hemorrhagic conjunctivitis.

J. Upper Respiratory Tract Infection

K. Gastroenteritis: Particularly seen in young infants.

Treatment
No specific therapies are available. Immune globulin may be beneficial for infections in immunodeficient hosts and, perhaps, in some neonatal infections.

Prophylaxis
Good hand washing can minimize spread of infection.

Prognosis
Prognosis is generally excellent. Paresis, when present, is usually transient. Myocarditis occasionally will lead to chronic heart failure or death. Severe neonatal disease has a high mortality.

VIRAL HEPATITIS

Viral hepatitis is an acute contagious disease often occurring in epidemics, always involving inflammation of the liver, and often accompanied by jaundice. Several viral etiologies are presently recognized, with distinct morphologic and antigenic characteristics.

Hepatitis A virus is transmitted by the fecal–oral route and by contaminated food or water. Daycare centers have been identified as an important source of hepatitis A virus spread. The incubation period is 15–50 days (average, 25–30 days).

Hepatitis B virus is transmitted via blood, mucous membrane secretions, and open wounds. Transmission may occur either from acutely infected patients or from chronically infected carriers. Perinatal transmission can occur prior to or, more commonly, at the time of birth, from a mother who is hepatitis B surface antigen (HBsAg) positive (especially if she is also hepatitis B e antigen positive). The incubation period of hepatitis B is 50–180 days (average, 120 days).

Hepatitis delta virus is a helper virus that, only in the presence of coinfection with hepatitis B virus, leads to accelerated acute or chronic hepatitis. It is transmitted via the same routes as hepatitis B virus, although perinatal transmission is unusual. The incubation period is approximately 28–56 days.

Non-A, non-B hepatitis is thought to include at least 2 agents, one transmitted by blood products and the other by the fecal–oral route, either directly from a shedding person or from contaminated water. Chronic carriage appears to occur with the bloodborne variety. Incubation periods have been estimated at 14–18 days. Hepatitis C virus has recently been identified as one of the etiologic agents of non-A, non-B hepatitis.

Clinical Findings

A. Symptoms and Signs:

1. Hepatitis A–This is most often asymptomatic or mild and nonspecific in infants and young children. It may produce acute clinical hepatitis with fever, jaundice, anorexia, nausea and vomiting, abdominal pain, and hepatomegaly; generally resolves within 2–4 weeks. Fulminant hepatitis rarely occurs.

2. Hepatitis B–This may also produce asymptomatic or mild anicteric illness in children. Hepatitis tends to be subacute; fever, jaundice, anorexia, nausea, malaise, and tender liver enlargement may be accompanied by rash or arthralgias/arthritis. Fulminant hepatitis, chronic hepatitis, or chronic asymptomatic viral carriage may occur.

3. Hepatitis delta–Can accelerate acute or chronic disease in patients with hepatitis B infection.

4. Non-A, non-B hepatitis–Tends to be mild and insidious; fulminant and/or chronic hepatitis may occur.

B. Laboratory Findings: Elevations in hepatic transaminases associated with elevated bilirubin levels are frequent. Specific serologic markers are available to diagnose infections by hepatitis A, hepatitis B, and hepatitis delta viruses.

Complications

Complications of acute severe hepatitis include hemorrhage, encephalopathy, ascites, renal failure, and hepatic necrosis. Chronic and/or recurring hepatitis, which may proceed to cirrhosis, can occur after acute infection with hepatitis B, delta, or non-A, non-B virus. Infection with hepatitis B virus, especially perinatal infection, may lead to chronic viral carriage, which is associated with an increased risk of cirrhosis and hepatocellular carcinoma.

Treatment

A. Specific Measures: None available. The use of antivirals such as interferon for complicated cases is under investigation.

B. General Measures: Rest as dictated by degree of illness and attention to dietary needs (including vitamins).

Prophylaxis

Standard immune globulin can prevent overt disease from hepatitis A infection but may not prevent infection. A dose of 0.02 mL/kg given within 2 weeks of exposure is recommended for household and daycare contacts. Travelers to endemic regions should receive 0.02 mL/kg for stays up to 3 months; 0.06 mL/kg every 5 months is recommended for longer stays.

Hepatitis B immune globulin (HBIG) is effective in preventing hepatitis B infection in exposed susceptible individuals, eg, those who have had contact with the blood of an infected person via a needle prick or a splash onto a mucosal surface. HBIG is given in a dose of 0.06 mL/kg as soon as possible after exposure (but within 7 days); the hepatitis B vaccine series should also be initiated. Perinatal exposure requires administration of 0.5 mL of HBIG as soon after birth as possible, preferably in the delivery room but within 48 hours, and initiation of hepatitis B vaccine (see below).

Inactivated hepatitis B vaccine, either plasma-derived or recombinant, is effective in the prevention of hepatitis B. The vaccine regimen consists of 3 doses administered intramuscularly; 0.5 mL per dose in persons under 10 years of age or 1.0 mL per dose in those 10 years or older (dose is doubled for immunosuppressed or dialysis patients). The first dose is followed in 1 month by the second and in 6 months by the third. In addition to use following blood exposure and to perinatal use, vaccination (and HBIG) is recommended for some household and sexual contacts of persons with hepatitis B and for other high-risk groups. Following the neonatal vaccine series, serum anti-HBs antibody and hepatitis B surface antigen should be measured at 9 months of age. If the antibody titer and surface antigen are negative, give another 0.5 mL dose of vaccine and retest antibody 1 month later; if surface antigen is positive, perform follow-up testing to determine whether chronic carriage has occurred.

Prognosis

Hepatitis A is usually a self-limited disease. In the absence of acute hepatic failure, the prognosis is good. Severe acute hepatitis or chronic progressive or recurrent liver disease may result from hepatitis B and hepatitis non-A, non-B infections and may lead to cirrhosis.

HERPES SIMPLEX INFECTIONS

Herpes simplex virus typically produces a subclinical or clinical primary infection, followed by latent persistence of the virus in a sensory ganglion. Recurrences are triggered by fever, trauma, stress, etc. Herpes simplex virus type 1 (HSV-1) occurs principally around the mouth and produces lesions on the face and upper part of the body; it is transmitted commonly by saliva or respiratory droplets. Herpes simplex virus type 2 (HSV-2) occurs principally on the genitals and the lower parts of the body and is often a sexually transmitted disease. It is the virus type more commonly implicated in neonatal herpes infection. The incubation period of genital HSV-2 infection is approximately 2–14 days.

Clinical Findings

A. Symptoms and Signs:

1. Acute herpetic gingivostomatitis–This is a typical primary infection of young children, with extensive vesicles and ulcers on the gums, palate, and buccal mucous membranes; pain, bleeding, and fever are common. It is self-limited and heals in 1–2 weeks. Primary oral infection is often subclinical.

2. Recurrent "cold sores"–These are most common at the mucocutaneous junctions of the lips or nose. They recur at the same site in a given person, with the virus latent in the trigeminal ganglion between recurrences. Individual vesicles develop 36–60 hours after a "trigger" (eg, sunburn), persist for 2–4 days, and then rupture, leaving an ulcer that crusts and heals without scarring.

3. Whitlow–This is a vesicular paronychia caused by primary or secondary infection of a finger with HSV.

4. Genital herpes–This is seen as vesicles and ulceration on the genitalia, with much surrounding inflammation. Recurrent lesions occur at the same site (penis, vulva, cervix), liberating virus and serving as a source of infection for sexual contact.

Primary episodes may be severe, while recurrent lesions may be associated with minimal inflammation and symptoms.

5. Keratoconjunctivitis–This may be a primary or recurrent infection, usually with HSV-1. Recurrent lesions often take the form of dendritic lesions or ulcers of the corneal epithelium. Sometimes the corneal stroma may be involved, leading to opacity and impairment of vision or to blindness.

6. Eczema herpeticum–Vesicular lesions concentrate in areas of eczematous dermatitis. Unless the child is immunodeficient, these widespread lesions usually heal.

7. Encephalitis–This may be a primary or a recurrent infection; it begins with headache, fever, impairment of the sensorium, seizures, or signs pointing to a lesion of the temporal lobe (aphasia, behavorial disorders, psychomotor convulsions). This necrotizing encephalitis is often fatal in untreated patients. Brain biopsy permits virus isolation, but cerebrospinal fluid findings are often negative. HSV-1 may also be responsible for 2–5% of cases of viral aseptic meningitis, with an almost universally favorable outcome.

8. Neonatal herpes–This is a primary infection transmitted from asymptomatically shed virus or lesions on the mother's genitalia to the child during or shortly before birth. Manifestations include cutaneous and oral vesicles; keratoconjunctivitis and chorioretinitis; meningoencephalitis; and/or multisystem disease affecting the liver, lungs, and other organs; disease usually occurs in the first month of life.

9. Infection in immunocompromised hosts–Herpes simplex may produce disseminated mucocutaneous and/or visceral disease. Pneumonia, hepatitis, or encephalitis may occur.

B. Laboratory Findings: Scrapings from ulcerations on the base of vesicles show multinucleated giant cells in Giemsa-stained smears. Swabs or aspirates from early lesions (first to fourth days) inoculated into cell cultures permit growth of the virus in 1–3 days.

Treatment

Several drugs can inhibit the herpes simplex virus replication. Idoxuridine, vidarabine, and trifluridine ophthalmic preparations, applied topically for herpetic keratitis, and local debridement will greatly accelerate corneal healing but will not affect the rate of recurrence.

Intravenous acyclovir is indicated for the treatment of neonatal HSV infection, HSV disease in immunocompromised hosts, HSV encephalitis, severe eczema herpeticum, and severe primary genital herpes infection.

Oral acyclovir may be used for treatment or prophylaxis of genital herpes and for treatment or prophylaxis of HSV infections in immunocompromised patients.

Prophylaxis

Susceptible individuals should avoid contact with open lesions. Transmission of genital herpes may be mimimized by the use of condoms. Cesarean section may prevent some neonatal infections when active genital lesions are present in the mother at the time of delivery. Cultures obtained from at-risk mothers and babies at the time of delivery may be useful in guiding management.

Prognosis

In most cases of mucocutaneous disease, the prognosis is excellent. In patients with central nervous system involvement and in newborns or other compromised hosts with systemic disease, the prognosis is poor.

INFECTIOUS MONONUCLEOSIS

Infectious mononucleosis is the prototype disease caused by Epstein-Barr (EB) virus, although EB virus produces a range of illnesses, from asymptomatic infection to severe, progressive disease. Infectious mononucleosis may occur at any age up to 30 years; it is rare in infancy and most common in the later years of childhood and early adult years. The incubation period ranges from approximately 30 to 50 days.

Clinical Findings

A. Symptoms and Signs: There is usually a gradual onset of malaise and fever to 38.9 °C (102 °F). A sore throat becomes apparent and sometimes becomes severe, with swelling of the neck and a membrane on the tonsils and pharynx. There is generalized lymphadenopathy, especially of the cervical nodes. The liver and spleen are characteristically enlarged, usually after the first week of symptoms. A morbilliform, scarlatiniform, or petechial rash may appear.

B. Laboratory Findings: A leukocytosis develops very early, with a predominant lymphocytosis, including large immature vacuolated lymphocytes. A rising titer of heterophil agglutinins usually appears in the serum by the second week; a slide agglutination test demonstrates the same antibody and can be used for diagnostic purposes. In uncertain cases, an EB virus serology panel can determine the timing of EB virus infection.

Complications

A secondary infection in the throat with group A streptococcus is the most common complication. Myocarditis, encephalitis, thrombocytopenia, hemolytic anemia, and agranulocytosis have been reported. Rupture of the spleen may occur from trauma to the abdomen. The role of EB virus in the chronic fatigue syndrome is being investigated.

Treatment

A. Specific Measures: None available.

B. General Measures: Pharyngitis complicated by group A streptococci should be treated with penicillin (see Chapter 15). Steroids may be useful for severe tonsillar swelling that threatens the airway. Contact sports and trauma should be avoided during the acute illness and convalescence.

Prognosis

The disease usually runs its course in 10–20 days. The prognosis is excellent in most cases. Rupture of the spleen is a serious complication requiring surgical intervention.

CYTOMEGALOVIRUS DISEASE

Cytomegalovirus disease is the cause of severe congenital infection as well as generally milder acquired infections. Routes of viral acquisition include transplacental, from cervical secretions during birth, from breast milk, via contact with saliva or urine, and by blood transfusion or tissue transplantation. While most infections are asymptomatic, certain clinical entities may result.

Clinical Findings

A. Symptoms and Signs:

1. Congenital cytomegalic inclusion disease–A minority of congenitally infected infants show evidence of this severe illness. In such babies there is onset of jaundice shortly after birth, with hepatosplenomegaly, purpura, and signs of encephalitis. Laboratory findings include thrombocytopenia, erythroblastosis, bilirubinemia, and marked lymphocytosis. Sequelae include intracranial calcifications, microcephaly, mental retardation, and chorioretinitis. The prognosis is poor. Fortunately, the majority of congenital infections cause only mild symptoms (hearing loss, mild developmental delay) or are asymptomatic.

2. Acute acquired disease–This resembles the syndrome of infectious mononucleosis (see above). There is a sudden onset of fever, malaise, joint pain, and myalgia. Pharyngitis is minimal, and respiratory symptoms are absent. Lymphadenopathy is generalized. The liver shows enlargement and often slight tenderness. Laboratory findings include the hematologic picture of momonucleosis as well as bilirubinemia. Heterophil antibody does not appear.

3. Generalized systemic disease–This occurs in immunosuppressed individuals, especially following organ transplant procedures, and in patients with acquired immunodeficiency syndrome (AIDS). Manifestations include pneumonitis, hepatitis, chorioretinitis, and leukopenia, often with a lymphocytosis. Generalized disease is occasionally fatal. Transplant patients without serologic evidence of previous infection are at especially high risk of serious disease.

B. Laboratory Findings: Infection may be diagnosed by virus culture of urine, saliva, leukocytes, or other secretions and tissues. Serologic tests are also available.

Treatment

Ganciclovir is a newly available drug that is being evaluated for the treatment of CMV-associated disease.

Prophylaxis

Good hand washing is the most effective way of preventing infection. Attempts should be made to avoid CMV-contaminated transfusions to high-risk groups (eg, premature newborns or immunosuppressed patients) by freezing blood in glycerol or by using blood from seronegative donors.

Prognosis

Ninety percent of survivors of the congenital cytomegalic inclusion disease are neurologically impaired, with microcephaly, mental retardation, and hearing loss. Acquired infection may be severe in immunocompromised hosts.

INFLUENZA

Influenza is an acute systemic viral disease that usually occurs in epidemics. It is caused by a distinct class of virus divided into 3 main serotypes (A, B, and C) based on the ribonucleoproteins. Further classification of each type is based on the surface proteins hemagglutinin and neuraminidase.

Clinical Findings

The onset is abrupt, with sudden fever to 39.4–40 °C (103–104 °F), extreme malaise, myalgia, headache, a dry, nonproductive cough, and nasal congestion. Small infants may exhibit only fever, cough, and marked irritability. Physical findings are minimal; they may include nasal congestion, pharyngitis, and myositis.

Complications

Primary complications are rare but may include pneumonia, croup, myocarditis, and toxic encephalopathy. Secondary complications due to bacterial agents include pneumonia and otitis media. The bacterial agent most often responsible is *Staphylococcus aureus*. Reye's syndrome is a rare complication of influenza B infection.

Treatment

Amantadine reduces symptoms of influenza A if begun early in the illness. Treatment for 2–5 days is recommended for children with severe disease and in those with underlying conditions that place them at high risk for severe infection.

Acetaminophen should be used for antipyresis; salicylates are to be avoided for fear of Reye's syndrome.

Prophylaxis

Immunization against influenza is recommended for high-risk children (and their close contacts), including those with chronic cardiopulmonary disease, immunocompromised patients, children with hemoglobinopathies, those with chronic metabolic or renal diseases, and children on chronic aspirin therapy.

Chemoprophylaxis with amantadine (against influenza A) is an alternative during an identified community outbreak. Rimantadine is a related drug that is being evaluated for prophylaxis (and treatment) against influenza A.

Prognosis

The prognosis of influenza is good in normal hosts. The course of illness may be severe in those with underlying diseases, especially those with preexistent cardiopulmonary disease and in those who develop primary complications such as myocarditis or secondary bacterial superinfections, eg, pneumonia.

KAWASAKI DISEASE
(Mucocutaneous Lymph Node Syndrome)

Kawasaki disease is a vasculitic illness of unknown etiology. It occurs primarily in children under 8 years of age.

Clinical Findings

A. Symptoms and Signs: The onset is abrupt, with fever as high as 40 °C (104 °F) and a diffuse rash over the body. The lips are very red, and the tongue has a bright "strawberry" appearance. The conjunctivae and the palms and soles are red and swollen. The lymph nodes in the neck are often enlarged. Fever usually subsides in 1–3 weeks, and there is a characteristic peeling of the skin, beginning around the fingertips and toenails. Associated symptoms or findings may include carditis, arthralgia, pyuria, gallbladder hydrops, and aseptic meningitis.

B. Laboratory Findings: Leukocytosis and elevated sedimentation rate are common, and the platelet count generally rises as the illness progresses.

Echocardiographic and electrocardiographic evaluations are critical both at the time of diagnosis and during follow-up.

Complications

Complications include carditis; arthritis; dilatation or aneurysms of coronary arteries; and aneurysms in other large arteries.

Treatment

Intravenous gamma globulin reduces the acute inflammatory signs of Kawasaki disease and also appears to reduce the frequency of coronary artery dilatation and aneurysm. Aspirin is generally used at high, anti-inflammatory doses during the acute phase of illness, followed by low-dose antiplatelet doses during the subacute and convalescent phases.

Prognosis

Patients with coronary artery involvement are at risk of coronary thrombosis, myocardial infarction, and/or sudden death. Mild coronary vessel dilatation often regresses over weeks or months.

ACQUIRED IMMUNODEFICIENCY SYNDROME (AIDS)

AIDS is caused by human immunodeficiency virus (HIV), a human retrovirus that infects the helper-inducer subset of T cells as well as other cells and tissues.

Adults and older children at risk include intravenous drug abusers, recipients of infected blood or blood products, and individuals with infected sex partners (homosexual or heterosexual). New pediatric infections with HIV most commonly (> 80%) occur in offspring of parents infected with HIV, whether or not either of the parents is symptomatic. Thirty-fifty percent of infants of HIV antibody–positive mothers will be infected.

Clinical Findings

A. Symptoms and Signs: Common findings in pediatric AIDS include failure to thrive, lymphadenopathy, hepatosplenomegaly, persistent thrush, recurrent bacterial infections, and lymphoid interstitial pneumonitis. Opportunistic infections occur, including *Pneumocystis carinii* pneumonia, cryptosporidiosis, and *Mycobacterium avium-intracellulare* infection. Developmental delay and encephalopathy are frequent.

B. Laboratory Findings: Frequent features include hypergammaglobulinemia, thrombocytopenia, lymphopenia, and decreased T4 (helper) lymphocytes. Diagnosis is generally made via serum ELISA and Western blot assays for antibody; other modalities include viral culture, antigen detection, and nucleic acid detection. Diagnosis is difficult in the first 15 months of life because of the presence of passively acquired maternal antibodies.

Complications

Although the full spectrum of HIV infection is not yet known, most cases of AIDS appear to be progressive, with a high fatality rate. Opportunistic infections, failure to thrive, malignancies, and encephalopathy are frequent.

Treatment

Azidothymidine (zidovudine) is an antiviral agent that has in vitro activity against HIV and has had some effectiveness in treating symptomatic adults. Trials studying the utility of this medication in infected children are underway. Intravenous immune globulin may benefit patients with recurrent bacterial infections; study of this therapeutic modality is continuing. Finally, treatment of typical bacterial and opportunistic infections is important in the total care of AIDS patients.

Prognosis

Children infected with HIV have displayed a spectrum of prognoses ranging from rapid death to survival for several years from the time of diagnosis. While most HIV infections are presumed to eventually produce progressive, symptomatic illness, the potential for prolonged asymptomatic infection and/or prolonged survival is still to be determined.

POLIOMYELITIS

Poliomyelitis is an acute viral infection of the spinal cord and brainstem. In its severe form, it leads to neuron destruction and irreversible muscular paralysis and, in 10% of the paralytic forms, to death. In countries where immunization is widely used, this disease is very rare.

The disease is caused by poliovirus serotypes 1, 2, and 3, which are enteroviruses. They are transmitted by the fecal–oral route and possibly by the respiratory route.

Clinical Findings

A. Symptoms and Signs: Poliovirus infection may be asymptomatic or produce a nonspecific febrile illness (abortive poliomyelitis). Other forms of infection include:

1. Nonparalytic poliomyelitis–Symptoms and signs are those of a febrile aseptic meningitis. Diagnosis can rarely be established except by inference in epidemics.

2. Paralytic poliomyelitis (spinal type)–Paralysis may occur without obvious antecedent illness, especially in infants. Paralysis usually begins and progresses during the febrile stage of the illness. Tremor upon sustained effort may be the first clue to diagnosis and may be present before weakness occurs. Muscle tightness and pain on stretching may cause malfunction and simulate paralysis. The cerebrospinal fluid white cell count may be normal in 10–15% of cases.

3. Bulbar polioencephalitis–This is paralytic poliomyelitis that includes involvement of the cranial nerves and brainstem. Significant lower spinal involvement may be absent. Any cranial nerve may be affected, but swallowing difficulties predominate. This form of poliomyelitis is more likely to occur in patients whose tonsils have been removed. Polioencephalitis is the term applied when there is impairment of cerebral function. It follows a fulminant course.

4. Respiratory difficulty in poliomyelitis–Respiratory difficulty may occur with paralysis of intercostal muscles, manifested by anxiety, increased respiratory rate, and reluctance to vocalize. The upper arm and shoulder muscles are often involved. Paralyses of the diaphragm, which are easily overlooked, are usually associated with intercostal paralysis. Weakness of the intercostal muscles and diaphragm is demonstrated by diminished chest expansion and decreased vital capacity. Damage to the medullary respiratory center may also occur, sometimes with severe symptoms of irregular, shallow, spasmodic breathing. Obstruction of the pharynx or trachea, due to aspiration of saliva secondary to pharyngeal or palatal paralysis (or both), may occur.

B. Laboratory Findings: Poliovirus can be grown from stool and throat specimens; it is rarely recovered from the cerebrospinal fluid. Serology can demonstrate seroconversion.

Treatment

A. Specific Measures: None available.

B. General Measures: Many patients with mild forms of poliomyelitis can be cared for at home. The need for isolation in special hospitals is questionable, since in epidemic conditions the virus is universally distributed. Special facilities and trained professional personnel are required for the more severely ill patient.

Bed rest is indicated, with careful observation for further paralysis during the first week of disease. Hot packs, hot soaks, bed boards, foot boards, and splints may be used. Physiotherapy is the most important single factor in recovery. During the acute stage passive motion is begun, to the point of pain only. All extremities must be exercised to prevent joint immobilization. Active motion is begun when pain subsides. Uncoordinated or unnatural function must be avoided as long as possible. Resistance-type exercises should be postponed until all tightness has subsided. Braces and surgery are indicated only after physiotherapy has been attempted.

C. Treatment of Respiratory Difficulties: Intercostal or diaphragm paralysis requires artificial ventilation before cyanosis appears. A tank respirator, operated by experienced personnel, may be used. The chest respirator (cuirass) is about 60% as efficient as the tank. It is useful in rehabilitation and simplifies the problem of nursing care. A positive-pressure ventilator may also be considered. Tracheostomy may be required in patients with paralysis of muscles of swallowing, weakness of muscles of respiration, or bulbar poliomyelitis.

Prophylaxis

The paralytic consequences of infection with poliomyelitis virus can be avoided by prophylactic use of oral vaccine (see Chapter 9). The vaccine should be administered to infants and children according to the routine schedule.

The oral, live attenuated vaccine has a very small risk of

causing paralytic poliomyelitis; this risk is increased in immuno-compromised hosts. Therefore, inactivated, intramuscular vaccine should be used for people with immune deficiency and for people who are in close contact with immunocompromised hosts. The inactivated vaccine is also the preferred vaccine for adults, as they have a slightly higher risk of developing vaccine-associated paralytic poliomyelitis than do children. Adults who are at increased risk for exposure to poliovirus, eg, those traveling to or residing in areas with endemic or epidemic disease, are candidates for immunization.

Prognosis

The prognosis with paralytic polio is guarded, although muscle function may improve within the first 2 years after infection. In the bulbar form, prognosis is good if complications are overcome. Patients with polioencephalitis usually have a poor prognosis for survival. If the respiratory center is severely involved, the prognosis is poor.

RESPIRATORY SYNCYTIAL VIRUS

Respiratory syncytial virus (RSV) is the most frequent cause of viral lower respiratory tract infection in infants. The incubation period ranges between 2 and 8 days. Annual epidemics in winter and early spring typically occur in temperate climates.

Clinical Findings

A. Symptoms and Signs: RSV typically causes bronchiolitis or pneumonia. Symptoms include fever, anorexia, lethargy, tachypnea, cough, and respiratory distress. Patients may have nasal flaring, retractions, rales, rhonchi, or wheezes. Apnea may be a presenting manifestation.

B. Laboratory Findings: Chest radiographs may show hyperexpansion, atelectasis, and/or scattered infiltrates. Blood gas or oximetry may reveal hypoxemia. Diagnosis can be made by viral isolation from nasopharyngeal secretions or rapid antigen detection (ELISA, immunofluorescence).

Complications

RSV infections in small infants may produce severe apnea and/or progressive pulmonary infection. Children at particular risk include premature babies, infants with congenital heart disease or chronic pulmonary disease (including bronchopulmonary dysplasia), and patients who are immunodeficient.

Treatment

Most infants require only supportive care. Oxygen is used for hypoxemia; mechanical ventilation may be required for significant apnea or pulmonary involvement. Ribavirin is an antiviral that may be delivered via aerosol to infants with RSV disease; it is generally reserved for those with severe disease or for those in high-risk groups.

Prognosis

The prognosis varies with the degree of illness and the presence of underlying risk factors. The majority of patients recover fully, although some may exhibit reactive airway disease in the future.

ROTAVIRUS

Rotaviruses are RNA viruses whose major clinical association is diarrheal illness. They are the most frequent cause of gastroenteritis worldwide.

Clinical Findings

A. Symptoms and Signs: Vomiting, watery diarrhea, and mild fever are frequent. Cough and rhinorrhea may also be present. Severe infection, particularly in infants, may induce dehydration and acidosis.

B. Laboratory Findings: Serum electrolytes may reflect dehydration and/or acidosis. Diagnosis may be made by detection of viral antigens in stool via ELISA or latex agglutination, or by visualization of virus in stool with electron microscopy.

Treatment

A. Specific Measures: None available.

B. General Measures: Fluid therapy, oral or parenteral, is essential to prevent and treat dehydration.

Prophylaxis

Hand washing and good hygiene are the major preventive measures. Live attenuated oral vaccines are being developed.

Prognosis

Prognosis is good if hydration is maintained. Some patients with severe diarrhea may malabsorb for a period after the acute enteritis subsides. Deaths are usually due to severe dehydration and/or electrolyte imbalance.

Table 14-2. Rickettsial diseases.

Disease	Agent	Natural Host	Vector	Geographic Prevalence
Epidemic typhus	*Rickettsia prowazekii*	Man	Body louse	Asia, Africa, Europe, Central & S. America
Endemic typhus	*R. typhi*	Rat	Rat flea	Worldwide, including Southeast US
Rocky Mtn. spotted fever	*R. rickettsii*	Tick, small animals, dogs	Tick	Americas, including southern & eastern US & upper Rocky Mtn. states
Q Fever	*Coxiella burnetii*	Farm & wild animals (including sheep, goats, cows)	—	Australia, Africa, Canada, Europe, Western US
Rickettsial pox	*R. akari*	House mouse	Mouse mite	US, Asia, Africa

Clinical Findings	Complications	Treatment	Prophylaxis
Nausea, vomiting fever, headache, maculopapular-hemorrhagic rash	Encephalopathy, myocarditis, renal failure, bacterial pneumonia	Tetracycline; chloramphenicol; pediculocides	Epidemic typhus vaccine (not available in US); delousing
Fever, headache, myalgia, macular rash	Unusual	Tetracycline, chloramphenicol	Insecticides; rat control
Fever, maculopapular-hemorrhagic rash, headache, myalgia, nausea, vomiting, conjunctivitis	Shock, disseminated intravascular coagulation, multisystem failure	Chloramphenicol; tetracycline; supportive care	Minimize tick exposure
Fever, malaise, headache, cough, weakness, hepatosplenomegaly	Pneumonia, endocarditis, hepatitis	Tetracycline; chloramphenicol	Reduce animal exposure, pasteurize milk
Papulovesicular rash, fever, headache, myalgia, photophobia. Eschar & lymphadenopathy at site of mite bite	Rare	Tetracycline, chloramphenicol	Insecticides & rodent control

RICKETTSIAL DISEASES

The rickettsiae are very small intracellular organisms that irregularly stain gram negative. They are divided immunologically into distinct groups and subgroups. While most groups stimulate the production in humans of agglutinins against strains of *Proteus vulgaris*, the determination of complement-fixing antibodies is a more accurate and acceptable serologic testing method (Table 14–2).

Infectious Diseases: Bacterial & Spirochetal | 15

Mark J. Abzug, MD

BACTERIAL DISEASES

STREPTOCOCCAL DISEASES

A variety of disease states directly or indirectly ascribed to streptococci are very important in the pediatric age groups. These are spread from person to person by droplets but may occasionally be transmitted by contact with soiled articles.

Etiology

Steptococci are gram-positive and characteristically appear in chains. They may be classified as follows:

A. β-Hemolytic Streptocci: These exhibit beta hemolysis on blood agar culture and are divided into a number of groups, of which A, B, and D are the principal pathogens. Group A infections most commonly occur in children and adults, and group B may cause severe disease in infants.

B. Non–β-Hemolytic Streptococci: These commonly exhibit alpha hemolysis or no hemolysis on blood agar culture. Viridans streptotocci and some group D streptococci are included in this category.

C. Peptostreptococci: These produce variable hemolysis, are found in the intestinal tract, and are sometimes pathogenic.

Clinical Findings

A. Symptoms and Signs: Streptococci produce a great variety of clinical diseases. Certain entities show a definite concentration in certain age groups.

1. Infection in neonates–Neonatal infections are principally caused by group B streptococci, especially type III. There are 2 clinical syndromes—early onset and late onset. In the early onset syndrome (at less than 5 days of age), infection is acquired from the maternal vagina. Symptoms of early onset disease include apnea, shock, pneumonia, and meningitis. There is a very high mortality rate. In the late-onset syndrome (between 2 weeks and 4 months), which may result from person-to-person transmission, meningitis, cellulitis, and osteomyelitis are common manifestations.

2. Infection in young children (< 3 years old)–In the early childhood type (group A) infection, the onset is insidious, with mild constitutional symptoms, mucopurulent nasal discharge, and suppurative complications (otitis media, lymphadenitis). Exudative tonsillitis is uncommon, and sore throat is apparently absent. Rheumatic fever, nephritis, and scarlet fever rarely occur in association with this form of the disease.

3. Infection in older children–In the middle childhood type (group A) infection, the onset is usually sudden, with temperature over 39°C (102.2°F). The throat is moderately sore and beefy red, with edema of anterior pillars and palatal petechiae. Exudative tonsillitis, with a white-yellow membrane, is relatively frequent. Anterior cervical lymph nodes are large and tender. Scarlet fever, which occurs in association with this form of disease, consists of streptococcal pharyngitis plus a rash due to host susceptibility to erythrogenic toxin. The rash appears 12–48 hours after the onset of fever; it begins in the areas of warmth and pressure, spreads rapidly to involve the entire body below the chin line, and reaches its maximum in 1 or 2 days (see Table 14–1). It is characterized by a diffuse erythema of the skin, with prominence of the bases of the hair follicles. It fades on pressure and does not involve the circumoral region. Transverse lines that do not fade on pressure are found at the elbow (Pastia's sign). The exanthem usually is followed by desquamation beginning in the second week, with peeling of the fingertips. The tongue may be coated but then desquamates and becomes beefy red.

4. Skin infection–In streptococcal disease of the skin (see Impetigo, Chapter 18), streptococci may enter the skin and subcutaneous tissues through abrasions or wounds and may produce impetigo; erysipelas, a superficially spreading infection with edema and erythema; or cellulitis. Wound infection with streptococci may result in "surgical scarlet fever" when the organism produces the erythrogenic toxin in a patient without antitoxin.

B. Laboratory Findings: The white blood cell count is usually elevated (12,000–15,000/μL) in patients with uncomplicated group A streptococcal upper respiratory tract infection; it may go to 20,000/μL or higher in patients with suppurative complications. An anti–group A streptococcal antibody screen (Streptozyme) will generally become positive, and antistreptolysin titers will rise above 150 units in the course of Group A streptococcal infection. A documented rise (or fall) in titer is a more reliable measure of recent streptococcal infection. Throat culture is generally positive for group A streptococci and is the diagnostic method of choice. Rapid agglutination tests for streptococci are now being used more extensively. Positive test results correlate well with culture results. Negative test results should be confirmed by culture, since rapid agglutination may fail to detect small numbers of streptococci.

Neonatal group B streptococcal infection may be identified by positive culture of blood, cerebrospinal fluid, or other involved body site or by positive latex agglutination of urine, serum, or cerebrospinal fluid for group B streptococcal antigen.

Complications
A wide variety of clinical conditions may result from the presence of streptococci in the upper respiratory tract, skin, or blood of the patient.

A. Otitis Media: This is commonly caused by streptococci as a complication of upper respiratory tract infection.

B. Adenitis: Streptococci are a common cause of adenitis (which is usually cervical) in children.

C. Septicemia: Septicemic occurs especially in the debilitated or the very young.

D. Pneumonia: Group A streptococcus is occasionally the cause of pneumonia, which may be severe and is frequently complicated by empyema.

E. "Metastatic Foci": These include meningitis, septic arthritis, osteomyelitis, and omphalitis (neonates).

F. Vaginitis and Perianal Cellulitis: Streptococci may cause vaginitis and perianal cellulitis.

G. Nonsuppurative Complications: These include rheumatic fever (see Chapter 19) and acute glomerulonephritis (see Chapter 24).

Treatment
A. Specific Measures:

1. Group B streptococcal infections–Parenteral penicillin or ampicillin is the therapy of choice. Combination therapy with an aminoglycoside is recommended until clinical stabilization and improvement have been observed. Treatment is ordinarily administered for 10–14 days.

2. Group A streptococcal infections–Oral penicillin V for 10 days or intramuscular benzathine penicillin are recommended for uncomplicated group A streptococcal infections. Alternatives for penicillin-allergic patients include erythromycin, cephalosporins, and clindamycin. Serve infections should be treated with parenteral antibiotics. Prompt therapy for group A streptococcal infections will prevent acute rheumatic fever in the majority of cases.

3. Group A streptococcal carriers–These usually do not require antibiotic therapy unless there is a personal or family history of acute rheumatic fever. However, illnesses accompanied by a positive throat culture require a course of antibiotic treatment.

Prophylaxis

Antibiotic prophylaxis against group A streptococcal infection is indicated for persons with a history of rheumatic fever, in order to prevent recurrent disease.

Prenatal identification and antibiotic treatment of mothers or neonates carrying group B streptococci may be effective in preventing infection of high-risk newborns. A vaccine for pregnant carriers is being investigated.

Prognosis

The prognosis for patients with early childhood and adult types of group A streptococcal infection is excellent with penicillin treatment. Uncomplicated cases of middle childhood–type infection subside in 4–5 days with or without specific treatment, but treatment is recommended for all children to prevent nonsuppurative complications. The prognosis for neonates with group B streptococcal infection varies with the severity of infection. The prognosis for patients with severe sepsis, pneumonia, or meningitis is guarded.

PNEUMOCOCCAL DISEASES

Streptococcus pneumoniae produces a number of disease entities principally in the respiratory tract. The organisms are gram-positive diplococci, and are divided into more than 83 types on the basis of specific capsular polysaccharides. Types 6, 14, 19, and 23 are more likely to cause disease in children than in adults. The disease is spread from person to person by respiratory droplets.

Clinical Findings
A. Symptoms and Signs:
1. Upper respiratory tract infection–This occurs commonly as a consequence of primary viral infections; otitis media and sinusitis are the most frequent manifestations.

2. Bacteremia–*S pneumoniae* is a frequent cause of bacteremia, with fever and leukocytosis occurring in children over 1 month of age. A presumptive diagnosis can be made when a characteristic gingival cystic swelling is found on the posterior buccal surface of the alveolar ridge. However, fever without any localizing signs may be the only presenting finding of "occult" bacteremia.

3. Pneumonia–Pneumonia is usually peribronchial in the child under 6 years of age. Typical lobar pneumonia occurs more commonly in older children.

4. Meningitis–Meningitis occurs usually as a result of pneumococcal bacteremia accompanying upper or lower respiratory tract disease.

5. Peritonitis–Peritonitis may occur, especially in patients with chronic glomerulonephritis and nephrosis.

6. Vaginitis–Vaginitis may occur in preadolescent girls.

B. Laboratory Findings: Leukocytosis is the rule in pneumococcal infection. Blood cultures should always be done when pneumonia, meningitis, or peritonitis is suspected; Gram's stain and culture of material from the site of infection should be obtained where possible. Rapid tests such as latex agglutination or counterimmunoelectrophoresis may also be helpful.

Complications

Localized pneumococcal infection may result from bacteremia or respiratory spread; infected sites may include joints, pericardium, pleural space, and bone.

Treatment

Penicillin is the drug of choice. In cases of penicillin allergy, patients may be treated with oral erythromycin, trimethoprim-sulfamethoxazole, clindamycin, or cephalexin. Severe infections should be treated parenterally; if partial or full penicillin resistance is observed, an alternative antibiotic, such as vancomycin, chloramphenicol, or cefotaxime may be preferable (particularly for meningitis).

Prophylaxis

Polyvalent polysaccharide vaccine is available and contains antigens of 23 different types of pneumococci, which account for more than 90% of strains producing bacteremic disease in adults and children. Experience in children is limited, but the vaccine is ineffective under 2 years of age. It is recommended for children over 2 years old who are in the following high-risk categories: children with functional (sicklemia), congenital, or surgical asplenia; nephrotic syndrome; antibody-deficient states (response is not ensured in this group, but some children may respond); Hodgkin's disease; and human immunodeficiency virus infection. Ordinarily, the vaccine is administered once; some individuals caring for children with sickle cell disease recommend 2 doses (at 2 years and again 3–5 years later). Otherwise, booster doses are not recommended and can cause severe reactions.

Antibiotic prophylaxis is recommended by many to prevent pneumococcal infections in patients with anatomic or functional asplenia (including sickle cell disease). Parents and patients should be advised that vaccine and antibiotics may not prevent acute infections and that they should report for medical care immediately if there is any febrile illness. Physicians seeing such children should treat them with therapeutic doses of penicillin (in the hospital, if necessary) if the illness is thought to be of potentially pneumococcal origin.

STAPHYLOCOCCAL DISEASES

The staphylococci are gram-positive organisms and are divided into several types. *Staphylococcus aureus*, which are coagulase-producing, are the most common pathogens. Coagulase-negative staphylococci, including *S epidermidis*, occasionally also cause invasive disease, particularly in compromised hosts and in patients with foreign bodies.

Staphylococci are common in the environment and are normally found in the nose and on the skin. In newborn infants, the umbilical stump is colonized, and a carrier state may produce endemic disease in the newborn nursery.

Clinical Findings

A. Symptoms and Signs:

1. Staphylococcus aureus–

a. Superficial infection–Pyoderma is the most common type of infection with this organism. Furuncles, folliculitis, carbuncles, and impetigo are discussed in Chapter 18.

b. Deep infection–Osteomyelitis or septic arthritis can occur following bloodstream spread from a local inoculation or a superficial infection. Pneumonia may occur, especially after a viral infection, eg, influenza; it tends to be severe and is usually associated with an empyema. Septicemia, with focal abscesses in the chest, abdomen, and brain, may be present. Enterocolitis in the small infant is often the result of intestinal flora being modified through use of broad-spectrum antibiotics.

c. Toxin disease–Food poisoning (see Table 15–1) may be the result of production of enterotoxin in contaminated foods, usually gravies or custards. The onset is abrupt, with vomiting, prostration, and diarrhea within 4 hours of ingestion. Staphylococcal scalded skin syndrome is an exfoliative skin disease caused by an exotoxin. Toxic shock syndrome, also caused by an exotoxin, may result from staphylococcal infection in surgical wounds, in the vagina during menstruation and with the use of tampons, in localized abscesses, and in fulminant staphylococcal sepsis. The onset is sudden with fever, vomiting, diarrhea, and hypotension, followed by a generalized erythroderma that desquamates.

2. Coagulase-negative staphylococci–

a. Bacteremia–Bacteremia with coagulase-negative staphylococci occurs in compromised patients, including premature infants and immunosuppressed patients. Bacteremia with these organisms frequently occurs as a consequence of indwelling vascular catheters.

b. Other foreign body infections–Coagulase-negative staphylococci are frequently the causative organisms of infections affecting ventriculoperitoneal shunts, peritoneal dialysis catheters, and other indwelling foreign bodies.

c. Urinary tract infections–*S saprophyticus* is a cause of urinary tract infections.

B. Laboratory Findings: Leukocytosis occurs in patients with deep infection. Culture of the blood yields positive results in many cases of deep infection. A Gram's stain and culture of pus from the local infection or a rectal smear in enterocolitis easily demonstrates the organism.

Treatment

Most *S aureus* are resistant to penicillin and require treatment with penicillinase-resistant penicillins, eg, nafcillin or oxacillin. Alternative agents include first-generation cephalosporins, clindamycin, or vancomycin. Vancomycin is the drug of choice for methicillin-resistant *S aureus* (infrequent) and methicillin-resistant coagulase-negative staphylococci (frequent). Deep infections may require several weeks of antibiotic therapy. Abscesses generally need to be drained and foreign bodies may need to be removed.

Prophylaxis

For prophylaxis of recurrent furunculosis, see Chapter 18. Prevent food poisoning by adequate refrigeration and sanitation. Cleanliness and antiseptic measures can control excessive

Table 15–1. Causes, characteristics, and treatment of acute foodborne gastroenteritis (food poisoning).

Cause	Source	Mechanism of Action	Incubation Period	Symptoms	Treatment
Bacillus cereus	Contaminated food.	Emetic and necrotizing toxins are produced.	1–12 h	Abrupt onset of vomiting and cramping; diarrhea follows; symptoms continue for 24 h.	Treatment nonspecific.
Clostridium botulinum	Anaerobic nonacid foods canned or processed at 115°C (239°F).	Absorbed toxin blocks neuromuscular junction.	24–96 h	See Chapter 25.	See Chapter 25.
Clostridium perfringens	Meat preparations.	Enterotoxin causes hypersecretion of fluid in small bowel.	8–18 h	Abrupt onset of profuse diarrhea; occasional vomiting.	Fluid and electrolyte replacement.
Escherichia coli (toxicogenic strains)	Contaminated food.	Organism grows in intestinal tract; toxin causes	24–72 h	Abrupt onset of diarrhea; rare vomiting.	Fluid and electrolyte replacement required in small infants.

	Source	Mechanism	Incubation period	Symptoms	Treatment
		hypersecretion of fluid in small bowel.			Neomycin, 100 mg/kg/d in 3 doses, may be useful. Dietary management.
Staphylococci	Meats, dairy products, gravy, cream preparations.	Enterotoxin produced in food acts on intestinal receptors that transmit to medulla.	1–18 h	Abrupt onset of violent vomiting; vomiting continues for 48 h. Occurs in groups eating same food.	Fluid and electrolyte replacement occasionally indicated.
Vibrio parahaemolyticus	Fish, shellfish, crabs.	Toxin causes hypersecretion of fluid in small bowel.	6–96 h	Abrupt onset of diarrhea; diarrhea continues for 1–3 d and is sometimes bloody. Occurs in groups eating same food.	Treatment nonspecific.

spread from draining lesions. Hand washing by attendants and other personnel is an important control measure.

Prognosis

In the typical case of local infection with adequate local treatment, the prognosis is excellent. In deep infections with sepsis, pneumonia, brain abscess, or other localization, the prognosis is guarded. Patients with osteomyelitis have an excellent prognosis if they are promptly treated by specific and general measures.

HAEMOPHILUS INFLUENZAE B DISEASES

Haemophilus influenzae B is the most important bacterial pathogen found in infants and young children and is the cause of the majority of bacterial meningitis in pediatrics. The organism is an encapsulated gram-negative pleomorphic rod. It generally infects children under the age of 6 years.

Clinical Findings

A. Symptoms and Signs: *H influenzae B* causes a wide spectrum of disease, including meningitis, pneumonia, empyema, bacteremia, epiglottitis, cellulitis (buccal, periorbital, or other), septic arthritis, osteomyelitis, pericarditis, and uvulitis. More than one of these processes may coexist. Patients usually present with fever and irritability and then develop specific localizing findings depending on the site of infection.

B. Laboratory Findings: Leukocytosis with a shift to the left is frequently present. Gram's stain of fluid obtained from the site of infection is frequently positive; latex agglutination or counterimmunoelectrophoresis of such fluid or urine is frequently positive. The organism can be cultured on chocolate agar from the blood or from fluid or swabs obtained from the site of localization.

Treatment

A. Specific Measures: Useful parenteral antibiotics for *H influenzae B* include ampicillin, chloramphenicol, cefotaxime, ceftriaxone, and cefuroxime. Antibiotic susceptibility testing will guide the choice of antibiotic; ampicillin resistance is common (up to 40%) and chloramphenicol resistance is occasional. Parenteral therapy is usually administered initially; oral agents that may be used to complete a course of therapy include amoxicillin, cefaclor, trimethoprim-sulfamethoxazole, amoxicillin-clavulanic acid, erythromycin-sulfisoxazole, cefuroxime axetil, and cefixime.

B. General Measures: Intensive support may be needed for severely ill patients, including those with meningitis, sepsis, pneumonia, pericarditis, and epiglottitis. Patients with epiglottitis require emergent tracheal intubation to assure an adequate airway. Patients with pericarditis, empyema, and arthritis generally benefit from aspiration or drainage of infected fluid.

Prophylaxis

Rifampin (20 mg/kg/d once daily for 4 days; adult dose 600 mg daily) is recommended for children who develop *H influenzae B* disease and for their household contacts. In addition, many experts recommend similar prophylaxis of daycare and nursery school contacts of index patients, particularly if there are attendees under 2 years of age. (Prophylaxis is indicated both for children vaccinated and unvaccinated against *H influenzae B*.) Children exposed to *H influenzae B* who develop a febrile illness should receive medical attention.

Immunization against *H influenzae B* disease is currently recommended for children at 18 months of age with a vaccine that conjugates *H influenzae B* capsular polysaccharide to a protein carrier. Children currently older than 18 months and younger than 60 months should also receive the vaccine. Children who have had invasive *H influenzae B* disease prior to the age of 24 months should be vaccinated with a conjugate vaccine; those with invasive disease after 24 months do not need to be vaccinated. Children older than 60 months of age who are in high-risk groups, eg, those with asplenia, sickle cell disease, or malignancy, should receive a conjugate vaccine.

Prognosis

Patients with mild to moderate disease who receive prompt therapy usually have a good prognosis. Patients with severe infections, including sepsis, pericarditis, meningitis, and epiglottitis, have a more guarded outlook, particularly if there is a delay in therapy.

MENINGOCOCCAL DISEASES

Neisseria meningitidis is a gram-negative diplococcus that is a common pathogen of children as well as adults.

Clinical Findings

A. Symptoms and Signs: Septicemia, or meningococcemia, presents with fever, irritability, lethargy, and, often, a maculopapular or petechial rash. In severe cases, hypotension, disseminated intravascular coagulation, and coma may occur (Waterhouse-Friderichsen syndrome). Meningococcal meningitis may also occur, with or without the signs of meningococcemia. Other meninococcal infections include bacteremia, pericarditis, arthritis, and pneumonia, alone or in combination. Chronic meningococcemia is a form of bacteremia that persists for less than 1 week and is associated with fever, rash, and arthralgias.

B. Laboratory Findings: Leukocytosis with a leftward shift is common; thrombocytopenia is present in severe meningococcemia.

The diagnosis may be made by Gram's stain identification in a culture of blood, cerebrospinal fluid, joint fluid, or petechiae. Latex agglutination or counterimmunoelectrophoresis of urine, serum, or cerebrospinal fluid may be positive, although sensitivity is lacking.

Treatment

A. Specifc Measures: The antibiotic of choice is penicillin G or ampicillin. Alternatives include chloramphenicol, cefotaxime, ceftriaxone, and cefuroxime.

B. General Measures: Intensive supportive care may be required for patients with meningococcemia or meningitis, particularly if shock and coagulopathy are present.

Prophylaxis

Prophylaxis is recommended for contacts of a patient with meningococcal disease, eg, household, daycare, and nursery contacts as well as any other people who have had contact with oral secretions of the index patient. Medical personnel involved with resuscitation or airway care should receive prophylaxis. The drug of choice for prophylaxis is rifampin (10 mg/kg every 12 hours for 2 days; adult dose 600 mg every 12 hours); sulfisoxazole is an alternative. Contacts who develop a febrile illness should receive medical attention.

Meningococcal vaccine is a quadrivalent polysaccharide vaccine. It is recommended for children 2 years of age and older who are in a high-risk group for meningococcal disease, eg, asplenic children or those with a deficiency of terminal complement. In addition, it is administered to people traveling to regions with hyperendemic or epidemic disease.

Prognosis

Patients with isolated focal disease who receive prompt therapy have a good prognosis. Patients with overwhelming meningococcemia have a guarded prognosis; features suggestive of a poor prognosis include hypotension, leukopenia, purpura, and absence of meningitis.

PERTUSSIS
(Whooping Cough)

Bordetella pertussis is a gram-negative bacillus. Transmission is by droplets during the catarrhal and paroxysmal stages of whooping cough. Pertussis is communicable from 1 week before to 3 weeks after onset of paroxysms. The incubation period is 7–10 days. A pertussis-like syndrome may be caused by *B parapertussis, Chlamydia trachomatis,* or several respiratory tract viruses.

Clinical Findings

A. Symptoms and Signs: Insidious onset of symptoms of a mild upper respiratory tract infection occurs, with rhinitis, sneezing, lacrimation, slight fever, and irritating cough (catarrhal stage). Within 2 weeks, the cough becomes paroxysmal; a repeated series of many coughs during one expiration is followed by a sudden deep inspiration with a characteristic crowing sound, or "whoop." Eating often precipitates paroxysms, which may also cause vomiting. Tenacious mucus may be coughed and vomited. The paroxysmal stage lasts 2–6 weeks, but a habit pattern of coughing may continue for many weeks (convalescent stage). Typical paroxysms and "whoops" may not be present in young infants or older children and adults.

B. Laboratory Findings: The white blood cell count may be very high, with predominant lymphocytosis. Cultures are best obtained by nasopharyngeal swab or washings. The nasopharyngeal culture on Bordet–Gengou medium yields positive results. Results are generally positive during the catarrhal stage and the first week or two of the paroxysmal stage. The fluorescent antibody test may give a rapid diagnosis. The sedimentation rate may be low.

Complications

Pneumonia accounts for 90% of the deaths due to pertussis. Atelectasis, emphysema, and bronchiectasis are other pulmonary complications. Neurologic complications include seizures, apnea, and encephalopathy.

Treatment

A. Specific Measures: Erythromycin will quickly eradicate organisms and reduce the possibility of spread of infection. It will not influence the course of the clinical disease unless begun during the catarrhal stage.

B. General Measures:

1. Respiration–Because of anoxic periods during paroxysms, infants may require constant attendance and such measures as insertion of an airway, artificial respiration, and suction of oropharynx. Oxygen should be administered to infants who have significant desaturation during coughing paroxysms. Bacterial superinfections of the respiratory tract require specific antimicrobial treatment.

2. Parenteral fluids–Severe paroxysms may prevent adequate intake of fluids and necessitate parenteral therapy.

3. Feedings–Frequent small feedings are less likely to cause vomiting than the usual 3-meals-a-day schedule. Thick feedings are often retained better than more fluid ones. If vomiting occurs during or immediately after a feeding, the child should be fed again. Paroxysms are less likely to occur at this time.

Prophylaxis

For active immunization in early infancy, see Table 9–3. Exposed household, daycare, and other close contacts of a patient with pertussis should receive a 14-day course of erythromycin.

Prognosis

Disease in infants under 1 year of age may be severe and is sometimes accompanied by a poor prognosis (especially if complications have occurred). The prognosis is good in patients over 1 year of age with uncomplicated infection.

DIPHTHERIA

Diphtheria is an actue febrile infection, usually of the throat, and is most common in the winter months in temperate zones. With active immunization in early childhood, the disease has become rare in the USA.

Diphtheria is caused by a gram-positive, pleomorphic rod, *Corynebacterium diphtheriae*. The disease is transmitted by droplets from the respiratory tract of a carrier or patient. The incubation period is 1–7 days (average, 3 days).

Clinical Findings

A. Symptoms and Signs:

1. Pharyngeal–Findings include mild sore throat, moderate fever to 38.5 °C (101.2–102.2 °F), rapid pulse, severe prostration, and exudate. A membrane forms in the throat and spreads from the tonsils to the anterior pillars and uvula. It is typically dirty gray or gray-green when fully developed but may be white early in the course. The edges of the membrane are slightly elevated, and bleeding results if it is scraped off. (This procedure is contraindicated as it will hasten absorption of toxin.)

2. Nasal–Nasal discharge is a potent source of spread of infection to others, and serosanguineous nasal discharge may excoriate the patient's upper lip. A membrane may be visible on turbinates; constitutional manifestations are slight.

3. Laryngeal–Findings of laryngeal involvement are the most serious and include hoarseness or aphonia, croupy cough, fever up to 39.5–40.0 °C (103–104 °F), marked prostration, cyanosis, difficulty in breathing, and, eventually, respiratory obstruction. Brawny edema of the neck may occur, and membrane formation may be visible in the pharynx.

4. Cutaneous, vaginal, and wound–Findings include ulcerative lesions with membrane formation. The lesions are persistent and often anesthetic.

B. Laboratory Findings:
The white blood cell count is normal, or there may be a slight leukocytosis. A smear of exudate stained with methylene blue shows rods with mid polar bars. Cultures on Loffler's medium yield positive results.

Complications

A. Myocarditis:
Myocarditis is a direct result of the effect of the toxin. Clinical diagnosis is discussed in Chapter 19. The ECG shows T-wave changes and partial or complete atrioventricular block.

B. Neuritis:
Neuritis is usually a late development. Both sensory loss and motor paralyses develop rapidly once neuritis becomes apparent. Complete recovery is usual.

1. Pharyngeal and palatal muscles–These are the earliest muscles to become involved. Manifestations include nasal voice, dysphagia, and nasal regurgitation of fluids.

2. Extrinsic eye muscles–Diplopia and strabismus are manifestations.

3. Skeletal muscles–Involvement of the legs and arms may end in quadriplegia.

C. Bronchopneumonia:

D. Proteinuria: Proteinuria usually clears as the temperature returns to normal, but nephritis may occur.

E. Thrombocytopenia

Treatment

A. Specific Measures: The following measures are for the treatment of all types of diphtheria.

1. Antitoxin–Diphtheria antitoxin in sufficient dosage must be given promptly. The longer the time between onset of disease and administration of antitoxin, the higher the mortality. Give antitoxin if disease is considered possible from clinical manifestations; do not wait for reports of cultures. The dosage is 20,000–100,000 units for patients of any age, depending on the site, severity, and duration of the disease. Always test for horse serum sensitivity before administration (see Administration of Animal Sera, Chapter 9); the preferred route is intravenous.

2. Antibiotics–Erythromycin (best) or procaine penicillin G for 14 days should be used in treatment and to shorten the carrier state. The administration of these antibiotics before specimens for culture are collected may prevent diagnosis of diphtheria by inhibiting growth of the organisms.

3. Toxoid–Diphtheria may not confer immunity. Patients recovered from diphtheria should receive a full primary course of immunization (see Chapter 9).

B. General Measures: Parenteral fluids, bed rest, and monitoring of the adequacy of the patient's airway are important elements of supportive care. Special measures for the treatment of patients with the laryngeal form of diphtheria include avoidance of sedation, suction of the larynx as necessary, tracheal intubation or tracheostomy for respiratory obstruction, and use of an atmosphere with high humidity.

C. Treatment of Complications:

1. Myocarditis–Treat with oxygen, antiarrhythmics, and blood pressure support as indicated.

2. Neuritis–Dysphagia may necessitate the use of an indwelling nasogastric tube. Intercostal paralysis may necessitate the use of a mechanical respirator.

Prophylaxis

Prophylactic measures include active immunization in early childhood (see Table 9–3), culture of close contacts and antibiotic treatment of identified culture-positive individuals, and booster immunization of contacts.

Prognosis

The prognosis is always guarded, varying with the day of disease on which antitoxin treatment is given. After 6 days without treatment, mortality is almost 50%. Myocarditis within the first 10 days is an ominous sign.

TETANUS

Tetanus is an acute disease characterized by painful muscular contractions. The causative organism of tetanus, *Clostridium tetani,* is an anaerobic, spore-forming, gram-positive organism that produces a very powerful neurotoxin. Bacilli and spores are widely distributed in soil and dust and are present in the feces of animals and humans. Inoculation of a wound with dirt or dust is most likely to occur with puncture wounds. In many cases, the original wound may have been very minor or overlooked entirely. In the newborn, transmission may occur by contamination of the umbilical cord, which, as it becomes necrotic, permits growth of the organism. The exotoxin acts upon the motor nerve endplates and anterior horn cells of the spinal cord and brainstem.

Clinical Findings

A. Symptoms and Signs: The incubation period varies from 3 days to 3 weeks, depending upon the size of the inoculum and the rapidity of its growth. The onset may be with spasm and cramplike pain in the muscles of the back and abdomen or about the site of inoculation, together with restlessness, irritability, difficulty in swallowing, and (sometimes) convulsions. A gradual increase in muscular tension occurs in the following 48 hours, with stiff neck, positive Kernig sign, tightness of masseters, anxious expression of the face, and stiffness of the arms and legs. Facial expression is modified by inability to open the mouth (trismus). Swallowing is difficult. Recurring tetanic spasms occur and last 5–10 seconds; they are characterized by agonizing pain, stiffening of the body, retraction of the head, opisthotonos, clenching of the jaws, and clenching of the hands. Fever is usually low-grade but may rarely be as high as 40 °C (104 °F). Auditory or tactile stimuli may initiate convulsions. Local tetanus, with muscle spasms only near the initial wound, may also occur.

B. Laboratory Findings: The white blood cell count is 8000–12,000/μL. Cerebrospinal fluid shows a slight increase in pressure, with a normal cell count. Anaerobic culture of excised necrotic tissue may yield positive results; however, the diagnosis is usually made on clinical presentation.

Treatment

A. Specific Measures:

1. Tetanus immune globulin (TIG) is preferred in doses of 500–3000 units, part delivered intramuscularly and part infiltrated locally around the wound (Table 15–2). If human TIG is not available, give tetanus antitoxin (equine), 50,000–100,000 units intravenously, after testing for horse serum sensitivity. The value of antitoxin treatment is questionable in mild cases and when treatment is delayed for several days after the appearance of symptoms.

2. Surgical exploration of the wound, with excision of necrotic tissue and cleaning and drainage, is indicated to eliminate a local source of infection.

3. Give parenteral penicillin or tetracycline for 10–14 days.

B. General Measures:

1. Keep the patient in a quiet, dark room. Minimize handling.

2. Give sedation as indicated; benzodiazopines and barbiturates are useful.

3. Gentle aspiration of secretions in the nasopharynx should be done as required.

4. Oxygen and intravenous fluids are given as required.

5. Airway maintenance may necessitate tracheal intubation or tracheostomy.

Table 15–2. Guide to tetanus prophylaxis in wound management.*

History of Tetanus	Clean, Minor Wounds		All Other Wounds	
Immunization	Td†	TIG‡	Td†	TIG‡
Uncertain, or < 3 doses	Yes	No	Yes	Yes
> 3 doses	No§	No	No‖	No

*Modified and reproduced, with permission, from *Report of the Committee on Infectious Diseases*, 21st ed. American Academy of Pediatrics, 1988, p 412.

†Td = tetanus toxoid and diphtheria toxoid, adult form. Use this preparation (Td adult) only in children over 7 years of age. Use DT or DTP in children < 7 years of age.

‡TIG = tetanus immune globulin.

§Yes, if more than 10 years since last dose.

‖Yes, if more than 5 years since last dose.

Prophylaxis

Active immunization (see Table 15–1) with a booster every 10 years will prevent tetanus in children and adults.

Adequate debridements of wounds is one of the most important preventive measures. In addition, administration of tetanus toxoid and/or tetanus immune globulin may be indicated depending on the type of wound and the immunization status (see Table 15–1).

Prognosis

The mortality rate in infants is 70%; in other age groups, mortality rates range from 10 to 60%.

BOTULISM

Classification

Three clinical syndromes due to the neuromuscular paralytic effects of the neurotoxins produced by *Clostridium botulinum* are now recognized:

A. Endogenous Toxin Syndrome: Infant botulism is the result of colonization of the infant's intestinal tract with *C botulinum,* probably from food sources other than milk. Contaminated honey has been implicated in several cases. Toxin is produced in the infant bowel and absorbed to produce symptoms.

B. Exogenous Toxin Syndrome: Poisoning from contaminated food, in which the organism has grown and produced toxin, may occur especially if the food is improperly processed or canned.

C. Wound Infection: Botulism may result from growth of *C botulinum* and toxin production in a colonized wound.

Clinical Findings

A. Symptoms and Signs:

1. Endogenous toxin syndrome–Onset of infant botulism occurs within the first 6 months of life. Manifestations include apathy, weakness, constipation, floppiness, sudden apnea (occasionally), and ocular palsies.

2. Exogenous toxin syndrome–Sudden onset of food poisoning occurs 12–36 hours after ingestion of contaminated food. Double vision, nystagmus, dry mouth, and dysphagia may occur. There may be progressive descending motor paralysis with no sensory impairment or meningeal signs.

3. Wound infection–Onset is 4–14 days after injury. Symptoms are similar to those found in patients with exogenous toxin syndrome.

B. Laboratory Findings: All possible food sources should be sampled for culture when botulism is suspected. Exogenous toxin can be demonstrated in the wound, vomitus, serum, stool, and/or implicated food. In infant disease, endogenous toxin may be found in the stool or serum. The organism can sometimes be cultured from the feces of the infant. Other laboratory findings are usually normal. Cerebrospinal fluid findings are normal. Electromyography shows responses characteristic of neuromuscular block.

Treatment

A. Specific Measures: Equine antitoxin should be given in the exogenous diseases after testing for hypersensitivity (see Table 15–3 regarding dosage and administration of the preparation). Endogenous disease in the infant does not require antitoxin. Antibiotic therapy (penicillin) is recommended only for wound botulism).

B. General Measures: Respiratory paralysis requires mechanical aids. Tracheal intubation or tracheostomy may be necessary to remove pooled secretions. Tube feeding may be necessary with prolonged paralysis. In infant disease, the possibility of sudden death due to respiratory arrest dictates constant and careful observation. The use of aminoglycoside antibiotics may exacerbate symptoms.

Prophylaxis

The best prophylaxis for exogenous disease is to assure proper food preservation, eg, use of a pressure cooker to kill *C botulinum* spores in home canned foodstuffs. Honey should not be given to small infants.

Prognosis

The mortality rate in exogenous disease is 20–50%. In endogenous disease, most infants recover after an illness that may last several weeks to months.

SALMONELLOSIS

Salmonellosis designates the group of disease states caused by organisms of the genus *Salmonella,* a gram-negative bacilli. Salmonellosis is spread from the feces of the infected person or fecal carrier to the mouths of other individuals. Epidemics have

Table 15-3. Treatment of exogenous botulism.*

Indication	Product	Dosage	Comments
Botulism	ABE polyvalent antitoxin, equine. (Hexavalent ABCDEF, bivalent AB, and monovalent E antitoxins are also available.)	One vial IV and 1 vial IM; repeat after 2–4 h if symptoms worsen, and after 12–24 h.	For treatment of botulism. Available from CDC.† Twenty percent incidence of serum reactions. Prophylaxis is not routinely recommended but may be given to asymptomatic persons with unequivocal exposure.

*Modified and reproduced, with permission, from Cohen SN: Immunization. Chapter 38 in: *Basic & Clinical Immunology*, 5th ed. Stites DP et al (editors). Lange, 1984.

†Centers for Disease Control (404)329-3356 during the day, (404)329-2888 nights, weekends, and holidays.

Note: Passive immunotherapy or immunoprophylaxis should always be administered as soon as possible after exposure to the offending agent. Immune antisera and globulin are always given IM unless otherwise noted. Always question carefully and test for hypersensitivity before administering animal sera (see text).

been traced to contaminated water, ice, milk, and various improperly prepared foods. Flies, ducks, turkeys, pet turtles, and egg preparations have been identified as sources of infection.

Etiology

There are more than 1500 serotypes of salmonellae pathogenic for humans; they are divided into groups A–E on the basis of somatic antigens. More recently, salmonellae have been divided into three groups: *S typhi* (the cause of typhoid fever), *S cholerasuis,* and *S enteritidis,* the latter including all nontyphi and noncholerasuis serotypes.

Clinical Findings

A. Symptoms and Signs: Salmonella infections are of 4 types:

1. Enteric fever–This type includes typhoid fever. After an incubation period of 8–16 days, fever to 40 °C (104 °F) appears and is accompanied by anorexia, vomiting, abdominal distention and tenderness, and extreme malaise. In many cases, these are the only symptoms. However, after about 5 days, a rash may appear, usually on the abdomen and consisting of red macules that blanch easily ("rose spots"). At this point, the patient is usually very ill, sometimes with coma or convulsions. Physical findings include hepatomegaly and splenomegaly and a relative bradycardia. Constipation may occur early; diarrhea is rarely prominent but may develop in the second or third week in untreated cases.

2. Bacteremia–Bacteremia is particularly common in infants. The onset is sudden, sometimes with seizures and spiking fever to 39.5–40.5 °C (103–105 °F). Bacteremia may accompany localized infectious processes (see below).

3. Gastroenteritis–Acute gastroenteritis and enterocolitis are probably the most common forms of salmonellosis. After an incubation period of 1–3 days, there is a sudden onset of vomiting, diarrhea, and fever to 49 °C (104 °F). Abdominal cramps and prostration are common. Stools usually contain pus and blood (see Table 22–2).

4. Localized infection–Salmonellae may cause localized infections in practically any part of the body. These include osteomyelitis, meningitis, appendicitis, peritonitis, and pneumonia. Children with sickle cell anemia and related hemoglobinopathies are particularly susceptible to salmonella osteomyelitis and other focal infections.

B. Laboratory Findings:

1. Enteric fever–Leukopenia occurs at the onset of typhoid fever. Blood, stool, urine, or bone marrow cultures may be positive. The serologic test for antibodies (Widal test, or "febrile agglutinans") is done with H and O antigens; however, this test is often unreliable.

2. Bacteremia–Blood cultures yield positive results during the febrile phase.

3. Gastroenteritis–Findings include moderate leukocytosis and white blood cells in the rectal smear. Stool culture often yields positive results. Multiple negative results on culture do not rule out this etiology.

4. Localized infection–Leukocytosis occurs. Cultures of specimens from involved areas are positive.

Complications

In the third week of typhoid fever, hemorrhage or perforation of the intestine may occur (rare in childhood). With septicemia, there may be a localized infectious process such as meningitis, osteomyelitis, pleural infection, or abscess in any organ. Gastroenteritis may be accompanied by dehydration and acidosis, as in any severe diarrhea.

Treatment

A. Specific Measures: For patients with enteric fever, bacteremia, or localized invasive infection, treatment is with ampicillin/amoxicillin or chloramphenicol. Alternative drugs, guided by susceptibility testing, include trimethoprim-sulfamethoxazole and third-generation cephalosporins. Patients with uncomplicated gastroenteritis do not require antibiotic therapy unless risk factors for invasive disease are present, eg, age less than 3 months, immunosuppression or malignancy, or hemoglobinopathy. Antibiotic therapy may promote a prolonged carrier state.

B. General Measures: Attention should be paid to hydration and nutritional status. Corticosteroids are indicated for patients with severe enteric fever. Transfusions for hemorrhage or surgery for perforations may be required.

Prophylaxis

Prophylactic measures include discovery and supervision of cases and carriers, sanitary disposal of excreta, protection and purification of food and water supplies, and supervision of food handlers. Active immunization against typhoid is recommended for travelers to areas in which typhoid fever is endemic (see Chapter 9).

Prognosis

In enteric fever, the prognosis is usually good with antibiotics. In bacteremia, the prognosis is guarded; local Salmonella infections are particularly difficult to treat. In gastroenteritis, the prognosis is usually good if adequate dietary measures are used to control diarrhea. The carrier state is common in young children. Treatment of the carrier is unsuccessful and not necessary. Family hygiene in such cases should be reviewed and improved by teaching.

SHIGELLOSIS

Shigella is spread from human feces of the infected person or fecal carrier to the mouths of other individuals. Epidemics have been traced to contaminated water, ice, milk, and various foods. Flies may serve as vectors in tropical regions.

Shigella are gram-negative rods; there are more than 40 serotypes. *Shigella sonnei* is the most common in the USA. *S dysenteriae* type 1 is common in Central and South America and Africa. The incubation period is 1–6 days (usually less than 4 days).

Clinical Findings

A. Symptoms and Signs: In severe and fulminant cases (bacillary dysentery), the onset is sudden, with prostration, fever to 39.5 °C (103 °F), vomiting, profuse bloody diarrhea, colic, and tenesmus. The patient may be in shock very early in the course of the illness. Meningismus, deep drowsiness, coma, or seizures may occur. Generalized abdominal tenderness is usually present and rigidity may be present at times. Patients with the mild form of the disease may show only a slight fever and a mild, watery diarrhea.

B. Laboratory Findings: An increase in the white blood cell count ($10,000-16,000/\mu L$) and the number of polymorphonuclear leukocytes occurs in most patients. Pus and blood may be seen in the smear of stool. Stool cultures usually yield positive results.

Complications

Complications may include fluid and electrolyte imbalance, seizures, and, rarely, hemolytic-uremic syndrome and Reiter's syndrome.

Treatment

A. Specific Measures: Most patients should be treated with antibiotics. Trimethoprim-sulfamethoxazole is recommended for organisms with unknown susceptibility or known to be ampicillin-resistant. Ampicillin is useful for susceptible strains (amoxicillin is ineffective). Tetracycline and chloramphenicol are alternative drugs.

B. General Measures: Parenteral hydration and correction of electrolyte disturbances are essential in all moderately or severely ill patients. Dietary measures (see Chapter 4) are most important.

Prophylaxis

Control of cases and general sanitation and personal hygiene are most important. No active immunizing agent is available.

Prognosis

When treatment is begun early in the disease, the prognosis is good. In infancy and old age, the mortality rate is highest if therapy is delayed. Relapse or reinfection occurs in 10% of cases. Prolonged carriage is unusual.

CAMPYLOBACTER

Campylobacter infections are caused by 3 species of small comma-shaped gram-negative rods, *Campylobacter jejuni, C fetus,* and *C pyloris. C jejuni* has emerged as an important cause of bacterial gastroenteritis. *C fetus* is an occasional cause of sepsis in neonates and other compromised hosts. *C pyloris* has been isolated from mucosa of patients with gastritis and peptic ulcer disease; its pathogenic role is not yet well defined. *C jejuni* may be spread by the fecal-oral route from infected people or animals (pets, farm animals, poultry) and via contaminated food and water.

Clinical Findings

A. Symptoms and Signs: Gastroenteritis caused by *C jejuni* presents with diarrhea, abdominal pain, fever, and, often, bloody stools. Less common findings include reactive arthritis and seizures (with fever).

B. Laboratory Findings: *C jejuni* can be presumptively identified by seeing motile rods in a wet-mount of stool; definitive identification is made by culture of stool.

Complications
Severe or prolonged enteric infection can mimic other gastrointestinal disease, eg, appendicitis, inflammatory bowel disease, etc.

Treatment
A. Specific Measures: Erythromycin is the drug of choice for campylobacter enteritis and will shorten the period of excretion of *C jejuni*.

B. General Measures: Rehydration and nutritional support during the period of diarrheal illness.

Prophylaxis
Hand washing after contact with animals and with persons with gastroenteritis is important. Proper cooking of meat and pasteurization of milk are also necessary.

Prognosis
The prognosis is excellent except in compromised hosts with systemic infection.

CHOLERA

The causative agent of cholera is *Vibrio cholerae*, a gram-negative, curved organism with a terminal flagellum that is actively motile in suspension. Transmission is by contaminated food or water; contaminated shellfish are frequently implicated sources.

Clinical Findings
A. Symptoms and Signs: During the incubation stage (1–3 days), mild diarrhea may be present. During the diarrheal stage, there is severe cramping and profuse diarrhea, the stools becoming almost clear fluid and albuminous ("rice water"). Vomiting is severe. In the collapse stage, diarrhea ceases and shock appears within 2–12 hours after onset of diarrhea. During the recovery stage, the stools become more normal within the course of a week. Infection may be mild or even symptomatic.

B. Laboratory Findings: There is a marked hemoconcentration, metabolic acidosis, and (often) elevation of urea nitrogen levels. The stools rarely show pus cells, but the vibrios can be easily cultured on appropriate media. Darkfield microscopy of fresh stool may suggest the diagnosis. The diagnosis may be confirmed by serologic tests.

Treatment

A. Specific Measures: Use of trimethoprim-sulfamethoxazole or furazolidone, or tetracycline in older children (see Chapter 8), may shorten the duration of disease.

B. General Measures: Give oral glucose/electrolyte solution as in other diarrheal conditions (see Chapter 22). The absorption of glucose and sodium occurs despite massive secretion by the intestine in patients with cholera. The solution need not be sterile and can be administered by nonprofessionals. Intravenous therapy with massive infusions of physiologic saline solution should be given when shock or coma prevents oral therapy. Potassium and bicarbonate supplements may be necessary.

Prophylaxis

Prophylactic measures include active immunization with killed whole-cell vaccine (50–70% effective for up to 1 year); boiling all water and potentially contaminated foods; and screening in endemic areas. Use of tetracycline or trimethoprim-sulfamethoxazole in full dosage (see Chapter 8) for 5 days may prevent infection in close contacts of cholera patients.

Prognosis

In untreated cases, the mortality rate is 25–50%. With early and adequate treatment, the prognosis is good.

GONORRHEA

Neisseria gonorrhoeae is a gram-negative, coffee bean–shaped diplococcus usually found both intracellularly and extracellularly in purulent exudate. The neonatal infection may be acquired during delivery by direct contact with infected material in the mother's vagina. In childhood, infection may be acquired by contact with infected vaginal or urethral discharge or, rarely, from household exposure.

Clinical Findings

A. Symptoms and Signs: For gonococcal conjunctivitis of the newborn, see Chapter 25. Urethritis with purulent discharge may occur in males, and gonorrheal vulvovaginitis may occur in prepubertal females. While the vaginal mucosa in adults is resistant to gonococcal infection, both the vagina and the vulva are readily infected before puberty, most commonly from birth to 5 years of age. The infection is spread by contact with contaminated articles or infected children or adults and is manifested by itching and burning of the vulva and vagina. The mucous membranes of the vulva and vagina are red and edematous, and there is a profuse yellow purulent discharge. Vulvovaginitis due to gonococci must be differentiated from nonspecific vulvovaginitis due to improper hygiene. Acute salpingitis (pelvic inflammatory disease) may develop suddenly after several weeks or months of inapparent infection; however, this is more common in postpubertal females. Nongonococcal salpingitis may have an indentical clinical picture. Perihepatitis in conjunction with salpingitis is characterized by right upper abdominal tenderness and, occasionally, abnormal results of liver function tests. Pharyngitis and proctitis are occasional manifestations of gonococcal disease.

B. Laboratory Findings: A smear of purulent exudate may show intracellular organisms. Cultures on Thayer–Martin medium should be carried out for any suspected case.

Complications

Complications of conjunctivitis include corneal ulceration and opacity. Vaginitis may spread to regional organs or (through the bloodstream) to joints. Bacteremia with purulent arthritis and distinctive skin lesions can occur. The skin lesions have an erythematous base, with central hemorrhage. They later become necrotic and vesicular. Nonpurulent polyarthritis also may occur, with low-grade fever, pain and swelling of joints, and redness and tenderness of areas over the wrist, ankle, knee, finger, foot, and other joints of the extremities. Tenosynovitis is also common.

Treatment

A. Specific Measures: The drugs useful for treating gonococcal infections include penicillin G and amoxicillin (often in combination with probenecid), tetracycline and doxycycline, aspectinomycin, and ceftriaxone and cefotaxime. Local resistance patterns as well as susceptibilities of individual isolates should be used to guide therapy. The dosage and duration of therapy vary with the site of infection.

B. General Measures:

1. Neonates with gonococcal infection should be hospitalized. In addition to parenteral antibiotics, frequent irrigation of the eyes is crucial.

2. Expectant therapy of potential copathogens, eg, *Chlamydia trachomatis,* is important for any patient with gonorrhea. In addition, serologic testing for syphilis should be performed.

3. Children who have gonococcal infections should be evaluated for the possibility of sexual abuse.

Prophylaxis

For prophylaxis of conjunctivitis, see Chapter 25. Pregnant women should undergo routine screening for gonorrhea. In addition, pregnant women with vaginitis should be examined and cultured prior to delivery. Examination, culturing, and treatment of sexual partners of any person with gonorrhea must be carried out. (Asymptomatic vaginal or urethral infection is common.)

Prognosis

The prognosis is excellent with prompt treatment. Untreated conjunctivitis may result in corneal scarring. Salpingitis as a result of spread from the vagina may be symptomatic and chronic and may lead to sterility.

TULAREMIA

The causative agent of tularemia is *Francisella tularensis*, a gram-negative coccobacillus. The infection is transmitted through direct contact with the blood of an infected rabbit, ground squirrel, or (more rarely) any one of many species of wild or domestic mammals; through bites of infected ticks or mosquitoes; or through ingestion of improperly cooked meat from wild mammals, usually rabbits, or of contaminated water. The incubation period is 1–21 days (average, 3–5 days).

Clinical Findings

A. Symptoms and Signs: Onset is sudden, with fever to 40–40.5 °C (104–105 °F), vomiting, chills in older children, and seizures in the rarely infected infant. Cutaneous eruptions of various types occur in about 10% of children. The clinical picture depends upon the portal of entry.

1. Ulceroglandular type–The lesion on the extremity where the bacteria enter the skin is at first papular but rapidly breaks down and becomes a punched-out ulcer. It is accompanied by enlargement and tenderness of regional lymph nodes and sometimes by nodules along the course of the lymphatics. Without therapy, suppuration of the lymph nodes frequently occurs. In some cases, there is lymphadenopathy, but no primary lesion can be detected (glandular type).

2. Oropharyngeal type–Ulceration and formation of a membrane on the pharynx and tonsils are accompanied by enlargement of the cervical lymph nodes.

3. Oculoglandular type–Infection is acquired when material is rubbed into the eye. Findings include acute conjunctivitis with edema; photophobia; itching and pain in the eye; swelling of the upper lid, which may show scattered small yellow nodules; and enlargement of lymph glands of the neck, axilla, and scalp.

4. Typhoidal type–The point of entry of the organisms cannot be recognized, and the symptoms are entirely systemic.

5. Pneumonia

B. Laboratory Findings: The white blood cell count may be normal, or there may be a slight leukocytosis. The serologic agglutinin test shows a positive rising titer, beginning around 7 days from onset. Culture of blood and material from other sites of infection may be positive (on special media); an indirect fluorescent antibody stain can also be done on potentially infected tissues or exudates.

Treatment

Give streptomycin or gentamicin for 7–10 days. Tetracyclines or chloramphenicol may be used as alternatives; they are associated with a greater chance of relapse.

Prophylaxis

Prophylactic measures include proper handling and cooking of meat from wild mammals, wearing rubber gloves in handling potentially infected animals, using extreme care in handling laboratory materials, and minimizing the chances of tick and mosquito bites. A live attenuated vaccine is recommended for persons with repeated exposures.

Prognosis

The mortality rate in patients with untreated ulceroglandular tularemia is 5%, and that in patients with the pneumonic type is 30%. Early chemotherapy eliminates fatalities. Skin tests and agglutinin tests suggest that the subclinical infection is common in endemic areas.

PLAGUE

Plague is a disease primarily of rats and other small rodents. It is transmitted to humans by a variety of rodent fleas, as well as by direct contact with infected rodents, rabbits, and domestic animals. The pneumonic form of the disease may be transmitted from person to person by the inhalation of infected droplets.

The causative agent is *Yersinia pestis,* a gram-negative, bipolar-staining, pleomorphic bacillus.

Clinical Findings

A. Symptoms and Signs: The incubation period is 2–6 days, and there are 3 clinical syndromes of the disease:

1. Bubonic plague–Onset is sudden, with chills, fever to 40 °C (104 °F), vomiting, and lethargy. There is tender, firm enlargement of the inguinal, axillary, and cervical lymph nodes (buboes) by the third day. Meningismus, seizures, and delirium may occur.

2. Pneumonic plague–Findings are as above but with the absence of buboes and onset of cough on the first day. Blood-tinged, mucoid or thin, bright-red sputum may be brought up. Clinical signs of pneumonia may be absent at first.

3. Fulminant (septicemic) plague–Onset is as above but with overwhelming bloodstream invasion before enlargement of nodes or pneumonia.

B. Laboratory Findings: Leukocytosis appears early, with counts as high as 50,000/μL (mostly polymorphonuclear leukocytes). Early blood cultures show positive results. Organisms can be cultured from lymph node contents, sputum, and sometimes from cerebrospinal fluid. The organism may also be identified in stains of blood smears, lymph node aspirates, cerebrospinal fluid, or sputum. Serologic testing may also indicate the occurrence of recent infection.

Treatment

A. Specific Measures: Streptomycin is the drug of choice. A tetracycline (for older children) or chloramphenicol may be used as an alternative, but these drugs are less reliable for treatment (see Chapter 8). Chloramphenicol should be included in the therapy of meningitis.

B. General Measures: Strict isolation of patients with pneumonic plague and disinfection of all secretions are mandatory.

Prophylaxis

Periodic surveys of rodents and their ectoparasites in endemic areas will provide guidelines for extensive rodent and flea control measures. Total eradication of plague from wild rodents in an endemic area is rarely possible. Active immunization in endemic areas and for those with occupational exposure may be indicated (see Chapter 9). Antibiotic prophylaxis with tetracycline or a sulfonamide may provide temporary protection for those exposed to plague infection, especially by the respiratory route.

Prognosis

If treatment can be started early enough in the disease, the prognosis is excellent. Delay in treatment may result in death from the fulminant form of disease. Without treatment, the prognosis is poor.

BRUCELLOSIS
(Undulant Fever, Malta Fever)

Brucellosis is caused by one of the 4 strains of gram-negative brucellae (*Brucella abortus*, *B melitensis*, *B canis*, and *B suis*). Although these varieties are most commonly found in cattle, goats, dogs, and hogs respectively, they have also been isolated in other species of animals. The incubation period ranges from a few days to greater than 1 month.

Transmission is by direct contact with diseased animals, their tissues, or unpasteurized milk or cheese from diseased cows and goats.

Clinical Findings

A. Symptoms and Signs: In the acute disease, the onset is gradual and insidious, with fever and loss of weight. Fever may at first be low-grade and present in the evening only, but in the course of days or weeks it may reach 40 °C (104 °F) and present a wavelike character over a period of 2–4 days. The chronic disease is manifested by low-grade fever, sweats, malaise, arthralgia, depression, hepatomegaly and splenomegaly, and leukopenia.

B. Laboratory Findings: The white blood cell count is usually normal to low, with a relative or absolute lymphocytosis. The organism can be recovered from the blood, bone marrow, urine, and local abscesses, usually with difficulty and requiring long incubation in a special medium. An agglutination titer greater than 1:160 or a rising titer will support the diagnosis. A prozone phenomenon in which the agglutination occurs in high dilutions but not in low ones is common. Skin tests are of no value and should not be carried out. Serologic tests may give a cross-reaction with tularemia, yersinia, and cholera.

Complications

Complications can include endocarditis, pneumonia, meningoencephalitis, and osteomyelitis.

Treatment

Tetracyclines are the drugs of choice. Continue treatment for 3 weeks. In severe illness, add streptomycin. Other drugs useful in treatment include rifampin and trimethoprim-sulfamethoxazole.

Prophylaxis
Milk and milk products should be pasteurized.

Prognosis
In patients with the acute form of infection, the prognosis is good with adequate treatment. In patients with the chronic form, response to treatment may be poor, although the disease generally is not fatal.

NOCARDIOSIS

Nocardia asteroides is a gram-positive filamentous aerobic bacterium causing chronic pulmonary and systemic disease or local infection of the skin. The organism exists in soil; infection is acquired via airborne particles, usually via the respiratory tract or by skin inoculation. Infection usually occurs in immunocompromised hosts.

Clinical Findings
Symptoms and Signs: The lungs are the most common site of initial infection, with systemic spread common in the course of a chronic febrile illness, especially in immunologically deficient children. Local skin infection or mycetoma (Madura foot) occurs by inoculation through an abrasion. Systemic disease includes multiple abscesses in the lungs, liver, brain, and lymph nodes.

B. Laboratory Findings: Partially acid-fast, branching gram-positive rods may be visible in smears of sputum, cerebrospinal fluid, pus, or tissue biopsies. The organism can also be cultured from these specimens.

Treatment
Trimethoprim-sulfamethoxazole or sulfadiazine are the drugs of choice; prolonged therapy is indicated. In case of poor response streptomycin or tetracycline may be added. In addition, surgical incision and drainage of abscesses may be useful.

Prognosis
Infections can usually be treated and controlled effectively, although this ability is influenced by the underlying immunodeficiency.

ACTINOMYCOSIS

Actinomyces israelii is a branching, anaerobic, filamentous bacterium that is found in the normal flora of the human tonsils and oropharynx.

Clinical Findings
A. Symptoms and Signs: After local trauma, organisms may invade tissues to form cervicofacial abscesses and draining sinuses. If organisms are aspirated, lesions may develop in the lung; after intestinal operations, abdominal lesions may occur. The lesions tend to be hard and painless, draining pus through sinuses. Fever and anemia are the systemic manifestations of infection.

B. Laboratory Findings: The diagnosis rests on either microscopic observation of beaded gram-positive rods and masses or filaments ("sulfer granules") in pus or growth of the organism in anaerobic culture.

Treatment
Administration of penicillin for prolonged periods (months) tends to be curative, but surgical drainage, excision, or revisions may also be required.

MYCOPLASMA PNEUMONIAE INFECTIONS

Mycoplasmas are free-living organisms without cell walls. The common clinical disease caused by *Mycoplasma pneumoniae* is pneumonia, which is most frequent in persons 5–18 years of age and especially in young adults. The incubation period is 2–3 weeks.

Clinical Findings
A. Symptoms and Signs: There is a gradual onset of moderate fever, with malaise and sore throat. Nonproductive cough occurs after 3–5 days. The cough becomes persistent and sometimes paroxysmal, resembling pertussis. Other findings include abdominal pain, vomiting, nausea, and dry rales occasionally accompanied by friction rub.

B. Laboratory Findings: The white blood cell count is normal early in the disease but later may show leukocytosis. Autohemagglutinins for type O human erythrocytes (cold agglutinins) appear usually after the first 10 days of disease. Complement fixation and other antibody tests are all useful, particularly when a 4-fold rise in titer is demonstrated. The organism may be grown on special media and will indicate either current or recent infection.

C. Imaging: The x-ray findings are those of pneumonitis, with infiltrates developing around the hilum and gradually spreading. Pleural effusion may be apparent.

Complications

Otitis media or bullous myringitis is common in younger individuals. Central nervous system disease, hemolytic anemia, exanthems, Stevens-Johnson syndrome, and arthritis have all been reported. Severe respiratory disease may be seen in immunocompromised hosts and in children with sickle cell disease.

Treatment

Erythromycin in young children or tetracycline in those over 9 years of age is the drug of choice (see Chapter 8).

Prognosis

With adequate treatment, the prognosis is excellent.

CHLAMYDIAL INFECTIONS

The species of the genus *Chlamydia* are obligate intracellular bacteria and are classified as *C trachomatis, C psittaci,* and TWAR agent *(C pneumoniae)*. These agents cause several disease entities.

Clinical Findings

A. Symptoms and Signs:

1. Inclusion conjunctivitis and trachoma–Neonatal inclusion conjunctivitis (inclusion blennorrhea) and trachoma are caused by *C trachomatis*. The neonatal infection is acquired during passage through the cervix and causes a purulent conjunctivitis within the first few weeks after birth (see Conjunctivitis, Chapter 25).

2. Pneumonitis–Neonatal pneumonitis, also a result of *C trachomitis* infection acquired during birth, is characterized by onset during early infancy, with progressive tachypnea, staccato cough, cyanosis, and vomiting. It is an afebrile illness. Chest x-ray shows bilateral infiltrates.

3. Lymphogranuloma venereum–Infection is caused by particular strains of *C trachomatis,* and there is inguinal and pelvic lymph node involvement after sexual contact with penile, vaginal, or rectal surfaces. The inguinal nodes in the male and the perirectal nodes in the female become infected, enlarge, and suppurate. This process is apparent as buboes in the male and proctitis in the female or in the homosexual male.

4. Urethritis and cervicitis–Infection is caused by *C trachomatis*. It is clinically similar to disease produced by gonococci and may be mistaken for penicillin-resistant gonococcal infection. Infection may be asymptomatic and it may be persistent.

5. Psittacosis–Psittacosis (ornithosis) is caused by *C psittaci* and is acquired by contact with parrots, parakeets, pigeons, chickens, ducks, and other wild birds. There is a sudden onset of fever, chills, and nonproductive cough, with clinical signs of pneumonia or bronchiolitis (see Chapter 21). Multisystem involvement rarely occurs.

6. TWAR Agent–A febrile respiratory illness consisting of pharyngitis, cough, cervical adenopathy, and penumonia has been described caused by this chlamydial agent, which is antigenically distinct from *C trachomatis* and *C psittaci*.

B. Laboratory Findings: Chlamydiae can be cultured, with difficulty, on special media. This test is generally available for *C trachomatis* and *C psittaci*. Characteristic inclusion bodies are found on Giemsa-stained smears of discharge in neonatal conjunctivitis and trachoma. Fluorescent antibody staining and enzyme-linked immunoassay tests are widely available for diagnosing *C trachomatis* infections. Complement fixation tests are diagnostic in lymphogranuloma venereum, psittacosis, and in TWAR agent infection.

Complications

Neonatal inclusion conjunctivitis (rarely) and trachoma (relatively commonly) may produce corneal scarring and vision problems if untreated. Untreated lymphogranuloma venerum in boys may produce extensive scarring around draining inguinal nodes; in girls, perirectal scarring may cause rectal stricture. Untreated urethritis in boys may cause chronic discharge and dysuria persisting for many weeks. Untreated cervicitis in girls may spread to cause salpingitis with resultant scarring and sterility. Untreated neonatal chlamydial pneumonia may produce chronic illness.

Treatment

A. Specific Measures:

1. Inclusion conjunctivitis–Therapy with oral erythromycin continued for 14 days (see Chapter 25) is the recommended treatment. Topical therapy is less effective.

2. Trachoma–Give oral tetracyclines (doxycycline) in addition to local treatment. Therapy may have to be continued for as long as 30 days.

3. Pneumonitis–Treat with oral erythromycin or sulfisoxazole for 14 days.

4. Lymphogranuloma venereum–Give tetracycline or sulfonamides orally for several weeks (see Chapter 8).

5. Urethritis and cervicitis–Oral tetracyclines or erythromycin may reduce symptoms but will not always eradicate the organisms.

6. Psittacocis–Give tetracyclines or erythromycin orally (see Chapter 8).

7. TWAR Agent–Erythromycin and tetracycline are the drugs of choice.

Prophylaxis

Topical erythromycin, tetracycline, or silver nitrate may prevent neonatal chlamydial conjunctivitis (as well as gonococcal ophthalmia). In addition, identification and treatment of pregnant women who are infected may prevent neonatal conjunctivitis and pneumonia. Sexual partners of patients with identified or probable chlamydial infections should be treated.

Prognosis

With early diagnosis and treatment, complications are minimal and the prognosis excellent.

CAT-SCRATCH FEVER
(Benign Lymphoreticulosis)

Cat-scratch fever is an acute illness probably due to a tiny pleomorphic gram-negative bacillus identified morphologically but not yet cultured.

Clinical Findings

A. Symptoms and Signs: Cat-scratch fever is characterized by low-grade fever, malaise, an erythematous papular or pustular cutaneous lesion at the site of contact, and regional lymphadenopathy occurring about 2–4 weeks later. The lymph nodes are usually not very painful, but they may become warm, fixed to surrounding tissue, and suppurative; the enlargement may persist for 1 week to several months. A history of cat scratch, cat bite, or contact with healthy cats before onset is characteristic.

B. Laboratory Findings: Heat-inactivated purulent material from enlarged and fluctuant lymph nodes has served as a skin test antigen under research conditions and produces a tuberculin-like reaction in convalescent cases. Warthin-Starry silver stain of lymph node tissue may reveal gram-negative bacilli.

Complications

An encephalopathy associated with cat-scratch fever has been reported, and a conjunctivitis associated with inoculation on the face has also been described. Other complications include osteomyelitis, thrombocytopenia, and erythema multiforme.

Treatment

No specific therapy is known; the illness is generally self-limited. Surgical removal or needle evacuation of the affected node will usually be followed by marked improvement.

Prognosis

Complete recovery usually occurs within a few months.

BACTERIAL INFECTIONS
OF THE CENTRAL NERVOUS SYSTEM

GENERAL CONSIDERATIONS IN MENINGITIS

The most important step in diagnosis of infection of the central nervous system is to suspect that it may be present.

The most frequent etiologic agents are group B streptococcus and gram-negative enterics in neonates and *Haemophilus influenza B, Streptococcus pneumoniae,* and *Neisseria meningitidis* in infants and children (Table 15–4).

Symptoms and Signs

A. "Meningeal" Signs: Signs include stiffness of the neck (inability to touch the chin to the chest), stiffness of the back (inability to sit up normally), a positive Kernig sign (inability to extend the knee when the leg is flexed anteriorly at the hip), and a positive Brudzinski sign (bending the head forward produces flexure movements of the lower extremity).

B. Increased Intracranial Pressure: Findings include bulging fontanelles in small infants, irritability, headache (may be intermittent), projectile vomiting (or vomiting may be absent), diplopia, "choking" of the optic disks, "cracked pot" percussion note over the skull (sometimes found in normal children also), slowing of the pulse, irregular respirations, and increase in blood pressure.

C. Change in Sensorium: Changes range from mild lethargy to coma.

D. Seizures: Seizures usually are generalized and are more common in infants.

E. Fever: Onset of high or low-grade fever may be sudden or insidious, or there may be a marked change in pattern during a minor illness.

F. Shock: Shock may appear in the course of many types of infection of the central nervous system.

G. Other: In the child under 2 years of age, irritability, persistent crying, poor feeding, diarrhea, or vomiting may be the *only* symptoms. Fever may be absent or low-grade, and meningeal signs as above may not be found. Therefore, the index of suspicion must be higher for infants.

Examination of Cerebrospinal Fluid

When infection of the central nervous system is suspected, lumbar puncture and examination of the cerebrospinal fluid must be performed to establish the diagnosis. The gross examination, cell count, chemistries, and microscopic examination for bacteria of a concentrated sediment may all be performed immediately after lumbar puncture. Latex agglutination and counterimmunoelectrophoresis are rapid and specific diagnostic tests that may be used to indentify capsular antigens of meningococci, pneumococci, or *Haemophilus influenzae* in cerobrospinal fluid.

Culture of Cerebrospinal Fluid & Blood

Cerebrospinal fluid must be cultured both aerobically and anaerobically. The organism causing the central nervous system infection may grow in a blood culture and not in cultures of the cerebrospinal fluid.

Differential Diagnosis

Bacterial meningitis must be differentiated from other types of central nervous system infection and disease (eg, granulomatous meningitis due to tuberculosis, coccidiomycosis, cryptococcosis, histoplasmosis, and syphilis) and from aseptic meningitis and viral encephalitis.

Leptospiral infection with meningeal involvement shows lymphocytic cellular response (see Leptospirosis, below).

Partially treated bacterial meningitis may present with the same course and same laboratory findings as aseptic meningitis following in adequate antimicrobial therapy.

Table 15—4. Bacterial meningitis: specific agents.

Organism	Epidemiology	Clinical Findings	Laboratory Findings	Complications	Treatment	Prophylaxis
Haemophilus influenzae B	Most frequent cause of pediatric meningitis; most frequent under 5 yrs, especially < 2 yrs.	May be of rapid or insidious onset, frequently follows URI. May have associated foci of infection, eg, arthritis, cellulitis.	Gram stain of CSF may show gram-negative pleomorphic rods (coccobacilli). CSF culture and, often, blood culture positive. Latex agglutination or counter-immunoelec-trophoresis (CIE) may be positive in CSF, serum, or urine.	Persistent or recurrent fevers; secondary sites of infection (arthritis, pericarditis; subdural effusions or empyemas. Long-term morbidity, especially hearing loss, may ensue.	Ampicillin, cefotaxime, ceftriaxone, chloramphenicol depending on susceptibilities. Ampicillin resistance ranges from 25–50%.	Rifampin prophylaxis of contacts; *Haemophilus influenzae B* vaccine.

Neisseria meningitidis	Most frequent in infants & young children. Increased risk in patients with terminal complement deficiency.	Morbilliform, petechial, or purpuric rash frequent. May present with shock.	Gram stain of CSF may show gram-negative diplococi. Organism may be grown from CSF, blood, & petechial lesions. Latex agglutination or CIE may be helpful, though lack sensitivity.	Secondary sites of infection may occur. DIC, myocarditis, pericarditis. Waterhouse–Friderichson syndrome, shock.	Penicillin G, ampicillin, chloramphenicol, cefotaxime, ceftriaxone.	Rifampin prophylaxis of contacts; meningococcal vaccine.
Streptococcus pneumoniae	Increased risk in children with deficiencies of humoral immunity or splenic function; common cause of posttraumatic meningitis.	Frequently follows URI or other infection (otitis, sinusitis, pneumonia).	Gram stain of CSF may show gram-positive diplococci. Organism often isolated from CSF and/or blood. Latex agglutination or CIE may be positive in CSF, serum or urine.	Secondary sites of infection may occur. Long-term morbidity common, including hearing loss, seizures, motor deficits, & intellectual impairment.	Penicillin G or ampicillin. If strain is not fully susceptible to penicillin, alternatives include vancomycin, chloramphenicol, & cefotaxime.	Antibiotic prophylaxis for asplenic patients; pneumococcal vaccine.

(continued)

503

Table 15-4. (Continued)

Organism	Epidemiology	Clinical Findings	Laboratory Findings	Complications	Treatment	Prophylaxis
Group B streptococcus	Neonates; increased risk with prematurity, prolonged rupture of membranes, maternal infection.	May present as early onset or late onset disease. Findings may be nonspecific.	Gram stain of CSF may show gram-positive cocci in chains; CSF & blood cultures usually positive. Latex agglutination or CIE frequently positive (urine, CSF, serum).	Long-term sequelae may include intellectual impairment, motor deficits, hearing loss, seizures.	Penicillin G, or ampicillin; an aminoglycoside may be added for possible synergy.	Antibiotic prophylaxis of pregnant women or neonates carrying group B streptococcus may be considered.
Gram-negative Enterics (*Escherichia coli, Klebsiella pneumoniae, Pseudomonas aeruginosa, Citrobacter diversus, Enterobacter* species)	Increased risk in premature neonates or other compromised hosts; may be associated with UTI, foreign body, other focus of infection, break in skin or mucosal integrity.	Usually acute onset, with systemic illness.	Gram stain of CSF may reveal gram-negative rods. Cultures of CSF, blood, often positive.	Tends to have severe course, with resultant morbidity. Brain abscess may occur.	Cefotaxime, ceftazidime, or an aminoglycoside, depending on susceptibilities.	

Organism					
Listeria monocytogenes	Neonates; patients with defective cell-mediated immunity.	May present as early onset or late onset disease in neonates. May be associated with maternal illness.	Gram stain of CSF shows gram-positive rods. Cultures of CSF & blood usually positive.	May have long-term morbidity if severe and/or treatment delayed.	Ampicillin plus an aminoglycoside.	Maternal avoidance of foods implicated in listeriosis outbreak; treat maternal infections when identified.
Mycobacterium tuberculosis	Infected contact can usually be identified; patient often in high-risk geographic or ethnic group.	Onset may be gradual; encephalopathic symptoms may predominate. Tuberculous pneumonia often present.	Positive tuberculin skin test; moderate CSF pleocytosis with very low CSF glucose. Acid-fast bacilli may be identified in or grown from CSF.	Long-term sequelae may develop as for other bacterial meningitis.	Prolonged antituberculous therapy with isoniazid, rifampin and usually a third drug (pyrazinamide, streptomycin, or ethambutol) depending on susceptibilities. Corticosteroids for increased intracranial pressure.	Prophylactic administration of isoniazid to contacts with active tuberculosis & to PPD converters. Use of BCG in rare circumstances.

505

The "neighborhood reaction" (ie, a response to a purulent infectious process in close proximity to the central nervous system) introduces elements of the inflammatory process—white cells or protein—into the cerebrospinal fluid. Such an infection might be brain abscess, osteomyelitis of the skull or vertebrae, epidural abscess, or mastoiditis.

Meningismus or noninfectious meningeal irritation may occur in such infections as pneumonia, shigellosis, salmonellosis, otitis media, and meningeal invasion by neoplastic cells. In the latter instance, there may be not only increased numbers of cells in the spinal fluid but also a lowered glucose level.

Complications

Central nervous system infection may produce fatality rates of up to 20% and long-term sequelae in up to 30% of survivors. Complications include hydrocephalus, especially in infants (uncommon since the advent of specific therapy); subdural accumulation of fluid, especially in a patient under 2 years of age; deafness; paralysis of various muscles; mental retardation; focal epilepsy; or psychologic residua. Persistent fever may be due to brain abscess, lateral sinus thrombosis, mastoiditis, drug reaction, continued sepsis, or simply to persistent inflammation.

Treatment

A. Emergency Measures: Treat shock (see Chapter 6). Avoid overhydration and aggravation of brain edema.

B. Specific Measures:

1. Infection with known organism–Treat with antibiotics appropriate for organism.

2. Suspected infection with undetermined bacterial organism–Obtain all possible diagnostic material before instituting antimicrobial therapy. Urgency depends on the presumed duration of disease, the presence and depth of coma, and the age of the patient, with infancy as an absolute indication for urgency. An additional factor of urgency is the degree of depression of the cerebrospinal fluid glucose level. Meningitis of unknown cause in premature infants and infants under 1 month of age should be treated with ampicillin plus cefotaxime or ampicillin plus gentamicin. Children over 1 month of age should be given cefotaxime, ceftriaxone, or chloramphenicol, usually in combination with ampicillin.

3. Increased intracranial pressure–Increased pressure may cause death before antimicrobial treatment takes effect. Treat as for encephalitis (see Chapter 27).

BRAIN ABSCESS

Brain abscess is usually caused by one of the common pyogenic bacteria: streptococci, oral anaerobes, pneumococci, staphylococci, or gram negatives. The source of infection is usually a septic focus elsewhere in the body (eg, oropharyngeal infection, sinusitis, otitis media, pneumonia, osteomyelitis, subacute infective endocarditis, furuncles). After skull fracture, organisms may enter through the sinuses or middle ear.

Clinical Findings

A. Symptoms and Signs: Findings may be few and diagnosis difficult. Onset is gradual, with fever, vomiting, lethargy, and coma. Increased intracranial pressure may be present, manifested by bulging fontanelles (infants) or papilledema (older children). Neurologic signs related to special areas of the brain may be present, and focal seizures may occur (see Convulsive Disorders, Chapter 27). A history of infection elsewhere in the body should be sought.

B. Laboratory Findings: Leukocytosis and cerebrospinal fluid changes may occur.

C. Imaging: Cranial sutures may be widened. CT scan, magnetic resonance imaging, radionuclide brain scan, and arteriography may give specific diagnosis and location.

Treatment

A. Specific Measures: Surgical aspiration and drainage, for diagnosis and therapy, are usually indicated. Identification of the pathogens will allow specific antibiotic therapy. Until this can be performed, broad-spectrum antimicrobial therapy should be initiated (eg, combinations of penicillin, nafcillin, chloramphenicol, cefotaxime, or metronidazole, as dictated by particular circumstances).

B. General Measures: Give anticonvulsants for seizures.

Prognosis

When the organism is known and is susceptible to antibiotics, and when treatment is initiated early, the prognosis is good. For extensive disease or delayed therapy, the prognosis is guarded. Brain damage may occur, with resultant cortical deficits.

SPIROCHETAL DISEASES

SYPHILIS

Syphilis is caused by *Treponema pallidum*. It occurs in congenital and acquired forms. Congenital syphilis is transmitted from mother to infant by direct inoculation into the blood through the placenta during the latter half of pregnancy. If infection of the mother has occurred recently, the infant is almost always affected. The longer the interval between infection of the mother and conception, the greater the likelihood that the infant will be free of the disease. Intrauterine infection may produce intrauterine fetal death or congenital syphilis.

Syphilis may be acquired in childhood by contact of an abrasion or laceration with infectious secretions, by contact with infected nipples, through kissing of infectious lesions, or by sexual contact.

Clinical Findings

A. Symptoms and Signs: Childhood syphilis may occur in early or late congenital forms or may be transmitted in the same way as the adult disease.

1. Early congenital syphilis–Signs generally appear before the sixth week of life. The more severe the infection, the earlier the onset. Rhinitis or "snuffles"—a profuse, persistent, mucopurulent nasal discharge—is usually the first symptom. The discharge may be blood-tinged. Skin rash follows onset of rhinitis and appears as a maculopapular or morbilliform eruption, heaviest on the back, buttocks, and backs of thighs. Bullous lesions on the hands and feet are suggestive. Other findings include bleeding ulcerations and fissures of mucous membranes of the mouth, anus, and contiguous areas; anemia, with erythroblasts often present in large numbers; osteochondritis or periostitis (or both), with pseudoparalysis, pathologic fractures, and a characteristic x-ray appearance of increased density, widening of the epiphyseal line, and scattered areas of decreased density; hepatomegaly and splenomegaly (jaundice may be prominent); pneumonia; and chorioretinitis, with eventual atrophy.

2. Late congenital syphilis–Symptoms do not usually occur until after the second year of life. There may be maldevelopment of bones of the nose (saddle nose) and legs (saber shins). Neurosyphilis may occur, with clinical evidence of meningitis, paresis, tabes, or a slowly developing hydrocephalus. Deciduous teeth are normal. Permanent dentition may show Hutchinson's teeth, in which upper central incisors have a characteristic V-shaped notch in a peg-shaped tooth. The first permanent molars may have multiple cusps ("mulberry molar"). Other findings include rhagades, or scars around the mouth and nose; interstitial keratitis, usually occurring in children between 6 and 12 years of age; and early conjunctivitis, which gradually infiltrates deeply into the cornea and produces opacity.

3. Acquired syphilis–Symptoms in children are similar to those in adults, with 3 stages: mucocutaneous ulcerative lesions, rash, and tertiary syphilis with its cardiovascular or neurologic changes.

B. Laboratory Findings: Darkfield microscopic examination of scrapings from mucocutaneous lesions and nasal discharge may show treponemal spirochetes.

Serologic tests for syphilis include nontreponemal tests (VDRL, RPR, ART) and treponemal tests (FTA-ABS, MHA-TP, TPI). The nontreponemal tests are useful for screening; positive tests need to be confirmed with the specific treponemal tests. The nontreponemal tests should be followed after therapy; a declining titer correlates with successful treatment while a persistent elevated titer suggests persistent infection. The nontreponemal tests generally become nonreactive within a year after adequate therapy, while the treponemal tests remain positive indefinitely.

The diagnosis of congenital syphilis is based on clinical findings as well as serologic tests. Positive nontreponemal and treponemal tests on neonatal serum may reflect neonatal infection or maternal infection (even a satisfactorily treated maternal infection). In some cases, the only way to define a neonatal infection is to follow the neonate's nontreponemal titer; a rising titer over the first few months suggests an active infection.

Children with suspected congenital syphilis or acquired syphilis of more than 1 year's duration should have their cerebrospinal fluid analyzed. Increases in protein or cell count, or a positive nontreponemal test (VDRL) on cerebrospinal fluid, suggest neurologic involvement by infection.

C. Imaging: Findings are characteristic in congenital syphilis. All of the long bones may be affected. Changes are apparent early in the disease. The epiphyseal line shows increased density, with decreased density proximal to it. In severe cases, destructive lesions occur near the ends of the long bones. Periostitis appears as a widening of the shaft of the long bones, with eventual calcification and distortion of the normal curvature.

Treatment

   A. Specific Measures:

   1. Congenital syphilis–Give aqueous penicillin G, 50,000 units/kg/d intramuscularly or intravenously in 2 divided doses, or procaine penicillin G, 50,000 units/kg/d intramuscularly in 1 dose for 10 days.

   Therapy should be provided for neonates with clinical syphilis and for newborns born to mothers who had syphilis during pregnancy but were untreated, had inadequate treatment, had unknown treatment, had nonpenicillin treatment, or had treatment during the last 4 weeks of pregnancy.

   Infants who are asymptomatic and are born to mothers who received appropriate treatment for syphilis during pregnancy do not need therapy; their nontreponemal test titer should be followed monthly until negative. Treatment should be provided if the titer is not negative by 6 months or if follow-up cannot be assured.

   2. Acquired syphilis–Give benzathine penicillin G, 50,000 units/kg up to 2.4 million units in intramuscular injections of 1.2 million units each, for disease of less than 1 year's duration. Infection of more than 1 year's duration should be treated with the same dosage given once a week for 3 weeks.

   3. Penicillin sensitivity–In individuals sensitive to penicillin, give tetracycline or erythromycin for 15 days. Penicillin should be used whenever safely possible during pregnancy.

   B. Complications of Specific Therapy: The Jarisch–Herxheimer reaction, with fever due to the sudden destruction of spirochetes by drugs, occurs within the first 24 hours and subsides within the next 24 hours. Treatment should not be discontinued unless aggravation of laryngitis, if present, obstructs the airway.

   C. Follow-up Treatment: Nontreponemal serologic tests should be done at intervals of 3 months for at least 1 year. Retreatment should be considered if titers do not fall to the negative range. For those with initially abnormal cerebrospinal fluid, cerebrospinal fluid examinations need to be performed at 6-month intervals for at least 3 years.

Prophylaxis

   All pregnant women should be screened for syphilis at least twice, once early in pregnancy and again at delivery. If syphilis is diagnosed early in pregnancy, treatment may be completed before delivery. The chances of preventing the disease in the newborn are excellent even if the mother is not treated until the seventh or eighth month of pregnancy.

Sexual contacts of patients identified as having syphilis should be tested and treated.

Prognosis

Rapid treatment of infants with early congenital syphilis or of older patients with early acquired disease will usually result in a cure and normal growth and development. In children with late congenital syphilis, the prognosis for cure of the spirochetal infection is good, but pathologic changes in the bones, nervous system, and eyes will remain throughout life.

LEPTOSPIROSIS

Leptospirosis is an acute febrile disease caused by *Leptospira* species or serovariants of *L interrogans*. The most common species (or serovariants) implicated are *L canicola, L icterohaemorrhagiae,* and *L pomona*. The infection is transmitted through the ingestion of food or water contaminated with the urine of the reservoir animal (dogs, rats, cattle, and swine). Ingestion may occur while bathing in contaminated water. Rat bites are also a source. The incubation period is 6–12 days.

Clinical Findings

A. Symptoms and Signs: Onset is abrupt, with fever to 39.5–40.5 °C (103–105 °F). Pharyngitis, cervical lymphadenopathy, and conjunctivitis accompany the first phase of the disease, which lasts 3–5 days and is followed by subsidence of fever and symptoms. The second phase of the disease appears after 2 or 3 days, with recurrence of fever and the onset of joint pain, vomiting, headache, and often a rash, which is morbilliform and sometimes purpuric. Meningitis and (more rarely) uveitis may develop at this phase of the disease.

B. Laboratory Findings: The white blood cell count usually is markedly elevated (as high as 50,000 μL), sometimes with immature forms. Cerebrospinal fluid may show 100–200 cells/μL. Leptospirae may occasionally be seen on darkfield examination, silver stain, or fluorescent antibody stain of blood, urine, or cerebrospinal fluid. The organism can be cultured (on special media) from these body fluids. Serum bilirubin levels may be elevated, and the AST (SGOT) level may be abnormal. The diagnosis is most often made serologically; antibody is detectable after the first 7 days of disease.

Complications

Renal involvement, with hematuria, proteinuria, and oliguria, occurs in about 50% of cases. Jaundice, with an enlarged and tender liver, is also common. Symptomatic meningitis with any of its findings may become apparent in the second phase of the disease. Myocarditis may infrequently occur.

Treatment

A. Specific Measures: Give procaine penicillin G intravenously for 7 days. In patients with penicillin sensitivity, give doxycycline.

B. Complications of Specific Therapy: The Jarisch–Herxheimer reaction may occur, as in the treatment of syphilis (see above).

Prophylaxis

Methods used to prevent leptospirosis include rodent control, protective clothing in occupational exposures, and prophylactic doxycycline.

Prognosis

In the absence of renal or hepatic involvement, recovery is complete after 10–21 days. With severe kidney and liver involvement, the mortality rate may be as high as 30%.

RELAPSING FEVER

Relapsing fever is endemic in many parts of the world, especially in mountainous areas. The causative organisms are *Borrelia recurrentis* and related borrelia species, and the reservoir is rodents, other small mammals, or human beings with relapsing fever. Transmission to humans occurs by lice or ticks and occasionally by contact with the blood of infected rodents.

Clinical Findings

A. Symptoms and Signs: After an incubation period of 2–14 days, the onset of disease is abrupt, with fever, chills, tachycardia, nausea, vomiting, headache, hepatosplenomegaly, arthralgia, and cough. A macular or morbilliform rash appears usually within the first 2 days over the trunk and extremities. Petechiae may also occur. Without treatment, the fever falls by crisis in 3–10 days. Relapse then characteristically occurs at intervals of 1–2 weeks, with relapses becoming progressively shorter and milder. As many as 10 such episodes may occur in the absence of treatment.

B. Laboratory Findings: Diagnosis depends upon the clinical course and the observation of spirochetes in the peripheral blood by darkfield examination or by use of Wright's stain, Giemsa stain, or acridine orange stain on thick smears or buffy coat smears. Aids to diagnosis include inoculation of blood in mice and proteus OX-K agglutinin serology.

Complications

Complications include meningitis, iridocyclitis, epistaxis, myocarditis, and intrauterine infection, which can lead to abortion or neonatal disease.

Treatment

Treatment with erythromycin, penicillin, tetracyclines, or chloramphenicol is successful. As with syphilis and leptospirosis, the Jarisch–Herxheimer reaction may occur in the first 24 hours of treatment.

Prophylaxis

Limiting contact with lice and ticks by good hygiene, appropriate clothing, and insect repellants is appropriate.

Prognosis

Prognosis is good except in debilitated patients.

LYME DISEASE

Lyme disease, caused by the spirochete *Borrelia burgdorferi*, is a multisystem disorder that is prevalent in the USA (upper Atlantic coast, Midwest, and West coast), Europe, and Australia. The major vectors are ticks, particularly *Ixodes* ticks.

Clinical Findings

A. Symptoms and Signs: The majority of patients develop an annular erythematous skin lesion—erythema chronicum migrans—at the site of a tick bite; the incubation period is 3–32 days. More extensive rashes, conjunctivitis, fever, malaise, or meningitis may also develop. Weeks to months later, involvement of several organ systems may occur: neurologic (Bell's palsy, cranial or peripheral neuritis, meningitis), cardiac (conduction block, myocarditis), or joints (chronic arthritis). These later findings may develop without the prior appearance of erythema chronicum migrans. Anecdotes of apparent intrauterine infection with adverse pregnancy outcome have been reported.

B. Laboratory Findings: The most widely available diagnostic test is the ELISA serology. Antibody may not be detectable for several weeks following onset of infection, and sensitivity and specificity may be lacking. Culture is not routinely available and lacks sensitivity.

Treatment

A. Specific Measures: Oral tetracycline, penicillin V, or erythromycin for 10–20 days is recommended for early disease (erythema chronicum migrans). High-dose intravenous penicillin G for 10 days is recommended once the later stages of disease have developed.

B. General Measures: Nonsteroidal anti-inflammatory agents may be useful for patients with arthritis.

Prophylaxis

The major preventive measure is to avoid tick exposure, eg, by wearing protective clothing in endemic areas, and to remove ticks promptly.

Prognosis

Patients treated early in the infection generally have a favorable course; patients with delayed therapy have more chronic courses.

Infectious Diseases: Protozoal & Metazoal | 16

Mark J. Abzug, MD

PROTOZOAL DISEASES

MALARIA

Malaria is an acute or chronic febrile disease caused by one of 4 types of plasmodia: *Plasmodium vivax, P malariae, P falciparum,* or *P ovale.* Transmission occurs through the bite of the female *Anopheles* mosquito, in which the sexual cycle of the parasite occurs. The asexual cycle occurs in humans.

Clinical Findings

In children, malaria does not always present the classic clinical picture seen in adults.

A. Symptoms and Signs: Sudden onset of paroxysms of fever to 39.5–40.5 °C (103–105 °F) may be accompanied by seizures in the very young. Chills are sometimes present, last at least 2–4 hours, and are followed by sweating. In young children, paroxysms may be continuous or very irregularly recurrent. In older children, recurrence of paroxysms varies with type of infection: 48 hours for *P vivax, P falciparum,* and *P ovale* infections and 72 hours for *P malariae* infection. Diarrhea and vomiting are frequent and splenomegaly is usually present. Hemolysis may lead to clinical jaundice and pallor. The child may be asymptomatic or have mild manifestations of illness between paroxysms.

B. Laboratory Findings: There is rapid onset of anemia, and serum bilirubin levels are increased. Thin and thick blood smears and bone marrow smears show parasites.

Complications

"Blackwater fever" is rare in childhood. It is usually associated with *P falciparum* infection and is characterized by hemoglobinuria and shocklike state. Coagulopathy, encephalopathy, and multiorgan failure may also result from *P falciparum* infection. Transplacental infection can occur. Nephrosis may complicate chronic *P malariae* infection.

Treatment

A. Specific Measures: Treatment is dictated in part by the malarial species involved and the region in which infection was contracted.

1. Chloroquine–Chloroquine phosphate (Aralen), given once daily orally for 3 days, is the drug of choice for *P vivax, P ovale, P malariae,* and nonresistant *P falciparum* infections.

If oral therapy is not possible, give intravenous quinine dihydrochloride (see below), and begin oral chloroquine as soon as possible.

2. Quinine, pyrimethamine, and sulfadiazine–In chloroquine-resistant *P falciparum* infection, fever will persist for more than 48 hours. Stop chloroquine; start concurrent oral quinine sulfate (3 days), pyrimethamine (3 days), and sulfadiazine (5 days).

Intravenous quinine dihydrochloride is used for patients who cannot tolerate oral medication. Oral therapy should be initiated once it becomes possible.

3. Primaquine phosphage–Use with chloroquine to prevent relapses in patients with *P vivax* and *P ovale* infections. Give orally once daily for 14 days. Patients should be screened for glucose-6-phosphate dehydrogenase (G6PD) deficiency before primaquine is begun.

B. General Measures: Fluid therapy is most important. Urge oral intake and, if not satisfactory, give parenteral fluids. Control high fever. Treat anemia with iron.

Prophylaxis

Pregnant women from nonendemic areas should be discouraged from traveling to malarial areas. Although chloroquine can be given safely in standard prophylactic doses during pregnancy, other antimicrobials may be fetotoxic.

Since true prophylaxis (prevention of infection by the destruction of sporozoites) is unavailable for travelers to endemic areas, a drug is given that suppresses schizogony and clinical symptoms. The most commonly used suppressive drug is chloroquine, given orally each week, beginning 1 week before travel to an endemic area and continued for 6 weeks after return from the endemic region. Travelers to areas where *P ovale* and *P vivax* are endemic should also generally be given primaquine phosphate for 14 days after departure from the endemic region, to prevent relapses (rule out G6PD deficiency before beginning primaquine).

Falciparum malaria resistant to chloroquine is widespread in Southeast Asia, Indonesia, some islands of the South Pacific (including the Philippines and Papua New Guinea), and South America and has been documented in the Indian subcontinent, East Africa, and parts of Panama. Chemoprophylaxis with chloroquine is not always effective in these areas. The combination of pyrimethamine and sulfadoxine (Fansidar) in a single tablet has been found to be effective against many but not all strains of chloroquine-resistant *P falciparum*. In recent years, there have been more deaths from complications of pyrimethamine–sulfadoxine use than chloroquine-resistant malaria in US travelers. Therefore, rather than receiving routine prophylaxis, travelers with short exposure (3 weeks or less) in high-risk areas for chloroquine-resistant falciparum malaria should carry a therapeutic dose to take if fever occurs and there is no access to medical help (in addition to taking routine chloroquine prophylaxis against nonfalciparum species).

Caution: Pyrimethamine–sulfadoxine is contraindicated in patients with a history of sulfonamide or pyrimethamine intolerance and in infants under 2 months of age. Severe, sometimes fatal, cutaneous reactions (such as Stevens–Johnson syndrome) have occurred; if any mucocutaneous signs or symptoms develop, the drug should be stopped immediately.

Daily doxycycline is an alternative for travelers to areas with chloroquine-resistant *P falciparum;* it is especially useful in areas where *P falciparum* is resistant to chloroquine and pyrimethamine–sulfadoxine.

Since most malarial vectors are night biters, mosquito nets to sleep in and mosquito repellants are important preventive measures. While chemoprophylaxis and environmental engineering or chemical control of mosquito populations currently represent the most feasible mass preventive measures, biologic control of mosquitoes and malarial vaccines are under study for future use.

People who have traveled to areas endemic for malaria should seek medical care if they develop fever after return from their travel—even if they have taken prophylactic medication.

Prognosis

In the majority of cases, the prognosis is excellent with proper therapy. In small infants and in the presence of malnutrition or chronic debilitating disease, the prognosis is more guarded.

AMEBIASIS

Amebiasis is an acute and chronic enteric infection with *Entamoeba histolytica*. Transmission from an infected person or a carrier is through the cysts, which are excreted in feces. The cyst may survive as long as 1 month in water. The disease is aquired by the oral route through contamination of food or drinking water or by person-to-person contact.

Clinical Findings

A. Symptoms and Signs: Amebic infection is most frequently asymptomatic or presents with mild gastrointestinal symptoms. Acute amebic dysentery is characterized by the sudden onset of diarrhea, which lasts about 1 week. The frequency of stools varies with the age of the child, being higher in infants and occurring only 2 or 3 times daily in older children. Stools are bloody and mucoid; other symptoms may include fever and abdominal pain. Atypical amebiasis, common in children, presents with mild recurrent diarrhea, irritability, anorexia, and slight abdominal pain (most often in the right upper quadrant).

B. Laboratory Findings: In the acute stage of infection, stool examination may show trophozoites. Cysts are excreted in cycles, and repeated stool examinations may be necessary. Biopsy of rectal mucosa sometimes provides a definitive diagnosis. Serologic testing is relatively sensitive for invasive disease but not for intestinal disease.

Complications

Amebic abscess of the liver is rare in early childhood but should always be considered. Early symptoms include relief of hunger by extremely small amounts of food and hiccupping as a result of diaphragmatic irritation. Liver scanning with radioisotopes and CT scans may provide useful diagnostic findings. Rarely, other sites may develop amebic abscesses via seeding from a primary hepatic or colonic focus.

Treatment

A. Specific Measures: Asymptomatic or mild infection is treated with a lumenal amebocide, either iodoquinol, diloxanide furoate, or paromomycin. More severe intestinal disease or hepatic abscess is treated with both a tissue and a lumenal amebocide, eg, with metronidazole and iodoquinol; emetine, chloroquine phosphate, and iodoquinol is an alternative regimen.

B. General Measures: Institute dietary measures for diarrhea (see Chapter 22) and take precautions with the disposal of stools and care of diapers.

Prognosis & Prophylaxis

The prognosis is excellent with adequate treatment and follow-up. Proper disposal of excreta and precautions in regard to drinking water are preventive measures.

GIARDIASIS

Giardiasis is caused by a flagellate, *Giardia lamblia*. Cysts are the infectious form and may be transmitted person to person or by ingestion of contaminated water or food.

Clinical Findings

A. Symptoms and Signs: The organism may infest the duodenum and jejunum without producing symptoms, or (especially in children) it may cause a chronic watery diarrhea or steatorrhea, abdominal cramping, and malaise. Failure to thrive may result from anorexia and malabsorption.

B. Laboratory Findings: The diagnosis is usually based on identification of cysts and trophozoites in the stool; multiple stool examinations may be needed. Duodenal aspiration or biopsy may be necessary to demonstrate the organisms if stools are repeatedly negative.

Treatment

A. Specific Measures: Furazolidone (Furoxone) is the drug of choice in young children because of its availability in suspension form and its good patient acceptance. Alternative drugs include metronidazole and quinacrine; the latter has a bitter taste and may cause skin discoloration and the former has an unknown safety profile in young children. Recurrence in 3 to 4 weeks is not unusual and should be an indication for repeat therapy.

B. General Measures: Rehydration, nutritional support, or both, may be required for children with more than mild disease.

Prophylaxis

Appropriate hand washing and other sanitary practices are essential, particularly in settings that are high-risk for transmission of giardia, eg, daycare centers. Water from streams used by campers should be boiled prior to use and municipal water supplies should be filtered.

Prognosis

The prognosis is good with appropriate diagnosis and therapy.

TRICHOMONIASIS

Trichomoniasis is caused by *Trichomonas vaginalis,* a flagellate protozoon. Infection is usually spread by sexual intercourse with an asymptomatic male carrier.

Clinical Findings
A. Symptoms and Signs: The symptoms are vaginitis and cervicitis with intense itching and a frothy discharge that is usually yellow-green with a characteristic "fishy" odor. Other symptoms may include abdominal pain and dysuria. Males may have urethritis or prostatitis. Trichomoniasis is very rare in patients before menarche.
B. Laboratory Findings: The diagnosis is usually made by visualization of the organism in a wet mount of vaginal secretions.

Treatment
Treatment with oral metronidazole is most effective. The male sexual partner should be treated concomitantly. Metronidazole should not be used in the first trimester of pregnancy; instead, clotrimazole may be used to reduce symptoms.

Prognosis
The prognosis for patients with vaginal trichomoniasis is excellent although reinfection or relapse may occur.

TOXOPLASMOSIS

Toxoplasma gondii, an obligate intracellular parasite, is found worldwide in humans and in many species of animals and birds. The parasite is a coccidian of cats, the definitive host. Human infection occurs by ingestion of oocysts from cat feces, by ingestion of cysts in raw or undercooked meat, by transplacental transmission, or, rarely, by direct inoculation of trophozoites, as in blood transfusion.

Clinical Findings
A. Symptoms and Signs:
1. Congenital toxoplasmosis–Congenital transmission occurs only as a result of acute infection *during* pregnancy and may occur in any trimester. Infection has been detected in up to 1% of women during pregnancy; about 45% of women who acquire the

primary infection during pregnancy and who are not treated will give birth to congenitally infected infants. Signs of congenital toxoplasmosis are present at birth in 10% of infected infants. The others may develop symptoms in the first months of life. Symptoms and signs of congenital toxoplasmosis include microcephaly, seizures, mental retardation, hepatosplenomegaly, jaundice, thrombocytopenia, pneumonitis, rash, fever, chorioretinitis, and cerebral calcification. Chorioretinitis is usually a late sequela of congenital infection, with symptoms being first noted in the second or third decade of life.

2. Toxoplasmosis in the immunocompromised host–Toxoplasmosis may present as a disseminated disease, particularly in patients given immunosuppressive drugs or patients with acquired immunodeficiency syndrome or lymphoreticular, hematologic, or other malignant diseases. Encephalitis and focal brain abscesses are the most common manifestations; pneumonitis and myocarditis may also occur.

3. Acquired toxoplasmosis–

a. There may be febrile lymphadenopathy resembling infectious mononucleosis but with a more prolonged course (sometimes 2–6 months) and with intermittent exacerbations.

b. There may be febrile disease without symptoms or signs of specific organ system involvement. Transient morbilliform rash may appear. A prolonged and recurrent course is not uncommon.

c. Chorioretinitis, with acute onset in children or young adults, may be recurrent and prolonged (almost pathognomonic of toxoplasmosis).

B. Laboratory Findings: The white blood cell count and differential count may resemble infectious mononucleosis (see Chapter 14) or may be entirely normal. The heterophil antibody titer is rarely elevated. The Sabin–Feldman dye test results become positive after initial infection and are positive in the mother of the child with congenital infection. Complement fixation, indirect hemagglutination, immunofluorescent antibody (IFA), and IgM-IFA tests are available in special laboratories and research institutes. A seroconversion or 4-fold rise in IgG titer, a very high single IgG titer, or a positive IgM test will confirm the clinical diagnosis. To diagnose congenital infection, maternal and neonatal sera should be analyzed simultaneously for IgG and IgM. A positive neonatal IgM or a very high or rising IgG level suggests the diagnosis of congenital toxoplasmosis. Toxoplasmosis can be diagnosed occasionally by histologic examination of tissue or by isolation of the parasite in bone marrow aspirates, cerebrospinal fluid sediment, sputum, blood, and other tissue and body fluids.

Only isolation from body fluids confirms acute infection; isolation from tissues could represent chronic infection.

C. X-Ray Findings: Skull x-rays or head CT scans show intracranial calcifications in recovered congenital infection.

Treatment

Treatment is indicated in immunocompromised patients, in pregnant women with acute infection, in congenitally infected infants with or without symptoms, and in patients with acquired disease whose symptoms persist for more than 2 weeks or who have active chorioretinitis.

A. Specific Measures:

1. Pyrimethamine, folinic acid, and sulfadiazine or trisulfapyrimidines–Treatment is with a combination of pyrimethamine (Daraprim), folinic acid (calcium leucovorin), and either sulfadiazine or trisulfapyrimidines (Terfonyl). The duration of therapy is determined by the severity of illness; treatment is usually administered for 1 to several months. Pyrimethamine should not be used during the first trimester of pregnancy as it is teratogenic in animals.

2. Prednisone–For patients with chorioretinitis, prednisone may be used if disease is progressive.

Prophylaxis in Pregnant Women

Since approximately 90% of women infected during pregnancy are asymptomatic, diagnosis in the pregnant woman can be made only by serologic (screening) methods. Pregnant women may have their serum examined for *Toxoplasma* IgG antibody, and an IgM-IFA test can be done (if facilities are available) when conventional IgG tests are positive at any titer. If the IgM-IFA test result is negative, no further evaluation is necessary. Women with negative IgG titers and pregnant women who do not know their toxoplasmosis status should take measures to prevent infection: (1) Avoid contact with or wear gloves when handling materials that are potentially contaminated (eg, cat litter boxes) or when gardening. (2) Avoid eating raw or undercooked meat. (3) Wash hands thoroughly after handling raw meat. (4) Wash fruits and vegetables before consumption. These same suggestions apply to the nonpregnant population, especially those who are immunosuppressed.

Prognosis

Nearly all children with congenital toxoplasmosis who are asymptomatic or have only mild abnormalities in the first year of life will subsequently develop untoward sequelae such as ophthalmologic and neurologic handicaps.

PNEUMOCYSTIS PNEUMONIA

Pneumocystis is an interstitial pneumonitis occurring in infants and children with low-resistance syndromes (eg, when receiving corticosteroids or cytotoxic drugs for neoplasms or transplants, from inborn or acquired immunodeficiency, or related to malnutrition and/or prematurity). It has emerged as a major problem in patients with acquired immunodeficiency syndrome (AIDS). The causative organism, *P carinii,* has not been classified definitively, although it is most commonly believed to be either a fungus related to the yeasts or a sporozoon.

Clinical Findings

X-rays show an interstitial pneumonitis, and physical signs may include tachypnea, dyspnea, cough, and fever. Hypoxemia is characteristically present. The diagnosis may be established by lung puncture biopsy or open lung biopsy, or by staining of bronchoscopic brush biopsy specimens or washes or of induced sputum specimens.

Treatment

A. Specific Measures: Trimethoprim–sulfamethoxazole is the treatment of choice, given intravenously or orally. Pentamidine isethionate, given by the intravenous or intramuscular routes, is also an effective therapy, but can have significant toxicities. New therapeutic regimens involving aerosolized pentamidine, oral trimetrexate, and other drugs are being studied.

B. General Measures: Oxygen, and, if needed, mechanical ventilation are important supportive measures. The cause of lowered resistance should be eliminated if known and possible.

Prophylaxis

Use of trimethoprim combined with sulfamethoxazole in subtherapeutic doses may prevent infection in patients at risk if administered throughout the period of increased susceptibility. Other potentially useful proplylactic regimens include aerosolized pentamidine and oral pyrimethamine–sulfadoxine (Fansidar).

CRYPTOSPORIDIOSIS

Cryptosporidium is a protozoan that has been implicated in diarrheal illnesses of normal and immunocompromised hosts. It is transmitted person to person and via ingestion of contaminated water.

Clinical Findings

A. Symptoms and Signs: Watery diarrhea, which may be associated with abdominal pain and anorexia, but usually is without systemic toxicity, is common. Untreated, the diarrhea resolves within several weeks in normal children; in immunocompromised patients, especially those with AIDS, diarrhea may be chronic and severe, resulting in malnourishment.

B. Laboratory Findings: Oocysts are identified in stool by staining with a modified acid-fast stain or a monoclonal antibody. Intestinal biopsy may also reveal the parasite.

Treatment

A. Specific Measures: No specific therapy is needed in normal hosts. Spiramycin and other medications are being studied for immunocompromised hosts.

B. General Measures: Rehydration and nourishment.

Prognosis

The prognosis is excellent in immunocompetent children; chronic enteritis may occur in immunodeficient patients. Dissemination outside of the gastrointestinal tract may occasionally occur in immunodeficient hosts.

METAZOAL DISEASES

Metazoal diseases are outlined in Table 16–1.

Table 16-1. Diseases caused by helminths.

Agent	Geographic Prevalence	Definitive Host (Mature Worms)	Intermediate Host (Larval Stages)	Route of Human Infection	Directly Communicable Human to Human	Eggs in Human Feces	Stage of Parasite Causing Disease	Pathology	Diagnostic Tests	Specific Treatment (Drugs Listed in Order of Preference)
Ancylostoma braziliense, A caninum (cat and dog hookworm)	Southern USA	Cats, dogs	Humans	Invasion of larvae in soil through skin	No	No	Larva	Cutaneous larva migrans, with serpiginous skin eruption at site of entry.	Clinical diagnosis	Self-limited; freezing, thiabenda-zole
Ancylostoma duodenale, Necator americanus (hookworm)	Tropics and subtropics, Europe, Asia	Humans	—	Larvae in soil enter through skin	Yes	Yes	Larva in skin and lungs; adult in bowel	Dermatitis and pneumonitis in larval stage; anemia, melena, anorexia from adult worm in bowel.	Detection of ova in stool	Mebendazole, pyrantel pamoate, bephenium hydroxynaph-thoate
Ascaris lumbricoides (roundworm)	Tropics and areas with poor sanitation	Humans	—	Ingestional of eggs in soil	Yes (via soil)	Yes	Larva in lungs; adult in bowel	Pneumonitis in larval stage; adult worm may cause intestinal obstruction, abdominal pain, peritonitis.	Detection of ova or adult worms in stool	Pyrantel pamoate, mebendazole, pyrvinium pamoate, piperazine

(continued)

525

Table 16-1. (continued)

Agent	Geographic Prevalence	Definitive Host (Mature Worms)	Intermediate Host (Larval Stages)	Route of Human Infection	Directly Communicable Human to Human	Eggs in Human Feces	Stage of Parasite Causing Disease	Pathology	Diagnostic Tests	Specific Treatment (Drugs Listed in Order of Preference)
Diphyllobothrium latum (fish tapeworm)	Worldwide	Humans, other mammals	Copepods, fish	Ingestion of fish containing larval worms	No	Yes	Adult	Vitamin B_{12} deficiency; intestinal irritation; anemia.	Identification of ova or proglottids in stool	Niclosamide, paromomycin, praziquantel
Dipylidium caninum (dog tapeworm)	Worldwide	Dogs, cats, humans	Fleas	Ingestion of fleas containing larval worms	No	Yes	Adult	Intestinal irritation.	Identification of ova in stool	Niclosamide, paromomycin
Echinococcus granulosus (unilocular hydatid cyst)	Scattered foci worldwide	Dogs, wolves	Domestic and wild herbivores, (including sheep), humans	Ingestion of worm eggs from canine feces	No	No	Larva (hydatid)	Circumscribed unilocular cysts in lung, liver, other viscera.	History, radiographs, serology, biopsies	Surgical removal, mebendazole, albendazole.
Echinococcus multilocularis (alveolar hydatid cyst)	Northern hemisphere	Foxes, dogs	Field rodents, humans	Ingestion of worm eggs from canine feces	No	No	Larva (hydatid)	Invasive multilocular cysts in liver.	History, radiographs, biopsies, serology	Surgical removal
Enterobius vermicularis (pinworm)	Worldwide	Humans	—	Ingestion of eggs on clothing, on food, in dust, etc	Yes	Yes	Adult female	Anal irritation and itching; vaginal inflammation; abdominal pain.	Scotch tape exam under microscope	Same as *Ascaris*

Hymenolepis diminuta (rat tapeworm)	Worldwide	Rodents, humans	Arthropods	Ingestion of arthropods containing larval worms	No	Yes	Adult	Intestinal irritation.	Detection of ova in stool	Niclosamide, paromomycin
Hymenolepis nana (dwarf tapeworm)	Worldwide in warm climates	Humans, rodents	Humans, rodents	Ingestion of worm eggs from human feces or infected insects	Yes	Yes	Adult	Intestinal irritation.	Detection of ova in stool	Niclosamide, paromomycin, praziquantel
Schistosoma mansoni, S japonicum, S haematobium (blood flukes)	S mansoni—tropics; S japonicum—Far East, SE Asia; S haematobium—Africa, Asia	Humans	Snails	Invasion of skin by cercariae in bodies of fresh water	No	Yes (S mansoni and S japonicum) (S haematobium in urine)	Adult	Maturation in veins draining intestines (S mansoni, S japonicum) or bladder (S haematobium), producing enteritis, hepatomegaly, portal hypertension, or hematuria and urinary symptoms.	Demonstration of eggs in stool or urine, tissue biopsies, serology	Praziquantel, oxamniquine (S mansoni), metriphonate (S haematobium), surgical removal
Strongyloides stercoralis (threadworm)	Tropics and subtropics	Humans, dogs, cats	—	Larvae enter through skin	Yes	Rare	Larva and adult	Penumonitis and intestinal irritation; disseminated disease in immuno-compromised host.	Identification of larvae in stool or duodenal aspirate; serology	Thiabendazole

(continued)

527

Table 16-1. (continued)

Agent	Geographic Prevalence	Definitive Host (Mature Worms)	Intermediate Host (Larval Stages)	Route of Human Infection	Directly Communicable Human to Human	Eggs in Human Feces	Stage of Parasite Causing Disease	Pathology	Diagnostic Tests	Specific Treatment (Drugs Listed in Order of Preference)
Taenia saginata (beef tapeworm)	Africa, Central and South America, Europe, Asia	Humans	Cattle	Ingestion of beef containing larval worms	No	Yes	Adult	Intestinal irritation with nausea, diarrhea.	Identification of ova or proglottids in stool, serology	Niclosamide, paromomycin
Taenia solium (pork tapeworm)	Africa, Asia, Central and South America, Europe	Humans	Hogs	Ingestion of pork containing larval worms	Yes	Yes	Adult	Intestinal irritation with nausea, diarrhea.	Identification of ova or proglottids in stool, serology	Niclosamide, paromomycin
			Humans	Ingestion of worm eggs from human feces	No	No	Larva (cysticercus)	Cysticercosis with lesions in muscles, brain, viscera, eyes. Seizures common.	Muscle biopsy; CT scan (head); serology	Surgical removal, praziquantel, corticosteroids
Toxocara canis, T cati (dog and cat roundworm)	North America, Europe	Dogs, cats	Humans	Ingestion of worm eggs in soil	No	No	Larva	Visceral larva migrans with fever, systemic symptoms, and infection of eyes, lung, heart, brain, liver.	Eosinophilia, organ biopsy, serology	Thiabendazole, diethyl-carbamazine, corticosteroids

Trichinella spiralis (trichina worm)	Worldwide	Hogs, bears, rats	Hogs, bears, rats, humans	Ingestion of larvae in meat	No	No	Larva in muscle, heart, and brain	Encystment of larvae in tissue (especially muscle) causes necrosis and inflammation. Symptoms produced include diarrhea, myalgia, fever, periorbital edema, urticaria, headache, myocardial failure.	Eosinophilia, serology, muscle biopsy, exam of suspect meat	Thiabendazole, mebendazole, corticosteroids
Trichuris trichiura (whipworm)	Worldwide	Humans	—	Ingestion of eggs in soil	Yes (via soil)	Yes	Adult	Adult worm in mucosa of colon usually produces no reactions or symptoms. Abdominal pain, colitis, and rectal prolapse may occur in severe infections.	Identification of ova in stool	Mebendazole

(continued)

529

Table 16–1. (continued)

Agent	Geographic Prevalence	Definitive Host (Mature Worms)	Intermediate Host (Larval Stages)	Route of Human Infection	Directly Communicable Human to Human	Eggs in Human Feces	Stage of Parasite Causing Disease	Pathology	Diagnostic Tests	Specific Treatment (Drugs Listed in Order of Preference)
Wuchereria bancrofti, Brugia malayi, B timori (filaria)	Tropics, subtropics	Humans	Humans, mosquitoes	Bite by infected mosquito	No	No	Adult	Inflammation or obstruction of lymphatics, producing lymphadenopathy, lymphangitis, edema of extremities and genitalia.	Demonstration of microfilariae in blood, tissue biopsies, serology	Diethylcarbamazine citrate, ivermectin, corticosteroids, surgical removal, treatment of superinfections

Infectious Diseases: Mycotic | 17

Mark J. Abzug, MD

Several systemic mycoses, including coccidioidomycosis, histoplasmosis, cryptococcosis, and paracoccidioidomycosis, share a number of characteristics. Infection of humans occurs through inhalation of free-living infectious spores of the fungus, which are present in the dust in endemic areas. Primary pulmonary infections are usually mild or asymptomatic, and most infections have a tendency to heal, mainly through cellular immune mechanisms. Results of specific skin tests become positive after primary infection and remain positive throughout life. In a few specifically predisposed persons, the disease progresses after primary infection, becomes disseminated and involves many organs, and may be fatal. Similar dissemination may occur years after primary infection if the person is immunosuppressed by disease (eg, lymphoma) or drugs.

COCCIDIOIDOMYCOSIS

Coccidioidomycosis is caused by inhalation of arthrospores of *Coccidioides immitis,* a fungus that grows in the soil of certain arid regions of the southwestern USA, Mexico, and Central and South America. Two-thirds of infections are subclinical and diagnosed only by positive skin test results.

Clinical Findings
A. Symptoms and Signs:
1. Primary infection–About 10–30 days after exposure, there may be symptoms of respiratory tract infection, with fever, headache, muscular aches and pains, nasopharyngitis, and bronchitis with cough. One to 2 weeks later, there may be arthralgia, erythema nodosum, or erythema multiforme. All of these tend to subside spontaneously, but a thin-walled pulmonary cavity develops in about 5% of pulmonary lesions. These may take months to close.
2. Disseminated disease–Dissemination occurs in 0.1% of white and 1% of nonwhite persons after primary infection. Racial susceptibility is high in Filipinos, Mexicans, and blacks, and

dissemination usually begins within 1–2 years after infection or following immunosuppression by disease or drugs. Pneumonia; empyema; involvement of bones, soft tissues (with abscesses and sinus tracts), and abdominal viscera; and meningitis (with a high mortality rate) may occur as a result of dissemination.

B. Laboratory Findings: In primary infection, the sedimentation rate is elevated, there may be mild leukocytosis, and chest x-ray examination may show parenchymal densities and enlarged hilar nodes. Precipitating antibodies develop within a few weeks and then decline as the patient recovers. At the same time, results of the coccidioidin skin test (1:100 dilution) become positive and remain so for many years in the well person. Antibody titers in the complement fixation (CF) test rise and fall more slowly. However, if dissemination occurs, the antibody titer in the CF test characteristically rises and remains high, while the coccidioidin skin test results are often negative. Culture of sputum, drainage fluid, cerebrospinal fluid, or biopsy specimens requires extreme caution. Laboratory-grown *Coccidioides* are *extremely* infectious. Smears of patient specimens (sputum, cerebrospinal fluid, biopsies, urine) may reveal spherules.

Treatment

A. Primary Infection: Primary coccidioidomycosis is usually a self-limited illness requiring no therapy. As the person recovers, substantial cellular immunity develops; results of the delayed-type skin test with coccidioidin are positive.

B. Disseminated Disease: In dissemination, cellular immunity is defective. Unrestrained multiplication of the fungus takes place, producing lesions in many organs. The most commonly used drug is amphotericin B intravenously, for progressive pulmonary disease, disseminated infection, and central nervous system infection. Intravenous amphotericin is supplemented by intrathecal or intraventricular amphotericin for central nervous system infections. Ketoconazole has also been used for coccidioidomycosis, supplemented by intraventricular miconazole in cases with neurologic involvement. Duration of therapy for serious infection is prolonged ($\geq$ 1 month), particularly if there is neurologic involvement.

Surgical excision of infected tissue may complement medical therapy. Shunting of cerebrospinal fluid is often needed to control hydrocephalus associated with central nervous system infection.

Prognosis

The prognosis is excellent in patients with primary infection, fair for prolonged survival in patients with disseminated disease who are intensively treated and show active cell-mediated reactions, and guarded for cure of patients with meningitis.

HISTOPLASMOSIS

Histoplasmosis is caused by inhalation of spores of *Histoplasma capsulatum* in dust. The organism grows profusely in bird feces, bat guano, and farm silos, and inhalation of dust from these sources causes massive infection. In the USA, most infections originate in the Central and Southern regions.

Clinical Findings
A. Symptoms and Signs:
1. Primary infection–Primary histoplasmosis is commonly asymptomatic or presents as a nonspecific influenzalike illness. Massive primary infection may produce pneumonitis with fever, cough, chest pain, and prostration. There may be enlargement of the lymph nodes, spleen, and liver. In most cases, all primary lesions heal.

2. Disseminated disease–Disseminated histoplasmosis develops in a small percentage of heavily exposed or immunodeficient persons, most commonly white males over 40 years of age and children under 2 years. Fever, anemia, diffuse lymphadenopathy, hepatomegaly, splenomegaly, pneumonitis, and severe prostration occur. Tumorlike granulomas in the skin may ulcerate, and there may be multiple bone lesions. The course is progressive and often fatal.

B. Laboratory Findings: Leukopenia is common and anemia marked in progressive disease. The erythrocyte sedimentation rate is commonly elevated during activity. Intracellular budding of yeast cells may be seen in biopsies of bone marrow, lymph nodes, or skin and (rarely) in sputum. The fungus can be cultured from such specimens. During primary infection, results of the histoplasmin skin test become positive and remain so for many years. Skin test results may be negative in disseminated disease. Repeated application of the histoplasmin skin test in nonreactors stimulates antibody development. Antibodies to histoplasmin can be demonstrated by immunodiffusion or complement fixation. A rising titer or a single high titer is associated with progressive disease.

C. Imaging: Chest x-rays may show scattered patches of consolidation. After healing of primary lesions, calcification may be visible on x-rays of lung.

Treatment

Most mild primary infections heal spontaneously and do not require therapy. In widespread or progressive histoplasmosis, treatment with amphotericin B has sometimes arrested the progress. Ketoconazole has also shown effectiveness. Medical treatment is usually continued for a period of several months. Surgical excision or drainage can be a valuable adjunct to treatment.

NORTH AMERICAN BLASTOMYCOSIS

The soil fungus *Blastomyces dermatitidis* causes a pulmonary/cutaneous syndrome and disseminated disease, principally in North, Central, and South America. Endemic areas in the USA include the central and southeastern regions. The disease is rare in children.

Clinical Findings
A. Symptoms and Signs: The cutaneous lesion is a papule that soon ulcerates and may be surrounded by very small abscesses. This is accompanied by pulmonary disease that appears on x-ray examination as massive densities radiating from mediastinal lymph nodes. The disseminated disease may follow the pulmonary/cutaneous syndrome and presents with cough, fever, spread of the cutaneous lesions, and sometimes central nervous system involvement with brain abscesses and coma. Abdominal viscera, bone, and muscles may also be involved.
B. Laboratory Findings: Diagnosis can be made by visualization of the yeast forms in secretions, culture, serology, and/or skin testing.

Treatment

Treatment usually includes amphotericin B; ketoconazole may be used for mild to moderate disease.

PARACOCCIDIOIDOMYCOSIS
(South American Blastomycosis)

Paracoccidioidomycosis is an infection caused by the soil organism *Paracoccidioides brasiliensis*. It occurs in Central and South America. In children, there are frequently skin and mucous membrane lesions that may disseminate to the lymph nodes, lung, and gut. The organism, seen as a yeast cell with multiple buds, can be cultured from biopsy material or pus. Serologic testing may also be useful.

Ketoconazole has proved effective; miconazole and amphotericin B have also been used.

CRYPTOCOCCOSIS

Cryptococcus neoformans lives in soil worldwide and grows profusely in bird feces. Inhalation of dust results in pulmonary infection.

Clinical Findings

A. Symptoms and Signs: Pulmonary infection is usually asymptomatic but sometimes causes an influenzalike illness, with pulmonary consolidation visible on x-ray. The most common clinical presentation is an indolent fungal meningitis in immunocompromised patients. The spinal fluid shows an increase in pressure, cell count, and protein content and a decrease in glucose content. Budding yeast cells with a large capsule can be seen in India ink preparations of the cerebrospinal fluid, and cryptococcal polysaccharide may be present in cerebrospinal fluid. Cryptococcal meningitis is typically characterized by exacerbations and remissions. There may also be bone or skin lesions and lymphadenopathy.

B. Laboratory Findings: Diagnosis may be made by identifying the yeast in smears of sputum, cerebrospinal fluid, or pus (India ink stain); culture; or latex agglutination testing.

Treatment

Mild pulmonary infection in normal hosts ordinarily does not require therapy. In patients with meningitis and other serious cryptococcal infections, treatment for months with amphotericin B intravenously, and with flucytosine orally, has induced protracted remissions. Intrathecal amphotericin B may help to speed the initial response. Miconazole may also be useful. Surgical removal of local tissue granulomas can be effective. Remissions for many years have occurred, but absolute eradication of the organism is difficult in immunocompromised patients.

CANDIDIASIS

Candida albicans and other *Candida* species are found in the normal flora of human mucous membranes, especially in the respiratory, gastrointestinal, and female genital tracts. In these locations, *Candida* may proliferate and produce local lesions.

Clinical Findings

A. Symptoms and Signs: Moist, warm, eroded skin in intertriginous areas, the diaper area, or nails are subject to chronic surface infection. Mucous membranes of the mouth (thrush) and vagina (vaginitis) are made more susceptible to overgrowth of *Candida* by use of antimicrobial agents that suppress normal flora or by use of corticosteroids. Rarely, *Candida* invades tissues or the bloodstream, as in patients with indwelling catheters, immunodeficiency, leukemia, parenteral drug abuse, or prematurity, and may then cause progressive systemic lesions, pneumonia, endocarditis, and involvement of other organs.

B. Laboratory Findings: Diagnosis is based on visualization of yeast and pseudohyphae in material from lesions or infected tissues or on culture of *Candida* from blood, cerebrospinal fluid, urine, or involved organs.

Treatment

Treatment consists of keeping local lesions dry and applying topical nystatin, clotrimazole, gentian violet, miconazole, or other antifungals. Ketoconazole has proved effective in many cases of esophageal candidiasis and chronic mucocutaneous disease. Treatment with amphotericin B intravenously is the approach of choice for systemic infections. Oral flucytosine is added for synergy in severe infections. Therapy is usually prolonged (weeks to months).

Prognosis

The prognosis is good for patients with local lesions but guarded for those with systemic dissemination.

SPOROTRICHOSIS

Sporothrix schenckii is a fungus that lives on plant matter. Human infection occurs when infected plant material is traumatically introduced into the skin.

Clinical Findings

A. Symptoms and Signs: Series of subcutaneous nodules or ulcers form along the lymph channels, but there is little systemic illness.

B. Laboratory Findings: Results of cultures from biopsy specimens or drainage of lesions will establish the diagnosis.

Treatment

The lesions often regress spontaneously or after treatment with oral potassium iodide solution. Amphotericin B is required in some cases.

ASPERGILLOSIS

Aspergillus is a fungus that is prevalent in soil and vegetable matter. It causes a number of clinical entities, particularly targeting patients with underlying pulmonary disease and those with immune deficiencies.

Clinical Findings
  A. Symptoms & Signs:
  1. Pulmonary disease–Allergic bronchopulmonary aspergillosis is an allergic reaction to airway colonization with *Aspergillus* that occurs in patients with underlying pulmonary disease, especially patients with cystic fibrosis. Findings include episodic fever, wheezing, eosinophilia, and fleeting pulmonary infiltrates.

Aspergillus may also form fungus balls, which grow in old lung cavities; this process is not invasive.
  2. Invasive disease–In patients with immune deficiencies, eg, those on cytotoxic chemotherapy or patients with malignancies, *Aspergillus* may be invasive, affecting the paranasal sinuses or lung most commonly. Infection may disseminate to bones, central nervous system, abdominal viscera, skin, orbit, etc.
  B. Laboratory Findings: The diagnosis of invasive disease is generally based on identification of typical branching septate hyphae in tissue specimens (potassium hydroxide, PAS, or silver stains) and/or growth of the organism from tissue specimens.

Diagnosis of allergic bronchopulmonary aspergillosis is supported by demonstration of airway colonization, elevated IgE and eosinophil levels, and serum precipitins to *Aspergillus*.

Treatment

Amphotericin B, sometimes with flucytosine, is the antifungal of choice for invasive disease. Prolonged therapy is usually required. Surgery of locally invasive lesions may be helpful.

Allergic bronchopulmonary aspergillosis usually responds to corticosteroids; antifungal therapy is not indicated.

Prophylaxis
Exposure of immunocompromised patients to *Aspergillus* should be minimized. Avoidance of construction sites and use of filtered air may be beneficial.

Prognosis
The prognosis for patients with invasive disease is guarded and is related to the degree of underlying immune deficiency.

Skin | 18

Jay Kincannon, MD, & William L. Weston, MD

Terminology

A. Primary Lesions (The First to Appear):

1. Macule–Any circumscribed color change in the skin that is flat. Examples: White (vitiligo), brown (café au lait spot), purple (petechia).

2. Papule–A solid, elevated lesion larger than 1 cm in diameter whose top may be pointed, rounded, or flat. Examples: Acne, warts, small lesion of psoriasis.

3. Plaque–A solid, circumscribed area less than 1 cm in diameter, usually flat-topped. Example: Psoriasis.

4. Vesicle–A circumscribed, elevated lesion greater than 1 cm in diameter and containing clear serous fluid. Example: Blisters of herpes simplex.

5. Bulla–A circumscribed, elevated lesion less than 1 cm in diameter and containing clear serous fluid. Example: Bullous erythema multiforme.

6. Nodule–A deep-seated mass with indistinct borders that elevates the overlying epidermis. Examples: Tumors, granuloma annular. If it moves with the skin on palpation, it is intradermal; if the skin moves over the nodule, it is subcutaneous.

7. Wheal–A circumscribed, flat-topped, firm elevation of skin resulting from tense edema of the papillary dermis. Example: Urticaria.

B. Secondary Changes:

1. Pustule–A vesicle containing a purulent exudate. Examples: Acne, folliculitis.

2. Scales–Dry, thin plates of keratinized epidermal cells (stratum corneum). Examples: Psoriasis, ichthyosis.

3. Lichenification–Dry, leathery thickening of the skin with deep and exaggerated skin lines and a shiny surface resulting from chronic rubbing of the skin. Example: Atopic dermatitis.

4. Erosion and oozing–A moist, circumscribed, slightly depressed area representing a blister base with the roof of the blister removed. Examples: Burns, bullous erythema multiforme. Most oral blisters present as erosions.

5. Crust–Dried exudate of plasma on the surface of the skin following acute dermatitis.

6. Fissure–A linear split in the skin extending through the epidermis into the dermis. Example: Angular cheilitis.

7. Scar–A flat, raised, or depressed area of fibrotic replacement of dermis or subcutaneous tissue. Examples: Acne, scar, burn scar.

8. Atrophy–Depression of the skin surface due to thinning of one or more layers of skin.

C. Color: The lesion should be described as red, yellow, brown, tan, or blue. Particular attention should be given to the blanching of red or brown lesions, eg, petechiae.

D. Configuration: Clues to diagnosis may be obtained from the characteristic morphologic arrangement of primary or secondary lesions.

1. Annular (circular)–Annular nodules represent granuloma annular; annular papules are more apt to be due to dermatophyte infections.

2. Linear (straight line)–Linear papules represent lichen striatus; linear vesicles, incontinentia pigmenti; linear papules with burrow, scabies.

3. Grouped–Grouped vesicles occur in herpes simplex or zoster.

E. Distribution: It is useful to note whether the eruption is generalized, acral (hands, feet, buttocks, or face), or localized to a specific skin region.

F. Description of Skin Lesions: Skin lesions are described in reverse order from that of their identification. One begins with distribution, followed by configuration, color, secondary changes, and then primary lesion; eg, guttate psoriasis could be described as generalized discrete, red, scaly papules.

GENERAL PRINCIPLES OF TREATMENT OF SKIN DISORDERS

Percutaneous Absorption & the Role of Water

Treatment should be simple and aimed at preserving or restoring the physiologic state of skin. It is essential to keep in mind that one is treating the child and not the anxious parent or grandparent. Topical therapy is often preferred because medication can be delivered in optimal concentrations at the exact site where it is needed.

Water is an important therapeutic agent that is often forgotten (it is the active ingredient in Burrow's solution, calamine lotion, potassium permanganate, and tannic acid soaks). When the skin is optimally hydrated, it is soft and smooth (Table 18–1). This occurs at approximately 60% environmental humidity. Since water evaporates readily from the cutaneous surface, the skin (stratum corneum of the epidermis) is dependent on the water concentration in the air, and sweating contributes little. However, if sweat is prevented from evaporating (eg, in the axilla or groin), the environmental humidity is increased and so is the hydration of the skin. As environmental humidity falls below 15–20%, the stratum corneum shrinks and cracks; the epidermal barrier is lost and allows irritants to enter the skin and induce an inflammatory response. Replacement of water will correct this if the water is not allowed to evaporate. Therefore, in treating dry and scaly skin, one would soak the skin in water for 5 minutes

Table 18–1. Bases used for topical preparations.

Base	Combined With	Uses
Liquids		Wet dressings: relieve pruritus, vasoconstrict.
	Powder	Shake lotions, drying pastes: relieve pruritus, vasoconstrict.
	Grease and emulsifier; oil in water	Vanishing cream: penetrates quickly (10–15 minutes) and thus allows evaporation.
	Excess grease and emulsifier; water in oil	Emollient cream: penetrates more slowly and thus retains moisture on skin.
Grease		Ointments: occlusive (hold material on skin for prolonged time) and prevent evaporation of water.
Powder		Enhances evaporation.

(1) Most greases are triglycerides (eg, Aquaphor, petrolatum, Eucerin).
(2) Oils are fluid fats (eg, Alpha Keri, olive oil, mineral oil).
(3) True fats (eg, lard, animal fats) contain free fatty acids that increase in amount upon standing and cause irritation.
(4) Ointments (eg, Aquaphor, petrolatum) should not be used in intertriginous areas such as the axillas, between the toes, and in the perineum, because they increase maceration. Lotions or creams are preferred in these areas.
(5) Oils and ointments hold medication on the skin for long periods of time and are therefore ideal for barriers or prophylaxis and for dried areas of skin. Medication gets into the skin more slowly from ointments.
(6) Creams carry medication into skin and are preferable for intertriginous dermatitis.
(7) Solutions, gels, or lotions should be used for scalp treatment.

and then add a barrier to prevent evaporation. Oils and ointments prevent evaporation for 8–12 hours. Thus, oils and ointments must be applied once or twice a day. In areas already occluded (axilla, diaper area), ointments or oils will merely increase retention of water and should not be used.

Overhydration (maceration) can also occur. As environmental humidity increases to 90–100%, the number of water molecules absorbed by the stratum corneum increases and the tight lipid junctions between the cells of the stratum corneum are gradually replaced by weak hydrogen bonds (water); the cells eventually become widely separated, and the epidermal barrier falls apart. This occurs in immersion foot, diaper areas, axillas, and other areas of the body exposed to excessive hydration. It is desirable to enhance evaporation of water in these areas. Exposure to less humidity and the use of powders (talcum) that take up extra water are indicated in maceration.

Evaporation of water is also cooling, vasoconstrictive ("gets the red out"), and antipruritic—all desirable objectives in the management of itchy, red skin. Water applied frequently to the skin and allowed to dry will result in drying of the skin surface.

Wet Dressing

By placing the skin in an environment where the humidity is 100% and allowing the moisture to evaporate to 60%, pruritus is relieved. Evaporation of water stimulates cold-dependent nerve fibers in the skin—thereby, theoretically, tying up the circuits so that the itching sensation coming through the pain fibers will not reach the central nervous system. Water also is vasoconstrictive, which helps reduce the erythema and decrease the inflammatory cellular response.

Gauze of 20/12 mesh is commonly used for wet dressings. Parke-Davis 4-in gauze comes in 100-yard rolls, and 5 yards is usually sufficient for application to the extremities. Curity 18-in gauze can be used for application to the trunk. An alternative is to use the "2 longjohns" technique, in which a pair of wet cotton long-sleeved and long-legged underwear is covered by a dry pair.

Warm but not hot water is used, and the gauze or longjohns are soaked in the water and then wrung out until no more drops come out. The dressings are then wrapped around the extremities and fastened with a safety pin. The wet dressing is then covered with dry flannel or dry longjohns, which will slow down the evaporation process but not completely retard it, so the wet dressings need only be changed every 3 or 4 hours.

Topical Glucocorticosteroids

Topical glucocorticosteroids (Table 18–2) can be used under wet dressings. Fluocinolone acetonide cream (Fluonid, Synalar 0.01%) is made specifically for this purpose. If these steroids are to be used, the wet dressings are removed completely and the medications replaced every 4–6 hours; this is usually sufficient to completely clear a severe generalized dermatitis. Prolonged use of this treatment will result in significant systemic absorption of steroids. Establishing a higher concentration of corticosteroid drugs in the skin by topical rather than systemic therapy will result in marked clearing. Because of the high concentration of steroids remaining in the skin, the mainstay of treatment of chronic forms of atopic dermatitis is application of topical glucocorticosteroid preparations twice daily (see Table 18–2).

DISORDERS OF THE SKIN IN NEWBORNS

Transient Diseases in the Newborn

No treatment is required for any of these disorders, although treatment may be given as noted below.

Table 18–2. Topical glucocorticosteroids.

	Concentrations (Percent)
Low potency = 1	
Hydrocortisone	1.0
Desonide	0.05
Moderate potency = 5–10	
Triamcinolone acetonide	0.025 and 0.1
Fluocinolone acetonide	0.01 and 0.025
Hydrocortisone valerate	0.2
Flurandrenolide	0.025
Flumethasone pivalate	0.03
Betamethasone valerate	0.1
Betamethasone acetate	0.2
Betamethasone dipropionate	0.05
Methylprednisolone acetate	0.25
Betamethasone benzoate	0.025
Desoximetasone	0.25
Diflorasone diacetate	0.05
High potency = 10–100	
Fluocinonide	0.05
Halcinonide	0.025 and 0.1

Milia

Multiple white papules 1 mm in diameter scattered over the forehead, nose, and cheeks are present in up to 40% of newborn infants. Histologically, they represent superficial epidermal cysts filled with keratinous material associated with the developing pilosebaceous follicle. Their intraoral counterparts are called Epstein's pearls and are even more common than facial milia. All these cystic structures spontaneously rupture and exfoliate their contents.

Sebaceous Gland Hyperplasia

Prominent yellow macules at the opening of each pilosebaceous follicle, predominantly over the nose, represent overgrowth of sebaceous glands in response to the same androgenic stimulation that occurs in adolescence.

Acne Neonatorum

Open and closed comedones, erythematous papules, and pustules identical in appearance to adolescent acne may occur in infants over the forehead, cheeks, and chin. The lesions may be present at birth but usually do not appear until 3–4 weeks of age. Spontaneous resolution occurs over a period of 6 months to a year. Rarely, neonatal acne may be a manifestation of a virilizing syndrome.

Harlequin Color Change

A cutaneous vascular phenomenon unique to neonates occurs when the infant (particularly one of low birth weight) is placed on one side. The dependent half develops an erythematous flush with a sharp demarcation at the midline, and the upper half of the body becomes pale. The color changes usually subside within a few seconds after the infant is placed supine but may persist for as long as 20 minutes.

Mottling

A lacelike pattern of dilated cutaneous vessels appears over the extremities and often on the trunk of neonates exposed to lowered room temperature. This feature is transient and usually disappears completely upon rewarming.

Erythema Toxicum

Up to 50% of term infants develop erythema toxicum. Usually at 24–48 hours of age, blotchy erythematous maculas 2–3 cm in diameter appear, most prominently on the chest but also on the back, face, and extremities. These are occasionally present at birth, and rarely have their onset after 4–5 days of life. The lesions vary in number from 2 to 3, up to as many as 100. Incidence is much higher in term infants than in premature ones. The macular erythema may fade within 24–48 hours or may progress to develop urticarial wheals in the center of the macules or, in 10% of cases, pustules. Examination of a Wright-stained smear of the lesion will reveal numerous eosinophils. This may be accompanied by peripheral blood eosinophilia of up to 20%. All the lesions fade and disappear by 5–7 days. A similar eruption in black newborns has a neutrophilic predominance and leaves hyperpigmentation.

Sucking Blisters

Bullae, either intact or in the form of an erosion representing a blister base without inflammatory borders, may occur over the forearms, wrists, thumbs, or upper lip. These presumably result from vigorous sucking in utero. They resolve without complications.

Miliaria

Obstruction of the eccrine sweat ducts occurs often in neonates and produces one of 2 clinical pictures depending upon the level of obstruction. **Miliaria crystallina** is characterized by tiny (1–2 mm) superficial grouped vesicles without erythema over intertriginous areas and adjacent skin (eg, neck and upper chest). Obstruction occurs in the stratum corneum portion of the eccrine duct. More commonly, obstruction of the eccrine duct deeper in the epidermis results in erythematous grouped papules in the same areas and is called **miliaria rubra.** Rarely, these may progress to pustules. Heat and high humidity predispose to eccrine duct port closure. Removal to a cooler environment is the treatment of choice.

Subcutaneous Fat Necrosis

Reddish or purple, sharply circumscribed, firm nodules occurring over the cheeks, buttocks, arms, and thighs and occurring between day 1 and day 7 in infants represent subcutaneous fat necrosis. Cold injury is thought to play an important role. These lesions resolve spontaneously over a period of weeks, although like all instances of fat necrosis they may calcify.

Sclerema

Premature newborns, especially those who suffer metabolic alterations (eg, metabolic acidosis, hypoglycemia, hypothermia) are susceptible to a diffused hardening of the skin that makes the skin look shiny and feel tight. Severe cold injury in undernourished infants is assumed to be the cause.

Treatment consists of protecting the infant from undue exposure to cold and repairing metabolic and nutritional deficiencies.

BIRTHMARKS

Birthmarks may involve an overgrowth of one or more of any of the normal components of skin: pigment cells, blood vessels, lymph vessels, etc. A nevus is a hamartoma of highly differentiated cells that retain their normal function.

1. PIGMENT CELL BIRTHMARKS

Mongolian Spot

A blue-black macule found over the lumbosacral area in 90% of American Indian, black, and Oriental infants is called a mongolian spot. These spots are occasionally noted over the shoulders and back and may extend over the buttocks. Histologically, they consist of spindle-shaped pigment cells located deep in the dermis. The lesions fade somewhat with time, but some traces may persist into adult life.

Café au Lait Spot

A café au lait spot is a light brown, oval macule (dark brown on black skin) that may be found anywhere on the body. Ten percent of white and 22% of black children have café au lait spots greater than 1.5 cm in their longest diameter. These lesions persist throughout life and may increase in number with age. The presence of 6 or more café au lait macules greater than 1.5 cm in their longest diameter may represent a clue to neurofibromatosis. Patients with Albright's syndrome also have increased numbers of café au lait macules. Although it has been suggested that the melanocytes of café au lait macules in neurofibromatosis contain giant pigment granules, this is not often the case in children, and their absence does not rule out neurofibromatosis.

Junctional Nevus & Compound Nevus

Dark brown or black macules, usually few in number at birth but becoming more numerous with age, represent junctional nevi. Histologically, these lesions are large clones of melanocytes at the junction of the epidermis and dermis. With aging, they may become raised (papules) and contain intradermal melanocytes, creating a compound nevus. Often the surface becomes irregular and roughened.

Lesions with variegated colors (red, white, blue), notched borders, and nonuniform, irregular surfaces should arouse a suspicion of melanoma. Ulceration and bleeding are advanced signs of melanoma.

If melanoma is a possibility, the treatment of choice is excisional biopsy for pathologic examination.

Intradermal Nevus & Blue Nevus

Brown to blue solitary papules with smooth surfaces represent intradermal nevi. When pigmentation is present deeper in the dermis, the lesions appear blue or blue-black and are called blue nevi.

Spindle & Epithelioid Cell Nevus (Juvenile Melanoma)

A reddish-brown solitary nodule appearing on the face or upper arm of a child represents a spindle and epithelioid cell nevus. The name melanoma is misleading because this tumor is biologically benign. Histologically, it consists of pigment-producing cells of bizarre shape with numerous mitoses.

Giant Pigmented Nevus (Bathing Trunk Nevus)

An irregular dark brown to black plaque over 10 cm in diameter represents a giant pigmented nevus. Often the lesions are of such size as to cover the entire trunk (bathing trunk nevi). Histologically, they are compound nevi. Transformation to malignant melanoma has been reported in as many as 10% of cases in some series, although the true incidence is probably somewhat less. Malignant change may occur at birth or at any time thereafter.

Because of the possibility of melanoma, it is currently recommended that the entire lesion be excised if feasible. The risk of melanoma and the potential for cosmetic improvement should be carefully evaluated for each patient.

2. VASCULAR BIRTHMARKS

Flat Hemangioma

Flat vascular birthmarks can be divided into 2 types: those that are orange or light red (salmon patch) and those that are dark red or bluish red (port wine stain).

A. Salmon Patch: The salmon patch (nevus flammeus) is a light red macule found over the nape of the neck, upper eyelids, and glabella. Fifty percent of infants have such lesions over their necks. Eyelid lesions fade completely within 3–6 months and glabella lesions by age 5 to 6; those on the nape of the neck fade somewhat but may persist into adult life.

B. Port Wine Stain: Port wine stains are dark red or purple maculas appearing unilaterally on the side of the face or an extremity. A port wine stain over the face may be a clue to **Sturge–Weber syndrome,** which is characterized by seizures, mental retardation, glaucoma, and hemiplegia. Most infants with unilateral port wine stains do not have Sturge–Weber syndrome, although if the angioma is in the distribution of the ophthalmic branch of the trigeminal nerve or hemihypertrophy of that side of the face exists, Sturge–Weber syndrome is more likely.

Similarly, a port wine hemangioma over an extremity may be associated with hypertrophy of the soft tissue and bone of that extremity (**Kippel–Trenaunay syndrome**).

The newest treatment consists of a pulse dye laser. Infants as young as 3–4 months of age have been successfully treated.

Strawberry Hemangioma

A red, rubbery nodule with a roughened surface is a strawberry nevus. The lesion is often not present at birth but is represented by a permanent blanched area on the skin that is supplanted at 2–4 weeks of age by red nodules. Histologically, these are often mixtures of capillary and venous elements, and although a deep nodule (cavernous hemangioma) may be part of this strawberry lesion, the biologic behavior is the same. Fifty percent resolve spontaneously by age 5; 70% by age 7; 90% by age 9; and the rest by adolescence.

Strawberry hemangiomas resolve, leaving only redundant skin, and uncomplicated ones are best treated by watchful waiting. Complications include superficial ulceration and secondary pyoderma, which are treated by topical antiseptics and observation.

Complications that require treatment are (1) thrombocytopenia due to platelet trapping within the lesion (**Kasabach–Merritt syndrome**); (2) airway obstruction (hemangiomas of the head and neck are often associated with subglottic hemangiomas); (3) visual obstruction (with resulting amblyopia); and (4) cardiac decompensation (high output failure). In these instances, the treatment of choice is prednisone, 1–2 mg/kg orally daily or every other day for 4–6 weeks.

Lymphangioma

Lymphangiomas are rubbery, skin-colored nodules occurring in the parotid area (**cystic hygromas**) or on the tongue. They often result in grotesque enlargement of soft tissue.

Surgical excision is the only treatment available, although the results are not satisfactory.

3. EPIDERMAL BIRTHMARKS

Nevus Unius Lateris & Ichthyosis Hystrix

Linear or groups of linear, warty, papular, unilateral lesions represent overgrowth of epidermis since birth. These areas may range from dirty yellow to brown or may be darkly pigmented. The histologic features of the lesions include thickening of the epidermis and elongation of the rete ridges and hyperkeratosis. Clinically, the lesions may be associated with focal motor seizures, mental subnormality, and skeletal anomalies.

Treatment once or twice daily with topical tretinoin 0.05% (retinoic acid [Retin-A]) will keep the lesions flat.

Nevus Comedonicus

The lesion known as nevus comedonicus consists of linear groups of widely dilated follicular openings plugged with keratin, giving the appearance of localized noninflammatory acne. The treatment of choice is surgical removal. If this is not feasible, topical retinoic acid is helpful.

Nevus Sebaceous

The nevus sebaceous of Jadassohn is a hamartoma of sebaceous glands and underlying apocrine glands that is diagnosed by the appearance at birth of a yellowish, hairless, smooth, plaque in the scalp or on the face. The lesion may be contiguous with an epidermal nevus on the face and constitute part of the linear epidermal nevus syndrome.

Histologically, nevus sebaceous represents an overabundance of sebaceous glands without hair follicles. At puberty, with androgenic stimulation, the sebaceous cells in the nevus divide, expanding their cellular volume, and synthesize sebum, resulting in a warty mass.

Because 15% of these lesions become basal cell carcinomas after puberty, excision before puberty is recommended.

4. CONNECTIVE TISSUE BIRTHMARKS

Connective tissue nevi are smooth, skin-colored papules 1–10 mm in diameter that are grouped on the trunk. A solitary, larger (5–10 cm) nodule is called a **shagreen patch** and is histologically indistinguishable from other connective tissue nevi that show thickened, abundant collagen bundles with or without associated increases of elastic tissue. Although the shagreen patch is a cutaneous clue to tuberous sclerosis, the other connective tissue nevi occur as isolated events.

These nevi remain throughout life, and no treatment is necessary.

HEREDITARY SKIN DISORDERS

The Ichthyoses

Ichthyosis is a term applied to several heritable diseases characterized by the presence of excessive scales on the skin. The nomenclature of this group of diseases is confusing. Major categories are listed in Table 18–3. X-linked ichthyosis is related to cholesterol sulfatase deficiency.

Control scaling with hydroxy acids, eg, 5% pyruvic, citric, lactic, or salicylic acid in petrolatum applied once or twice daily. Restoring water to the skin is also very helpful.

Epidermolysis Bullosa

The diagnostic feature of this group of diseases is the formation of hemorrhagic blisters in response to slight trauma. They can be divided into scarring and nonscarring types (Table 18–4).

Treatment usually consists of systemic antibiotics for infection, protective dressings of petrolatum or zinc oxide, and cooling the skin. If hands and feet are involved, reducing skin friction with 5% glutaraldehyde every 3 days is helpful. In recessive dystrophic epidermolysis bullosa, phenytoin (Dilantin), 3 mg/kg/d, has reduced new blister formation in most cases.

Incontinentia Pigmenti

Linear blisters in the newborn represent incontinentia pigmenti. These are replaced by hypertrophic, linear, warty bands within several months, followed by swirling brown hyperpigmentation. Most cases are thought to be X-linked dominant, lethal to the male. Mental retardation and seizures were reported in as many as 30% of cases in one series, but the true incidence is probably much less.

Table 18–3. Four major types of ichthyosis.*

Name	Age at Onset	Clinical Features	Histology	Inheritance
Ichthyosis with normal epidermal turnover				
Ichthyosis vulgaris	Childhood	Fine scales, deep palmar and plantar markings	Decreased to absent granular layer, hyperkeratosis	Autosomal dominant
X-linked ichthyosis	Birth	Palms and soles spared; thick scales that darken with age; corneal opacities in patients and carrier mothers	Hyperkeratosis	X-linked
Ichthyosis with increased epidermal turnover				
Epidermolytic hyperkeratosis	Birth	Verrucous, yellow scales in flexural areas and palms and soles	Hyperkeratosis, vacuolated reticular spaces in epidermis	Autosomal dominant
Lamellar ichthyosis	Birth; collodion baby	Erythroderma, ectropion, large coarse scales; thickened palms and soles	Hyperkeratosis, many mitotic figures	Autosomal recessive

*Reproduced, with permission, from Frost P, Weinstein GD: Ichthyosiform dermatoses. In: *Dermatology in General Medicine.* Fitzpatrick TB (editor). McGraw-Hill, 1971.

Table 18–4. Types of epidermolysis bullosa.

Name	Age at Onset	Clinical Features	Histology	Inheritance
Nonscarring types				
Epidermolysis bullosa simplex	Birth	Hemorrhagic blisters over the lower legs; cooling prevents blisters	Disintegration of basal cells	Autosomal dominant
Recurrent bullous eruption of the hands and feet (Weber–Cockayne syndrome)	First few years of life	Blisters brought out by walking	Cytolysis of suprabasal cells; keratotic cells	Autosomal dominant
Junctional bullous epimatosis (Herlitz disease)	Birth	Erosions on legs, oral mucosa; severe perioral involvement	Separation between plasma membrane of basal cells and PAS-positive basal lamina	Autosomal recessive
Scarring types				
Epidermolysis bullosa dystrophica, dominant	Infancy	Numerous blisters on hands and feet; milia formation	Separation of PAS-positive basal lamina; anchoring fibrils lost	Autosomal dominant
Epidermolysis bullosa dystrophica, recessive	Birth	Repeated episodes of blistering, secondary infection and scarring—"mitten hands and feet"	Separation below PAS-positive basal lamina; anchoring fibrils lost	Autosomal recessive

552

COMMON SKIN DISEASES IN INFANTS, CHILDREN, & ADOLESCENTS

ACNE

Clinical Findings

The common forms of acne in pediatric patients occur at 2 ages: in the newborn period and in adolescence. Neonatal acne is a response to maternal androgen, first appearing at 4–6 weeks of age and lasting until 4–6 months of age. It is characterized by inflammatory papules with all lesions in the same stage at the same time. The lesions are seen primarily on the face, upper chest, and back, in a distribution similar to that seen in adolescent acne. It has been hypothesized but not proved that infants who have severe neonatal acne will develop severe adolescent acne.

The onset of adolescent acne is between ages 8 and 10 in 40% of children. The early lesions are usually limited to the face and are primarily closed comedones (whiteheads; see below). Eventually, 85% of adolescents will develop some form of acne.

Acne occurs in sebaceous follicles, which, unlike hair follicles, have large, abundant sebaceous glands and usually lack hair. They are located primarily on the face, upper chest, back, and penis. Obstruction of the sebaceous follicle opening produces the clinical lesion of acne. If the obstruction occurs at the follicular mouth, the clinical lesion is characterized by a wide, patulous opening filled with a plug of stratum corneum cells. This is the open comedo, or blackhead. Open comedones are the predominant clinical lesion seen in early adolescent acne. The black color is due not to dirt but to oxidized material within the stratum corneum cellular plug. Open comedones do not often progress to inflammatory lesions. Closed comedones, or whiteheads, are caused by obstruction just beneath the follicular opening in the neck of the sebaceous follicle, which produces a cystic swelling of the follicular duct directly beneath the epidermis. The stratum corneum produced accumulates continuously within the cystic cavity. The resultant lesion is an enlarging sphere just beneath the skin surface. Most authorities believe that closed comedones are precursors of inflammatory acne. If open or closed comedones are the predominant lesions on the skin in adolescent acne, it is called **comedonal acne.**

In typical adolescent acne, several different types of lesions are present simultaneously, eg, open and closed comedones and inflammatory lesions such as papules, pustules, and cysts.

Inflammatory lesions may also rarely occur as interconnecting, draining sinus tracts. Adolescents with cystic acne require prompt medical attention, since ruptured cysts and sinus tracts result in severe scar formation. New acne scars are highly vascular and have a reddish or purplish hue. Such scars return to normal skin color after several years. Acne scars may be depressed beneath the skin level, raised, or flat to the skin. In adolescents with a tendency toward keloid formation, keloidal scars can occur following acne lesions, particularly over the sternal area.

Treatment

A. Topical Keratolytic Agents: Two classes of potent keratolytic agents are available: retinoic acid and benzoyl peroxide gel. These have been found to be the most efficacious agents in the treatment of acne. Either agent may be used once daily, or the combination of retinoic acid cream applied to acne-bearing areas of the skin once daily in the evening and a benzoyl peroxide gel applied once daily in the morning may be used. This regime will control 80–85% of cases of adolescent acne.

B. Topical Antibiotics: Topical antibiotics are less effective than systemic antibiotics and at best are equivalent in potency to 250 mg of tetracycline orally once a day. One percent clindamycin phosphate solution is the most efficacious of all topical antibiotics; 1.5% and 2% topical erythromycin solutions are effective; while 1% topical tetracycline solution is minimally effective.

C. Systemic Antibiotics: Antibiotics that are concentrated in sebum, such as tetracycline and erythromycin, are very effective in inflammatory acne. The usual dose is 0.5–1 g taken once or twice daily on an empty stomach (nothing to eat 1 hour before or after the medication). Tetracycline or erythromycin should be continued for 2–3 months until the acne lesions are suppressed.

D. Oral Retinoids: An oral retinoid, 13-cis-retinoic acid (isotretinoin; Accutane), offers the most efficacious treatment of severe cystic acne. The precise mechanism of its action is unknown, but decreased sebum production, decreased follicular obstruction, decreased skin bacteria, and general anti-inflammatory activities have been described. The initial dosage is 40 mg once or twice daily. This drug is not effective in comedonal acne or other mild forms of acne. Side effects include dryness and scaliness of the skin, dry lips, and, occasionally, dry eyes and dry nose. Up to 10% of patients experience mild, reversible hair loss. Elevated liver enzymes and blood lipids have been described. Isotretinoin is teratogenic. Use in young women of childbearing age is not recommended.

E. Other Acne Treatments: There is no convincing evidence that dietary management, mild drying agents, abrasive scrubs, oral vitamin A, ultraviolet light, cryotherapy, or incision and drainage have any beneficial effects in the management of acne.

F. Avoidance of Cosmetics and Hair Spray: Acne can be aggravated by a variety of external factors that result in further obstruction of partially occluded sebaceous follicles. Discontinuing the use of oil-base cosmetics, face creams, and hair sprays may alleviate the comedonal component of acne within 4–6 weeks.

Patient Education & Follow-up Visits

It is important to explain the mechanism of acne and the treatment plan to adolescent patients. Time should be set aside at the first visit to answer the patient's questions. Explain that there will not be much improvement for 4–8 weeks. Establish guidelines for ideal control, and explain that the best the patient might achieve is one or two new pimples a month. A written education sheet is most useful.

BACTERIAL INFECTIONS OF THE SKIN

Impetigo

Erosions covered by honey-colored crusts are diagnostic of impetigo. Staphylococci and group A streptococci are important pathogens in this disease, which histologically consists of superficial invasion of bacteria into the upper epidermis, forming a subcorneal pustule.

Although topical antibiotics may effect a clinical cure, parenteral penicillin or oral penicillin for 10 days is necessary to eradicate streptococci. The risk of nephritogenic strains varies considerably from area to area, but active treatment of patients and contacts with systemic penicillin will significantly reduce the incidence of acute glomerulonephritis in endemic areas. Dicloxacillin or other antistaphylococcal antibiotics are used when staphylococcal infection is suspected.

Ecthyma

Ecthyma is a firm, dry crust, surrounded by erythema, that exudes purulent material. It represents deep invasion by the streptococcus through the epidermis to the superficial dermis.

Cellulitis

Cellulitis is characterized by erythematous, hot, tender, ill-defined plaques accompanied by regional lymphadenopathy. Histologically, this disorder represents invasion of microorganisms into the lower dermis and sometimes beyond, with obstruction of local lymphatics. *Haemophilus influenza, Streptococcus pneumoniae,* and *S pyogenes* are the most common offending organisms, although a bluish cellulitis is diagnostic of hemophilus influenzae.

Septicemia is common, and treatment with the appropriate systemic antibiotic is indicated.

Folliculitis

A pustule at the follicular opening represents folliculitis. If the pustule occurs at eccrine sweat orifices, it is correctly called **poritis.** Staphylococci and streptococci are the most frequent pathogens.

Treatment consists of measures to remove follicular obstruction—either cool wet compresses for 24 hours or keratolytics such as are used for acne.

Abscess

An abscess occurs deep in the skin, at the bottom of a follicle or an apocrine gland, and is diagnosed as an erythematous, firm, acutely tender nodule with ill-defined borders. Staphylococci are the most common organisms.

Treatment consists of incision and drainage and systemic antibiotics.

Scalded Skin Syndrome

This entity consists of the sudden onset of bright red, acutely painful skin, most obvious periorally, periorbitally, and in the flexural areas of the neck, the axillas, the popliteal and antecubital areas, and groin. The slightest pressure on the skin results in severe pain and separation of the epidermis, leaving a glistening layer (the stratum granulosum of the epidermis) beneath. The disease is due to a circulating toxin (exfoliation) elaborated by group II staphylococci.

Scalded skin syndrome includes **Ritter's disease** of the newborn, toxic epidermal necrolysis, and the mildest form, staphylococcal scarlet fever. (See also Bullous Impetigo, below). In all the forms of this entity, the causative staphylococci may not be isolated from the skin but rather from the nasopharynx, an abscess, blood culture, etc.

Treatment consists of systemic administration of anti-staphylococcal drugs, eg, dicloxacillin, 25–50 mg/kg/d orally, or methicillin, 200–300 mg/kg/d intravenously. No topical therapy is necessary or warranted except in the newborn, where silver sulfadiazine or other burn therapy is used.

Bullous Impetigo

A fourth form of scalded skin syndrome is bullous impetigo. All impetigo is bullous, with the blister forming just beneath the stratum corneum, but in "bullous impetigo" there is, in addition to the usual erosion covered by a honey-colored crust, a border filled with clear fluid. Staphylococci may be isolated from the lesions, and systemic signs of circulating exfoliation are absent. "Bullous varicella" is a disorder that represents bullous impetigo in varicella lesions.

Treatment with dicloxacillin, 25–50 mg/kg/d orally for 5–6 days, is effective. Application of cool compresses to debride crusts is a helpful symptomatic measure.

FUNGAL INFECTIONS OF THE SKIN

1. DERMATOPHYTE INFECTIONS

Essentials of Diagnosis
• Red, scaly, round lesions.
• Hair loss with or without scaling in tinea capitis.

General Considerations

Dermatophytes become attached to the superficial layer of the epidermis, nails, and hair, where they proliferate. They grow mainly within the stratum corneum and do not invade the lower epidermis or dermis. Release of toxins from dermatophytes, especially those whose natural host is animals or soil, eg, *Microsporum canis* and *Trichophyton verrucosum,* results in dermatitis. Fungal infection should be suspected with any red and scaly lesion.

Diagnosis

A. Tinea Capitis: Thickened, broken-off hairs with erythema and scaling of underlying scalp are distinguishing features (Table 18–5). Pustule formation and a boggy fluctuant mass on the scalp occur in *M canis* and *T tonsurans* infections. The mass, called a **kerion,** represents an exaggerated host response to the

Table 18–5. Clinical features of tinea capitis.

Most Common Organisms	Clinical Appearance	Microscopic Appearance in KOH
Trichophyton tonsurans (60%)	Hairs broken off 2–3 mm from follicle; "black dot"; no fluorescence	Hyphae and spores within hair
Microsporum canis (39%)	Thickened broken-off hairs that fluoresce yellow-green with Wood's lamp*	Small spores outside of hair; hyphae within hair
Microsporum audouini (1%)	Thickened broken-off, hairs that fluoresce yellow-green with Wood's lamp*	Small spores outside of hair; hyphae within hair

*Select fluorescent hairs for examination in KOH and culture.

organism. Fungal culture should be performed in all cases of suspected tinea capitis.

B. Tinea Corporis: Tinea corporis presents either as annular marginated papules with a thin scale and clear center or as an annular confluent dermatitis. The most common organisms are *T mentagrophytes* and *M canis.* The diagnosis is made by scraping thin scales from the border of the lesion, dissolving them in 20% KOH, and examining for hyphae.

C. Tinea Cruris: Symmetric, sharply marginated lesions in inguinal areas are seen with tinea cruris. The most common organisms are *T rubrun, T mentagrophytes,* and *Epidermophyton floccosum.* Scrapings taken from the border should be examined under the microscope with 20% KOH for dermatophytes.

D. Tinea Pedis: The diagnosis of tinea pedis in a prepubertal child must always be regarded with skepticism; atopic feet or contact dermatitis is a more likely diagnosis in this age group. Tinea pedis is seen most commonly in postpubertal males with blisters on the instep of the foot. Fissuring between the toes is occasionally seen. Microscopic examination of thin scales or the undersurface of the blister roof confirms the diagnosis.

E. Tinea Unguium (Onychomycosis): Loosening of the nail plate from the nail bed (onycholysis), giving a yellow discoloration, is the first sign of fungal invasion of the nails. Thickening of the distal nail plate then occurs, followed by scaling and a crumbly appearance of the entire nail plate surface. *T rubrum* and *T mentagrophytes* are the most common causes. The diagnosis is confirmed by KOH examination. Usually one or 2 nails are involved. If every nail is involved, psoriasis or lichen planus is a more likely diagnosis than fungal infection.

Treatment

The treatment of dermatophytosis is quite simple: If hair or nails are involved, griseofulvin is the treatment of choice. Topical antifungal agents do not enter hair or nails in sufficient concentrations to clear the infection. The absorption of griseofulvin from the gastrointestinal tract is enhanced by a fatty meal; thus, whole milk or ice cream taken with the medication increases absorption. The dosage of griseofulvin is 10–20 mg/kg/d. With hair infections, it should be continued for a minimum of 6 weeks; in nail infections, for a minimum of 3 months. It is supplied in capsules containing 250 mg or as a suspension containing 125 mg/5 mL. The side effects are few, and the drug has even been used successfully in the newborn period.

The treatment of kerion includes suppression of the exaggerated inflammatory response with corticosteroids. Prednisone, 1.5 mg/kg/d orally for 7–10 days, is recommended for prevention of scarring and alopecia.

Tinea corporis, tinea pedis, and tinea cruris can be treated effectively with topical medication after careful inspection to make certain that the hair and nails are not involved. Treatment with clotrimozole (Lotvimin), miconazole (Micatin), econazole (Spectazol) or haloprosin (Halotex), applied twice daily for 3–4 weeks, is recommended.

2. TINEA VERSICOLOR

Tinea versicolor is a superficial infection caused by *Pityrosporon orbiculare* (also called *Malassezia furfur*), a yeastlike fungus. It characteristically causes polycyclic connected hypopigmented maculas and very fine scales in areas of sun-induced pigmentation. In winter, the polycyclic maculas appear reddish-brown.

Treatment consists of application of selenium sulfide (Selsun), full-strength suspension, or 25% sodium thiosulfate (Tinver). Selenium sulfide should be applied to the whole body and left on overnight. Treatment can be repeated again in a week and then monthly thereafter. It tends to be somewhat irritating, and the patient should be warned about this difficulty.

3. *CANDIDA ALBICANS* INFECTIONS

In addition to being a frequent invader in diaper dermatitis, *Candida albicans* also infects the oral mucosa, where it appears as thick white patches with an erythematous base (**thrush**); the angles of the mouth, where it causes fissures and white exudate (**perleche**); and the cuticular region of the fingers, where thickening of the cuticle, dull red erythema, and distortion of growth of the nail plate suggest the diagnosis of candida paronychia. *C albicans* is able to penetrate the stratum corneum layer and locally activate the complement system.

Nystatin (Mycostatin) is the drug of first choice for *C albicans* infections. It is supplied as an ointment or a cream, as an oral suspension, and as vaginal tablets. In diaper dermatitis, the cream form can be applied every 3–4 hours. In oral thrush, the suspension should be applied directly to the mucosa with the finger or a cotton-tipped applicator, since it is not absorbed and acts topically. In candida paronychia, nystatin is applied over the area, covered with an occlusive plastic wrapping, and left on overnight after the application is made airtight.

Haloprogin, miconazole, econazole nitrate, or clotrimazole is an effective alternative.

VIRAL INFECTIONS OF THE SKIN

Herpes Simplex

Grouped vesicles or grouped erosions suggest herpes simplex. The microscopic findings of epidermal giant cells after scraping the vesicle base with a No. 15 blade, smearing on a slide, and staining with Wright's stain (Tzank smear) suggests herpes simplex or varicella zoster. In infants, lesions due to herpes simplex type 1 are seen on the gingiva and lips, periorbitally, or on the thumb in thumb suckers. Recurrent erosions in the mouth are usually aphthous stomatitis rather than recurrent herpes simplex. Herpes simplex type 2 is seen on the genitalia and in the mouth in adolescents. Cutaneous dissemination of herpes simplex occurs in patients with atopic dermatitis (**eczema herpeticum, Kaposi's varicelliform eruption**).

In severe disseminated infection, oral acyclovir may be helpful.

Varicella Zoster

Grouped vesicles in a dermatome on the trunk or face suggest herpes zoster. Zoster in children is not painful and usually has a mild course. In patients with compromised host resistance, the appearance of an erythematous border around the vesicles is a good prognostic sign. Conversely, large bullae without a tendency to crusting imply a poor host response to a virus. Varicella zoster and herpes simplex lesions undergo the same series of changes: papule, vesicle, pustule, crust, slightly depressed scar. Varicella appears in crops, and many different stages of lesions are present at the same time.

Itching is usually the only symptom, and cool baths as frequently as necessary or drying lotions such as calamine lotion are sufficient to relieve symptoms. In immunosuppressed children, intravenous or oral acyclovir should be considered.

Virus-Induced Tumors

A. Molluscum Contagiosum: Molluscum contagiosum consists of umbilicated white or whitish-yellow papules found in groups on the genitalia or trunk. They are common in sexually active adolescents as well as in infants and preschool children. Crushing a lesion between glass slides followed by microscopic examination after staining with Wright's stain will demonstrate epidermal cells with inclusions. Molluscum contagiosum is a poxvirus that induces the epidermis to proliferate, forming a pale papule.

Removal of the lesion with a sharp curet or knife is curative. This therapy may leave a small scar, and one must weigh the advantage of removal of lesions that will disappear in 2 or 3 years.

B. Warts: Warts are skin-colored papules with irregular (verrucous) surfaces. They are intraepidermal tumors caused by infection with human papilloma virus. This DNA virus induces the epidermal cells to proliferate, thus resulting in the warty growth. If the wart virus stimulus is small, the result is a flat wart. If the stimulation is great, the cells proliferate and thicken, causing the skin to fold upon itself and giving rise to an irregular (verrucous) surface—as seen on the isolated wart on the body (verruca vulgaris), the plantar wart (verruca plantaris), and, often, the venereal wart (condyloma acuminatum).

No therapy for warts is ideal, and some types of therapy should be avoided because the recurrence rate of warts is high. Flat warts generally require no treatment. They may be considered a mild wart virus infection, and since they usually disappear within 6–9 months they are best left alone. The holds true especially for all flat warts on the face. A good response to 0.05% tretinoin (Retin-A) cream, applied once daily for 3–4 weeks, has been reported.

The best treatment for the solitary **common ("vulgaris")** **wart** is to freeze it with liquid nitrogen. The liquid nitrogen should be allowed to drip from the cotton-tipped applicator onto the wart without pressure. Pressure amplifies the cold injury by causing vasoconstriction and may produce a deep ulcer and scar. Liquid nitrogen is applied by drip until the wart turns completely white and stays white for 20–25 seconds. Small plantar warts usually need not be treated. Large and painful ones are treated most effectively by applying 40% salicylic acid paste cut with a scissors to fit the lesion. The sticky brown side of the plaster is placed against the lesion, taped on securely with adhesive tape, and left on for 5 days. The plaster is then removed, and the white necrotic warty tissue can be gently rubbed off with the finger and a new salicylic acid plaster applied. This procedure is repeated every 5 days, and the patient is seen every 2 weeks. Most plantar warts resolve in 2–4 weeks when treated in this way.

Sharp scalpel excision, electrosurgery, and radiotherapy should be avoided, since the resulting scar often becomes a more difficult problem than the wart itself and there may be recurrence of the wart in the area of the scar.

Condyloma acuminatum is best treated with 25% podophyllum resin (podophyllin) in alcohol. This should be painted on the lesions and then washed off after 4 hours. Retreatment in 7–10 days may be necessary. A condyloma not on the vulvar mucous membrane but on the adjacent skin should be treated as a common wart and frozen.

For isolated warts and periungual warts, cantharidin (Cantharone) is effective and painless in children. It causes a blister and sometimes is difficult to control. An undesirable complication is the appearance of warts along the margins of the cantharidin blister. Cantharidin is applied to the skin, allowed to dry, and covered with occlusive tape such as Blenderm for 24 hours.

No wart therapy is immediate and definitive, and recurrences are reported in 20–30% of cases even with the best care.

HIV INFECTIONS

The onset of skin lesions in perinatally acquired AIDS is 4 months; it is 11 months in transfusion acquired AIDS. Persistent oral candidiasis and recalcitrant candida diaper rash are the most frequent cutaneous manifestations of infantile HIV infection. Severe herpetic gingivostomatitis, herpes zoster, and molluscum contagiosum are seen. Recurrent staphylococcal pyodermas, tinea of the face, and onychomycosis are also observed. A generalized dermatitis with features of seborrhea is extremely common. In general, persistent, recurrent or extensive skin infections should make one suspicious of AIDS.

INSECT INFESTATIONS
(Zoonoses)

Essentials of Diagnosis
- Discrete red papules, nodules, and S-shaped burrow on skin.
- Hand and foot involvement common.

Scabies
Scabies is suggested by the appearance of linear burrows about the wrists, ankles, finger webs, areolas, anterior axillary folds, genitalia, or face (in infants). Often, there are excoriations, honey-colored crusts, and pustules from secondary infection. Identification of the female mite or her eggs and feces is necessary to confirm the diagnosis. Slice off an unscratched papule or burrow with a No. 15 blade and examine it microscopically in either immersion oil or 10% KOH to confirm the diagnosis. In a child who is often scratching, scrape under the fingernails. Examine the parent for unscratched burrows.

Lindane (gamma benzene hexachloride; Kwell) is an excellent scabicide. However, since lindane is concentrated in the central nervous system, and central nervous system toxicity from systemic absorption in infants has been reported, the following restricted use of this agent is recommended: (1) For adults and older children, one treatment of lindane lotion or cream applied to the entire body and left on for 4 hours, followed by a shower, is sufficient. (2) Infants tend to have more organisms and many more lesions and may have to be retreated in 7–10 days. All family members should be treated simultaneously. Crotamiton (Eurax) may be substituted for lindane in infants.

Pediculoses (Louse Infestations)
Excoriated papules and pustules with a history of severe itching at night suggest infestation with the human body louse. This louse may be discovered in the seams of underwear but not on the body. In the scalp hair, the gelatinous nits of the body louse adhere tightly to the hair shaft. The pubic louse may be found crawling among pubic hairs, or blue-black macules may be found dispersed through the pubic region (maculae ceruleae). The pubic louse is often seen in the eyelashes of newborns.

Lindane (gamma benzene hexachloride; Kwell) has been the treatment of choice. Since this agent is concentrated in the central nervous system and central nervous system toxicity from systemic absorption in infants has been reported, the following modification in its use is recommended: For head lice, a shampoo preparation is left on the scalp for 5 minutes and rinsed out thoroughly. The hair is then combed with a fine-tooth comb to remove nits. This may be repeated in 7 days. Lindane cream or lotion applied to the body for 4 hours may be necessary for body lice, but washing the clothing in boiling water followed by ironing the seams with a hot iron usually eliminates the organisms. Permethrin 1% cream rinse is also efficacious for lice.

Lindane cream or lotion applied to the pubic area for 24 hours is sufficient to treat pediculosis pubis. It may be repeated in 4–5 days.

Papular Urticaria

Papular urticaria is characterized by grouped erythematous papules surrounded by an urticarial flare and distributed over the shoulder, upper arms, and buttocks in infants. These lesions represent delayed hypersensitivity reactions to stinging or biting insects and can be reproduced by patch testing with the offending insect. Dog and cat fleas are the usual offenders. Less commonly, mosquitoes, lice, scabies, and bird and grass mites are involved. The sensitivity is transient, lasting 4–6 months.

The logical therapy is to remove the offending insect. Topical corticosteroids and oral antihistamines will control symptoms.

DERMATITIS (Eczema)

Essentials of Diagnosis
- Red skin with disruption of skin surface.
- Vesicles, crusting, or lichenification may be present.

Atopic Dermatitis

Atopic dermatitis is not a clearly defined clinical entity but rather a general term for chronic superficial inflammation of the skin that can be applied to a heterogeneous group of patients. Many (not all) patients go through 3 clinical phases. In the first, infantile eczema, the dermatitis begins on the cheeks and scalp and frequently expresses itself as oval patches on the trunk, later involving the extensor surfaces of the extremities. The usual age at onset is 2–3 months, and this phase ends at age 18 months to 2 years. Only one-third of all infants with atopic eczema progress to phase 2—childhood or flexural eczema—in which the predominant involvement is in the antecubital and popliteal fossae, the neck, the wrist, and sometimes the hands or feet. This phase lasts from age 2 years to adolescence. Some children will have involvement of the soles of their feet only, with cracking, redness, and pain—the so-called atopic feet. Only a third of children with typical flexural eczema will progress to adolescent eczema, which is usually manifested by hand dermatitis only. Atopic dermatitis is quite unusual after age 30.

Atopic dermatitis has no known cause, and despite the high incidence of asthma and hay fever in these patients (39%) and their families (70%), evidence for allergy beyond this hereditary association is limited to testimonials. The evidence for food and inhalant allergens as causes of atopic dermatitis is not specific.

A few patients with atopic dermatitis have immunodeficiency with recurrent pyodermas, unusual susceptibility to herpes simplex and vaccinia virus, hyperimmunoglobulinema E, defective neutrophil and monocyte chemotaxis, and impaired T lymphocyte function.

A faulty epidermal barrier may predispose the patient with atopic dermatitis to itchy skin. Inability to hold water within the stratum corneum results in rapid evaporation of water, shrinking of the stratum corneum, and "cracks" in the epidermal barrier. Such skin forms an ineffective barrier to the entry of various irritants—and, indeed, it may be clinically useful to regard atopic dermatitis as a primary irritant contact dermatitis and simply tell the patient, "You have sensitive skin." Chronic atopic dermatitis is frequently secondarily infected with *Staphylococcus aureus* or *Streptococcus pyogenes*.

A. Treatment of Acute Stages: Application of wet dressings and topical corticosteroids is the treatment of choice for acute, weeping atopic eczema. Topical steroid is applied 4 times daily and covered with wet dressings as outlined at the beginning of this chapter. Systemic antibiotics chosen on the basis of appropriate skin cultures may be necessary, since lesions in the acute stages are often secondarily infected with *S aureus* or streptococci.

B. Treatment of Chronic Stages: Treatment is aimed at avoiding irritants and restoring water to the skin. No soaps or harsh shampoos should be used, and the patient should avoid woolen clothing or any rough clothing. Restoring water to the skin is important in atopic dermatitis. This can be accomplished by 2 "drip-dry" baths daily, less than 5 minutes each, after which lubricating oils or ointments are applied. Moisturel is a useful lubricant. Plain petrolatum and lards are often too greasy and may cause considerable sweat retention. Liberal use of Cetaphil lotion as a soap substitute 3 or 5 times a day is also satisfactory as a means of lubrication. A bedroom humidifier is often helpful. Topical corticosteroids should be limited to the less potent ones. Hydrocortisone ointment, 1% twice daily, is often sufficient. There is never any reason to use high-potency corticosteroids in atopic dermatitis. In superinfected atopic dermatitis, systemic antibiotics for 10–14 days (erythromycin, 40 mg/kg/d; dicloxacillin, 50 mg/kg/d) are necessary.

Treatment failures in chronic atopic dermatitis are most often due to patient noncompliance. This is a frustrating disease for parent and child.

Nummular Eczema

Nummular eczema is characterized by numerous symmetrically distributed coin-shaped ("nummular") patches of dermatitis, principally on the extremities. These may be acute, oozing, and crusted or dry and scaling. The disease lasts 9 months to 2 years. The differential diagnosis should include tinea corporis and atopic dermatitis.

The same topical measures should be used as for atopic dermatitis, though treatment is often more difficult.

Primary Irritant Contact Dermatitis (Diaper Dermatitis)

Contact dermatitis is of 2 types: primary irritant and allergic eczematous. Primary irritant dermatitis develops within a few hours, reaches peak severity at 24 hours, and then disappears. Allergic eczematous contact dermatitis (see below) has a delayed onset of 18 hours, peaks at 48–72 hours, and often lasts as long as 2 or 3 weeks, even if exposure to the offending antigen is discontinued.

Diaper dermatitis, the most common form of primary irritant contact dermatitis seen in pediatric practice, is due to prolonged contact of the skin with urine and feces, which contain irritating chemicals such as urea and intestinal enzymes. The diagnosis of diaper dermatitis is based on the picture of erythema and thickening of the skin in the perineal area and the history of skin contact with urine or feces. In 80% of cases of diaper dermatitis lasting more than 4 days, the affected area is colonized with *Candida albicans* even before the classic signs of a beefy red, sharply marginated dermatitis with satellite lesions appear.

Treatment consists of changing diapers frequently. Because rubber or plastic pants serve as occlusive dressings and prevent the evaporation of the contactant and enhance its penetration into the skin, they should be avoided as much as possible. Air drying is useful. Streptococcal infection should be included in the differential diagnosis.

Treatment of long-standing diaper dermatitis should include application of nystatin (Mycostatin) cream with each diaper change. In extremely inflammatory diaper dermatitis, 1% hydrocortisone cream may be alternated with nystatin cream at every other diaper change.

Lichen Simplex Chronicus (Localized Neurodermatitis)

Lichen simplex chronicus is a sharply circumscribed single patch of lichenification, usually found on the back of the neck in adolescent girls. The patients produce the morphologic skin changes by chronic rubbing and scratching.

Treatment of the thickened lesions is with topical corticosteroids. Because the epidermal barrier has thickened, penetration of topical corticosteroids is poor. Penetration can be enhanced in several ways. Airtight occlusion with plastic dressings (eg, Saran Wrap) overnight over topical corticosteroids is useful, or flurandrenolide (Cordran) tape impregnated with corticosteroids will penetrate the lesion. Covering the lesion will also prevent scratching the area.

Allergic Eczematous Contact Dermatitis (Poison Ivy Dermatitis)

Children often present with acute dermatitis with blister formation, oozing, and crusting. Blisters are often linear and of acute onset. Plants such as poison ivy, poison sumac, and poison oak cause most cases of allergic contact dermatitis in children. Allergic contact dermatitis has all the features of delayed type (T lymphocyte–mediated) hypersensitivity. Although many substances may cause such a reaction, nickel sulfate (metals), potassium dichromate, and neomycin are the most common causes. The true incidence of allergic contact dermatitis in children is not known.

Treatment of contact dermatitis in localized areas is with topical corticosteroids. In severe generalized involvement, prednisone, 1–2 mg/kg/d orally for 14–21 days, can be used.

Dry Skin (Asteatotic Eczema, Xerosis)

Newborns and older children who live in arid climates are susceptible to dry skin, characterized by large cracked scales with erythematous borders. The stratum corneum is dependent upon environmental humidity for its water, and below 30% environmental humidity the stratum corneum loses water, shrinks, and cracks. These cracks in the epidermal barrier allow irritating substances to enter the skin, predisposing to dermatitis.

Treatment consists of increasing the water content of the skin's immediate external environment. House humidifiers are very useful. Two 5-minute baths a day with immediate application of oil; or ointments (petrolatum, Aquaphor) after the bath will allow the skin to retain water. Frequent soaping of the skin impairs its water-holding capacity and serves as an irritating alkali, and all soaps should therefore be avoided. Frequent use of emollients (eg, Moisturel, Cetaphil, Eucerin, Lubriderm) should be a major part of therapy.

Keratosis Pilaris

Follicular papules containing a white inspissated scale characterize keratosis pilaris. Individual lesions are discrete and may be red. They are prominent on the extensor surfaces of the upper arms and thighs and on the buttocks and cheeks. In severe cases, the lesions may be generalized. Such lesions are seen frequently in children with dry skin and have also been associated with atopic dermatitis and ichthyosis vulgaris.

Treatment is with keratolytics such as topical retinoic acid cream followed by skin hydration.

Pityriasis Alba

White, scaly macular areas with indistinct borders are seen over extensor surfaces of extremities and on the cheeks in children. Suntanning exaggerates these lesions. Histologic examination reveals a mild dermatitis. These lesions may be confused with tinea versicolor.

There is no satisfactory treatment.

Polymorphous Light Eruption

The appearance of vesicular, eczematous, or urticarial lesions in sun-exposed areas (cheeks, nose, chin, dorsum of the hands and arms) in the springtime should suggest a diagnosis of polymorphous light eruption. Confirmation can be made by skin biopsy demonstrating dense lymphocytic infiltrates in the dermis or by reproducing the lesion by daily exposure to artificial ultraviolet light. In American Indians, it is inherited as an autosomal dominant trait. Onset is usually at age 5 or 6, and spontaneous improvement occurs at puberty. The first rays of sunlight of sufficient energy reaching the earth's surface in early spring induce the disease. As summer progresses, the skin thickens in response to sunlight. Less ultraviolet energy enters the skin, and the disease subsides. The differential diagnosis includes erythropoietic protoporphyrin, in which patients experience severe pain and itching after 5 or 10 minutes of exposure to the sun but do not develop significant skin lesions except for small papules over the dorsum of the hand; and photodermatitis from plants (psoralens) or drugs, eg, thiazide diuretics, antihistamines, phenothiazine tranquilizers, tetracyclines, and sulfonamides.

Treatment of the dermatitis with topical corticosteroids, eg, 1% hydrocortisone cream to the face 3 times daily, and daily use of a sunscreen applied at bedtime and each morning are sufficient.

COMMON SKIN TUMORS

If the skin moves with the nodule on lateral palpation, the tumor is located within the dermis; if the skin moves over the nodule, it is subcutaneous. Table 18–6 lists the tumors according to these categories.

Granuloma Annulare

Circles or semicircles of nontender interdermal nodules found over the lower legs and ankles, the dorsum of the hands and wrists, and the trunk, in that order, suggest granuloma annulare. Histologically, the disease appears as a central area of tissue death (necrobiosis) surrounded by macrophages and lymphocytes.

No treatment is necessary. Lesions resolve spontaneously within 1 or 2 years.

Pyogenic Granuloma

Rapid growth of a dark red papule with an ulcerated and crusted surface 1–2 weeks following skin trauma suggests pyogenic granuloma. Histologically, this represents excessive

Table 18–6. Common skin tumors.

Intradermal	Intradermal (cont'd)
Granuloma annulare	Lymphangioma
Dermatofibroma	Hemangioma
Epidermal inclusion cyst	Hair and sweat gland hamartomas
Neurofibroma	**Subcutaneous**
Neuroma	Lipoma
Leiomyoma	Rheumatoid nodule
Calcifying epithelioma	Osteoma
Melanocytic nevus	
Pyogenic granuloma	

new vessel formation with or without inflammation (granulation tissue). It is neither pyogenic nor granulomatous but should be regarded as an abnormal healing response.

Excision is the treatment of choice.

Epidermal Inclusion Cysts

Epidermal inclusion cysts are smooth, dome-shaped nodules in the skin that may grow to 2 cm in diameter. In infants they may be found about the eyes and in older children and adolescents on the chest, back, and scalp. They are the most common superficial lumps in children.

Treatment, if desired, is surgical excision.

Keloids

Keloids are scars raised above the skin surface with many radial projections of scar tissue. They continue to enlarge over several years. They are often found on the face, earlobes, neck, chest, and back. Keloids show no racial predilection. Treatment includes intralesional injection with triamcinolone acetonide, 20 mg/mL, or excision and injection with glucocorticosteroids.

PAPULOSQUAMOUS ERUPTIONS
(See Table 18–7)

Pityriasis Rosea

Erythematous papules that coalesce to form oval plaques preceded by a large oval plaque with central clearing and a scaly border (the herald patch) establish the diagnosis of pityriasis rosea. The herald patch has the appearance of ringworm and is often treated as such. It appears 1–30 days before the onset of the generalized papular eruption. The oval plaques are parallel in their long axis and follow Langer's lines of skin cleavage. In whites, the lesions are primarily on the trunk, accentuated in the

Table 18–7. Papulosquamous eruptions in children.

Psoriasis
Pityriasis rosea
Secondary syphilis
Lichen planus
Chronic parapsoriasis
Pityriasis rubra pilaris
Tinea corporis
Dermatomyositis
Lupus erythematosus

axillary and inguinal areas. In blacks, lesions are primarily on the extremities. This disease is common in school-age children and adolescents and is presumed to be viral in origin. It lasts 6 weeks and may be pruritic for the first 7–10 days. The major differential diagnosis is secondary syphilis, and a VDRL test should be done if syphilis is suspected. A chronic variant of this disase may last 2 or 3 years and is called **chronic parapsoriasis** or **pityriasis lichenoides chronicus.**

Exposing the skin to sunlight until a mild sunburn occurs (slight redness) will hasten the disappearance of lesions. Ordinarily, no treatment is necessary.

Psoriasis

Psoriasis is characterized by erythematous papules covered by thick white scales. Guttate (droplike) psoriasis is a common form in children that often follows an episode of streptococcal pharyngitis by 2–3 weeks. The sudden onset of small (3–8 mm) papules, which are seen predominantly over the trunk and quickly become covered with thick white scales, is characteristic of guttate psoriasis. Chronic psoriasis is marked by thick, large (5–10 cm), scaly plaques over the elbows, knees, scalp, and other sites of trauma. Pinpoint pits in the nail plate are seen as well as yellow discoloration of the nail plate resulting from onycholysis. Thickening of all 20 fingernails and toenails is an uncommon feature. The sacral and seborrheic areas are commonly involved. Psoriasis has no known cause and demonstrates active proliferation of epidermal cells with a turnover time of 3–4 days, versus 28 days for normal skin. These rapidly proliferating epidermal cells produce excessive stratum corneum, giving rise to thick opaque scales. Papulosquamous eruptions that present problems of differential diagnosis are listed in Table 18–7.

All therapy is aimed at diminishing epidermal turnover time. Sunlight or artificial ultraviolet light (UVL) alone will produce some improvement. Coal tar enhances the effect of UVL and hastens the disappearance of psoriatic lesions. Bathing with a bath product containing tar (eg, Balnetar) at night, followed by UVL the next day, may be sufficient in mild cases. In more severe psoriasis, 2% crude coal tar in petrolatum should be applied after the bath. The newer tar gels (Estar gel, psoriGel) do not cause staining and are most effacious. They are applied twice daily for 6–8 weeks.

Crude coal tar therapy is messy and stains bed clothes, and patients may prefer to use topical corticosteroids. Penetration of topical corticosteroids through the enlarged epidermal barrier in psoriasis requires that more potent preparations be used, eg, fluocinonide (Lidex, Topsyn) 0.05%, or triamcinolone (Aristocort, Kenalog), 0.05%, 4 times daily. A successful alternative is to add a keratolytic agent to the topical corticosteroid to help remove scales and enhance penetration of the steroid. A cream consisting of salicylic acid, 2%, in fluocinonide, 0.05%, 4 times daily, is effective.

Anthralin therapy is also useful. Anthralin is applied to the skin for a short contact time (eg, 20 minutes once daily) and is then washed off with a neutral soap (eg, Dove). A 6-week course of treatment is recommended.

Scalp care using a tar shampoo (Polytar, Zetar, many others) requires leaving the shampoo on for 5 minutes, washing it off, and then shampooing with commercial shampoo to remove scales. It may be necessary to shampoo daily until scaling is reduced.

More severe cases of psoriasis are best treated by a dermatologist using the Goeckerman regimen.

Lichen Planus

Lichen planus consists of pruritic, light-purple, flat-topped, many sided papules, predominantly on the lower legs, penis, wrist, and arms. A white lacy pattern in the buccal mucosa is often seen. Pruritis may be severe.

If pruritus is mild, no treatment is necessary, and the disease will disappear in 6–12 months. With severe pruritus, a trial of antihistamines, eg, diphenhydramine, 5 mg/kg/d, or hydroxyzine, 2 mg/kg/d orally, is warranted. Rapid relief of pruritus and disappearance of the lesions can be achieved by administering prednisone, 1 mg/kg/d orally for 3–4 weeks.

HAIR LOSS
(Alopecia)

Hair loss in children (Table 18–8) imposes great emotional stress on the parent and doctor—often more so than on the child. A 60% hair loss in a single area is necessary before hair loss can be detected clinically. Examination should begin with the scalp to determine if there are color changes or infiltrative changes. Hairs should be examined microscopically for breaking and structural defects and to see if growing or resting hairs are being shed. Placing removed hairs in mounting fluid (Permount) makes them easy to examine. Three diseases account for most cases of hair loss in children: alopecia areata, tinea capitis, and trichotillomania.

Table 18–8. Causes of hair loss in children.*

Hair loss with scalp changes
  Nodules and tumors
    Nevus sebaceus
    Epidermal nevus
  Thickening
    Linear scleroderma
      (morphea) (en coup de sabre)
    Burn
  Atrophy
    Lupus erythematosus
    Lichen planus
Hair loss with hair shaft defects (hair fails to grow out enough to require haircuts)
  Monilethrix—alternating bands of thin and thick areas
  Trichorrhexis nodosa—nodules with fragmented hair
  Trichorrhexis invaginata (bamboo hair)—intussusception of one hair into another
  Pili torti—hair twisted 180 degrees, brittle
  Pili annulati—alternating bands of light and dark pigmentation

*Price VH: Office diagnosis of hair shaft defects. *Cutis* 1975;**15**:231.

REACTIVE ERYTHEMAS

Erythema Multiforme

Erythema multiforme begins with fixed papules for 7–10 days that later develop a dark center and then evolve into lesions with central blisters and the characteristic target lesions (iris lesions) with 3 concentric circles of color change. Primary injury is to endothelial cells, with later destruction of epidermal basal cells and blister formation. Erythema multiforme has sometimes been diagnosed in severe mucous membrane involvement, but **Stevens–Johnson syndrome** is the usual term for severe involvement of conjunctiva, oral cavity, and genital mucosa.

Many causes are suspected, particularly herpes simplex virus, drugs, and mycoplasma infections. Recurrent erythema multiforme is usually associated with reactivation of herpes simplex virus. Stevens–Johnson syndrome is more likely to be associated with a drug, especially nonsteroidals, anticonvulsants, and sulfonamides. In the mild form, spontaneous healing occurs in 10–14 days, but Stevens–Johnson syndrome may last 6–8 weeks if untreated.

Treatment is symptomatic in uncomplicated erythema multiforme. Removal of offending drugs is an obvious necessary measure. Oral antihistamines such as hydroxyzine, 2 mg/kg/d orally, are useful. Cool compresses and wet dressings will relieve pruritus.

Erythema Nodosum

Erythema nodosum consists of painful erythematous nodules on the anterior lower legs. In streptococcal infections, coccidioidomycosis, histoplasmosis, and tuberculosis, the onset of erythema nodosum parallels the appearance of cell-mediated immunity. Streptococcal infections and birth control pills are the most common causes of this panniculitis in the USA.

Treatment consists of removal of the offending drug or eradication of infection. Topical corticosteroids afford some relief, but prednisone, 1–2 mg/kg/d orally, may be necessary for 2–3 weeks.

Drug Eruptions

Drugs may produce urticarial, morbilliform, scarlatiniform, or bullous skin eruptions. Urticaria may appear within minutes after drug administration, but most reactions begin 7–14 days after the drug is first administered. Drugs commonly implicated in skin reactions are listed in Table 18–9.

NAIL DISORDERS

Nail biting and candida paronychia are the two most common nail disorders. Onychomycosis is uncommon. Nail pitting is seen in psoriasis and alopecia areata.

MISCELLANEOUS SKIN DISORDERS ENCOUNTERED IN PEDIATRIC PRACTICE

Aphthous Stomatitis

Recurrent erosions on the gums, lips, tongue, palate, and buccal mucosa are often confused with herpes simplex. A smear of the base of such a lesion stained with Wright's stain will aid in ruling out herpes simplex by the absence of epithelial giant cells. A culture for herpes simplex is also useful in this difficult differential diagnosis problem. It has been shown that recurrence of aphthous stomatitis correlates positively with lymphocyte-mediated cytotoxicity.

There is no specific therapy for this condition. Rinsing the mouth with liquid antacids will provide relief in most patients. Topical corticosteroids in a gel base that adheres to mucous

Table 18–9. Common skin reactions associated with frequently used drugs.

Drug	Common Reactions
Aspirin	Urticaria rarely; purpuric eruptions.
Anti-infective agents Erythromycin	Urticaria.
Griseofulvin	Exanthematous eruptions; rarely, cold urticaria or photodermatitis.
Lincomycin (Lincocin)	Urticaria or exanthematous eruptions.
Penicillin and synthetic penicillins	Serum sickness, urticaria, exanthematous eruptions, anaphylactic shock. Ampicillin causes a high incidence of exanthematous eruption in patients with infectious mononucleosis.
Streptomycin	Exanthematous eruptions, urticaria, stomatitis.
Sulfonamides	Urticaria, erythema multiforme, exanthematous eruptions, Stevens–Johnson syndrome, photodermatitis.
Tetracycline	Exanthematous eruptions, urticaria; rarely, bullous eruptions. Demeclocycline (Declomycin) can cause phototoxic reactions.
Antihistamines	Exanthematous eruptions, urticaria, photodermatitis.
Barbiturates	Maculopapular eruptions, urticaria, erythema multiforme, Stevens–Johnson syndrome, bullous eruptions.
Chlorothiazides	Exanthematous eruptions, urticaria, photodermatitis, hemosiderosis of the lower extremities, leading to development of petechiae with resultant pigmentation (Schamberg's phenomenon).
Cortisone and derivatives	Acneiform drug reactions on trunk—pustular, purpuric eruptions.
Insulin	Urticaria, erythema at injection site.
Iodides (cough syrups, antiasthma preparations)	Acneiform pustules over trunk, granulomatous reaction.
Phenytoin	Exanthematous eruptions usually in first 3 weeks of treatment; gingival hyperplasia, hypertrichosis; pseudolymphoma syndrome.
Prochlorperazine	Urticaria, pruritus, photosensitive dermatitis.

Table 18–10. Cutaneous signs of systemic disease in infants and children.

Sign	Disease
Acnelike erythematous papules in mid face and white ash-leaf macules on trunk, shiny thickened patch on back, subungual fibromas	Tuberous sclerosis
Pruritic blisters on buttocks, elbows, knees, and scapula	Dermatitis herpetiformis (celiac disease)
Café au lait macules	Neurofibromatosis, Albright's disease
"Chicken skin"—yellow rows of soft papules with wrinkled valleys in between in neck, axillas, groin	Pseudoxanthoma elasticum
"Dirty" neck and axillas (hyperpigmented, velvety flexural papules)	Acanthosis nigricans and obesity (endocrinopathies)
Eczematous erosions around the mouth, eyes, perineum, fingers, and toes; alopecia and diarrhea	Acrodermatitis enteropathica (zinc deficiency)
Erythematous isolated papules on elbows, knees, buttocks, face	Papular acrodermatitis (antigen-positive hepatitis)
Erythematous truncal macules with central pallor	Juvenile rheumatoid arthritis

Erythematous flat-topped papules over knuckles	Dermatomyositis
Hemorrhagic (1–2 mm) macules on lips, tongue, palms (epistaxis, gastrointestinal bleeding)	Hereditary hemorrhagic telangiectasia (Osler–Weber–Rendu syndrome)
Hyperpigmentation in palmar creases, knuckles, scars, buccal mucosa, linea alba, scrotum	Addison's disease
Linear or oval vesicles on hands or feet, erosions on soft palate, tonsillar pillars	Hand, foot, and mouth syndrome (Coxsackie A16 and others)
Palpable purpura	Vasculitis
Pigmented macules on oral mucosa	Peutz–Jeghers disease (benign small intestinal polyps)
Purpuric lakes	Purpura fulminans—disseminated intravascular coagulation
Purpuric pustules on hands and feet	Gonococcemia
Purpuric (petechiae) seborrheic dermatitis	Histiocytosis X
Sebaceous (multiple) cysts on face and trunk	Gardner's syndrome (premalignant polyps of colon and rectum)
Stretchy skin; healing with large purple scars	Ehlers–Danlos syndrome

(continued)

Table 18–10 (cont'd). Cutaneous signs of systemic disease in infants and children.

Sign	Disease
Tight, hard skin, telangiectases, hypo- and hyperpigmentation	Scleroderma
Ulcers with undermined, liquifying borders	Pyoderma gangrenosum (ulcerative colitis, regional enteritis, rheumatoid arthritis)
Vitiligo (completely depigmented macules with hyperpigmented borders)	Pernicious anemia, Hashimoto's thyroiditis, Addison's disease, diabetes mellitus
Yellow papules (lower eyelids, joints, palms)	Xanthomas, hyperlipidemias

membrane (eg, Lidex gel) may provide some relief. In severe cases that interfere with eating, prednisone, 1 mg/kg/d orally for 3–5 days, will suffice to abort an episode.

Morphea (Linear Scleroderma)

Morphea is characterized by the appearance, anywhere on the body, of well-circumscribed, shiny, white, firmly adherent skin. It is particularly cosmetically deforming on the face. A light purple border is indicative of an early lesion or continuing activity. Skin biopsy reveals replacement of subcutaneous fat with thickened collagen fibers. The lesions tend to burn themselves out in 3–5 years. It may be difficult to differentiate morphea from lichen sclerosis et atrophicus, which has similar white patches that occur primarily on the upper back and genitalia. Histopatholgic differentiation is often necessary and may be difficult. It has been noted that linear scleroderma in children may progress to severe systemic lupus erythematosus after several years. Borrelia infections have recently been implicated in morphea.

Lesions that are not cosmetically disturbing should not be treated. Lesions on the face may be cleared by injections of repository corticosteroids, eg, triamcinolone acetonide diluted 1:4 with saline to make 2.5 mg/mL and injected through a 30-gauge needle. Less than 1 mL should be injected. Complications of local corticosteroid injection include atrophy, depigmentation, ulceration, and infection; therefore, this therapy should be reserved for unusual circumstances.

CUTANEOUS SIGNS OF SYSTEMIC DISEASE

Cutaneous signs of systemic disease in infants and children are outlined in Table 18–10.

19 | Heart

Lee Ann Pearse, MD, & Michael S. Schaffer, MD

Cardiovascular disease in children is a significant cause of morbidity and mortality throughout the world. Congenital heart defects are a major cause of these illnesses, while acquired heart diseases also play an important role. We also recognize that the precursors of adult heart disease begin in childhood and its prevention needs to be addressed at these early ages.

DIAGNOSTIC EVALUATION

History

The history provides valuable clues that suggest the presence of heart disease. The prenatal history should probe for any exposure to teratogens in the first trimester, a crucial period in cardiac development. The perinatal history should include questions concerning the labor and delivery, the APGAR scores, and the estimated gestational age. Cyanosis in a term infant without a difficult delivery suggests heart disease. In the older neonate and infant the parents should be questioned about feeding intolerance, diaphoresis, failure to thrive, and inability to keep up with their peers, all behaviors suggestive of congestive heart failure. Hypercyanotic spells (''tetralogy'' spells) or squatting may indicate tetralogy of Fallot or similar lesions. In the older child, they can tell you themselves if they have had any ''skipped beats'' or syncopal episodes, possibly indicating a dysrhythmia. Finally, the family history should be investigated for the presence of heart disease since congenital heart defects are frequently familial or associated with hereditary syndromes (Table 19–1).

Physical Examination

The general physical examination, with specific attention paid to activity level, growth parameters, vital signs, state of perfusion, and other congenital malformations, will identify the presence of heart disease. The cardiac examination will usually pinpoint the exact nature of the problem.

The temperature, heart rate, respiratory rate, blood pressure, and growth parameters should be obtained. Hypothermia can cause cyanosis while fever causes tachycardia and tachypnea. Hypertension in the upper extremity may be secondary to coarctation of the aorta or an interrupted aortic arch, in which case 4 extremity blood pressures should be obtained. Failure to thrive is often seen in congenital heart disease. Congestive heart failure will affect primarily the weight, while genetic or hereditary syndromes frequently involve all the growth parameters.

An orderly approach to the examination is important to ensure completeness. Following the plan of inspection, palpation, percussion, and auscultation is helpful. Upon inspection, does the child appear healthy or chronically ill? Are there any dysmorphic features such as the stigmata of Down syndrome or a webbed neck? The presence or absence of cyanosis should be determined, keeping in mind that the child may appear more ashen and hypoperfused than cyanosed. If the patient is cyanotic, is it peripheral or central, peripheral involving the skin and extremities, and central involving the tongue? Examination of the chest will reveal the presence of enlargement of either hemithorax (seen in cardiac enlargement). Clubbing and peripheral edema, along with desquamation and hemorrhagic areas, may be found in the extremities.

Palpation of the precordium detects the location of the point of maximal impulse (PMI) and the presence or absence of thrills, right or left ventricular heaves, or palpable heart sounds. The intensity of the pulses in the upper and lower extremities is

Table 19–1. Genetic and environmental associations.*

A. CHROMOSOMAL ABNORMALITIES	
Autosomal	
Trisomy 13	VSD, PDA, dextrocardia
Trisomy 18	VSD, PDA, PS
Trisomy 21	Endocardial cushion defect, VSD, ASD
Pericentric inversion of chromosome 8	TOF, DORV, PDA
Sex Chromosome	
XO (Turner's)	Coarctation of the aorta, AS, ASD
XXXXY	PDA, ASD
Fragile X	Aortic root dilatation, MVP

(continued)

Table 19–1 (cont'd). Genetic and environmental associations.*

B. GENE ABNORMALITIES

Autosomal Recessive

Ellis–van Crevald	ASD, single atrium
Friedreich ataxia	Cardiomyopathy
Glycogen storage disease, type II	Cardiomyopathy
Jervell–Lange–Nielson	Prolonged QT interval
Hurler	Coronary artery disease, AI, MR, conduction defects
Seckel	VSD, PDA
Smith–Lemli–Opitz	VSD, PDA

Autosomal Dominant

Ehlers–Danlos	Rupture of the large blood vessels
Holt–Oram	ASD, VSD
Marfans	Great artery aneurysm, AI, MR
Neurofibromatosis	PS, coarctation of the aorta
Osler–Weber–Rendu	Pulmonary AV fistulas
Romano–Ward	Prolonged QT interval
Tuberous sclerosis	Myocardial rhabdomyoma, aortic aneurysm
Ullrich–Noonan	PS, ASD, IHSS

X-Linked Recessive (X-R) and X-Linked Dominant (X-D)

Hunter (X-R)	Coronary artery disease, valve disease
Duchenne muscular dystrophy (X-D)	Cardiomyopathy

C. TERATOGENS

Alcohol	VSD, PDA, ASD
Phenytoin	PS, AS, coarctation of the aorta, PDA
Trimethadione	TGA, TOF, HLHS
Lithium	Ebstein's anomaly, TGA, ASD
Thalidomide	TOF, VSD, ASD, truncus arteriosus
Rubella	PPS, PDA, VSD, ASD
Maternal DM	ASH, TGA, VSD, coarctation of the aorta
Maternal phenylketonuria	TOF, VSD, ASD
Maternal SLE	Complete heart block

*AI, aortic insufficiency; AS, aortic stenosis; ASD, atrial septal defect; ASH, assymetric septal hypertrophy; AV, arteriovenous; DORV, double outlet right ventricle; HLHS, hypoplastic left heart syndrome; IHSS, idiopathic hypertrophic subaortic stenosis; MR, mitral regurgitation; MVP, mitral valve prolapse; PDA, patent ductus arteriosus; PPS, peripheral pulmonic stenosis; PS, pulmonary stenosis; SLE, systemic lupus erythematosus; TGA, transposition of the great arteries; TOF, tetralogy of Fallot; VSD, ventricular septal defect.

determined, along with the presence of any pulse lag. Diaphoresis, as seen in congestive heart failure, will be noted during palpation if present, as will the state of perfusion. Examination of the abdomen is important in determining hepatic and splenic size and engorgement.

Percussion is helpful in determining the liver span. It may also be helpful in assessing the extent of pleural effusion.

Auscultation should include not only the heart and lungs but also the head, neck, and abdomen since arteriovenous malformations and arterial stenoses may create a bruit. The cardiac rate and rhythm are assessed. Is the rhythm regular, regular-irregular, or irregular-irregular?

The location, quality and timing of the heart sounds are evaluated next. S1 represents mitral and tricuspid valve closure and is usually single, being loudest at the lower left sternal border. S2 has two components—A2 and P2—which represent aortic and pulmonic valve closure, respectively. A2 is best heard at the mid left sternal border, whereas P2 is loudest at the left upper sternal border. P2 follows A2 normally and the degree of splitting varies with respiration, increasing with inspiration. Increased P2 intensity suggests pulmonary hypertension, and fixed splitting suggests an atrial septal defect with volume overload of the right ventricle. Wide but variable splitting indicates ventricular conduction delay. A single S2 may be heard in semilunar valve atresia and often in transposition of the great vessels and tetralogy of Fallot. S3, heard at the apex, represents passive ventricular filling, is mid diastolic and low pitched, and may be a normal finding. S4 is caused by the atrial contribution to ventricular filling and occurs in late diastole. It is not a normal finding and implies a noncompliant ventricle. Clicks are abnormal extra sounds that are heard throughout the precordium, indicating valvular dysfunction.

When evaluating murmurs it is important to list where they are maximal; where they radiate; and their timing, intensity, and quality. Murmurs can occur in early, mid, or late systole, diastole, or continuously. Systolic murmurs are graded from I to VI/VI with increasing intensity, with grade IV–VI associated with a precordial thrill. Diastolic murmurs are graded from I to IV. The quality may be harsh, soft, blowing, musical, vibratory, or high or low pitched.

It is important to realize and to inform parents that all murmurs are not necessarily indicative of heart disease. Some murmurs are heard in normal growing children and may be accentuated during times of increased cardiac output, such as fever, hypovolemia, anemia, etc. These murmurs are referred to as innocent or functional murmurs and are benign (Table 19–2).

Table 19-2. Functional (innocent) murmurs.*

Name	Grade	Timing	Quality	Location	Etiology	Natural Course
1. Newborn or "baby" murmur	I/VI	Short systolic	Nondescript	Mid-LLSB	Unknown	Usually disappears by 2–3 wk
2. Transient PPS	I–II/VI	Short or long systolic	High pitched	LUSB—both axillae, back	Secondary to turbulent developing pulmonary arteries	Neonatal period through 6 mo of age; more common in prematures
3. Pulmonary outflow ejection murmur	I–II/VI	Short systolic	Mid to high pitched	Mid LUSB	Secondary to exaggeration of normal turbulence of RVOT, MPA	Anytime throughout childhood; increases with elevated cardiac output

4. Still's	I–II/VI	Mid systolic	Low pitched; vibratory or "groaning" or musical	LLSB	Turbulence in LVOT	Usually 2 yr to adolescence, increasing with cardiac output
5. Venous hum	I–II/VI	Continuous	Nondescript	Periclavicular; right or left	Turbulence from upper body venous return	Throughout childhood
6. Innominate or carotid bruit	II–III/VI	Systolic ejection	Harsh	Supraclavicular, neck	Turbulence within carotids	Throughout childhood
7. Hemic	I–III/VI	Systolic ejection	High pitched	RUSB, LUSB	Increased cardiac output secondary to anemia	Throughout childhood

*LLSB, left lower sternal border; LUSB, left upper sternal border; LVOT, left ventricular outflow tract; MPA, main pulmonary artery; PPS, peripheral pulmonic stenosis; RUSB, right upper sternal border; RVOT, right ventricular outflow tract.

LABORATORY INVESTIGATION

Electrocardiography

The electrocardiogram (ECG) is a graphic representation of myocardial electric activity: the P wave represents atrial depolarization, the QRS wave represents ventricular depolarization, and the T wave represents ventricular repolarization. The QRS wave is a summation of both left and right ventricular activity. Throughout childhood, the heart continues to mature with a shift from right to left ventricular predominance. Thus, normal electrocardiographic criteria are dependent on the age of the subject (Figure 19–1). Increased myocardial muscle mass creates an imbalance of forces and is depicted as ventricular hypertrophy. In the presence of hypoplastic chambers, the balance of forces will be shifted and represented as hypertrophy of the opposite ventricle (eg, right ventricular hypertrophy in hypoplastic left heart syndrome).

Chest Radiography

The chest x-ray is critical for evaluating heart size and pulmonary blood flow. The cardiothoracic ratio is increased in neonates, with 0.55 being the upper limit of normal in neonates and 0.5 the maximum in normal older children. The presence of increased and enlarged pulmonary arteries or the paucity of pulmonary vascular markings suggests increased or decreased pulmonary blood flow, respectively (Figure 19–2).

Cardiac Ultrasound

M-mode and two-dimensional echocardiography now produce accurate and precise representations of the intracardiac and great vessel structure and function. However, the distal pulmonary vasculature is still not well visualized (see Figure 19–2).

Doppler ultrasound measures blood flow characteristics. The assessment of laminar or turbulent flow patterns and flow velocities permits the calculation of cardiac outputs and transvalvular gradients. In the presence of ventricular septal defect, patent ductus arteriosus, or tricuspid regurgitation, pulmonary artery pressure can now be calculated with precision.

Cardiac Catheterization

The role of cardiac catheterization is rapidly evolving from a diagnostic tool to one of therapeutic intervention. Anatomic definition and intracardiac pressures are evaluated via catheterization when noninvasive means fail to produce the desired information.

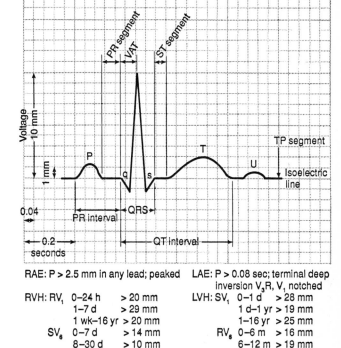

RAE: P > 2.5 mm in any lead; peaked

LAE: P > 0.08 sec; terminal deep inversion V_3R, V_1 notched

RVH:	RV_1	0–24 h	> 20 mm
		1–7 d	> 29 mm
		1 wk–16 yr	> 20 mm
	SV_6	0–7 d	> 14 mm
		8–30 d	> 10 mm
		1–6 mo	> 7 mm
		0.5–16 yr	> 5 mm

LVH:	SV_1	0–1 d	> 28 mm
		1 d–1 yr	> 19 mm
		1–16 yr	> 25 mm
	RV_6	0–6 m	> 16 mm
		6–12 m	> 19 mm
		1–16 yr	> 21 mm

Figure 19–1. The pediatric electrocardiogram. LAE, left atrial enlargement; LVH, left ventricular hypertrophy; RAE, right atrial enlargement; RVH, right ventricular hypertrophy; VAT, ventricular activation time.

Balloon dilatation valvuloplasty has become the treatment of choice for pulmonary valve stenosis and recoarctation of the aorta. Transvascular dilatation of the aortic, mitral, and tricuspid valves is still experimental, as is dilatation of native coarctation. Catheter occlusion of patent ductus arteriosus and atrial septal defect is also favored over the surgical approach in selected cases.

Intracardiac electrophysiologic studies are now performed during cardiac catheterization on infants and older children.

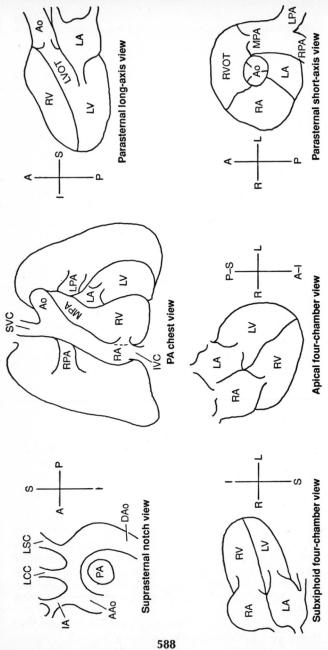

Parasternal long-axis view

Ao
LA
LVOT
RV
LV

S / A—P / I

PA chest view

SVC
Ao
LPA
LA
MPA
LV
RPA
RV
RA
IVC

Suprasternal notch view

S / A—P

LCC
LSC
IA
AAo
PA
DAo

Parasternal short-axis view

MPA
LPA
Ao
RPA
RVOT
LA
RA

A—P / R—L

Apical four-chamber view

LV
LA
RV
RA

P—S / R—L / A—I

Subxiphoid four-chamber view

RV
LV
RA
LA

I—S / R—L

Complex dysrhythmias can be evaluated and their mechanism defined.

Transcatheter ablation of the atrioventricular (AV) node or accessory pathways can now be performed and obviate the need for surgical ablation in resistant dysrhythmias.

CONGESTIVE HEART FAILURE

Congestive heart failure (CHF) is a clinical syndrome in which the heart cannot generate sufficient cardiac output to supply the needs of the body. The syndrome is the result of one of 4 circumstances: 1) dysfunctional myocardium, eg, myocarditis or cardiomyopathy; 2) congenital cardiac malformations that decrease systemic perfusion, eg, critical aortic stenosis or large left to right shunts with pulmonary overcirculation; 3) normal cardiovascular systems in the face of an abnormal demand, eg, thyrotoxicosis or severe anemia and; 4) dysrhythmias that fail to produce an adequate cardiac output.

Clinical Findings

Tachycardia, tachypnea, and hepatomegaly characterize the clinical findings in CHF. Despite the numerous underlying mechanisms, the clinical findings are surprisingly similar in all cases. Additional clinical findings include diaphoresis, jugular venous distention, peripheral edema (periorbital edema in infants), cardiomegaly and, in severe, advanced cases, cyanosis.

Treatment

The treatment of CHF should be directed at the underlying cause; however, nonspecific treatment will generally improve the patient's condition. 1) Oxygen should be administered even in the absence of cyanosis as it will increase systemic oxygen

Figure 19–2. Standard chest x-ray and echocardiographic views. A, anterior; AAo, ascending aorta; Ao, aorta; DAo, descending aorta; I, inferior; IA, innominate artery; IVC, inferior vena cava; L, left; LA, left atrium; LCC, left common carotid artery; LPA, left pulmonary artery; LSC, left subclavian artery; LV left ventricle; LVOT, left ventricular outflow tract; MPA, main pulmonary artery; P, posterior; PA, pulmonary artery; R, right; RA, right atrium; RPA, right pulmonary artery; RV, right ventricle; RVOT, right ventricular outflow tract; S, superior; SVC, superior vena cava.

delivery and also reduce reactive pulmonary vasoconstriction. 2) Digitalization will improve myocardial contractility and increase cardiac output and produce a diuresis. 3) Diuretics decrease preload and reduce pulmonary edema. 4) Afterload reduction will decrease systemic vascular resistance and increase cardiac output (for medication doses, see Table 19–3).

HYPERCYANOTIC SPELLS

Hypercyanotic or "tetralogy spells" are sudden episodes of increasing irritability, tachypnea, and intense cyanosis that may progress to syncope and seizures. They may last from minutes to hours and are frequently seen in patients with tetralogy of Fallot, tricuspid atresia, or any cardiac anomaly with reduced pulmonary blood flow and unobstructed intracardiac communication. The spells are caused by 1) infundibular hypercontractility, 2) decreased systemic vascular resistance, or 3) decreased systemic venous return.

Treatment of the spells is directed at correcting the underlying problem. Frequently, soothing the child or placing the child in a knee–chest position to stop the irritability and increase systemic venous return will break the cycle. Morphine sulfate 0.1–0.2 mg/kg subcutaneously will quiet the child and reduce the tachypnea. Intravenous propranolol 0.05–0.10 mg/kg may be given in acute cases and oral propranolol 1.0–4.0 mg/kg/d may be used chronically until palliative or definitive surgery can be arranged.

CONGENITAL HEART DISEASE

Congenital heart disease (CHD) occurs in approximately 6–8/1000 live births; in the USA alone 25,000–35,000 children with CHD are born each year. Palliative or corrective surgery is now available for well over 90% of these children, with successful intervention dependent upon an early, accurate diagnosis. When a child presents with cyanosis or CHF, a rapid, orderly sequence of evaluation and intervention must begin immediately (Figure 19–3).

Table 19-3. Commonly used medications.*

Drug	Route	Dose	Onset	Mechanism of Action†	Precautions/ Complications
Diuretics					
Bumetanide	PO	0.015–0.1 mg/kg/d	30–60 min	Inhibits sodium reabsorption in the ascending loop of Henle	Hypotension, hypokalemia, hypocalcemia, hyperuricemia
	IV	Dose not established	15–30 min		
Ethacrynic acid	PO	25 mg/dose max 2–3 mg/kg/d	30 min	Inhibits sodium reabsorption in the ascending loop of Henle and proximal and distal tubules	Hypotension, hypokalemia
	IV	1 mg/kg/dose; repeat dose not recommended	5 min		
Furosemide	PO	2 mg/kg/dose	30–60 min	Inhibits sodium reabsorption in the ascending loop of Henle	Ototoxicity in renal disease, hypokalemia, hypocalcemia, dehydration, nephrocalcinosis in premature infants
	IV	1 mg/kg/dose	Minutes		
Hydrochlorothiazide	PO	2–3 mg/kg/d	1–2 h	Inhibits renal tubular absorption of sodium	Hyperbilirubinemia, hypokalemia, hypoglycemia, hyperuricemia
Spironolactone	PO	1–3 mg/kg/d	4–5 d	Aldosterone inhibitor	Hyperkalemia, GI distress

(continued)

591

Table 19–3 (cont'd). Commonly used medications.*

Drug	Route	Dose	Onset	Mechanism of Action†		Precautions/ Complications
Inotropic Agents						
Digoxin Therapeutic Level: 0.6–2.0 ng/ml	PO	Total digitalizing dose (TDD) 1/2, 1/4, 1/4 q 6–8 hr) Premature, 20–40 μg/kg Newborn–2 yr, 50 μg/kg 2 yr, –40 μg/kg	1–2 h	CHF - contractility Dysrhythmia - atrial conduction, AV node refractoriness		Anorexia, nausea, vomiting, headache, diarrhea, excitement, disorientation, abdominal pain, bradycardia, atrial fibrillation, ventricular tachycardia
	IV	Maintenance: 1/4 TDD divided bid 75–80% po dose	15–60 min			
	IM	75–80% po dose	5–15 min			
Dobutamine	IV	2.5–20 μg/kg/min	Minutes	Low dose:	alpha + beta₁ ++ beta₂ ++	Tachydysrhythmias, ectopy, hypertension; contraindicated in hypertrophic cardiomyopathy
				Medium dose:	alpha ++ beta₁ ++ beta₂ +++	
				High dose:	alpha ++ beta₁ + beta₂ +	
Dopamine	IV	1–4 μg/kg/min	Minutes	Dopaminergic ++++ alpha + beta₁ + beta₂ +		Tachydysrhythmias, hypertension
		4–8 μg/kg/min		Dopaminergic ++++ alpha + beta₁ + beta₂ +		

Drug	Route	Dose	Onset	Action	Side Effects
		8–20 µg/kg/min		Dopaminergic ++++ alpha +++ beta$_1$ +++ beta$_2$ +++	
Epinephrine	IV	0.1–0.5 µg/kg/min	Minutes	Alpha, beta$_1$, beta$_2$	Tachycardia, hypertension, headaches, nausea, vomiting
Isoproterenol	IV	0.05–0.5 µg/kg/min	Minutes	Beta agonist	Tachycardia, ventricular ectopy
Antihypertensives					
Captopril	PO	1–4 mg/kg/d divided q 8–12h 1/10 dose for premature infants, increasing with caution	1 hr	Angiotensin converting enzyme inhibitor	Hypotension, decreased renal perfusion
Diazoxide	IV	3–5 mg/kg/dose	1–2 min	Arterial vasodilator	Hypotension, hyperglycemia
Hydralazine	PO	0.75–7.0 mg/kg/d divided q 6–8 hr	Hours to days	Arterial vasodilator	Hypotension, tachycardia lupuslike syndrome
	IV	0.8–3.0 mg/kg/d divided q 4–6 hr	10–30 min		
Nitroprusside	IV	0.5–6.5 µg/kg/min IV drip	Minutes	Peripheral vasodilator (arterial and venous)	Hypotension, cyanide toxicity (discontinue if thiocyanate level >12 mg/dL)

(continued)

593

Table 19-3 (cont'd). Commonly used medications.*

Drug	Route	Dose	Onset	Mechanism of Action†	Precautions/ Complications
Propranolol	PO	0.5–1.0 mg/kg/dose q 6 hr	30 min	Beta blockade	Decreased cardiac output, bradycardia, hypoglycemia, asthma
	IV	0.01–0.1 mg/kg/dose q 6–8 hr	2–5 min		
Antidysrhythmics					
Atropine	IV	0.01–0.03 mg/kg/dose q 4–6 hr, maximum dose 0.4 mg/dose	Seconds	Parasympathetic blockade	Tachycardia
Bretylium tosylate	IV	5 mg/kg then 1–2 mg/min	Minutes	Inhibits norepinephrine release	Hypotension
Digoxin (see above)					
Lidocaine Therapeutic Level: 2–5 μg/mL	IV	1.0 mg/kg then 30–50 μg/kg/min	15–90 sec	Local anesthetic Decreases myocardial irritability	Dysrhythmia
Phenytoin Therapeutic Level: 10–20 μg/mL	PO	2–5 mg/kg/d, divided q 8–12 hr	2–4 hr	Elevates fibrillation threshold	Bradycardia, hypotension with rapid IV infusion, blood dyscrasias, gingival hyperplasia
	IV	3–5 mg/kg loading dose	5–10 min		
Procainamide Therapeutic Level: 4–10 μg/mL	PO	40–60 mg/kg/d divided q 6–8 hours	30–60 min	Slows myocardial conduction and prolongs repolarization	Hypotension, blood dyscrasias, lupuslike syndrome, acquired long QT syndrome, GI upset
	IV	10–20 mg/kg/dose	1–5 min		

594

	Route	Dose	Onset	Action	Side Effects/Comments
Propranolol (see above)					
Quinidine gluconate Therapeutic Level: 1–6 μg/mL	PO	10–30 mg/kg/d divided q 12 hr	Minutes	Slows myocardial conduction and prolongs repolarization	Hypotension, blood dyscrasia, tinnitus, GI upset
Verapamil	PO IV	3–6 mg/kg/d divided tid 0.1–0.15 mg/kg over 1 min	Minutes	Calcium antagonist	Exacerbates heart failure; have colloid and calcium available during rapid infusion
Ductal-Related					
Indomethacin	IV	0.2 mg/kg q 12 hr (0.1 mg/kg for 2nd and 3rd dose if infant < 48 hr old)	Minutes	Prostaglandin inhibitor	GI bleeding, infection, transient renal impairment; discontinue if urine output < 0.6mL/kg/hr
Prostaglandin E$_1$	IV	0.01–0.1 μg/kg/min	Minutes	Smooth muscle relaxation especially ductal tissue Maintain systemic or pulmonary perfusion in ductal-dependent CHD	Apnea, fever, hypotension

*AV, atrioventricular; CHD, congenital heart disease; CHF, congestive heart failure; TDD, total digitalizing dose.
†Plus signs indicate degree of activity.

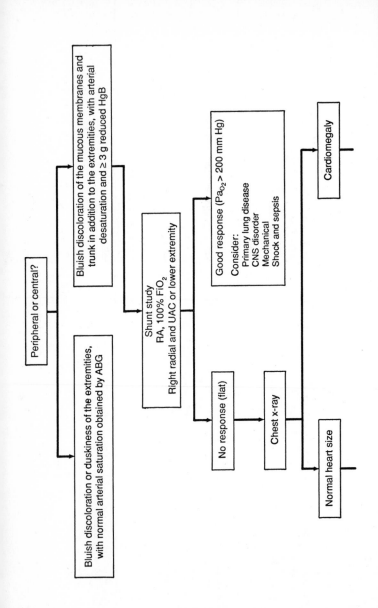

Peripheral or central?

Bluish discoloration of the mucous membranes and trunk in addition to the extremities, with arterial desaturation and ≥ 3 g reduced HgB

Bluish discoloration or duskiness of the extremities, with normal arterial saturation obtained by ABG

Shunt study
RA, 100% FiO₂
Right radial and UAC or lower extremity

Good response (Pa$_{O_2}$ > 200 mm Hg)

Consider:
Primary lung disease
CNS disorder
Mechanical
Shock and sepsis

No response (flat)

Chest x-ray

Cardiomegaly

Normal heart size

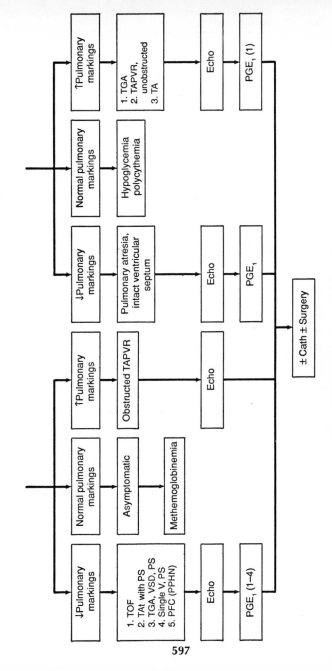

597

ACYANOTIC HEART DISEASE

Ventricular Septal Defect (VSD)

A. General Considerations: VSD is the most common form of CHD, excluding bicuspid aortic valves. It occurs in 25% of all cases of CHD, and is more common in males than in females. It is the most common lesion found in chromosomal abnormalities.

B. Anatomy: The most common location is in the peri-membranous ventricular septum. VSDs can also be found in the muscular septum and in the supracristal region. The size ranges from pinpoint to involving most of the septum.

C. Symptoms and Signs: The physical presentation depends largely on the size of the defect and on the pulmonary pressure plus the presence of associated lesions. In a small to moderate sized defect there will be a normal P2 and a grade II–VI/VI harsh, pansystolic murmur (PSM) at the lower left sternal border. In a large shunt without pulmonary hypertension the P2 is normal, a grade II–III/VI PSM is heard at the lower left sternal border, a mid diastolic flow rumble is appreciated at the apex, and CHF is present. In the presence of marked pulmonary hypertension, a right ventricular lift is present, P2 is loud, a short systolic ejection murmur is present along the left sternal border, and the patient may be cyanotic if Eisenmenger's syndrome has developed.

D. Laboratory Findings: In a small shunt, the heart size will be normal on the chest x-ray and the ECG will be normal. In moderate-sized defects, the chest x-ray may show mild cardiac enlargement and increased pulmonary blood flow, and the ECG will be variable. Large defects result in marked cardiomegaly with increased pulmonary vascularity; the ECG demonstrates right ventricular hypertrophy (RVH), left ventricular hypertrophy (LVH), or both. The echocardiogram is helpful in locating the VSD, with color flow imaging especially useful for small defects.

Figure 19–3. Evaluation of the cyanotic neonate. ABG, arterial blood gas; CNS, central nervous system; CoA, coarctation of the aorta; FiO$_2$, 90% inspired oxygen; PFC, persistent fetal circulation; PGE, prostaglandin; PPHN, persistent pulmonary hypertension of the newborn; PS, pulmonary stenosis; RA, room air; TAt, tricuspid atresia; TA, truncus arteriosus, TAPVR, total anomalous pulmonary venous return; TGA, transposition of the great arteries, TOF, tetralogy of Fallot; UAC, umbilical artery catheter; V, ventricle; VSD, ventricular septal defect.

E. Treatment: Small defects rarely need any surgical or medical management other than subacute bacterial endocarditis (SBE) prophylaxis. There is a significant spontaneous closure rate indirectly related to the size of the defect. Anticongestive heart failure medications are used in the presence of CHF. Surgery is recommended for patients with refractory CHF, failure to thrive in spite of adequate medical and nutritional management, repeated episodes of pneumonia or reversible pulmonary hypertension.

Patent Ductus Arteriosus (PDA)

A. General Considerations: PDA is a common form of CHD, accounting for 12% of all cases of CHD; it occurs in 20–60% of all premature infants. Females are affected twice as often as males and there appears to be an increased incidence at higher altitudes.

B. Anatomy: The ductus arteriosus is a vessel located between the pulmonary artery and the descending aorta, found in all fetuses and generally closing shortly after birth in full-term infants. It is commonly located on the left side but may be right-sided or occasionally bilateral.

C. Symptoms and Signs: In premature infants, depending on the size of the PDA, the precordium may be hyperactive and a variable systolic murmur may be present. The absence of a murmur does not correlate with the absence of a PDA. The pulses are often bounding. In the older child a continuous murmur can be heard at the left upper sternal border below the clavicle, with radiation to the back. The pulses are bounding.

D. Laboratory Findings: In a small PDA the chest x-ray and ECG are normal. Moderate to large PDAs will show LVH on the ECG with cardiomegaly and increased pulmonary markings on the chest x-ray. If pulmonary hypertension is present the ECG will show RVH or biventricular hypertrophy. The two-dimensional and doppler echocardiogram can demonstrate the PDA. In large shunts, the left atrium will be enlarged secondary to increased pulmonary venous return.

E. Treatment: Premature infants are urgently treated either medically (indomethacin) or surgically. In the absence of pulmonary vascular obstructive disease, effective surgical ligation or transvenous occlusion in the catheterization lab is indicated for older children.

Atrial Septal Defect (ASD)

A. General Considerations: There are 3 types of ASDs—ostium secundum, ostium primum, and sinus venosus. Ostium secundum make up 10% of cases of CHD and have a 2:1 female:male ratio. Ostium primum defects comprise 2% of cases of CHD and occur approximately equally among males and females. Five percent of ASDs are made up of sinus venosus ASDs.

B. Anatomy: Ostium secundum defects involve the area around the fossa ovalis. Ostium primum anomalies result from deficiencies in the atrial septum primum during the embryonic period. This defect is the most common type of partial endocardial cushion defect. The sinus venosus defect is located posteriorly to the fossa ovalis and is often associated with partial anomalous pulmonary venous return of the right upper pulmonary veins.

C. Symptoms and Signs: In general, there is a right ventricular heave and the S2 is widely split and fixed. A grade II/VI systolic ejection murmur is heard at the left upper sternal border, followed by a mid diastolic flow rumble in the tricuspid valve region.

D. Laboratory Findings: The chest x-ray demonstrates cardiomegaly with increased pulmonary markings. The ECG shows RVH with an rsR' in V1. Left axis deviation (LAD) and RVH with an rsR' in V1 is seen in ostium primum defects. The echocardiogram reveals a dilated right atrium and right ventricle plus paradoxical septal motion. The defect itself can be visualized in the atrial septum.

E. Treatment: Spontaneous closure has been reported, although it is not as common as in VSDs. Anticongestive medications are used for CHF. Where there is a large left to right shunt, CHF, or pulmonary congestion, surgical closure is recommended. Transvenous closure in the catheterization lab with an occluding device is now an alternative to surgical closure.

Pulmonary Stenosis (PS)

A. General Considerations: PS occurs in 10% of cases of CHD, with a male predominance.

B. Anatomy: The valve is conical or dome-shaped and is formed by fusion of the valve leaflets. Twenty percent of autopsy cases show bicuspid valves and 10–15% of cases have dysplastic valves.

C. Symptoms and Signs: In mild to moderate PS the P2 is soft and there is a systolic ejection click. The click is followed by a grade I–III/VI systolic ejection murmur at the left upper sternal border that radiates to the back. In severe PS, P2 becomes silent and the murmur becomes longer and louder and peaks later in systole.

D. Laboratory Findings: The chest x-ray in mild PS shows a normal-sized heart and dilatation of the main pulmonary artery. The degree of pulmonary artery dilatation does not correlate with the severity of the stenosis. The ECG is normal. In moderate to severe pulmonary stenosis, the ECG shows RVH and RVH with strain in critical PS. The echocardiogram demonstrates the abnormal pulmonary valve and the associated degree of right ventricular hypertrophy. Doppler echocardiography defines the transvalvular gradient precisely.

E. Treatment: Transcatheter balloon valvuloplasty is the recommended procedure for moderate and severe cases. It is now being performed in small infants, thus avoiding the high risks of neonatal surgery.

Coarctation of the Aorta (CoA)

A. General Considerations: CoA accounts for 6% of cases of CHD, with a 1.7:1 male predominance. CoA is commonly seen in association with Turner's syndrome.

B. Anatomy: CoA is defined as a constriction of the aorta typically in the region adjacent to the ductus arteriosus (juxtaductal). It may involve a discrete narrowing or a long segment. Bicuspid aortic valves are associated in 50% of cases. The CoA syndrome consists of coarctation, PDA, tubular hypoplasia of the aortic isthmus, and VSD and is frequently complicated by CHF.

C. Symptoms and Signs: Hypertension and decreased femoral pulses with a brachial–femoral pulse lag herald the diagnosis. In neonates the decreased femoral pulses can be masked in the presence of a large PDA.

D. Laboratory Findings: The chest x-ray shows cardiomegaly with pulmonary venous congestion in infants with CHF. The ECG will show RVH (LV hypoplasia). In older children the chest x-ray may be normal or show rib notching or poststenotic dilatation of the aorta. LVH is seen on the ECG. The echocardiogram shows a dilated right ventricle and possibly a hypoplastic left ventricle during infancy. The aortic arch and coarctation site can be visualized; in addition, aortic doppler studies will demonstrate the disturbed arterial flow.

E. Treatment: Infants with CHF need stabilization and urgent surgery. In neonates, administration of PGE_1 to reopen the ductus arteriosus will improve systemic perfusion and resolve acidosis. Asymptomatic patients should have their hypertension controlled medically and undergo elective surgery during the first 3 years of life.

Aortic Stenosis (AS)

A. General Considerations: AS accounts for 5% of cases of CHD, with a 2:1 male predominance. AS can be classified as valvar, subvalvar, or supravalvar. Supravalvar AS is associated with William's syndrome (elfin facies and hypercalcemia of infancy).

B. Anatomy: In valvar AS, the valve is usually bicuspid and the leaflets are dysplastic and thickened with decreased mobility. In severe cases the anulus itself is frequently hypoplastic.

C. Symptoms and Signs: Infants may present with CHF. Older children are usually asymptomatic. A systolic ejection click will be heard at the apex and a grade II–VI/VI systolic ejection murmur will be heard at the upper right sternal border with radiation to the carotids. In moderate to severe disease a thrill is often palpable at the suprasternal notch and the base. The click is absent in subvalvar and supravalvar disease. Subaortic stenosis is frequently associated with aortic regurgitation.

D. Laboratory Findings: The chest x-ray shows a normal heart size and a dilated aortic root. The ECG is similar to CoA with RVH in infancy and LVH in older children. Echocardiography demonstrates the abnormal aortic valve and the left ventricular outflow tract abnormalities. Doppler flow studies can precisely estimate the pressure gradient.

E. Treatment: The gradient can be relieved by balloon valvuloplasty or surgery. Indications for surgery are symptoms, a gradient greater than 60 mm Hg, an abnormal blood pressure response to exercise, or electrocardiographic evidence of myocardial strain.

Endocardial Cushion Defect

A. General Considerations: This disorder, common in Down syndrome, is found in approximately 4% of patients with CHD. Males and females are affected equally. Pulmonary hypertension and irreversible pulmonary vascular obstructive disease are major risks.

B. Anatomy: In complete endocardial cushion defect, there is a large AV septal defect and a common AV valve that arises from both the right and left atria. The partial form has an ostium primum ASD and an abnormal mitral valve, with mitral regurgitation.

C. Symptoms and Signs: In the newborn period the murmur may be inaudible and P2 will be loud. A nonspecific systolic murmur along with a mid diastolic flow rumble at the apex is usually heard in later infancy.

D. Laboratory Findings: The chest x-ray demonstrates cardiomegaly and increased pulmonary vascular markings. The ECG will show LAD with RVH, LVH, or both. Fifty percent of cases will have first-degree heart block. The echocardiogram is useful in assessing the AV valve structures and the atrial and ventricular septal defects.

E. Treatment: Anticongestive medication is used to control CHF. Surgery is performed prior to the development of irreversible pulmonary vascular disease, usually before 6–12 months.

Mitral Valve Prolapse (MVP)

A. General Considerations: The incidence of MVP is from 2–20% and most often occurs in slender females over the age of 6 years. Significant symptoms are rare.

B. Anatomy: Focal or diffusely redundant (myxomatous) valve tissue exists involving one or both leaflets with or without associated lengthening of the chordae tendinea.

C. Symptoms and Signs: A mid systolic click is heard at the apex and possibly the left sternal border. A mid to late systolic murmur may follow the click if mitral regurgitation is present.

D. Laboratory Findings: The chest x-ray is normal. Electrocardiographic findings vary from normal to nonspecific ST–T wave changes and/or dysrhythmias. The echocardiogram demonstrates abnormal posterior displacement of the mitral valve leaflets in systole.

E. Treatment: SBE prophylaxis is recommended if mitral regurgitation is present. Patients with significant chest pain are treated with beta blockade.

Hypoplastic Left Heart Syndrome (HLHS)

A. General Considerations: HLHS occurs in 1.5% of patients with CHD, with a male predominance. Without surgery it is virtually 100% fatal.

B. Anatomy: Aortic and mitral atresia with small left ventricular cavity.

C. Symptoms and Signs: The patients usually present in the first week of life with CHF and weak pulses. There is a single S2, and a pulmonary ejection click is associated with a nonspecific systolic ejection murmur at the left sternal border.

D. Laboratory Findings: The chest x-ray shows cardiomegaly and interstitial pulmonary edema. The ECG shows RVH with absence of left-sided forces. The echocardiogram demonstrates the hypoplastic left ventricle and aorta.

E. Treatment: Stabilization with prostaglandins and management of CHF can maintain these patients until surgery. With the development of the Norwood surgical approach and neonatal cardiac transplantation, a substantial number of these children now survive.

CYANOTIC HEART DISEASE

Cyanotic heart disease describes those children who have right to left shunts and are *usually,* but not always, cyanotic. Cyanosis is determined by the presence of at least 4–5 grams of unsaturated hemoglobin in the capillary bed. With this in mind, therefore, a child with a cyanotic heart lesion with anemia may not appear cyanotic. It is important to also remember that cyanotic infants may appear ashen in color rather than blue.

Tetralogy of Fallot (TOF)

A. General Considerations: TOF is the most common form of cyanotic cardiac malformation, accounting for 10–15% of all cases of CHD. There is a slight predominance of males over females.

B. Anatomy: TOF consists of infundibular PS, a large unrestrictive VSD, an aorta overriding the VSD, and RVH. Associated anomalies may include a right aortic arch in 25%, an ASD in 15%, absent pulmonary valve, pulmonary atresia, endocardial cushion defect, and a left superior vena cava to the coronary sinus.

C. Symptoms and Signs: Depending on the degree of left-to-right shunting, the patient may either be acyanotic (ie, pink tetralogy) or cyanotic. The degree of right ventricular outflow tract obstruction largely determines the degree of cyanosis. Auscultation reveals a single S2 and a grade I–III/VI systolic ejection murmur at the mid to high left sternal border. During a hypercyanotic spell the murmur diminishes in intensity and the patient becomes more cyanotic and irritable.

D. Laboratory Findings: The ECG commonly shows right axis deviation and RVH. The chest x-ray reveals a normal or small heart, often with the apex upturned, and a narrow mediastinum. The pulmonary markings are normal to decreased. The aortic arch is right sided in approximately 25% of cases. The echocardiogram demonstrates the overriding aorta, VSD, pulmonary infundibular stenosis, and the hypertrophied right ventricle. An arterial blood gas demonstrates a normal pH and P_{CO2} at rest, with a variable degree of hypoxemia.

E. Treatment: Beta blockade may prevent hypercyanotic spells. Surgical palliation is provided with creation of a systemic artery to pulmonary artery anastomosis to increase pulmonary blood flow (Blalock–Taussig shunt). Later, total correction is completed with VSD closure and patch augmentation of the right ventricular outflow tract or the placement of a conduit from the right ventricle to the pulmonary artery.

Transposition of the Great Arteries (TGA)

A. General Considerations: TGA is the second most common cyanotic heart lesion and accounts for 5–7% of all cases of CHD. There is a 3:1 male predominance.

B. Anatomy: The aorta arises from the right ventricle and the pulmonary artery arises from the left ventricle. Associated anomalies may include a VSD (30–35%), PS and VSD (10%), PS alone (5%), or CoA (5%).

C. Symptoms and Signs: The infants are cyanotic at birth and generally comfortable appearing and well developed. The first heart sound is normal and S2 is single. The systolic murmur of PS or VSD is heard when those associated lesions are present.

D. Laboratory Findings: The ECG may be entirely normal or show right-axis deviation and RVH. In the first few days of life, the chest x-ray can be normal or show the diagnostic triad of an oval or egg-shaped cardiac silhouette, a narrow mediastinum, and increased pulmonary markings. The echocardiogram will demonstrate the aorta arising from the right ventricle and the pulmonary artery from the left ventricle. Associated anomalies such as VSD and PS can be ascertained. The arterial blood gas shows Pa_{O2} rarely higher than 35 mm Hg with little or no response to supplemental oxygen and a normal P_{CO2}.

E. Treatment: Medically, the infant is started in PGE_1. At cardiac catheterization, a balloon atrial septostomy is performed to enlarge an ASD and improve systemic and venous mixing. Surgically, the systemic and pulmonary venous return may be rerouted at the atrial level (Mustard or Senning procedure) or a supravalvar arterial switch with coronary artery relocation may be performed.

Total Anomalous Pulmonary Venous Return (TAPVR)

A. General Considerations: TAPVR describes a group of disorders in which no pulmonary venous return enters directly into the left atrium. This heart lesion accounts for 2% of cases of CHD and is seen equally in males and females except when the veins enter the portal system, in which case there is an approximate 3:1 male predominance.

B. Anatomy: The pulmonary veins generally form a confluence and then enter the heart (1) via a vertical vein into the left innominate vein; (2) directly into the coronary sinus, the right atrium, or the right superior vena cava; or (3) across the diaphragm and into the inferior vena cava or the portal system. They may or may not be obstructed.

C. Symptoms and Signs: Patients without pulmonary venous obstruction are usually mildly cyanotic and asymptomatic at birth; CHF develops later. A right ventricular heave may be present. S1 is loud, followed by a widely split S2 and usually an S3 at the apex. A grade II/VI systolic ejection murmur is usually, but not always, heard in the pulmonic region, with a mid diastolic flow rumble in the tricuspid valve region. Patients with obstruction to pulmonary venous return usually develop signs and symptoms within 24 hours of birth, including respiratory distress, feeding problems, and cardiac failure. They are cyanotic. S1 is normal and S2 splits with an increased P2. A murmur may be barely audible.

D. Laboratory Findings: In unobstructed TAPVR, the ECG shows right-axis deviation, right atrial enlargement (RAE), and RVH. The chest x-ray will demonstrate increased pulmonary flow, an enlarged right heart, and occasionally a "snowman" figure when the return is supracardiac. The echocardiogram shows an enlarged right atrium and ventricle. The anomalous pulmonary veins can usually be demonstrated. With obstructed pulmonary venous return the ECG will show RVH. The chest x-ray reveals a normal heart size and diffuse interstitial edema. The echocardiogram shows a large right ventricle, and doppler flow studies will demonstrate the pulmonary venous obstruction.

E. Treatment: Surgical correction with reanastomosis of the pulmonary veins to the left atrium is mandatory in early infancy and is emergent when the veins are obstructed.

Tricuspid Atresia

A. General Considerations: This lesion occurs in 2% of cases of CHD and is slightly more common in males.

B. Anatomy: There is complete atresia of the tricuspid valve and, therefore, no direct communication between the right atrium and the right ventricle. The right ventricle has varying degrees of hypoplasia. There is a mandatory ASD. The great vessels may be normally related or transposed and a VSD may or may not be present. The pulmonary valve is normal, stenotic, or atretic.

C. Symptoms and Signs: The infants are cyanotic at birth. S1 is normal and S2 is single. A grade I–III/VI harsh systolic ejection murmur is heard along the lower left sternal border and there may be CHF when the pulmonary blood flow is increased.

D. Laboratory Findings: The ECG shows LAD, RAE, and LVH. The chest x-ray reveals a slightly to markedly enlarged heart with variable pulmonary artery markings, depending on the associated lesions. The echocardiogram demonstrates the absence of the tricuspid valve and the right ventricular hypoplasia. The relationship of the great vessels can be determined and the status of the pulmonary valve and ventricular septum identified.

E. Treatment: A balloon atrial septostomy is performed in the catheterization lab to allow unobstructed flow to the left heart. For those patients with high pulmonary blood flow, anticongestives are utilized followed by an atriopulmonary anastomosis (Fontan procedure) at a later date. Pulmonary artery banding may be required to protect the pulmonary vascular bed prior to the Fontan repair. Low pulmonary blood flow indicates the need for a systemic-to-pulmonary shunt followed later by the Fontan procedure.

Pulmonary Atresia, Intact Ventricular Septum
    A. General Considerations: Pulmonary atresia with an intact ventricular septum accounts for approximately 1% of cases of CHD.

    B. Anatomy: The pulmonary valve does not form and the right ventricle is either small with a hypertrophied wall or of relatively normal size. The ventricular septum is intact. The tricuspid valve shows varying degrees of hypoplasia. Fistulous communication between the right ventricle and coronary arteries may occur.

    C. Symptoms and Signs: The infants are cyanotic from birth. S1 is normal and S2 is single. A grade I–II/VI continuous murmur (PDA) may be heard at the left upper sternal border as may a grade I–III/VI harsh pansystolic murmur at the left lower sternal border (tricuspid regurgitation).

    D. Laboratory Findings: The ECG shows a normal axis, RAE, and LVH. The chest x-ray reveals a large heart with decreased pulmonary blood flow. The echocardiogram shows the atretic pulmonary valve plus an intact ventricular septum. The size of the right ventricular cavity can be ascertained as well as the presence and degree of tricuspid regurgitation.

E. Treatment: Prostaglandins are utilized to keep the ductus arteriosus open while awaiting intervention. A balloon atrial septostomy is performed in the catheterization lab. If the right ventricle is small a systemic-to-pulmonary shunt procedure is created. If the right ventricle is of adequate size a pulmonary valvulotomy is performed. Right ventricular outflow tract reconstruction is performed at a later date if necessary.

Truncus Arteriosus

A. General Considerations: Approximately 0.7% of children with CHD have truncus arteriosus, which is equally distributed between males and females. DiGeorge's syndrome with thymic aplasia is frequently present.

B. Anatomy: One large vessel giving rise to the aorta, pulmonary artery, and coronary arteries arises from the heart. It overrides a VSD. The truncal valve may be stenotic and/or incompetent. A right aortic arch is common.

C. Symptoms and Signs: When there is unobstructed pulmonary blood flow the child presents with CHF. If there is decreased flow to the lungs the infant will be cyanotic. S1 and S2 are loud, and a systolic ejection click is present. A grade II–IV/VI systolic ejection murmur is heard at the left lower sternal border. A diastolic decrescendo murmur of truncal valve insufficiency may be audible.

D. Laboratory Findings: ECG usually demonstrates right ventricular or biventricular hypertrophy and ST–T wave depression. The chest x-ray reveals a large boot-shaped heart with absence of the pulmonary artery segment, often a right aortic arch, and variable pulmonary markings. The echocardiogram identifies the single truncal root and the large VSD.

E. Treatment: Anticongestive medications are needed for patients with high pulmonary blood flow. Early total correction is performed by closing the VSD to include the truncal root. The pulmonary arteries are detached from the root and then reanastomosed to the right ventricle, with or without an interposed conduit.

ACQUIRED HEART DISEASE

Acquired heart disease includes infectious, immunologic, and metabolic involvement of the endocardium, myocardium, or pericardium. It frequently presents in all age groups as a life-threatening illness.

ACUTE RHEUMATIC FEVER (ARF)

A. General Considerations: ARF is a disease occurring in susceptible people following a group A β-hemolytic streptococcal infection of the respiratory tract. It is more common in the 5–15-year-old age group, females, and blacks. Two major, or one major and 2 minor, criteria from the list of Jones' criteria plus positive evidence of a streptococcal infection are required to make the diagnosis.

B. Symptoms and Signs: The physical examination varies, depending on which of the criteria are present. The major criteria include:

1. Cardiac–The new onset of a mitral regurgitation or aortic regurgitation murmur, pericarditis, or CHF.

2. Polyarthritis–Inflammation of 2 or more joints, typically the larger joints. Inflammation is often migratory.

3. Subcutaneous nodules–Nontender, mobile nodules located just beneath the skin.

4. Erythema marginatum–Macular erythematous rash on the trunk and the extremities, generally sparing the face.

5. Sydenham's chorea–Emotional instability and an involuntary, usually unilateral, motion disorder. The minor criteria include fever, polyarthralgia, prolonged PR interval, acute phase reactants [elevated C-reactive protein (CRP), erythrocyte sedimentation rate (ESR), or white blood count (WBC)], and a history of previous acute rheumatic fever.

C. Laboratory Findings: There *must* be positive evidence of streptococcal infection, either elevated ASO titers or positive throat cultures. The chest x-ray will often show cardiomegaly and the ECG will show first-degree heart block or nonspecific ST–T wave changes. The echocardiogram demonstrates the presence of a pericardial effusion, valvular regurgitation, and decreased contractility.

D. Treatment: During the acute period penicillin should be administered to eradicate the streptococcal infection. Aspirin is given for 2–6 weeks and steroids may be added in severe cases. Limited activity is prescribed, the degree of which is determined by the severity of the disease. Long-term treatment includes penicillin prophylaxis, anticongestive medications when indicated, and valve replacement if necessary.

KAWASAKI DISEASE

A. General Considerations: Kawasaki disease, or mucocu-taneous lymph node syndrome, is an inflammatory disorder of unknown etiology; it has multisystem involvement, most notably the heart. Eighty percent of the cases involve children less than 4 years of age, with a 1.5:1 male to female ratio. Asians are affected more frequently than blacks, who are more frequently affected than whites.

B. Symptoms and Signs: As with acute rheumatic fever, the physical findings depend on the particular criteria present, 5 of which are needed to make the diagnosis.

1. Fever–longer than 5 days, not responsive to antibiotics.

2. Mucous membrane involvement–cracked, fissured lips and tongue–"strawberry tongue."

3. Conjunctivitis–nonpurulent.

4. Polymorphous rash–generally involving the trunk and extremities.

5. Lymphadenopathy

6. Digital swelling and desquamation

Examination of the cardiovascular system may reveal findings consistent with myocarditis, pericarditis, and peripheral arteritis.

C. Laboratory Findings: The WBC, ESR, and CRP will be elevated, as will the platelet count. A normochromic anemia can be present, as can a sterile pyuria. The ECG often shows a prolonged PR interval, ST–T wave changes, and low voltage. The chest x-ray may show cardiomegaly. The echocardiogram is vital in Kawasaki disease since 20% of patients will develop coronary artery aneurysms or dilatation. A pericardial effusion may be present.

D. Treatment: Current therapy includes aspirin and intravenous gamma globulin. Serial ECGs and echocardiograms should be obtained since Kawasaki disease has acute and chronic phases and some findings, most notably coronary involvement, may not be present on the initial examination.

ENDOCARDITIS

A. General Considerations: Infective endocarditis is an infection of the endocardium in patients with structural heart disease or in immunocompromised hosts. It is rarely seen in a normal population. The most common organisms include *Strep-*

tococcus viridans and *Staphylococcus aureus,* along with fungal infections.

B. Symptoms and Signs: The patient may have a history of persistent fever and weight loss. The physical examination will be positive for changing murmurs and splenomegaly (70%), petechiae, and peripheral embolic phenomenon.

C. Laboratory Findings: The ESR and WBC are often elevated and the urine can be heme positive. Cultures of the blood may or may not be positive. Cardiomegaly will be present on the chest x-ray and heart block will be seen on the ECG when the aortic anulus is involved. The echocardiogram will identify large endocardial vegetations, but may be normal.

D. Treatment: Appropriate antibiotics should be administered for both culture-positive and culture-negative endocarditis. Treatment for CHF and valve replacement may be necessary.

MYOCARDITIS

A. General Considerations: In a majority of cases the cause is unknown. Viral etiologies are common and include Coxsackie A & B, rubella, cytomegalovirus, mumps, adenovirus, and herpes.

B. Symptoms and Signs: In the newborn period the onset is rapid with CHF and vascular collapse. Mitral and tricuspid regurgitation may also be present. The onset is more insidious in the older child.

C. Laboratory Findings: The WBC is variable and both bacterial and viral cultures are usually negative. A chest x-ray will show cardiomegaly with moderate to marked venous congestion and possibly pneumonia. Decreased voltage, ST–T wave changes, and dysrhythmias may be seen on the ECG. Decreased contractility and dilation of the heart are seen by echocardiography.

D. Treatment: CHF is treated with digitalis, diuretics, and afterload reduction. Care is taken with digitalization, using two-thirds the total digitalizing dose owing to an increased risk of toxicity.

PERICARDITIS

A. General Considerations: Pericarditis may be nonpurulent, secondary to rheumatic fever, viral infection, collagen vascular disease, and uremia; or purulent, caused by *Haemophil-*

us influenzae, S aureus, and streptococcus pneumoniae. It is rarely an isolated event. Tamponade may occur and may lead to rapid deterioration and death.

B. Symptoms and Signs: Fever is present along with retro-sternal chest pain. Dyspnea and grunting respirations may be present in infants. There may be jugular venous distention and pulsus paradoxus. Cardiac examination may reveal muffled heart sounds and a pericardial friction rub.

C. Laboratory Findings: In nonpurulent pericarditis, the WBC and ESR may be elevated with negative blood cultures. In purulent pericarditis the blood culture is positive and the WBC and ESR may be elevated. In the presence of an effusion, the cardiac silhouette has a "water-bottle" shape. ST–T wave changes can be seen on the ECG. The echocardiogram can document the presence of a pericardial effusion and evidence of purulent loculation.

D. Treatment: Aspirin and other anti-inflammatories are used for nonpurulent pericarditis. Antibiotics and pericardiectomy are indicated in purulent pericarditis. Cardiac tamponade requires an emergent pericardiocentesis.

DYSRHYTHMIAS

Recognition and management of cardiac dysrhythmias in childhood is growing rapidly. This growth is due partly to increased awareness secondary to the availability and improving technology in cardiac monitoring equipment, eg, continuous heart rate monitoring in intensive care units and the 24-hour Holter monitor. Also, there is a true increase in the incidence and prevalence of dysrhythmias as more patients are surviving open heart surgery, and dysrhythmias are frequently seen in these survivors. Understanding the basic underlying mechanism of dysrhythmias helps in establishing a diagnostic and treatment approach.

SINUS DYSRHYTHMIAS

Sinus Arrhythmia
Sinus rhythm with a variable heart rate. This is a normal variant with an increase in rate with inspiration and a decrease with expiration. No treatment is required.

Sinus Bradycardia

Sinus heart rate less than the lower limits of normal for age (60 BPM in newborns, 40 BPM in older children). This may be a normal finding in athletes and at rest. Other causes include sick sinus syndrome, hypertension, and central nervous system abnormalities. Asymptomatic patients need only to be watched, while treatment should be directed at correcting the underlying cause.

Sinus Tachycardia

Sinus heart rate greater than the upper limits of normal for age (220 BPM in newborns, 190 BPM in older children). This is found in fever, anemia, hypovolemia, and CHF. Treatment should be directed at the underlying cause.

CONDUCTION ABNORMALITIES

First-degree Heart Block

Prolonged PR interval that is greater than the upper limits of normal for age. No treatment is required.

Second-degree Heart Block

Mobitz Type I (Wenckebach) is progressive lengthening of the PR interval until a nonconducted P wave occurs. Mobitz Type II has a consistent PR interval with an occasional nonconducted P wave. Type I may be seen in normal persons while Type II implies advanced conduction system disease. Type I seldom requires treatment, while Type II may need temporary or permanent pacing.

Third-degree Heart Block (Complete AV Block)

This may be congenital or acquired after cardiac surgery, myocarditis, or drug ingestion. Seventy-five percent of patients with congenital third-degree block *without structural heart disease* have mothers with systemic lupus erythematosus.

Treatment of acute complete block includes isoproterenol or temporary pacing. Long-term treatment requires a permanent pacemaker if the patient is symptomatic, has exercise intolerance, or has a sleeping heart rate less than 40.

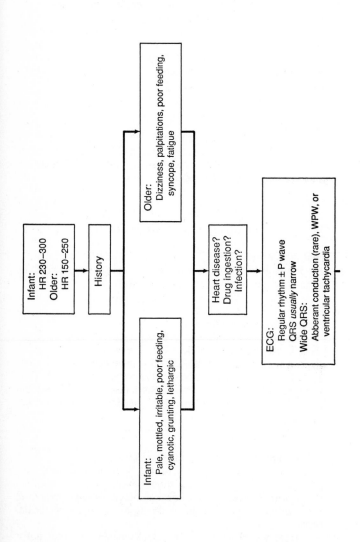

Infant:
HR 230–300
Older:
HR 150–250

History

Infant:
Pale, mottled, irritable, poor feeding,
cyanotic, grunting, lethargic

Older:
Dizziness, palpitations, poor feeding,
syncope, fatigue

Heart disease?
Drug ingestion?
Infection?

ECG:
Regular rhythm ± P wave
QRS *usually narrow*
Wide QRS:
Aberrant conduction (rare), WPW, or
ventricular tachycardia

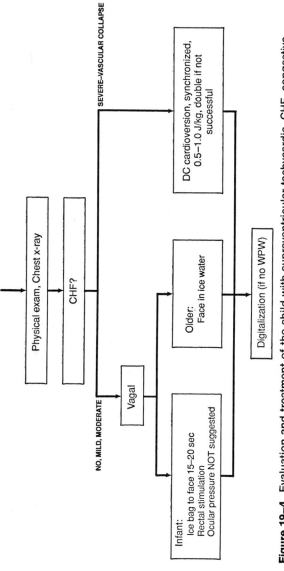

Figure 19–4. Evaluation and treatment of the child with supraventricular tachycardia. CHF, congestive heart failure; CXR, chest x-ray; DC, direct current; ECG, electrocardiogram; HR, heart rate; WPW, Wolff–Parkinson–White syndrome.

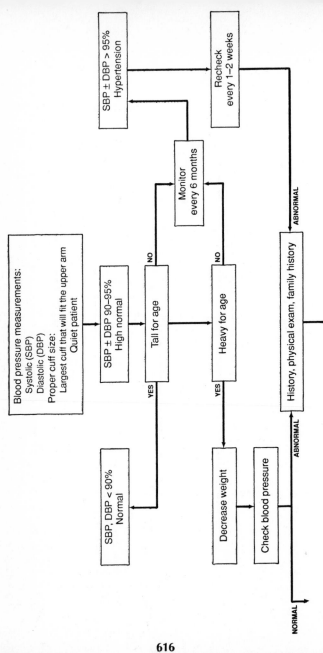

Blood pressure measurements:
Systolic (SBP)
Diastolic (DBP)
Proper cuff size:
Largest cuff that will fit the upper arm
Quiet patient

SBP ± DBP 90–95%
High normal

SBP, DBP < 90%
Normal

Tall for age

YES

NO

Heavy for age

YES

NO

Decrease weight

Check blood pressure

Monitor every 6 months

SBP ± DBP > 95%
Hypertension

Recheck every 1–2 weeks

History, physical exam, family history

ABNORMAL

ABNORMAL

NORMAL

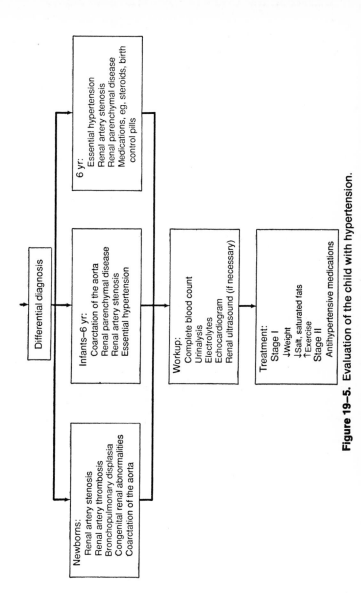

Figure 19–5. Evaluation of the child with hypertension.

Differential diagnosis

Newborns:
Renal artery stenosis
Renal artery thrombosis
Bronchopulmonary dysplasia
Congenital renal abnormalities
Coarctation of the aorta

Infants–6 yr:
Coarctation of the aorta
Renal parenchymal disease
Renal artery stenosis
Essential hypertension

6 yr:
Essential hypertension
Renal artery stenosis
Renal parenchymal disease
Medications, eg, steroids, birth
control pills

Workup:
Complete blood count
Urinalysis
Electrolytes
Echocardiogram
Renal ultrasound (if necessary)

Treatment:
Stage I
↓Weight
↓Salt, saturated fats
↑Exercise
Stage II
Antihypertensive medications

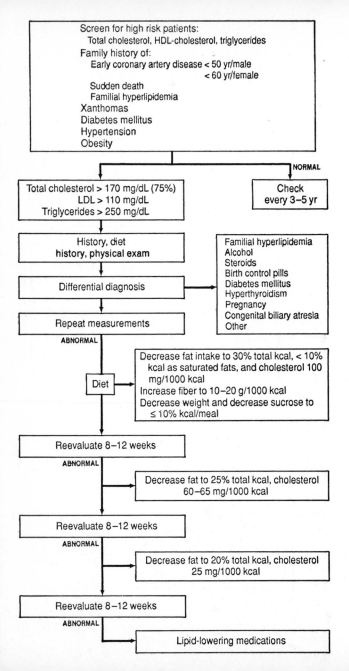

Screen for high risk patients:
    Total cholesterol, HDL-cholesterol, triglycerides
Family history of:
    Early coronary artery disease < 50 yr/male
                                    < 60 yr/female
    Sudden death
    Familial hyperlipidemia
Xanthomas
Diabetes mellitus
Hypertension
Obesity

NORMAL → Check every 3–5 yr

Total cholesterol > 170 mg/dL (75%)
LDL > 110 mg/dL
Triglycerides > 250 mg/dL

History, diet history, physical exam

Differential diagnosis →
    Familial hyperlipidemia
    Alcohol
    Steroids
    Birth control pills
    Diabetes mellitus
    Hyperthyroidism
    Pregnancy
    Congenital biliary atresia
    Other

Repeat measurements

ABNORMAL

Diet →
    Decrease fat intake to 30% total kcal, < 10% kcal as saturated fats, and cholesterol 100 mg/1000 kcal
    Increase fiber to 10–20 g/1000 kcal
    Decrease weight and decrease sucrose to ≤ 10% kcal/meal

Reevaluate 8–12 weeks

ABNORMAL →
    Decrease fat to 25% total kcal, cholesterol 60–65 mg/1000 kcal

Reevaluate 8–12 weeks

ABNORMAL →
    Decrease fat to 20% total kcal, cholesterol 25 mg/1000 kcal

Reevaluate 8–12 weeks

ABNORMAL →
    Lipid-lowering medications

PREMATURE DEPOLARIZATIONS

Premature Atrial Contraction (PAC)

Premature atrial depolarizations—P waves—that may or may not be conducted through the AV node. It is usually idiopathic (normal variant) but may be secondary to hypokalemia, hypoxia, hypoglycemia, atrial enlargement, or digitalis toxicity. No treatment is required unless supraventricular tachycardia (SVT) is present.

Premature Junctional Contraction (PJC)

Premature QRS waves of normal morphology not preceded by a P wave. The beats originate in the AV nodal region and have the same significance as PACs.

Premature Ventricular Contraction (PVC)

Premature QRS complex with a prolonged duration and a morphology different from the preceding normal QRS complex. It is not preceded by a P wave. PVCs may be found in a normal heart or may be secondary to hypokalemia, hypocalcemia, cardiomyopathy, or myocarditis. In asymptomatic patients with no underlying heart disease, no treatment is necessary. Treatment should be directed at correcting the underlying cause. Suppression with antidysrhythmic agents should be initiated in a hospital setting.

TACHYDYSRHYTHMIAS

Supraventricular Tachycardia (SVT) (Figure 19–4)
Atrial Flutter

Saw-tooth configuration of atrial flutter waves with atrial rates varying from 300 to 600. There may be variable AV node conduction. This rhythm is seen in right or left atrial enlargements, sick-sinus syndrome, hypokalemia, hypoxia, hypoglycemia, atrial septal aneurysm, and following cardiac surgery. Acute treatment includes DC cardioversion, overdrive atrial pacing, and intravenous digitalis or procainamide.

Figure 19–6. Screening and evaluation of the child with hyperlipidemia. HDL, high density lipoproteins; Hx, history; LDL, low density lipoproteins; PE, physical examination.

Atrial Fibrillation

Rapid irregularly-irregular atrial rate with irregular QRS rhythm. This is a rare entity in children but can occur in right and left atrial enlargement, hypokalemia, hypoxia, hypoglycemia, hyperthyroidism, and following atrial surgery. Acute treatment includes DC cardioversion and intravenous digitalis.

Ventricular Tachycardia

Three or more consecutive PVCs at rates of greater than 120. The PVCs may be unifocal and multifocal. The ventricular origin of the tachycardia is substantiated by the presence of fusion beats. Ventricular tachycardia can be seen in myocarditis, cardiomyopathy, digitalis toxicity, long QT syndrome, hypertrophic cardiomyopathy, myocardial tumors, and following cardiac surgery. Treatment includes DC cardioversion when the patient is hemodynamically unstable. Antidysrhythmic agents are used to suppress recurrences and must be initiated in a hospital setting.

PREVENTIVE CARDIOLOGY

Hypertension (Figure 19–5) and hyperlipidemia (Figure 19–6) are well recognized as risk factors for atherosclerotic heart disease. Long-range population-based studies have shown elevations of these risk factors to persist from childhood throughout adolescence and adulthood. Screening and intervention programs are now being offered in most pediatric centers.

Stephen Berman, MD

DISEASES OF THE EAR

OTITIS MEDIA

Otitis media, defined as an inflammation of the middle ear, is usually associated with an effusion or collection of fluid in the middle ear space. Otitis media with effusion is classified by its duration (acute if present for less than 6 weeks; subacute if present from 6 weeks to 3 months; and chronic if present for longer than 3 months) and by the characteristics of the effusion. The effusion is purulent in acute otitis media, is a transudate in serous otitis media, and is thick and tenacious in mucoid (secretory) otitis media. Chronic effusions may be purulent, serous, or mucoid, and it is often difficult to identify the type of effusion by otoscopy. Recurrent otitis media is defined as 3 episodes within a 6-month period.

The diagnosis of otitis media with effusion is based on specific otoscopic findings, which include the appearance of the tympanic membrane and an assessment of its mobility.

1. ACUTE OTITIS MEDIA

General Considerations

Bacteriologic findings in middle ear aspirates can be summarized as follows: *Streptococcus pneumoniae*, 30% of cases; *Haemophilus influenzae*, 21%; *Branhamella catarrhalis*, 12%; group A streptococci, 3%; *Staphylococcus aureus*, 2%; and others (including enteric gram-negative organisms and anaerobic organisms), 4%. In 20% of cases, aspirates are sterile and 18% grow presumed nonpathogens such as *S epidermidis* and diptheroids.

Recently, *B catarrhalis* has been more commonly recognized as a causative agent of acute purulent otitis media. *H influenzae* remains an important pathogen in cases throughout childhood and into early adulthood. In many areas, the prevalence of beta-lactamase–producing isolates for *H influenzae* is 30% and for *B catarrhalis* is 80%. This means that one in 4 cases of acute otitis may be resistant to amoxicillin.

Attempts to isolate respiratory viruses or *Mycoplasma pneumoniae* from ear aspirates have generally been unsuccessful.

In about 3% of cases, multiple pathogens are isolated from a single specimen of middle ear effusion. In children with bilateral acute otitis media, different pathogens can be recovered from each ear in 5–10% of cases.

The microbiologic causes of acute otitis media in early infancy differ from those in later life. The risk of gram-negative enteric infection is especially high in infants who are under 6 weeks of age and have been hospitalized in a neonatal intensive care nursery. In normal infants seen during the first 3 months of life, acute otitis media can often be caused by *S aureus* and *Chlamydia trachomatis*, as well as *S pneumoniae*, *H influenzae*, and *B catarrhalis*.

Clinical Findings

A. Symptoms and Signs: Acute otitis media often presents with pain in association with symptoms of upper respiratory tract infection (eg, rhinorrhea, stuffy nose, and cough) or purulent conjunctivitis. While older children may complain of earache, young children demonstrate pain by crying, increased irritability, or difficulty in sleeping. Irritability may be related to hearing loss as well as pain. Tugging at the ears, sometimes a useful sign, is often falsely positive. Fever is present in less than half of cases. Facial palsy or ataxia may occur in a rare case.

The tympanic membrane appears either red or yellow, depending on the degree of inflammation and the amount of purulent material in the middle ear space. White exudate may be visible on the membrane. In early cases, bulging may be limited to the pars flaccida. Later, the entire eardrum bulges outward, giving a doughnutlike appearance. Tympanic membrane mobility is absent or markedly diminished. If the eardrum has spontaneously ruptured, cloudy to purulent discharge will be present in the ear canal, making examination of the tympanic membrane difficult.

Occasionally, bullae form between the outer and middle layers of the tympanic membrane and produce acute bullous myringitis. This entity should be considered a form of acute purulent otitis media.

Treatment

A. Specific Measures:

1. Systemic antibiotics–In areas where beta-lactamase–producing pathogens are common, the initial treatment for acute otitis media should be 10 days of trimethoprim, 10 mg/kg/dose with sulfamethoxazole, 50 mg/kg/d in 2 divided doses; or erythromycin, 40 mg/kg/dose plus sulfisoxazole, 150 mg/kg/dose in 4 divided doses. Otherwise, the drug of choice for acute otitis media in children of all ages is amoxicillin, 50 mg/kg/d in 3 divided doses, continued for 10 days.

Patients allergic to penicillin can be treated adequately with erythromycin plus sulfisoxazole, or trimethoprim plus sulfamethoxazole. Tetracyclines are contraindicated for ear infections, because about 50% of pneumococci and streptococci are resistant to these drugs and because they cause staining of the tooth enamel. Trimethoprim–sulfamethoxazole is not effective against *S pyogenes* and should not be used if streptococcal pharyngitis is suspected.

If symptoms such as fever, earache, irritability, vomiting, or lethargy persist beyond 48 hours of therapy, the patient should be reevaluated. After 2–3 weeks, about 50% of children are cured, 40% still have residual middle ear effusion, and 10% still have persistent acute infection.

Children with persistent infection after a 10-day course of amoxicillin should receive a full 14-day course of trimethoprim plus sulfamethoxazole or erythromycin plus sulfisoxazole. If the physician is concerned about compliance, the patient can be treated with intramuscular injection of penicillin G benzathine and procaine combined (Bicillin C-R) and oral sulfisoxazole. Children with persistent infection after a course of trimethoprim plus sulfamethoxazole or erythromycin plus sulfisoxazole should receive amoxicillin plus, 40 mg/kg/d in 3 divided doses, amoxicillin plus clavulanate, 40 mg/kg/d in 3 divided doses, or a third-generation oral cephalosporin. If the acute symptomatic infection still persists after this second course of antibiotics, myringotomy or tympanocentesis should be performed and middle ear secretions cultured to determine the most appropriate antibiotic therapy. Failure of acute otitis media to resolve after a third course of antibiotic therapy requires referral to an otolaryngologist for possible placement of tympanostomy tubes.

Acute otitis media in infants less than 6 weeks of age with a complicated neonatal course requiring prolonged hospitalization is often caused by gram-negative enteric organisms. These patients should have a tympanocentesis, blood culture, and lumbar puncture and receive intravenous ampicillin plus either gentamicin or cefotaxime in the hospital pending culture results. Acute otitis in infants under 3 months without additional risk factors or signs of serious illness can be treated with erythromycin plus sulfamethoxazole, a third-generation cephalosporin, or Augmentin as an outpatient. These children should be reexamined at 24 and 48 hours. If their condition worsens during this time period, they should be hospitalized.

2. Antibiotic ear drops–If the eardrum has been perforated, there is usually a cloudy to watery material in the ear canal, and antibiotic ear drops are not required. However, the child with considerable purulent drainage from the ear may profit from this adjunctive therapy. The purulent material can be removed by gentle suction, using a syringe and short plastic tubing such as can be made by cutting a scalp vein needle set. Normal saline solution can be instilled without force and then removed. After this type of cleansing has eliminated the pus, antibiotic corticosteroid ear drops (eg, Cortisporin Otic Suspension) can be instilled 3 times a day. The child should be held with the head sideways and stationary for a few minutes after drops are instilled. Cotton plugs are contraindicated.

3. Unwarranted measures–Antihistamine–decongestant combinations are ineffective in the treatment of otitis media. Vasoconstrictor nose drops are of no value, since it is nearly impossible to deliver them to the entrance of the auditory tube. Analgesic ear drops have not proved effective for the relief of pain and have the disadvantage of obscuring the field of vision if the tympanic membrane needs to be reexamined.

4. Myringotomy and tympanocentesis–Myringotomy is indicated if the patient has severe pain (as evidenced by inconsolable screaming) or if recurrent vomiting or ataxia is associated with the ear infection. In these circumstances, myringotomy is more effective than analgesics or antiemetics. Unfortunately, myringotomy does not appear to prevent the development of persistent residual effusions.

Prognosis

With treatment, suppurative complications such as mastoiditis are rare. Temporary hearing loss is common, permanent conductive hearing loss is less common, and permanent sensorineural hearing loss is rare.

2. ACUTE BULLOUS MYRINGITIS

In acute bullous myringitis, bullae form between the outer and middle layers of the tympanic membrane. In the past, this was considered to be always due to viral infections. Studies demonstrate that 50–75% of affected patients have an underlying acute purulent otitis media. The organisms isolated in cases of acute bullous myringitis are similar to those found in acute otitis media. A causative role for *M pneumoniae* or viruses in cases of bullous myringitis has not been confirmed.

The patient usually complains of ear pain on the involved side. Examination of the ear reveals 1–3 bullae that may cover 20–90% of the drum surface. They are thin-walled and often sagging in appearance, and they often contain a straw-colored fluid. There is minimal erythema.

Antibiotics are prescribed as for acute otitis media. Analgesics are sometimes indicated. The bullae do not have to be opened unless they are causing significant pain. They can be easily opened by nicking them with a myringotomy knife or spinal needle.

Follow-up care is the same as that described for acute purulent otitis media.

3. PERSISTENT MIDDLE EAR EFFUSION

General Considerations

Residual serous otitis media following appropriate antibiotic therapy for acute otitis media occurs in 40–50% of children. These residual effusions clear spontaneously within 2 months in 85% of cases. Effusions that fail to clear are called persistent. The effusion may be serous or mucoid (secretory).

Persistent serous effusions may be associated with a low-grade bacterial infection, especially infection with beta-lactamase–producing organisms such as *H influenzae*, *B catarrhalis*, *S aureus*, and penicillin-resistant *S pneumoniae*.

Clinical Findings

Children with serous otitis media are usually asymptomatic and have hearing loss. The patient may complain of a feeling of fullness in the ear. An older patient may compare the feeling with "talking inside a barrel." In the preverbal child, hearing loss should be suspected if irritability, inattentiveness, or increased behavior problems are noted. Unlike acute purulent otitis media, there is minimal pain.

The tympanic membrane may appear mildly injected and dull or have a normal appearance. Mobility is diminished or absent. When fluid levels or air bubbles are visualized, the effusion is in a stage of resolution, with eustachian tube function improving. When eustachian tube dysfunction results in persistent negative pressure in the middle ear space, the tympanic membrane appears retracted, and the position of the short process of the right malleus changes from 7 o'clock to 9 o'clock. Tympanic membrane mobility is altered; ie, the membrane may move only when negative pressure is applied.

The most common complication of a persistent effusion is conductive hearing loss, which may adversely affect language development, intellectual functioning, and academic performance. The presence of an effusion predisposes the child to another episode of acute otitis media.

Treatment

A. Medical Measures: If a residual effusion has persisted longer than 8 weeks, despite 2 courses of antibiotic therapy, consider a trial of prednisone, 0.5 mg/kg/dose in 2 divided doses for 7 days combined with a 21–28 day course of one of the following regimens to treat beta-lactamase–producing organisms: trimethoprim plus sulfamethoxazole; erythromycin plus sulfisoxazole; erythromycin plus sulfisoxazole; cefaclor alone; or ampicillin plus clavulanic acid.

Oral decongestants and antihistamines have not proved to be effective for treatment.

B. Surgical Treatment: If manifestations of a persistent effusion (ie, documented effusion, hearing loss > 20 dB, and abnormal findings on tympanogram) have failed to resolve after a 3-month period despite a trial of antibiotics plus prednisone, the patient should be referred to an otolaryngologist for insertion of tympanoplasty tubes. A child with signs of partial resolution noted on otoscopy, audiogram, or tympanogram should be followed for another month prior to referral. A child whose tympanic membrane is severely retracted and whose tympanogram shows a peak at negative pressure should be followed for the development of persistent retraction pockets. Persistent retraction pockets should also be treated with tympanoplasty tubes.

Myringotomy followed by insertion of tympanoplasty tubes (polyethylene flanged ventilation tubes) has given excellent results in this disorder as long as the tubes are in place. The tubes permit pressure equalization and drying of the middle ear cavity without a functional eustachian tube. The hearing returns to normal with the tube in place. This procedure can be done in an outpatient surgical setting by an otolaryngologist. The long-term efficacy of tympanoplasty tubes has not been well evaluated.

Removal of the adenoids is rarely helpful. Adenoidectomy should be reserved for patients who have not benefited from ventilating tubes or who have signs of upper airway obstruction. Apparently, benefit is not related to adenoid size, so it is not possible to identify accurately which patients will benefit from this surgery.

4. RECURRENT OTITIS MEDIA WITH EFFUSION
(The "Otitis-Prone Condition")

Antibiotic Prophylaxis

Prophylaxis should be started following the resolution of the third episode within a 6-month period. Antibiotics shown to be effective include sulfisoxazole, 70 mg/kg/d, amoxicillin, 20 mg/kg/d, or erythromycin, 20 mg/kg/d, given in 2 divided doses. One daily dose may also be effective. Sulfisoxazole should be continued for 3 months. During the next 3–6 months, it is often helpful to advise parents to restart the antibiotic at the first sign of a cold and give it for a minimum of 2 weeks or until cold symptoms resolve. This program of prophylaxis has reduced the frequency of recurrent acute otitis by 50%. Failure to prevent a second breakthrough infection on continuous prophylaxis is an indication for referral to an otolaryngologist for insertion of ventilating tubes. Occasionally, patients with ventilating tubes continue to have recurrent acute otitis media and benefit from antibiotic prophylaxis.

OTITIS EXTERNA
(Inflammation of the External Ear Canal)

The most common cause of otitis externa is maceration of the ear canal lining due to frequent swimming or shower bathing. Trauma, reactions to foreign bodies, and accumulation of cerumen are other contributing factors. Pyogenic (especially *Pseudomonas* or staphylococcal) and mycotic superinfections are common.

Recurrent otitis externa is usually caused by the frequent use of cotton-tipped applicators or frequent swimming in chlorinated pools (or both).

Treatment

A. Pyogenic Infections: Treatment is aimed at keeping the external ear canal clean and dry and protecting it from trauma. Debris should be removed from the ear canal by gentle irrigation. Topical antibiotics combined with a corticosteroid applied as ear drops are essential. Give systemic antibiotics (usually penicillin) in full doses for 10 days if there is evidence of extension of the infection beyond the skin of the ear canal (fever, adenopathy, or cellulitis of the pinna). During the acute phase, swimming should be avoided if possible.

B. Removal of Foreign Bodies: Removal should always be done under direct vision and never done blindly. A stream of lukewarm saline directed past the foreign body into the external canal may float it out. Vegetable matter, such as peas and beans, swells in the presence of water and should instead by removed with a wire loop; care should be taken not to push the object farther into the canal. If the object is large or is wedged in place, the patient should be referred to an otolaryngologist.

C. Removal of Impacted Cerumen: Cerumen in the external ear must be removed before the examination can continue. It may be removed with a wire loop or with cotton on the end of a thin wire applicator. Cerumen may be softened, if necessary, by instilling mineral oil or Cerumenex. (*Caution:* Cerumenex can cause contact dermatitis if left in the ear canal for over 30 minutes.) It may also be washed out with warm water or saline, using a syringe. Irrigation is contraindicated if any possibility of a perforated eardrum exists.

Prognosis

After removal of a foreign body, rapid improvement occurs.

CHRONIC PERFORATION OF THE EARDRUM

Clinical Findings

A. Symptoms: Recurrent or persistent ear drainage may be present. Chronic otitis may be painless, and the child may be afebrile in the intervals between acute exacerbations.

B. Signs: The eardrum is perforated. Peripheral perforations provide a greater risk of cholesteatoma formation. Marked scarring of the drum signifies previous perforations. Mastoid tenderness may be present. A conductive type hearing loss will be present.

C. Laboratory Findings: Secondary invaders following perforations are frequent causes of chronic drainage and are much more resistant to therapy. These include *Pseudomonas, Escherichia coli, Klebsiella pneumoniae,* and staphylococci.

D. Imaging: X-ray studies for evidence of mastoid involvement are indicated in selected cases.

Complications

Complications include hearing loss, mastoiditis, brain abscess, meningitis, and labyrinthitis (with dizziness).

Treatment

Keep water out of the ear by plugging the ear with cotton impregnated with petrolatum when washing or bathing. Swimming should be forbidden. Instill appropriate antibiotic drops containing polymyxin for any serious drainage; systemic antibiotics are also indicated for purulent drainage or systemic signs.

Myringoplasty or tympanoplasty is performed when the child is about age 10 or older. Cholesteatoma is a pocket of skin that invades the middle ear and mastoid spaces from the edge of a perforation. This type of chronic otitis should be treated surgically when diagnosed.

Course & Prognosis

With massive and prolonged antibiotic treatment and surgical drainage of the mastoid bone when indicated, the prognosis is good. If no treatment is given, hearing loss is certain.

MASTOIDITIS

Infection of the mastoid antrum and air cells may follow an episode of untreated or improperly treated acute otitis media. The most common etiologic agents are *S pyogenes, S pneumoniae,* and *S aureus. H influenzae* causes mastoiditis much less frequently than expected. Other agents that can cause this disease include *Pseudomonas, Mycobacterium,* enteropathic gram-negative rods, and *B catarrhalis.* Anaerobic organisms appear to play a role in chronic mastoiditis; however, there are no data on how frequently they cause acute mastoiditis.

Clinical Findings

The principal complaints are postauricular pain and fever. On examination, the mastoid area is often swollen and reddened. In the late stage, it may be fluctuant. The earliest finding is severe tenderness upon mastoid percussion. Late findings are a pinna that is pushed forward by postauricular swelling and an ear canal that is narrowed in the posterior superior wall because of pressure from the mastoid abscess.

Mastoiditis is a clinical diagnosis. It cannot be diagnosed on the basis of x-rays alone. In the acute phase, there is diffuse inflammatory clouding of the mastoid cells as in every case of acute purulent otitis media. Only later is there evidence of bony destruction and resorption of the mastoid air cells.

Complications

Meningitis is a complication in about 9% of cases of acute mastoiditis. Brain abscess occurs in 2% of cases and may be associated with persistent headache, recurring fever, or changes in sensorium.

Treatment & Prognosis

The patient must be hospitalized because this disorder represents osteitis. Before therapy is initiated, myringotomy should be performed in order to obtain material for culture and also to relieve the pressure in the middle ear–mastoid space.

The initial management of uncomplicated acute mastoiditis includes intravenous antibiotic therapy and possibly surgery. Results of gram-stained smears taken during tympanocentesis may help in the choice of antibiotics. Ampicillin and nafcillin are a reasonable initial choice. Indications for immediate surgery include the clear evidence of a major complication such as meningitis, brain abscess, cavernous sinus thrombosis, acute suppurative labyrinthitis, or facial palsy. Some otolaryngologists consider the destruction of septal bone (osteitis) and resorption of the mastoid air cells an indication for surgery.

Oral antibiotics should be continued for 4–6 weeks after the patient is discharged.

The prognosis is good if treatment is started early and continued until the process is inactive.

DETECTION & MANAGEMENT OF HEARING DEFICITS

Hearing deficits are classified as conductive, sensorineural, or mixed (Table 20–1). Conductive hearing loss results from a

Table 20–1. Causes and types of hearing loss.

Source	Cause	Type	Degree of Loss
Congenital Endogenous	Hereditary (recessive, X-linked, or dominant)	Sensorineural (usually organ of Corti)	Moderate to profound

(Continued)

Table 20–1. (cont'd) Causes and types of hearing loss.

Source	Cause	Type	Degree of Loss
Exogenous	Asphyxia	Sensorineural (organ of Corti)	Moderate (high-frequency deficits)
	Erythroblastosis	Sensorineural (brainstem)	Mild to severe (high-frequency deficits)
	Maternal rubella and other viruses	Sensorineural (organ of Corti)	Moderate to severe
	Ototoxic drugs (aminoglycosides)	Sensorineural (usually organ of Corti)	Moderate to profound
Either endogenous or exogenous	Congenital atresia, stenosis, or ossicular deformity	Conductive (may be unilateral)	Moderate
Acquired	Labyrinthitis	Sensorineural (cochlear)	Mid to profound
	Measles	Sensorineural (usually cochlear)	Moderate to profound
	Meningitis	Sensorineural (cochlear and 8th nerve)	Moderate to profound
	Mumps	Sensorineural (usually cochlear and unilateral)	Profound
	Trauma	Conductive, sensorineural, or mixed	Moderate to profound
	Tumors	Sensorineural (8th nerve)	Moderate to profound
	Cerumen	Conductive	Mild to moderate
	Cholesteatoma		
	Foreign bodies		
	Otosclerosis		
	Perforated tympanum		
	Purulent otitis media		
	Repeated loud noise		
	Serous otitis media		

blockage of the transmission of sound waves from the external auditory canal to the inner ear and is characterized by normal bone conduction and reduced air conduction hearing. In children, conductive losses are most often caused by middle ear effusion. Sensorineural hearing loss occurs when the auditory nerve or cochlear hair cells are damaged. Mixed hearing loss is characterized by components of both conductive and sensorineural loss. The criteria for normal hearing levels in children are lower than those in adults, since children are in the process of learning language. In children, a hearing loss of 15–30 dB is considered mild, 31–50 dB moderate, 51–80 dB severe, and 81–100 dB profound.

Conductive Hearing Loss

The greatest number of conductive hearing losses during childhood are caused by otitis media and its sequelae. Other causes include atresia, stenosis, or collapse of the ear canal; furuncle, cerumen, or foreign body in the ear; aural discharge; bony growths; otitis externa; perichondritis; middle ear anomalies (eg, stapes fixation, ossicular malformation); and cleft palate.

The average hearing loss due to middle ear effusion (whether serous, purulent, or mucoid) is 27–31 dB, which is a mild hearing loss. This loss may be intermittent in nature and may occur in one or both ears, which accounts for the wide variability of the effects of ear disease on language development in children.

The American Academy of Pediatrics recommends that hearing be assessed and language development skills be monitored in children who have frequently recurring acute otitis media or middle ear effusion persisting longer than 3 months. The effects of hearing loss may be insidious and may not be discernible until the explosive phase of expressive language development occurs betwen 16 and 24 months of age; therefore, the optimal times for screening very young children are 18 and 24 months. An acceptable tool for language screening at these ages is the Early Language Milestone (ELM) scale. Children 3, 4, and 5 years of age should also be screened for language delays.

To mitigate the likelihood of a communication disorder developing, the physician should inform the parents of a child with middle ear disease that the child's hearing may not be normal and should instruct the parents to (1) turn off sources of background noise (eg, televisions, radios, dishwashers) when speaking to the child; (2) focus on the child's face and gain his or her direct attention before speaking; (3) speak slightly louder than usual; and (4) place the child in the front of the classroom.

Sensorineural Hearing Loss

Sensorineural hearing loss arises from a lesion in the cochlear structures of the inner ear or in the neural fibers of the auditory nerve (cranial nerve VIII). Most sensorineural losses in children are congenital, with an incidence of one in 750 live births. Causes of congenital deafness include perinatal infections, problems related to premature birth, and autosomal recessive and dominant inheritance of various deafness syndromes.

CONGENITAL MALFORMATIONS OF THE EXTERNAL EAR

Congenital malformation of the auricle is a cosmetic problem; associated abnormalities of the urogenital system or inner ear may be present. In children with congenital malformation, hearing should be tested by 6 months of age.

A small skin tag, fistula, or cystic mass in front of the tragus is a characteristic remnant of the first branchial cleft. These are best treated surgically.

Protruding auricles are a dominant hereditary characteristic. If the defect is severe, otoplasty should be performed for cosmetic purposes when the child is 5–6 years of age.

Agenesis of the external auditory canal or ear can be corrected surgically. If agenesis is bilateral, a hearing aid is fitted when the child is 2–4 weeks of age so that the child is not deprived of auditory stimulation during early development. Surgery is performed before school age in patients with bilateral agenesis and after childhood in patients with unilateral agenesis.

DISEASES OF THE NOSE & SINUSES

COMMON COLD

Nonbacterial upper respiratory tract infections are exceedingly common in the pediatric age group; about 2–4 such infections per year (6–8 in younger children) are considered usual in the USA.

A number of viruses are specific agents. Secondary bacterial invaders (beta-hemolytic streptococci, pneumococci, *H influenzae*) frequently contribute to prolongation of illness (beyond 4 days).

Clinical Findings

A. Symptoms: Malaise, sneezing, "stuffiness" of head, sore throat, and cough may be present.

B. Signs: Signs include serous nasal discharge and moist and boggy nasal mucous membranes. Fever is variable and may be high in an infant.

C. Laboratory Findings: The white blood cell count is normal or low.

Treatment

A. General Measures: Usually, no medications are needed. Give acetaminophen for pain or fever. Humidifying the air (vaporizer or bathroom shower water) is helpful in relieving nasal and pharyngeal discomfort and cough.

B. Local Measures: Topical vasoconstrictors, nose drops, or nasal sprays may provide symptomatic relief of nasal congestion but should not be used for more than 1 week. Overuse of any topical medication may result in irritation and "rebound" congestion. Oral decongestants cause jitters, and oral antihistamines cause lethargy; their use for treatment of the common cold is questionable.

Course & Prognosis

The usual course is of 4 days' duration. Continuation of rhinitis, regardless of whether it is serous or purulent, considerably beyond this period suggests bacterial complications or sinusitis that might respond to antibiotic therapy. Prognosis is excellent, but reinfections occur throughout life.

RECURRENT RHINITIS

A child with a chief complaint of "constant colds" is not uncommonly seen in office practice.

Differential Diagnosis & Treatment

A. Common Cold: The most common cause of recurrent runny nose is repeated viral upper respiratory tract infection. The onset is usually after 6 months of age. The bouts of rhinorrhea are usually accompanied by fever. Cultures are negative for bacteria. There is usually some evidence of contagion within the family.

Serum immunoelectrophoresis is an excessively ordered test. Children with immune defects do not have an increased number of colds.

Treatment consists of specific reassurance. The parents can be told that their child's general health is good; that the child will not have a great number of colds for more than a few years; that exposure to colds is building up the body's supply of antibodies; and that the child's problem is not the parents' fault.

B. Allergic Rhinitis: The onset of "hay fever" usually occurs after 2 years of age, ie, after the child has had adequate exposure to allergens. There is no fever or contagion among close contacts. The attacks include frequent sneezing, rubbing of the nose, and a profuse clear discharge. The nasal mucosa is pale and boggy. Smear of nasal secretions demonstrates over 20% of the cells to be eosinophils. Oral decongestants and antihistamines should be prescribed.

C. Chemical Rhinitis: Prolonged use of vasoconstrictor nose drops (beyond 7 days) results in a rebound reaction and secondary nasal congestion. The nose drops should be discontinued.

D. Vasomotor Rhinitis: Some children react to air pollution, tobacco smoke, or sudden changes in environmental temperature by manifesting prolonged congestion and rhinorrhea. Oral decongestants can be used periodically to give symptomatic relief.

PURULENT RHINITIS

Purulent rhinitis caused by pathogenic bacteria is an occasional aftermath of nonbacterial upper respiratory tract infection. In children with persistent rhinitis, consider underlying sinusitis.

Etiology & Clinical Findings

Pyogenic infection is usually due to group A hemolytic streptococci, *H influenzae,* or pneumococci. Infection with these organisms is characterized by purulent nasal discharge, dried pus about the nares, and inflamed nasal mucous membranes.

Nasal diphtheria is characterized by chronic serosanguineous nasal discharge.

Foreign bodies usually cause mucopurulent discharge from one nostril only, and that discharge often has a foul odor.

Treatment

If purulent rhinitis is due to infection, an appropriate antibiotic in the adequate dosage (see Chapter 8) should be given. For treatment of nasal diphtheria, see Chapter 15. Cases of rhinitis due to foreign bodies should usually be referred to a specialist if removal is not possible.

Prognosis

The prognosis is excellent. Improvement is prompt with specific therapy.

SINUSITIS

1. ACUTE SINUSITIS

General Considerations

Acute inflammation of the paranasal sinuses or sinusitis may complicate up to 5% of upper respiratory tract infections. The maxillary and ethmoid sinuses are most commonly involved because of poor drainage related to anatomic features. When mucociliary clearance and drainage is further compromised by an upper respiratory infection, the risk of secondary bacterial infection increases. Sinusitis is also commonly seen during pollen season in children with allergic rhinitis. In cases in which superinfection occurs, the organisms are *S pneumoniae, H influenzae* (nontypable), *B catarrhalis,* and beta-hemolytic streptococci. Rarely, anaerobic bacterial infections can cause fulminant frontal sinusitis. Viruses can be isolated in 10% of sinus aspirates but their pathogenic role is unclear. Anerobic and staphylococcal organisms are often responsible for chronic sinusitis.

The ethmoid sinus is the only one that is significantly developed at birth. The maxillary sinus is rudimentary at birth and visible on x-ray by 6 months. The frontal sinus is not visible until 3–9 years of age. Clinical ethmoiditis does not usually occur until 6 months of age. Maxillary sinusitis is seen clinically after 1 year of age. Frontal sinusitis is unusual before 10 years of age.

Clinical Findings

A. Symptoms and Signs: The most common clinical presentation of children is persistance of nasal discharge or postnasal drip and daytime cough lasting longer than 7–10 days. Persistent low-grade fever is often present. Malodorous breath or intermittent painless morning periorbital swelling is often noted. Older patients may complain of acute onset of headache, a sense of fullness, or facial pain overlying the involved sinus. Ethmoiditis causes retroorbital pain; maxillary sinusitis causes upper molar or zygomatic pain; and frontal sinusitis causes pain above the eyebrow. These signs are often associated with a high fever.

Physical examination reveals injected nasal mucosa, usually associated with nasal or postnasal mucopurulent discharge. Occasionally there is percussion tenderness overlying the sinusitis.

B. Laboratory Findings: Sinus aspiration should be performed for diagnostic purposes in patients with complications and in those with an immunosuppressive disease. Gram stain and culture of nasal discharge is unnecessary as the type of discharge (thin, mucoid, or purulent) is not a useful predictor of sinusitis and does not correlate with cultures of sinus aspirates. If the patient is hospitalized because of complications, a blood culture should be obtained.

C. Imaging: In most cases, the clinical findings are so classic that x-rays are not needed. Positive x-rays in children over 1 year will show opacification of the involved sinus, air-fluid levels if the obstruction is intermittent, or mucosal thickening of greater than 5 mm. It is notable that x-ray findings positive for sinusitis may be found in asymptomatic patients with colds or nasal allergies. Sinus views include the anteroposterior (Caldwell) for the frontal and ethmoid sinuses, occipitomental (Waters) for the maxillary sinuses, and submento vertex and lateral for the sphenoid sinus. A Waters view is usually sufficient. Sinus x-rays are mainly indicated in children with facial swelling of unknown cause; acute sinusitis that is unresponsive to 48 hours of therapy; undocumented chronic or recurrent sinusitis; and chronic asthma. A CT scan should be performed if bony erosions are present. Ultrasonography can also be used to document sinusitis.

Complications

The most frequent complication of paranasal sinusitis is preseptal periorbital cellulitis secondary to ethmoiditis. Less frequently, orbital cellulitis or abscess develops associated with decreased extraocular movement, proptosis, edema, and altered visual acuity. The most common complication of frontal sinusitis is osteitis of the frontal bone, called "Potts puffy tumor." Additional serious intracranial complications include cavernous sinus thrombosis, subdural empyema, brain abscess, and meningitis. The most common maxillary complication is cellulitis of the cheek. Rarely osteomyelitis of the maxilla can develop.

Treatment

A. Oral Antibiotics: Treat acute sinusitis with oral antibiotics for 10–14 days to achieve more prompt relief of symptoms and more rapid resolution of inflammation. The usual antibiotic should be amoxicillin 15 mg/kg/dose 3 times a day. In areas where beta-lactamase–positive pathogens are common or when the patient is allergic to penicillin, use trimethoprim plus sulfamethoxazole, 0.5 mL/kg/dose in 2 divided doses or erythromycin plus sulfamethoxazole 10 mg(eryth)/kg/dose in 4 divided doses. Continue antibiotic treatment for another week if the patient has improved but is not totally asymptomatic. Failure to improve after 48 hours suggests a resistant organism or potential complication. Assess the patient for a central nervous system complication. If none is found, switch antibiotics to an agent effective against beta-lactamase–producing pathogens.

B. Decongestants and Antihistamines: Topical decongestants and oral combinations are frequently used in acute sinusitis to promote drainage. Their effectiveness has not been evaluated and concern has been raised about potential adverse effects related to impaired ciliary function, decreased blood flow to the mucosa, and reduced diffusion of antibiotic into the sinuses. Patients with underlying allergic rhinitis may benefit from intranasal Cromolyn or corticosteroid nasal spray. Vasoconstrictor nose drops and sprays are all associated with rebound edema if used for more than 5 days.

Follow-up Care

The patient should be seen in 48 hours if there is no improvement with antibiotic therapy and at the end of the 2-week course. Obtain a confirmatory x-ray if symptoms persist at 2 weeks. Chronic or recurrent sinus infections suggest an underlying anatomic malformation, an allergy, cystic fibrosis, immotile cilia syndrome (Kartagener's syndrome), or an immunodeficiency disorder.

EPISTAXIS

Etiology

The most common cause of epistaxis during childhood is trauma to the nose due to nose picking or nose rubbing, which results in abrasion of the anterior inferior part of the nasal septum (Kiesselbach's area). Trauma to the nose may also be due to falls or blows. Bleeding diseases such as hemophilia, leukemia, von Willebrand's disease, and hereditary hemorrhagic telangiectasia (Rendu-Osler-Weber disease) may present as epistaxis. Other causes include presence of infection (a bloody, purulent nasal discharge is found in syphilis and diphtheria), foreign bodies, and allergic rhinitis. Severe epistaxis may occur with many tumors (eg, angiofibroma, lymphoma, sarcoma).

DISEASES OF THE THROAT

ACUTE STOMATITIS

Recurrent Aphthous Stomatitis ("Canker Sore")

The main finding is multiple (1–4) small (3–10 mm) ulcers on the inside of the lips and throughout the remainder of the mouth. There is usually no associated fever or cervical adenopathy. The ulcers are very painful and last 1–2 weeks. The cause is not known, although an allergic or autoimmune basis is suspected.

Treatment consists of topical corticosteroids, either in a dental paste—eg, triamcinolone acetonide, 0.1% (Kenalog in Orabase)—or in a mouthwash administered 4 times a day. Pain can be symptomatically improved by a bland diet, avoiding salty or acid foods, switching from a bottle to a cup in infants, 2% viscous lidocaine (Xylocaine) prior to meals, and aspirin or even codeine at bedtime. In children not old enough to expectorate the lidocaine, it must be used sparingly to prevent side effects.

Herpes Simplex Gingivostomatitis

Approximately 1% of children who have their first encounter with the herpes simplex organism develop multiple (10 or more) small (1–3 mm) ulcers of the buccal mucosa, anterior pillars, inner lips, tongue, and especially the gingiva, with associated fever, tender cervical nodes, and generalized inflammation of the mouth. The children are commonly under 3 years of age. This disorder lasts 7–10 days. Severe dysphagia interferes with eating and drinking. The primary disorder does not recur; herpes simplex recurs only in the form of cold sores that are found mainly at the labial mucocutaneous juncture. A throat culture is recommended to rule out streptococcal infection and a white blood cell count to rule out agranulocytic mucosa lesions.

Treatment is symptomatic as described for recurrent aphthous stomatitis (see above), with the exception that corticosteroids are contraindicated because they may result in spread of the infection. The patient must be followed closely. Dehydration occasionally ensues despite liberal offerings of cold fluids, in which case the patient must be hospitalized so that intravenous fluids can be administered. Herpetic laryngotracheitis is a rare complication.

Thrush of the Mouth

Oral candidiasis mainly affects bottle-fed infants and occasionally older children in a debilitated state. *Candida albicans* is a saprophyte that normally is not invasive unless the mouth is abraded. The use of broad-spectrum antibiotics may be a contributing factor. The symptoms include soreness of the mouth and refusal of feedings. Lesions consist of white curdlike plaques predominantly on the buccal mucosa. These plaques cannot be washed away after a water feeding.

Specific treatment consists of use of nystatin (Mycostatin) oral suspension, 1 mL 4 times a day for 1 week. This should be preceded by attempts to remove any large plaques with a moistened cotton-tipped applicator. The child should be fed temporarily with a spoon and cup to eliminate pain, continued abrasion, and possible contamination from nipple feedings.

ACUTE VIRAL PHARYNGITIS & TONSILLITIS

Over 90% of cases of sore throat and fever in children are due to viral infections. Most children develop associated rhinorrhea and mild cough and in fact are having a cold and nothing more. The findings seldom give any clue to the particular viral agent, but 6 types of viral pharyngitis are sufficiently different to permit the clinician to make an educated guess about the specific cause.

Clinical Findings

A. Infectious Mononucleosis: The findings are an exudative tonsillitis, generalized cervical adenitis, and fever, usually in a teenage patient. A palpable spleen or axillary adenopathy adds weight to the diagnosis. The presence of more than 20% atypical lymphocytes on a peripheral blood smear or a positive mononucleosis spot test (Monospot) confirms the diagnosis. This diagnosis is often not considered until a patient with a presumptive diagnosis of streptococcal pharyngitis has failed to respond to 48 hours of treatment with penicillin.

B. Herpangina: Herpangina ulcers, 2–3 mm in size, are found on the anterior pillars and sometimes on the soft palate and uvula. There are no ulcers in the anterior mouth as seen in herpes simplex. Fever is present. The disease lasts up to a week. Herpangina is caused by several members of the coxsackie A group of viruses, and a patient can have up to 5 bouts of herpangina in a lifetime.

C. Lymphonodular Pharyngitis: The classic finding is small, yellow-white nodules in the same distribution as the small ulcers in herpangina. In this condition, which is caused by coxsackievirus A10, the nodules do not ulcerate.

D. Hand, Foot, and Mouth Disease: This entity is caused by coxsackieviruses A5, A10, and A16. Ulcers occur on the tongue and oral mucosa. Vesicles, which usually do not ulcerate, are found on the palms, soles, and interdigital areas.

E. Pharyngoconjunctival Fever: This disorder is caused by an adenovirus. Exudative tonsillitis, conjunctivitis, and fever are the main findings.

F. Rubeola: The prodrome of measles looks like any nonspecific viral respiratory infection until one closely examines the buccal mucosa and the inner aspects of the lower lip. Small white specks the size of salt granules on an erythematous base (Koplik's spots) found at these sites are pathognomonic of measles.

Treatment

The treatment of acute viral pharyngitis is strictly symptomatic. Older children can gargle with warm hypertonic salt solution. Younger children can suck on hard candy (especially butterscotch). Analgesics and antipyretics are sometimes helpful. Antibiotics are contraindicated.

ACUTE STREPTOCOCCAL PHARYNGITIS & TONSILLITIS

Approximately 10% of children with sore throat and fever have a streptococcal infection. Untreated streptococcal pharyngitis can result in acute rheumatic fever, glomerulonephritis, and suppurative complications (eg, cervical adenitis, peritonsillar abscess, otitis media, cellulitis, and septicemia). Vesicles and ulcers are suggestive of viral infection, whereas cervical adenitis, petechiae, a beefy-red uvula, and a tonsillar exudate are suggestive of streptococcal infection; the only way to make a definitive diagnosis is by obtaining a throat culture.

Other bacterial causes of acute pharyngitis are *Corynebacterium diphtheriae, Neisseria gonorrhoeae,* group C streptococci, meningococci, *Chlamydia,* and *M pneumoniae. S aureus* and *S pneumoniae* may play a role in debilitated patients (eg, patients with cystic fibrosis).

Treatment is with a single dose of benzathine penicillin G (Bicillin), 0.6–1.2 million units intramuscularly, or oral phenoxymethyl penicillin (penicillin V), 125–250 mg every 6 hours between meals for 10 days. Parenteral therapy is indicated if there is vomiting or sepsis. Ampicillin, nafcillin, oxacillin, cloxacillin, and dicloxacillin are also effective in the treatment of streptococcal infections.

PERITONSILLAR ABSCESS
(Quinsy)

Tonsillar infection occasionally penetrates the tonsillar capsule, spreads to the surrounding tissues, and causes peritonsillar cellulitis. If untreated, necrosis occurs and a tonsillar abscess forms. This can occur at any age. The most common cause is beta-hemolytic streptococci. Other pathogens are group D streptococcus, alpha streptococcus, *S pneumoniae,* and anaerobes.

The patient complains of a severe sore throat even before the physical findings become marked. A high fever is usually present. The process is almost always unilateral. The tonsil bulges medially, and the anterior pillar is prominent. The soft palate and uvula on the involved side are edematous and displaced medially toward the uninvolved side. In severe cases, there is trismus, dysphagia, and, finally, drooling. The quality of the voice is severely impaired by the fixation of the soft palate. On palpation, the tonsil is firm and exquisitely tender.

Aggressive treatment in early cases of peritonsillar cellulitis may abort the process and prevent suppuration. The treatment of choice is penicillin. Daily follow-up is critical to detect possible abscess. If the initial swelling is marked, fluctuation develops, a neck mass develops, the patient appears toxic, or symptoms fail to respond to 48 hours of antibiotics, the patient should be hospitalized for intravenous penicillin or clindamycin. An otolaryngologist should be consulted to perform incision and drainage.

RETROPHARYNGEAL ABSCESS

Retropharyngeal nodes drain the adenoids and nasopharynx and can become infected. The most common cause is beta-hemolytic streptococci; less common pathogens are *S aureus* and oral anaerobes. If this pyogenic adenitis goes untreated, a retropharyngeal abscess forms. The process occurs almost exclusively during the first 2 years of life. Beyond this age, retropharyngeal abscess usually results from superinfection of a penetrating injury of the posterior wall of the oropharynx.

The diagnosis should be strongly suspected in an infant with fever, respiratory symptoms, and neck hyperextension. Dysphagia, dyspnea, and gurgling respirations are also found and are due to the impingement by the abscess. Prominent swelling on one side of the posterior pharyngeal wall confirms the diagnosis. Swelling usually stops at the midline because a medial raphe divides the prevertebral space. Lateral neck soft tissue films provide additional confirmation if needed.

Retropharyngeal abscess is a surgical emergency. Immediate hospitalization is required. A surgeon should incise and drain the abscess to prevent its extension. The head should be kept down during incision to prevent aspiration of purulent material. Intravenous hydration and antibiotics should be instituted before surgery. A penicillinase-resistant penicillin should be given. Clindamycin is an alternative.

ACUTE CERVICAL ADENITIS

General Considerations

Local infections of the ear, nose, and throat can spread to the regional node and cause a secondary inflammation there. The most commonly involved node is the jugulodigastric node, which drains the tonsillar area. The problem is most prevalent among preschool children.

A classic case involves a large, unilateral, solitary, tender node. About 70% of these cases are due to beta-hemolytic streptococci, 20% are due to staphylococci, and the remainder may be due to other bacteria and viruses.

The most common site of invasion is from pharyngitis or tonsillitis. Other entry sites for pyogenic adenitis are periapical dental abscess (usually producing a submandibular adenitis), facial impetigo (infected cuts or bug bites), infected acne, and otitis externa (usually producing a preauricular adenitis).

Clinical Findings

A. Symptoms and Signs: The patient is brought in with the chief complaint of a swollen neck or face. There is usually sustained high fever, especially in staphylococcal infections. The mass is often the size of a walnut or even an egg. It is taut, firm, and exquisitely tender. If left untreated, it may develop an overlying erythema. The exact size of the node should be measured for future follow-up. Each tooth should be examined for a periapical abscess and precussed for tenderness. A protective torticollis is sometimes present.

B. Laboratory Findings: The white blood cell count is usually about 20,000/μL with a shift to the left. The combination of leukocytosis and a positive throat culture or an elevated ASO titer identifies streptococci in about two-thirds of streptococcal cases. A tuberculin skin test should be given. Aspirated material from fluctuant nodes should be gram-stained and cultured.

Differential Diagnosis

The causes of cervical adenopathy are numerous. Five general categories can be distinguished on the basis of the clinical findings.

A. Acute Unilateral Cervical Adenitis: See above.

B. Acute Bilateral Cervical Adenitis: Painful and tender nodes are present on both sides, and the patient usually has fever.

1. Infectious mononucleosis–This diagnosis can be aided by the findings of splenomegaly, over 20% atypical cells on the white blood cell smear, and a positive mononucleosis spot test (Monospot). Toxoplasmosis and cytomegalovirus infections can imitate this disorder.

2. Tularemia–There will be a history of wild rabbit or deerfly exposure.

3. Diphtheria–This only occurs in nonimmunized children.

C. Subacute or Chronic Adenitis: In this condition, an isolated node usually exists, but it is smaller and less tender than the acute pyogenic adenitis described previously.

1. Nonspecific viral pharyngitis–This accounts for about 80% of cases in this category.

2. Beta-hemolytic streptococcal infection–Streptococci can occasionally cause a low-grade cervical adenitis; staphylococci never do.

3. Cat-scratch fever–The diagnosis is aided by the finding of a primary papule in approximately 60% of cases. Cat contact or scratches are present in over 90% of cases. The node is usually mildly tender. The cat-scratch skin test is helpful and relatively safe.

4. Atypical mycobacterial infection–The node is generally nontender and submandibular (occasionally preauricular). The nodes become fluctuant after several months. Affected patients are usually 1–5 years of age. A history of drinking unpasteurized milk is helpful. A mildly positive PPD is suggestive. A PPD-standard gives 5–10 mm of induration.

D. Cervical Node Tumors: Malignant tumors usually are not suspected until the adenopathy persists despite treatment. Classically, the nodes are painless, nontender, and firm to hard in consistency. They may occur as a single node, unilateral multiple nodes in a chain, bilateral cervical nodes, or generalized adenopathy. Cancers that may present in the neck are Hodgkin's disease, lymphosarcoma, fibrosarcoma, thyroid cancer, leukemia, and cancers with an occult primary in the nasopharynx (eg, rhabdomyosarcoma). One benign tumor that presents as enlarged cervical nodes is sinus histiocytosis.

E. Imitators of Adenitis: Several structures in the neck can become infected and resemble a node. The first 3 masses are of congenital origin and are listed in order of frequency.

1. Thyroglossal duct cyst–When superinfected, this congenital malformation can become acutely swollen. Helpful findings are the fact that it is in the midline, located between the hyoid bone and suprasternal notch, and moves upward on sticking out the tongue or swallowing. Occasionally, the cyst develops a sinus tract and opening just lateral to the midline.

2. Branchial cleft cyst–When superinfected, this can become a tender mass, 3–5 cm in diameter. Aids to diagnosis are the fact that the mass is located along the anterior border of the sternocleidomastoid muscle and is smooth and fluctuant as a cyst should be. Occasionally, it is attached to the overlying skin by a small dimple or a draining sinus tract.

3. Cystic hygroma–Most of these lymphatic cysts are located in the posterior triangle just above the clavicle. The mass is soft and compressible and can be transilluminated. Over 60% are noted at birth, and the remainder usually present by 2 years of age. If cysts become large enough, they can compromise swallowing and breathing.

4. Mumps–Mumps crosses the angle of the jaw, is associated with preauricular percussion tenderness, and is bilateral in 70% of cases; there is frequently a history of exposure to mumps. Submandibular mumps can present a diagnostic dilemma.

5. Sternocleidomastoid muscle hematoma–This cervical mass is noted at 2–4 weeks of age. On close examination it is found to be part of the muscle body and not movable. An associated torticollis is usually confirmatory.

Treatment

A. Specific Measures: Unless the patient has recently been exposed to beta-hemolytic streptococci, dicloxacillin or erythromycin is usually started initially. The antibiotic can be changed to penicillin if the original antibiotic is not well tolerated and the throat culture is positive for streptococci. The patient should be referred to a dentist if a periapical abscess is suspected.

B. General Measures: Analgesics (even codeine) are necessary during the first few days.

C. Surgical Treatment: Early treatment with antibiotics prevents many cases of pyogenic adenitis from progressing to suppuration. However, once fluctuation occurs, antibiotic therapy alone is not sufficient treatment. When fluctuation or pointing is present, the primary physician should incise and drain the abscess. Hospitalization is required only if the patient is toxic, dehydrated, dysphagic, dyspneic, or less than 6 months of age.

D. Follow-up Care: The patient must be seen daily. A good response includes resolution of the fever and improvement in the tenderness after 48 hours of treatment. Reduction in size of the nodes may take several more days. The antibiotic should be continued for 10 days. If there is no improvement in 48 hours and the PPD test is negative, the node should be aspirated with an 18-gauge needle and 0.5 mL of normal saline in the syringe to obtain material for gram-stained smear, culture, and sensitivity tests. Aspirated material should be cultured aerobically and anaerobically.

The patient with a cervical node that has been enlarging for more than 2 weeks despite treatment or is still large and unchanged in size for more than 2 months should be referred to a surgeon for biopsy.

TONSILLECTOMY & ADENOIDECTOMY

Very few children require tonsillectomy and adenoidectomy. If possible, surgery should be deferred for 2–3 weeks after an acute attack has subsided.

Indications for surgery include persistent nasal obstruction, persistent oral obstruction, cor pulmonale, recurrent peritonsillar abscess, recurrent pyogenic cervical adenitis, suspected tonsillar tumor, persistent snoring, and sleep apnea syndrome. Snoring and hyponasal speech may be indications for adenoidectomy.

Contraindications to surgery include tonsillitis in the acute phase, bleeding disease, and polio epidemics. Great care must be taken in evaluating the child with cleft palate, submucous cleft palate, or bifid uvula for adenoid and tonsil surgery, because there is a risk of aggravating the defect of the short palate. Tonsillectomy and adenoidectomy do not significantly affect the later occurrence of otitis media.

Invalid reasons for surgery include "large" tonsils, recurrent colds and sore throats, recurrent streptococcal pharyngitis, parental pressure, school absence, and "chronic" tonsillitis. Over 95% of tonsillectomies and adenoidectomies are performed for these unjustified reasons.

ORAL CONGENITAL MALFORMATIONS

Cleft Lip & Cleft Palate

Cleft lip, cleft palate, or both conditions are found in one in 800 live births. They are readily diagnosed in the newborn nursery. Treatment requires a multidisciplinary team approach— plastic surgeons, otolaryngologists, audiologists, speech therapists, orthodontists, and prosthodontists. Cleft lip repair is usually withheld until the child weighs over 5 kg. Cleft palate repair is usually performed at 18 months of age; this is essential to permit normal speech development, which should begin at this time. Occasionally, the palate is short and results in nasal speech.

Cleft palate causes eating problems and poor weight gain due to nasal regurgitation or lung aspiration of milk. Best results are obtained by feeding the baby with a cup or special compressible feeder. Approximately 90% of children with cleft palate have chronic otitis media and must be carefully followed for this problem.

Pierre Robin Syndrome

This congenital malformation is characterized by the triad of micrognathia, cleft palate, and glossoptosis. Affected children present as emergencies in the newborn period because of infringement on the airway by the tongue. The main objective of treatment is to prevent asphyxia until the mandible becomes large enough to accommodate the tongue. In some cases, this can be achieved by leaving the child in a prone position while unattended. In severe cases, a custom-fitted oropharyngeal airway or large suture through the base of the tongue that is anchored to the soft tissue in front of the mandible is required. The child requires close observation until the problem is outgrown.

21 | Respiratory Tract

Steven H. Abman, MD

ACUTE RESPIRATORY EMERGENCIES

ACUTE RESPIRATORY FAILURE (ARF)

ARF is the inability of the respiratory system to provide sufficient Pao_2 or remove enough CO_2 to meet the metabolic needs of the body, because of the presence of either severe lung or airway disease or inadequate respiratory effort. In pediatrics, cardiopulmonary arrests are more commonly due to respiratory causes than to primary cardiac abnormalities. Several anatomic and physiologic factors [smaller airway diameters, easy fatigability of the diaphragm and other respiratory muscles, high chest wall compliance, and decreased intra-alveolar connections (pores of Kohn)] make young children more vulnerable than adults to ARF. ARF occurs in a wide variety of clinical settings (including all the disorders discussed in this chapter), and presents with variable physical findings depending on the exact etiology and physiologic response.

In general, early recognition of the high risk of ARF in various clinical settings is important, in order to anticipate and therefore initiate appropriate therapy prior to cardiopulmonary arrest (Tables 21–1, 21–2, and 21–3). Often the clinical severity of respiratory insufficiency may not be appreciated without arterial blood gas measurements of arterial oxygen tension (Pa_{O2}), carbon dioxide tension (Pa_{CO2}), and pH. Although the use of pulse oximeter and transcutaneous P_{O2} monitoring is helpful to demonstrate noninvasively serial changes in oxygenation, measurements of arterial blood gas tensions are necessary for a full assessment of acid–base balance and ventilation. Pa_{CO2} is a direct reflection of alveolar ventilation; as Pa_{CO2} rises, effective ventilation decreases proportionately. Determination of pH will help sort out the relative contributions of respiratory and metabolic causes of acidemia or alkalemia. A change in Pa_{CO2} of 10 torr will cause a change in arterial pH of 0.08 unit in the opposite

Table 21–1. Systematic approach to acute respiratory failure.

1. Anticipate high-risk clinical setting for early monitoring and intervention prior to cardiopulmonary arrest.
2. Assessment of respiratory distress prior to arrest:
   A. *Physical examination:* mentation, cyanosis, apnea, respiratory rate, severity of distress (use of accessory muscles, grunting, retractions, paradoxical respiratory effort, breath sounds, response to oxygen administration).
   B. *Laboratory examination:* chest x-ray, monitoring with pulse oximeter and serial arterial blood gas studies.
3. Therapy dependent on clinical setting, severity of clinical findings: Intubation, ventilation, pharmacologic therapy, chest postural drainage, etc.
4. Initiate basic CPR with arrest:
   A. Airway patent? Head-tilt/chin tilt or jaw thrust; oropharyngeal/ nasopharyngeal airway; endotracheal tube; cricothyrotomy.
   B. Adequacy of oxygenation? Supplemental oxygen (100%) by nasal cannula, head hood, or face mask.
   C. Adequacy of ventilation? Self-inflating bag-ventilation by face mask or through endotracheal tube.
   D. Circulation? Chest compressions if cardiac activity ineffective or absent; vascular access for fluid, drug administration; arterial and/or central venous access for monitoring.

direction. Similarly, a change in HCO_3 of 10 meq/L will cause a change in pH of 0.15 unit. The clinical approach to the patient with ARF begins with the same assessments used in CPR training: airway, breathing (effort), and circulation, with further monitoring and therapeutic interventions dependent upon the severity of distress.

Table 21–2. General indications for intubation with acute respiratory failure.

Cardiopulmonary arrest, severe shock

Apnea—frequent or prolonged episodes

Rising Pa_{CO_2} (especially if > 50 mm Hg, with changes in mentation, fatigue, or in face of marked respiratory effort)

Falling Pa_{O_2} despite supplemental oxygen therapy (especially if < 60 mm Hg while breathing high fraction of inspired oxygen (FiO_2)

Marked lethargy, fatigue, encephalopathy, coma

Loss of gag reflex, inability to protect airway

Severe upper airway obstruction

Table 21–3. Age-dependent changes in pediatric sizes of endotracheal tubes, laryngoscope blades, tracheostomy tubes, and chest tubes.

Age	Internal Diameter of Endotracheal Tube (mm)	Size of Laryngoscope Blade for Intubation	Tracheostomy Size (Shiley)	Chest Tube Size (French)
Premature				
1000 g	2.5	Miller 0	Neonatal 00	10
1000–2500 g	3.0	Miller 0	Neonatal 0	10–14
Newborn–6 mo	3.0–3.5	Miller 1	Pediatric 1	12–18
6 mo–1 yr	3.5–4.0	Miller 1	Pediatric 1–2	14–20
1–2 yr	4.0–5.0	Miller 1	Pediatric 3	14–24
2–6 yr	$\dfrac{\text{Age (yr)} + 16}{4}$	Miller 1–2	Pediatric 3,4	20–32
6–12 yr	Same as above	Miller/Macintosh 2	Pediatric 4	28–38
> 12 yr	Same as above	Miller/Macintosh 3	Pediatric 6	

ADULT RESPIRATORY DISTRESS SYNDROME (ARDS)/ PULMONARY EDEMA

ARDS is a clinical syndrome characterized by the progressive development of respiratory failure associated with acute lung injury due to indirect (septic or hemorrhagic shock, head trauma, burn injury, pancreatitis, others) or direct (smoke or chemical inhalation, pneumonia, aspiration, emboli) causes. Its pathophysiologic hallmark is the presence of nonhydrostatic, or permeability, edema owing to injury to the alveolar–capillary network. This is in contrast to the pulmonary edema secondary to elevated pulmonary venous pressures more typical of congestive heart failure.

Clinical Findings

ARDS typically progresses from tachypnea, cyanosis, and retractions to ARF within 6–48 hours of an acute catastrophic event. Although the rate of progression and the severity of illness vary, early chest x-rays often appear normal. However, serial studies will reveal patchy alveolar infiltrates, air bronchograms, and loss of lung volume. Diminished breath sounds and rales are typical auscultatory findings. Although initially responsive to supplemental oxygen, hypoxemia often becomes refractory to treatment because of severe ventilation–perfusion mismatch, requiring mechanical ventilation with high mean airway pressures. Physiologically, lung compliance is low, and pulmonary artery wedge pressure (as measured with a pulmonary artery catheter) is normal.

Treatment

Therapy is currently supportive only. Along with treating the underlying disorder, the early recognition of at-risk patients allows initiation of appropriate monitoring for progressive respiratory distress, thus decreasing the risk for sudden cardiopulmonary arrest. Monitoring generally includes a systemic arterial line for frequent arterial blood gas and continuous blood pressure measurements. Pulse oximetry provides continuous assessments of oxygenation. Assessment of fluid status often requires the placement of a Foley catheter. Dependable peripheral and central venous lines provide access for administration of blood products, fluids, and medications, and for assessing volume status. In some cases, placement of a pulmonary artery catheter will allow essential measurements of cardiac output, pulmonary artery and wedge pressures, and mixed venous oxygen tension and saturation. The overall goal of therapy is to maximize tissue oxygen delivery, which is determined by the arterial oxygen content and the cardiac index. Treatment typically includes maintaining the hematocrit above 40%, cardiac index over 4.5 L/min, and oxygen saturation above 90–92%. Volume ventilators are required to ensure delivery of sufficient tidal volume in the face of changing respiratory compliance. High levels of mean airway pressure and peak end-expiratory pressures are often needed to correct the hypoxemia. Steroids have not been shown to improve the clinical course or outcome of ARDS.

Prognosis

Mortality rates of 50–60% are commonly reported, with death often due to multiple organ-system failure associated with secondary infection and progressive respiratory failure. Some patients require prolonged ventilator support and develop chronic lung disease. Most survivors, however, appear to have little sequelae at follow-up.

ACUTE AIRWAY OBSTRUCTION

The most common causes of acute airway obstruction in children include foreign body aspiration, viral croup, epiglottitis, bacterial tracheitis, peritonsillar abscess, marked adenoidal or tonsillar hypertrophy due to infection, allergy, and trauma (most commonly postextubation).

1. FOREIGN BODY OBSTRUCTION OF THE UPPER AND LOWER AIRWAY

Foreign body aspiration contributes significantly to the morbidity and mortality of early childhood, with over 3000 deaths from this cause occurring each year. Children between 6 months and 4 years are at greatest risk.

Clinical Findings

A. Symptoms and Signs: Upper airway obstruction presents as the acute onset of cyanosis and choking, with drooling, cough, and stridor (if partial) or inability to vocalize or cough (if complete). If untreated, progressive cyanosis, loss of consciousness, seizures, and cardiopulmonary arrest follow. Onset is abrupt, with a history of a small child running with food, a small toy, or other object in the mouth. Poor household "childproofing" or an older sibling feeding the younger child age-inappropriate food are common findings.

Lower respiratory tract obstruction generally presents with the abrupt onset of cough, wheezing, or respiratory distress. These signs may decrease or disappear over time, however, and if left untreated may lead to bronchiectasis. Lower respiratory tract obstruction should be suspected in any child with chronic cough or recurrent "pneumonias." Physical examination may reveal asymmetric breath sounds or localized wheezing or rales.

B. Laboratory Findings: Foreign body obstruction is generally a medical emergency without the need for laboratory studies. If obstruction is incomplete, lateral neck x-rays may be helpful, although it generally does not replace visualization. When lower respiratory tract foreign body aspiration is suspected, inspiratory and forced expiratory (manual abdominal compression) chest x-rays should be obtained. The initial chest x-ray may show asymmetric hyperinflation or atelectasis. A positive forced expiratory film will show mediastinal shift away from the side of the obstruction.

Treatment

The emergency treatment of partial upper airway obstruction due to a foreign body includes allowing the child to use his or her own cough reflex to extrude the foreign body. Acute intervention in infants less than 1 year old includes placing the child in a face-down position over the rescuer's arm, with the head positioned below the trunk. Four measured back blows are delivered rapidly between the scapulae. If still obstructed, the infant should be rolled over, and 4 chest compressions (as performed in CPR) delivered. This sequence should be repeated until the obstruction is relieved. Blind probing of the airway to attempt to dislodge the foreign body is discouraged. If the foreign body can be visualized, careful removal with the fingers or available instruments (Magill forceps) can be attempted. The abdominal thrust technique ("Heimlich maneuver") is recommended in older children.

Lower respiratory tract foreign body aspiration requires rigid bronchoscopy for removal, followed by beta-adrenergic nebulization with chest physiotherapy treatments in children with persistent symptoms.

2. INFECTIOUS CAUSES
OF UPPER AIRWAY OBSTRUCTION

Several infectious agents can cause the acute onset of upper airway obstruction, and although many causes have a distinctive clinical presentation, the overlap of clinical findings must be appreciated (Table 21–4). For example, viral croup may present with high fever and marked distress, as more typically seen with epiglottitis. Upper airway obstruction from a foreign body must be considered in the differential diagnosis (see above).

STATUS ASTHMATICUS

Status asthmaticus is defined as an acute asthma attack during which respiratory distress persists despite multiple therapeutic interventions. Marked bronchospasm, increased mucus secretions, and mucosal edema lead to increased airways resistance and hyperinflation, which clinically present as cough, retractions, and cyanosis. Although marked wheezing is most often present, diminished air entry with severe obstruction may lead to decreased wheezing. Hyperinflation, peribronchial cuffing, and atelectasis are common radiologic findings. Initial management includes the immediate administration of supplemental oxygen by face mask, and treatment with beta-adrenergic nebulization [terbutaline (0.1–0.3 mg/kg), albuterol (0.1 mg/kg), or metaproterenol (0.3 mg/kg)]. If the patient is on long-term theophylline therapy, a blood level should be checked and intravenous aminophylline administered. Steroid (methylprednisolone, 1–2 mg/kg intravenously) is given early during the course of treatment. The response to acute bronchodilator treatment is determined by frequent physical assessments (mentation, fatigue, degree of distress, changes in breath sounds, and pulsus paradoxus) and serial arterial blood gas measurements. Serial changes in Pa_{CO2} is a reliable indicator of impending respiratory failure. Disease progression or exhaustion due to prolonged or marked respiratory distress, despite multiple nebulizations and related interventions, can lead to respiratory failure, necessitating mechanical ventilation. Many intensive-care specialists will treat poorly responsive disease with continuous infusions of isoproterenol or terbutaline. Side effects, however, can be significant, and include marked tachycardia, dysrhythmias, myocardial ischemia or infarction, and worsening ventilation–perfusion mismatch.

Table 21–4. Infectious causes of upper airway obstruction.

Disease	Clinical Signs	Ages	Season	Causes	Diagnosis and Therapy
Croup	Stridor, barky cough, mild fever, hoarseness, URI, worse at night	6 mo–3 yr	Late fall–winter	Parainfluenza (other viruses)	Cool mist, racemic epinephrine (IPPB),* ± brief steroid use
Epiglottitis	Abrupt onset, toxic, anxious, high fever, drooling, dysphagia, rare cough	3–7 yr	None	H influenzae B	Direct visualization,† nasotracheal intubation, IV antibiotics, ICU admit
Retropharyngeal abscess	Acute pharyngitis, high fever, toxic, dysphagia, hyperextension of head, drooling	Variable	None	Group A strep, S aureus, anaerobic bacteria	Visualization,† lateral neck x-rays, IV antibiotics, surgery
Bacterial tracheitis	Crouplike illness, high fever, toxic	< 6 yr	Late fall–winter	S aureus	Visualization,† lateral neck x-ray, racemic epinephrine, IV antibiotics

*IPPB, intermittent positive pressure breathing.
†Visualization should be performed by experienced personnel under controlled settings (usually in the PICU or under general anesthesia). The use of lateral neck x-rays are often helpful, but do not replace direct visualization, and should not be obtained without the patient being observed by a physician capable of managing the airway in case of an abrupt obstruction.

655

PLEURAL EFFUSIONS AND EMPYEMA

Pleural effusions in pediatrics are most often parapneumonic, ie, associated with a concomitant bacterial, mycoplasmal, viral, fungal, or mycobacterial lung infection. However, effusions are also associated with nephritis or nephrosis, cirrhosis, ascites, liver abscess, congestive heart failure, collagen vascular disease, pancreatitis, drug-induced lung injury, malignancy, and other causes. Clinical findings are dependent upon the underlying condition and the size of the effusion. Cough and dyspnea are common, with a secondary rise in fever often heralding the development of pleural effusion. Breath sounds are decreased, with dullness to percussion over the involved area. Chest x-ray may show mediastinal shift; lateral decubitus or chest ultrasound studies help demonstrate the presence or absence of fluid loculation and the amount of fluid present. Thoracentesis provides helpful fluid samples for diagnostic and often therapeutic benefit. Studies should include pH determination (obtained in a small heparinized syringe, placed immediately on ice); stains and cultures for aerobic, anaerobic, and acid-fast organisms; cell count and differential; determination of glucose, lactate dehydrogenase (LDH), protein, specific gravity, hematocrit, and amylase; and cytologic examination. Serum samples from simultaneously drawn blood should be sent for protein, glucose, amylase, and LDH. These tests help differentiate transudate from exudate and may aid in providing a specific diagnosis for the source of the effusion and the potential need for early chest tube drainage (in the presence of a complicated parapneumonic empyema with pH < 7.15, LDH > 1000, protein > 4.5 gm/dL, and/or glucose < 40 mg/dL; Table 21–5).

APPARENT LIFE-THREATENING EPISODES (ALTE)

Marked controversy exists regarding the clinical management of infants with apnea or ALTE. As suggested by the long list of potential causes of ALTE or apnea (Table 21–6), these children are a heterogeneous group. Typically, infants with an ALTE present with an acute episode consisting of a combination of apnea (central or obstructive) with or without cyanosis or pallor, changes in muscle tone, or choking or gagging. The episode is felt to be life-threatening by the observer, with resuscitative efforts usually initiated. Whether some children truly represent "aborted" or "near-miss" sudden infant death syndrome is not known; however, there are reports of subsequent sudden

Table 21–5. Pleural effusions: transudate or exudate?

Type	White Blood Cell Count	Protein (g/dL)	Ratio, Pleural Fluid:Serum Protein	Ratio, Pleural Fluid:Serum LDH*	Glucose	pH
1. Transudate (CHF, nephrosis, cirrhosis)	< 1000 (mononuclear)	< 1	< 0.5	< 0.6	= serum	> 7.40
2. Exudate (parapneumonic, inflammatory, collagen vascular diseases, etc)						
A. Uncomplicated	10,000	1.4–6.1	> 0.5	> 0.6	= serum	> 7.30
B. Complicated†	20,000 (PMNs)	> 4.5	> 0.5	> 0.6	< 40 g/dL	< 7.10

*LDH, lactic dehydrogenase.

†"Complicated" parapneumonic effusions are believed to require early chest tube drainage for an improved clinical response and minimize potential sequelae.

Table 21–6. Causes of apparent life-threatening episodes.

Infectious
  Viral (RSV, other respiratory pathogens)
  Bacterial sepsis (Group B *Streptococcus*, pertussis, others)

Gastrointestinal
  Reflux
  Aspiration

Respiratory
  Airway anomalies
  Infection

Neurologic/Metabolic
  Seizure
  Central hypoventilation
  Infection
  Leigh's syndrome
  Tumor
  Carnitine deficiency
  Medium-chain acyl dehydrogenase deficiency

Cardiac
  Cardiomyopathy
  Endocardial fibroelastosis
  Arrhythmia
  Malformations

Nonaccidental Trauma

Unknown
  (Apnea of infancy)

death in such infants. Clinical evaluation includes obtaining a clear description of the event to determine whether the episodes are associated with being awake or asleep, with feedings, with crying, or with signs of acute infection. The duration of the episode, the resuscitative efforts, and the infant's subsequent responses are critical. Further history of developmental delays, neurologic abnormalities, signs of chronic disease, or nonaccidental trauma or neglect ("Munchausen's by proxy") are helpful. Physical examination may help direct the laboratory evaluation, which includes sleep studies to assess respiratory pattern and oxygenation (oximetery), chest x-ray, ECG, barium swallow, esophageal pH study, air laryngotracheogram, EEG, determination of serum electrolytes and hematocrit. A thorough psychosocial assessment is also an important part of the evaluation. Therapy is directed toward the identified cause. Indications for the use and duration of home apnea monitoring and respiratory stimulants, including caffeine, doxapram, and theophylline, remain controversial.

SUDDEN INFANT DEATH SYNDROME (SIDS)

SIDS, or "crib death," is a tragic but common cause of infant mortality, with an estimated frequency of 1–2 per 1000. Although its cause is unknown, SIDS generally occurs in children between 1 and 6 months of age (peak incidence, 2 months), with most deaths occurring between midnight and 8 AM. Mild upper respiratory tract infection symptoms may be present, but whether infection plays an important role is not known. Risk factors include low birth weight; teenage, drug addicted, or smoking mothers; and a family history of previous SIDS deaths. There are still no known predictors to identify at-risk newborns. The diagnosis is based on the clinical setting and a postmortem examination that rules out other causes of death, and may include such findings as intrathoracic petechiae, mild respiratory tract congestion, brainstem gliosis, and extramedullary hematopoiesis. Therapy is directed toward providing family support during the immediate crisis as well as follow-up counseling by local resources. The National SIDS Foundation is an excellent resource for providing this support.

ACUTE BRONCHIOLITIS

Bronchiolitis is one of the most common causes of acute hospitalizations in young infants, especially during the winter months. Although respiratory syncytial virus (RSV) is the most common cause, other agents include parainfluenza, influenza, adenovirus, *Mycoplasma,* and *Chlamydia.*

Clinical Findings
A. Symptoms and Signs: The usual course of RSV-bronchiolitis is 1–2 days of fever, rhinorrhea, and cough, followed by tachypnea, wheezing, and retractions. Some young infants, especially preterm newborns, may present with apnea and few auscultatory findings, but may later develop rales, rhonchi, and wheezing. Otitis media and superimposed bacterial pneumonia (especially pneumococcus may develop).

B. Laboratory Findings: Chest x-ray findings include hyperinflation with mild interstitial infiltrates or segmental atelectasis. The peripheral white blood cell count may be normal or show a mild lymphocytosis.

Treatment

Although most children infected with RSV are readily managed as outpatients, hospitalization is frequently required for children less than 2 years of age. Indications for admission include hypoxemia in room air, apnea, moderate tachypnea with feeding difficulties, or marked respiratory distress. Admission is more frequent in children with underlying chronic cardiopulmonary disorders, such as congenital heart disease, bronchopulmonary dysplasia, or cystic fibrosis. Arterial blood gas assessments or noninvasive measurements of oxygenation with a pulse oximeter or transcutaneous P_{O2} monitor should be used to assess oxygen requirements and the response to therapy. Supportive therapy includes supplemental oxygen, intravenous hydration, beta-adrenergic nebulization, theophylline, or steroids. Mechanical ventilation may be required in infants with apnea or marked distress. Ribavirin therapy is currently recommended for children with coexistent cardiopulmonary disease or immunodeficiency (eg, recent transplant recipients and children undergoing chemotherapy for malignancy). Its efficacy, however, remains unproven.

Prognosis

Whereas the acute outcome is generally excellent, children with pulmonary hypertension, bronchopulmonary dysplasia, or cystic fibrosis may have prolonged courses with high morbidity and mortality. In addition, recurrent episodes of wheezing may follow acute infection in almost half of hospitalized patients, suggesting either a predisposition to acute bronchiolitis or an important role in the pathogenesis of chronic reactive airways disease.

CHRONIC RESPIRATORY DISORDERS

General Considerations

The diagnostic evaluation of children with chronic respiratory disease can be approached in a staged work-up, which includes consideration of the age at onset of symptoms, the predominant clinical respiratory signs, and related findings (Table 21–7). Because of the wide diversity of etiologies, the pace of the work-up should be based on the severity or rate of progression of clinical findings. In addition, since normal, healthy children often have 6–8 respiratory infections during infancy, it is

Table 21–7. Work-up of chronic lung disease.*

Initial Laboratory Studies
1. Review previous course, lab data, and radiologic studies.
2. Obtain: Chest x-ray (PA and lateral)
   CBC with differential
   Sweat test (pilocarpine iontophoresis)
   Skin testing (TB, coccidioidomycosis, histoplasmosis, etc, depending on history)
   Pulmonary function testing (if age-appropriate)
   Sputum or nasal washings for culture

Follow-up ("Second Stage") Studies
1. More extensive pulmonary function testing (response to bronchodilator, exercise, or methacholine challenge).
2. Additional imaging studies:
   Air laryngotracheogram
   Barium swallow
   Chest CT or ultrasound
3. Serologic studies.
4. Screening immunologic testing (serum immunoglobulin levels, including IgE and IgG subclasses, antistreptolysin, isohemagglutinin, and titers assessing response to past immunizations, T cell subsets, HIV status, etc).

"Third Stage" Studies
1. Flexible or rigid laryngoscopy/bronchoscopy (with or without bronchoalveolar lavage, brush sampling, biopsy, or bronchography).
2. More specialized immunologic or serologic testing.
3. Esophageal pH monitoring.
4. Cardiac catheterization, angiography.
5. Lung biopsy.

*Reproduced, with permission, from Taussig LM, Lemen RJ: Chronic obstructive lung disease. In: *Advances in Pediatrics.* Year Book, 1979.

important to distinguish several different infections in a thriving child from a chronic lung disorder in which there are intermittent exacerbations superimposed on persistent respiratory signs. Also, evaluations should seek to determine whether exposure to environmental factors, such as passive smoking, gas heat and stoves, wood-burning stoves, or pollution, plays any role.

ASTHMA

Many childhood lung disorders, such as cystic fibrosis, bronchopulmonary dysplasia, chronic aspiration, and others, can often be characterized by airways hyperreactivity ("reactive airways disease"), or by the presence of wheezing that improves with bronchodilator therapy. However, asthma may be characterized by reversible airflow obstruction in the absence of other disease. Other factors supporting the diagnosis of asthma include a strong family history of allergy or asthma, improvement with decreased exposure to suspected allergens, positive skin tests, nasal or systemic eosinophilia, normal serum immunoglobulins except for an elevated IgE, and a negative sweat test. Although most commonly manifested by wheezing, chronic cough without wheezing (or "cough-equivalent asthma"), "chronic bronchitis," "recurrent pneumonias," and right middle lobe atelectasis are common presenting signs.

BRONCHOPULMONARY DYSPLASIA (BPD)

BPD is a significant chronic lung disease that may be defined clinically by the following criteria. (1) Acute respiratory distress in the first week of life (mostly in preterm infants with hyaline membrane disease). (2) Past or ongoing treatment with mechanical ventilation and oxygen therapy. (3) Persistent signs of chronic respiratory distress, including physical signs, chest x-ray findings, and oxygen requirement after the first month of life. Immaturity, oxygen toxicity, barotrauma, and inflammation are considered to be the major risk factors for developing BPD. The exact definition and cause of BPD remain controversial. Factors such as excessive fluid administration, patent ductus arteriosus, pulmonary interstitial emphysema, pneumothorax, infection, and inflammatory stimuli appear to play important roles in its pathogenesis and pathophysiology. The differential diagnosis based on radiographic findings includes Wilson–Mikity disease, meconium aspiration syndrome, congenital infection (especially cytomegalovirus and perhaps *Ureaplasma*), cystic fibrosis, cystic adenomatoid malformation, recurrent aspiration, pulmonary lymphangiectasia, total anomalous pulmonary venous return, overhydration and idiopathic pulmonary fibrosis.

Clinical Course & Treatment

The clinical course of BPD is widely variable, ranging from patients with mild oxygen requirements who improve steadily over a few months to more severely affected children who require chronic tracheostomy and mechanical ventilation. Airways hyperreactivity is common in infants with BPD, leading to frequent treatment with beta-adrenergic agonists (such as terbutaline, salbutomol, and metaproterenol), theophylline, steroids and cromolyn. Part of the rationale for steroids use is to decrease lung inflammation and enhance responsiveness to the beta-nebulization treatments. Recurrent atelectasis, tracheomalacia, subglottic stenosis, and other structural airway problems frequently contribute to the severity of the underlying BPD. Recurrent pulmonary edema, perhaps owing to increased vascular permeability, pulmonary hypertension, left ventricular dysfunction, or fluid overload, leads to the frequent use of long-term diuretic therapy, including furosemide, hydrochlorothiazide, and aldactone. Severe volume contraction, hypokalemia, hyponatremia, and alkalosis are common side effects of the diuretics. To minimize the development or progression of pulmonary hypertension, infants with BPD are carefully monitored with serial pulse oximeter and blood gas tension measurements to maintain Pao_2 or O_2 saturations above 55–60 torr or 92%, respectively. Serial ECG and echocardiogram studies monitor for the development of right ventricular hypertrophy (cor pulmonale) and left ventricular hypertrophy. Along with the cardiopulmonary abnormalities of BPD, clinical management requires close monitoring of growth, nutrition, metabolic status, development, neurologic status, and related problems.

Prognosis

Although mortality is high for advanced ("stage 4") BPD, the long-term outlook is generally favorable for most infants with BPD. However, more time and further study are needed to better determine the long-term impact of such sequelae as persistent airways hyperreactivity (asthma), exercise intolerance, and perhaps abnormal lung growth.

CYSTIC FIBROSIS (CF)

CF is the most common lethal genetic disease occurring in Caucasians, with an estimated incidence of 1 in 2000 births. Although CF is found in black (1:17,000) and oriental children (1:100,000), the incidence is far less than in Caucasians. Genetic linkage studies have demonstrated the CF gene to be on human chromosome 7. Although the basic defect remains unknown, it appears to involve an abnormality in the regulation of the chloride channel in secretory epithelial cells. This defect is believed to cause the characteristic abnormalities in sweat electrolytes and secretions in the lung, pancreas, intestine, liver, and other sites, which subsequently cause multiple organ dysfunction. The clinical manifestations of CF are diverse, and children with CF may present with a wide variety of clinical abnormalities (Table 21–8). The leading cause of morbidity and mortality, however, is progressive respiratory failure due to chronic endobronchial infection and inflammation. *Pseudomonas aeruginosa,* especially in its mucoid form, is the major bacterial pathogen of CF; *Staphylococcus aureus* and nontypable *Haemophilus influenzae* are other common isolates. Although clinical courses are variable, recurrent hospitalizations for respiratory exacerbations and gastrointestinal and nutritional problems are common. Prognosis has improved over the past decade but is variable; the current median age of survival is 26 years.

Table 21–8. Presenting signs of patients with cystic fibrosis.

1. Respiratory
  Chronic cough, wheezing
  Persistent atelectasis
  "Recurrent pneumonia"
  Staphylococcal pneumonia
  Pseudomonas aeruginosa pneumonia, sinusitis, or bronchitis
  Clubbing
  Bronchiectasis
  Nasal polyps
  Hemoptysis

2. Gastrointestinal/nutritional
  Meconium ileus or plug syndrome
  Small bowel atresia
  Meconium peritonitis
  Direct hyperbilirubinemia
  Unexplained hepatomegaly, cirrhosis
  Failure to thrive
  Steatorrhea
  Chronic diarrhea
  Rectal prolapse
  Bowel obstruction
  Hypoalbuminemia
  Vitamin A, E, or K deficiency

3. Other
  Family history of CF
  Aspermia
  "Tastes salty"
  Metabolic alkalosis
  Hypoelectrolytemia
  Heat stroke, exhaustion
  Elevated intracranial pressure (vitamin A deficit)
  Intracranial hemorrhage (vitamin K deficit)

RECURRENT ASPIRATION

Although a history of breathing difficulties that occur during or shortly after a feeding, awake apnea, or vomiting can be elicited in patients with chronic aspiration, some patients present with recurrent wheezing, "recurrent pneumonia," or chronic cough, in the absence of such a history. Disorders associated with recurrent aspiration include abnormal sucking or swallowing owing to neuromuscular immaturity, brain injury, or other primary neurologic and muscle abnormalities; structural lesions of the mouth, tongue, pharynx, or jaw; esophageal dysfunction owing to vascular ring, severe reflux, achalasia, hiatal hernia, or other causes; or aspiration owing to tracheoesophageal fistula or cleft. Chest x-ray findings of migratory asymmetric infiltrates are suggestive of recurrent aspiration. Barium swallow, esophageal pH studies, and the presence of significant numbers of lipid-laden alveolar macrophages in tracheal aspirates or bronchial washings may help with the diagnostic evaluation. The decision to undergo surgical (fundoplication) intervention depends upon the severity and frequency of aspiration, as well as on its underlying cause.

INTERSTITIAL LUNG DISEASES

Pediatric interstitial lung diseases include a diverse group of clinical disorders (Table 21–9), which can be characterized by persistent inflammation and edema of the lung interstitium, alveoli, and bronchiolar walls, which may lead to mild dysfunction or cause progressive pulmonary fibrosis.

The clinical presentation is highly variable, but generally tachypnea is the earliest manifestation, with cough, dyspnea, retractions, and cyanosis often found. Weight loss, clubbing, hemoptysis, chest pain, and other signs may be present. Often respiratory symptoms develop insidiously. Fine rales and diminished breath sounds are heard on chest auscultation. Chest x-ray findings are highly variable, with diffuse reticular, reticulonodular, or nodular infiltrates present. Peribronchial cuffing, hilar adenopathy, and other abnormalities are present depending on the underlying cause. Pulmonary function tests often indicate a restrictive pattern, with low lung volumes and compliance and a widened gradient of alveolar–arterial oxygen tensions, especially with exercise. Diagnostic assessments include bronchoalveolar lavage and lung biopsy. Treatment and prognosis depend on the specific abnormality.

Table 21–9. Causes of pediatric interstitial lung disease.

Infectious
  Viral (CMV, HIV, RSV, adenovirus, influenza, parainfluenza, measles, EBV, varicella)
  Mycoplasma
  Protozoal (*Pneumocystis carinii*)
  Mycobacterial
  Fungal
  Bacterial (*Haemophilus influenzae, Legionella, Bordetella pertussis*)

Postinfectious
  Bronchiolitis obliterans

Inhalational
  Inorganic dusts (silica, asbestos, talcum powder)
  Organic dusts (hypersensitivity pneumonitis)
  Fumes (sulfuric acid, hydrochloric acid)
  Gases (chlorine, nitrogen dioxide, ammonia)
  Aerosols

Drug-induced
  Cytotoxic (cyclophosphamide, BCNU, CCNU, methotrexate, azothioprine, vinblastine, bleomycin, cytosine arabinoside)
  Others (nitrofurantoin, penicillamine, gold salts)

Radiation

Neoplastic
  Leukemia
  Lymphoma
  Histiocytosis

Lymphoproliferative disorders
  Pseudotumor
  Others

Metabolic
  Cystic fibrosis
  Lipidoses
  Storage disorders

Idiopathic interstitial fibrosis

Associated with collagen vascular disease, systemic vasculitis

Associated with neurocutaneous syndromes

Sarcoidosis

Pulmonary hemosiderosis

Pulmonary alveolar proteinosis

Pulmonary infiltrates with eosinophilia

Cardiac failure

Renal disease

BRONCHIECTASIS

Bronchiectasis generally refers to chronic, irreversible airways injury that leads to fixed dilatation. It is most commonly due to recurrent lower respiratory tract infections, often in association with a primary chronic disease, including CF, immune deficiency, immotile cilia syndrome, anatomic airway obstruction, congenital deficiency of bronchial cartilage, foreign body, chronic aspiration pneumonitis, or sequelae of severe acute infections (including such agents as tuberculosis, pertussis, adenovirus, measles, influenza, or *Staphylococcus aureus*). Bronchiectasis can be classified as cylindric, varicose, or saccular, depending on its radiologic, bronchographic, or histologic appearance. With cylindric lesions, there is slight but uniform dilatation of the larger bronchi. Varicose bronchiectasis has irregular dilatation and constriction of bronchi, and the saccular form is described as having a progressively larger bronchial diameter, with gross destruction of more peripheral airways.

Clinical Findings

A. Symptoms and Signs: In 80–95% of patients with bronchiectasis, a chronic suppurative cough is present, which is generally worse in the early morning or with exercise. Purulent sputum production, hemoptysis, wheezing, and severe sinusitis can be present. Auscultation frequently reveals localized wheezing or moist rales over the bronchiectatic lung. Digital clubbing may be present.

B. Laboratory Findings: Although chest x-ray findings are often insensitive and not specific for the presence of bronchiectasis, the typical appearance of "tram lines," increased localized bronchovascular markings, or cystic changes may be found. The left lower lobe, right middle lobe, and lingula are the most common sites. Chest CT scan may be helpful to confirm the presence of bronchiectasis, as well as to evaluate the rest of the lung for diffuse lesions. Bronchography can be performed in centers with experience in this technique if surgical removal is under consideration. Diagnostic evaluation depends on the clinical setting, but often includes sweat test; immunologic work-up; PPD skin test, sputum cultures and stains for bacteria, fungi, and mycobacteria; barium swallow and esophageal pH study; CBC; and bronchoscopy.

Treatment

In addition to specific therapy to treat an underlying primary disease, aggressive chest physiotherapy after beta-adrenergic nebulization therapy is undertaken for at least 2–4 weeks. Antibiotics (based on culture results) are often used. Indications for surgical resection include the presence of localized disease producing severe symptoms or pulmonary hemorrhage. In the presence of diffuse lung involvement, surgery is generally not indicated.

HEMOPTYSIS, PULMONARY HEMORRHAGE, & HEMOSIDEROSIS

Acute pulmonary hemorrhage can occur with or without overt hemoptysis, and is usually accompanied by alveolar infiltrates on chest x-ray. Hemosiderin-laden macrophages are found within the sputum and tracheal and gastric aspirates. Many cases are secondary to infection (bacterial, mycobacterial, parasitic, viral, or fungal), lung abscess, bronchiectasis (CF, immune deficiency), foreign body, coagulopathy, elevated pulmonary venous pressure (congestive heart failure), structural lesions (arteriovenous fistula, telangiectasia, sequestration, bronchogenic cyst), lung contusion, tumor, pulmonary embolus, or collagen-vascular diseases (lupus, Wegener's granulomatosis, rheumatoid arthritis, polyarteritis nodosa, Shönlein–Henoch purpura, Goodpasture's syndrome, others). Idiopathic pulmonary hemosiderosis refers to the accumulation of hemosiderin in the lung (alveolar macrophage). It may be related to cow's milk allergy ("Heiner's syndrome").

Clinical findings are often nonspecific, and include cough, tachypnea, retractions, hemoptysis, poor growth, and fatigue. Some patients may present with massive hemoptysis. Auscultation reveals decreased breath sounds, wheezing, or rales. The presence of iron-deficiency anemia and hematuria should be sought. Chest x-ray findings are variable; fluffy alveolar or interstitial infiltrates may be transient, with or without atelectasis and mediastinal adenopathy. Pulmonary function testing generally reveals restrictive impairment with low lung volumes and poor compliance. Diagnostic evaluation depends upon the age of the patient and the associated signs (for example, serum precipitins to cow's milk proteins in infants and young children). Treatment and prognosis are dependent on the underlying etiology. Steroids or cytotoxic agents are frequently used.

CONGENITAL STRUCTURAL LESIONS

Congenital extrathoracic respiratory abnormalities cause inspiratory stridor or poor air movement despite increased respiratory effort from birth or within the first months of life. Congenital causes of airway obstruction that present in early infancy include choanal atresia; macroglossia; micrognathia (Pierre–Robin); laryngeal atresia, cleft, web, stenosis, or cyst; subglottic hemangioma; and others. Laryngomalacia is one of the most common causes, accounting for perhaps more than half the cases. The epiglottis and arytenoid cartilages collapse into the airway during inspiration, causing laryngeal stridor. Diagnosis is readily made by flexible laryngoscopy. Although tracheostomy may be required, most children resolve their stridor within the first 2 years of life.

Congenital intrathoracic lesions are diverse and have variable clinical presentations, ranging from severe neonatal respiratory distress to mild chronic cough in older adolescents.

Tracheomalacia

Tracheomalacia consists of dynamic collapse of the trachea, often associated with other conditions, such as vascular rings, tracheoesophageal fistula, BPD, and others. It may be primary. Diagnosis can be made by air laryngotracheogram or flexible bronchoscopy.

Vascular Rings

The clinical signs of vascular rings or slings vary considerably, depending on the type of lesion and the severity of compression of central airways or the esophagus. Most commonly, stridor, wheezing, or obstructive apnea are the initial presenting signs within the first months of life. Some children may have a more delayed presentation after long-term therapy for presumed asthma. The most common type of vascular abnormality is double aortic arch, in which persistence of left- and right-sided embryologic fourth aortic arches leads to esophageal and tracheal compression. Aberrant innominate artery, right aortic arch with aberrant left subclavian and left ligamentum arteriosum, and pulmonary sling (distal take-off of the left pulmonary artery) are other common vascular anomalies. Laboratory evaluation includes a chest x-ray, especially noting which side the aortic arch is on and the tracheal caliber. Barium swallow may reveal persistent indentation of the esophagus, suggesting an aortic arch anomaly (posterior esophageal compression) or pulmonary vascular sling or aberrant subclavian artery (anterior esophageal compression). A normal barium esophagogram is found with aberrant innominate artery compression; however, anterior tracheal compression about 2 centimeters above the carina may be noted on lateral chest film in these patients. Further evaluation generally includes bronchoscopy to assess tracheal or bronchial compression, and, often, angiography to more precisely define the anatomy. Surgical intervention is required for children with significant airway obstruction. Tracheomalacia may persist at the site of compression following surgery.

Mediastinal Masses

Mediastinal masses present with stridor, wheezing, chronic cough, or as incidental findings on chest x-rays obtained for other purposes. The differential diagnosis is dependent upon the mediastinal compartment in which the mass is located (Table 21–10). Although some of the lesions are congenital, others develop later in childhood. Work-up includes barium swallow, chest CT scan, bronchoscopy, or exploratory thoracotomy. Skin testing for mycobacterial disease with related controls should be performed as well.

Table 21–10. Mediastinal masses.

Compartment	Cause
Superior	Cystic hygroma
	Hemangioma
	Thymic tumors
	Teratoma
Anterior	Thymoma
	Thymic hyperplasia
	Thymic cyst
	Teratoma
	Intrathoracic thyroid
	Lymphoma
	Pericardial cyst
Posterior	Neurogenic tumors
	Neurenteric anomaly
	Anterior meningocele
	Bronchogenic cyst
Middle	Lymphoma
	Lymphadenopathy
	Bronchogenic cyst
	Pericardial cyst
	Cardiac tumors
	Anomalies of the great vessels

Tracheoesophageal Fistulas (TEF)

Tracheoesophageal fistulas are caused by the failure of septation of the esophagus and trachea. Distal TEF with esophageal atresia is the most common type (90%), and includes a proximal esophagus that ends in a blind pouch, with the distal esophagus connected to the trachea. Clinically, TEF may be associated with polyhydramnios, and with congenital abnormalities (35%), such as vertebral anomalies, imperforate anus, congenital heart disease, and genitourinary lesions. Cough, choking, and respiratory distress present shortly after birth. Lung injury can occur from gastric secretions entering the airway. Diagnosis is suggested by attempts to pass an esophageal catheter. Chest x-ray will confirm the position of the nasogastric tube curled in the proximal esophagus. Treatment includes suctioning secretions from the esophageal pouch to prevent aspiration; ultimate treatment is surgical repair in the newborn period. Tracheomalacia often persists as a clinical problem after surgical repair. Late complications include leakage at the anastomosis site, mediastinitis, esophageal stricture, diaphragm paralysis, hiatal hernia, poor esophageal motility, and recurrent fistulas.

Pulmonary Hypoplasia

Pulmonary agenesis or hypoplasia represent imcomplete lung development, generally reflecting an intrauterine interruption or alteration of the normal sequence of embryologic events. It may be associated with other congenital anomalies. Lungs are considered hypoplastic when their size is decreased as assessed by weight (ratio of lung to body weight is below 0.15 in premature infants less than 28 weeks' gestation, or 0.012 in older newborns). Etiologies include the presence of an intrathoracic mass resulting in the lack of space for lung growth (eg, diaphragmatic hernia, fetal hydrops, extralobar sequestration, thoracic neuroblastoma), decreased size of the thoracic cage (eg, asphyxiating thoracic dystrophy, achondrogenesis), decreased fetal breathing movements or diaphragmatic elevation (eventration, phrenic nerve agenesis, fetal ascites, abdominal masses), oligohydramnios (urinary outflow tract obstruction, polycystic kidneys, prolonged amniotic fluid leak); trisomies 13, 18 and 21; severe musculoskeletal disorders (arthrogryposis, osteogenesis imperfecta), and cardiac lesions (Ebstein's anomaly, pulmonic stenosis, hypoplastic right heart, scimitar syndrome). Clinical presentation is highly variable, and is related to the severity of hypoplasia as well as to associated abnormalities. Some newborns present with spontaneous pneumothorax, perinatal stress, and persistent pulmonary hypertension. Children with milder degrees of hypoplasia may present with tachypnea and related chronic respiratory signs. Chest x-ray findings include variable degrees of volume loss with a small hemithorax and mediastinal shift. Ventilation-perfusion scans, angiography, and bronchoscopy are often helpful with the clinical evaluation. Outcome is dependent on the severity of hypoplasia or related clinical problems.

Pulmonary Sequestrations

Pulmonary sequestrations are localized masses of pulmonary parenchyma that may be anatomically separate from the lung. Extralobar sequestrations have a distinct pleural investment and intralobar are located within the lung pleura. Extralobar sequestration receives its blood supply from the systemic circulation, pulmonary vessels, or both, and rarely communicates with the stomach or esophagus. The arterial supply to intralobar lesions is from the aorta or systemic branches. Intralobar lesions are often found in lower lobes (98%), are rarely associated with congenital lesions (less than 2% versus 50% with extralobar), are rarely seen in the newborn period (unlike extralobar), and may represent acquired lesions (ie, postinfectious). Clinically, sequestrations can present as chronic cough, wheezing, recurrent pneumonias, or hemoptysis. Treatment is by surgical resection.

Congentital Lobar Emphysema

This usually presents in the newborn period as severe respiratory distress, or during the first year of life as progressive respiratory impairment. Rarely, there is a delayed diagnosis because of mild or intermittent symptoms in older children. Chest x-ray shows overdistention of the affected lobe, with wide separation of bronchovascular markings, collapse of adjacent lung, shift of the mediastinum away from the affected side, and a depressed diaphragm on the affected side. Diagnostic studies often include fluoroscopy, ventilation–perfusion scans, chest CT, angiography, and exploratory thoracotomy. Bronchoscopy may be helpful to examine whether extrinsic or intrinsic compression of the bronchus is present. The differential diagnosis includes pneumothorax, pneumatocele, ateletasis with compensatory hyperinflation secondary to ball-valve mechanism, and cystic adenomatoid malformations. Management is usually surgical resection.

Cystic Adenomatoid Malformations (CAM)

These are unilateral hamartomatous lesions that generally present with marked respiratory distress within the first days of life. This lesion accounts for 95% of cases of congenital cystic lung disease. These space-occupying lesions are gland-like ("adenomatoid"), and have intercommunicating cysts of various sizes. Classification of the 3 types of CAM is based on the size of the cysts. Type 1 consists of large cysts; it is the most common (75%), and has the best survival (98%). Type 2 lesions consist of smaller cysts, and are often associated with other congenital anomalies (renal, cardiac, intestinal), leading to a lower (40%) survival. Type 3 CAM presents as a bulky, firm mass, and has a 50% survival rate. Treatment is by surgical resection.

Bronchogenic Cysts

These are middle mediastinal masses of variable sizes, which are usually located near the carina and major bronchi. These cysts usually do not communicate with the airway, and can present with acute respiratory distress and chronic cough and wheezing, or may be incidental findings on chest x-ray. Chest CT scan or ultrasound can differentiate solid from cystic mediastinal mass. Surgical excision is required.

Pulmonary Lymphangiectasia

This is a rare and usually fatal disorder that presents as acute or persistent respiratory distress in the newborn period. It may be accompanied by generalized lymphangiectasis, Noonan syndrome, asplenia, cardiovascular lesions (especially total anomalous pulmonary venous return), chylothorax, or renal malformations. Chest x-ray findings include a "ground glass" appearance, prominent interstitial markings, and hyperinflation. Therapy is largely supportive, and prognosis is poor, with most deaths occurring within the first months of life. There are isolated reports of its diagnosis and survival later in childhood.

22 | Gastrointestinal Tract

Judith M. Sondheimer, MD

RECURRENT ABDOMINAL PAIN

Recurrent abdominal pain of childhood is characterized by at least 3 discrete episodes of abdominal pain in a 3-month period in a child whose physical examination is normal. It occurs in 10–15% of children between 4 and 12 years of age. The pain may be severe, is sometimes associated with pallor and emesis (30%), and frequently interferes with school attendance. Less than 10% of such children will prove to have organic disease. The incidence of organic disease increases in children under 3 years and in the presence of other symptoms such as diarrhea, weight loss, dysuria, fever, or neurologic symptoms. The pain is variable in intensity, duration, and sometimes location. The presence of nighttime pain does not rule out the diagnosis. Headache, constipation, and limb pains are common findings. Overt emotional stress related to family or school may be found in 30–50%. Laboratory evaluations are usually negative and should be used sparingly. Abdominal examination is usually negative except for voluntary guarding, which may be out of proportion to the apparent pain.

Treatment is directed toward relieving anxiety surrounding the symptom by providing both parent and child with a clear explanation of the frequency and benign nature of the complaint. Return to school is important. Antispasmodics and fiber supplements are sometimes used. A lactose-free diet is occasionally helpful in the child with associated lactase deficiency.

VOMITING

Vomiting is a common symptom throughout childhood and may be associated with a wide variety of diseases of all degrees of severity. Organic disease must always be considered if vomiting is protracted or severe. Bilious emesis must always be investigated. A list of the causes and characteristics of vomiting is given in Table 22–1.

Table 22–1. Causes and characteristics of vomiting.

	Emesis	Other Characteristics
Gastric Outlet Obstruction:		
Pyloric stenosis	Forceful emesis, gastric contents.	4–12 wk infant; alkalosis, weight loss, palpable mass in right upper quadrant (see Pyloric Stenosis section).
Gastric web, duplication, annular pancreas	Emesis of variable force, usually gastric contents.	Presents at any age; x-ray diagnosis.
Duodenal stenosis/atresia	Emesis of variable force depending upon severity of obstruction; usually gastric contents.	Duodenal atresia presents at birth; common in Down's syndrome.
Malrotation with mesenteric bands	Often bilious.	May be associated with intestinal volvulus.
Intestinal Obstruction:		
Volvulus	See Malrotation section.	See Malrotation section.
Intussusception	See Intussusception section.	See Intussusception section.
Superior mesenteric artery syndrome	Emesis of variable force; may be bilious.	Associated with sudden weight loss; often follows body casting after scoliosis repair; x-ray shows obstruction of transverse duodenum.
Peptic Disease:		
Gastric, duodenal ulcer, gastritis, esophagitis	Emesis is especially common in young infants; may contain bright red or dark blood.	Pain, irritability; weight loss in small infants; endoscopy most accurate diagnostic test.

(Continued)

Table 22–1 (cont'd). Causes and characteristics of vomiting.

	Emesis	Other Characteristics
Motility:		
Hypokalemia	Distention, ileus and emesis.	Generalized weakness.
Hypercalcemia, hypermagnesemia	Forceful emesis, constipation.	
Pseudo obstruction	Distention, ileus, emesis of gastric contents and bile.	Cause unknown; may be present at birth or present later; sometimes familial; may spare segments.
Irritants:		
Aspirin, alcohol	Gastric contents; may contain gross blood.	History of ingestion but not necessarily overdose.
Erythromycin, theophylline	Gastric contents.	Many drugs are direct gastric irritants.
Opiates	Gastric contents.	Stimulation of medullary vomiting center.
Infections:		
Gastroenteritis	Usually precedes diarrhea.	Mediated by toxin or secondary to ileus.
UTI and obstructive uropathy	Usually gastric contents, sometimes bilious.	Common in infants; probably centrally mediated.
Otitis media	Usually gastric.	Common in infancy; probably centrally mediated.
Pneumonia, pertussis bronchiolitis	Usually gastric; often post tussive.	
Central Nervous System:		
Meningitis, tumor, pseudotumor; vascular anomalies	Usually gastric; often upon change of position.	Stimulation of medullary vomiting center.
Metabolic:		
Galactosemia, fructosemia, hyperammonemia, congenital adrenal hyperplasia, organic acidemia, phenylketonuria	Usually gastric, occasionally bilious.	Ill infant; seek specific diagnostic indicators for these diseases.
Gastroesophageal Reflux:	Gastric contents; variable force; often postprandial.	Most common under 6 months.

DIARRHEA
(See Tables 22–2, 22–3.)

Diarrhea (> 20 mL of stool/kg/d) is a common symptom in children. When it occurs acutely, it is usually infectious. In the infant under 2 years of age, it may be the first or only symptom of infection outside the gastrointestinal tract, eg, pneumonia, sepsis, or meningitis. The physician should always consider diarrhea seriously because of the risk of dehydration, and must begin general treatment measures as soon as diagnostic studies are obtained. Because diarrhea may gradually become severe, the patient should be under careful observation. If the child is being kept at home, parents should be instructed to observe and report signs of dehydration.

The following information should be routinely obtained: (1) Duration, frequency, and description (consistency and color) of diarrheal stools. The parents may interpret watery stool as urine. (2) Incidence and character of vomiting. (3) Incidence, volume, and frequency of urination. Dehydration will decrease the volume and frequency of urination. (4) Estimate of weight loss. In the infant or young child, weighing at the onset of diarrhea will provide an index with which subsequent weights can be compared. (5) Incidence of other cases of diarrhea or vomiting in the family, nursery, or school.

Examine the abdomen for tenderness and abnormal masses. Examine rectally for further localization and to obtain stool for microscopic examination and culture.

GENERAL TREATMENT MEASURES FOR DIARRHEA

General Considerations

Loss of more than 5% of body weight through emesis or diarrhea must be replaced immediately. Dehydration from acute viral gastroenteritis is often accompanied by metabolic acidosis (decreased serum HCO_3) and sometimes by hyper- or hyponatremia, depending upon the concentration of electrolyte in the stool. Potassium content of stool may be as high as 30–40 meq/L, and the dehydrated infant may be depleted of intracellular potassium with normal serum potassium. Serum electrolytes should be checked in any child with more than 5% dehydration.

Table 22-2. Causes, characteristics, and treatment of acute enteritis.

Cause	Stool Examination	Symptoms	Treatment
Bacterial:			
Salmonella	Liquid, foul, + WBC + gross or occult blood.	Fever, abdominal pain.	None unless signs of extra-intestinal infection or sepsis; ampicillin, amoxicillin, amoxicillin + trimethoprim-sulfamethoxazole.
Shigella	Small, grossly bloody, frequent.	Fever, tenesmus, abdominal pain.	None or trimethoprim-sulfamethoxazole.
Campylobacter jejuni	Gross blood and mucus.	Few systemic symptoms.	None or erythromycin.
Yersinia enterocolitica	Similar to *Salmonella*.	Similar to *Salmonella*.	
Aeromonas hydrophilia	Watery; mild to moderate.	Nausea, vomiting; probably enterotoxin-mediated.	Usually self-limited; trimethoprim-sulfamethoxazole.
Pleisiomonas shigelloides	Watery.	Nausea, vomiting; possible enterotoxin.	Usually self-limited; trimethoprim-sulfamethoxazole.
Escherichia coli			
Invasive	Small, grossly bloody, + WBC.	Abdominal pain, tenesmus.	Trimethoprim-sulfamethoxazole; ampicillin; gentamicin.
Enterotoxic	Liquid, green, voluminous.	Nausea, vomiting; heat labile toxin–mediated.	Usually self-limited.
Enteropathogenic	Liquid, green, voluminous.	Nausea, vomiting; adherence factors important.	Usually self-limited.
Hemorrhagic 0157:H7	Small, grossly bloody, + WBC.	Fever, tenesmus, organism produces shigella-type toxin;	Trimethoprim-sulfamethoxazole.

Viral:			
Rotavirus	Liquid, few WBC.	Emesis, nausea.	None; fluid management.
Others—Norwalk, enteric, adenovirus, enteroviruses	Same as above.	Same as above.	None; fluid management.
Parasitic:			
Giardia lamblia	Very foul, liquid; cysts present in 30–60%.	Vomiting, nausea, abdominal distension, gas.	Furazolidone (5 mg/kg/d × 7 d); Metronidazole (15 mg/kg/d × 5 d); Quinacrine (6 mg/kg/d × 5 d).
Entamoeba histolytica	Blood and mucus, trophozoites on fresh stool exam.	Abdominal pain, tenesmus.	Metronidazole (35–50 mg/kg/ d × 10 d).
Cryptosporidium	Watery or bloody depending upon site of infestation.	Often in immunodeficient patients but occasionally in healthy children; history of animal exposure.	Spiramycin or metronidazole may be tried.
Other Toxic Diarrhea:			
E coli (see above)		may precede hemolytic-uremic syndrome.	
Clostridium difficile	Bloody, + WBC, cytotoxin present in stool.	Abdominal pain, fever, history of prior antibiotic use is typical.	Vancomycin (30–40 mg/ kg/d × 7 d); metronidazole (25 mg/kg/d × 7 d); oral bacitracin (1500 U/ kg/d × 7 d).
Staphylococcus aureus	Explosive, watery, + WBC.	Nausea, emesis, history of group outbreaks.	Fluid management.
Clostridium perfringens	Explosive, watery, + WBC.	Emesis, abrupt onset, history of meat ingestion.	Fluid management.

679

Table 22–3. Chronic diarrhea—guide to differential diagnosis.

	Age	Type of Diarrhea	Associated Features
Disease:			
Bacterial infections	Any age	Mucoid bloody stool.	Rarely chronic except in immunocompromised hosts; *Salmonella* and *Yersinia* most likely.
Viral infection	Any age	Watery.	Rarely chronic except in immunocompromised hosts; CMV, adenovirus, rotovirus.
Parasitic infestation	Any age	Depends on organism.	Amoeba, giardia, cryptosporidium.
Dietary Factors:			
Overfeeding—especially starches	< 6 m	Watery.	Colicky behavior without weight loss.
Protein allergy	< 2 m	Watery ± malabsorption of fat; at times blood and mucus.	Colic, emesis, anemia, hypoproteinemia.
Acrodermatitis enteropathica	< 12 m	Voluminous with steatorrhea.	Malnutrition, skin rash; low serum Zn; usually genetic; sometimes secondary to severe dietary Zn deficiency.
Primary bile acid malabsorption	< 1 m	Voluminous with steatorrhea.	Malnutrition; defective ileal transport of bile acids.
Irritable colon/chronic nonspecific diarrhea	6–36 m	Watery, frequent, with mucus, undigested food; no steatorrhea.	Healthy child; often starts with bout of gastroenteritis.
Toxic diarrhea (antibiotics, cancer chemotherapy, radiation)	Any age	Loose; sometimes steatorrhea, occult blood or pus.	Vomiting; anorexia.
Functional tumors (neuroblastoma, carcinoid, pancreatic	Any age	Secretory diarrhea, watery, persists when patient fasting.	Hypokalemia; other symptoms depend upon tumor.

cholera, Zollinger–
Ellison syndrome)
Carbohydrate
malabsorption:

Sucrase–isomaltase	< 6 m	Watery; low pH; reducing substance positive after acid hydrolysis; volume varies with sucrose intake.	Abdominal distension; poor growth; deficiency present in 0.8% North Americans, 10% Alaskan natives.
Glucose galactose malabsorption	< 1 m	Intractable diarrhea with feeding; stool pH low; watery; reducing substances present.	Poor growth; defect in glucose transport.
Genetic Deficiencies:			
Lactase	< 4 yr	Watery diarrhea with lactose; low pH; reducing substances present.	Deficiency develops in 100% Orientals, 80% American blacks, 15% American whites.
Acquired Deficiencies:			
Lactase and sucrase	Any age	Watery; low pH; reducing substances present.	Follows intestinal injury or infection.
Monosaccharide transport	< 6 m	Watery; low pH; reducing substances present.	Rare; follows infection; made worse by malnutrition.
Pancreatic Disorders:			
Cystic fibrosis	< 6 m	Steatorrhea; bulky, foul, pale.	Respiratory infection; poor weight gain.
Shwachman syndrome	< 2 yr	Steatorrhea; bulky, foul, pale.	Neutropenia; short stature; bacterial infections; metaphyseal dysostosis.

(Continued)

681

Table 22–3 (cont'd). Chronic diarrhea—guide to differential diagnosis.

	Age	Type of Diarrhea	Associated Features
Chronic pancreatitis	Any age	Steatorrhea; bulky, foul, pale.	Rare in children; usually associated with alcoholism.
Celiac disease	< 12 m	Steatorrhea; bulky, foul, pale.	Emesis, distention, irritability, anorexia.
Intestinal lymphangiectasia	3 m	Voluminous, steatorrhea.	Lymphedema, lymphopenia, hypoalbuminemia.
Immune Defects:			
Hypogammaglobulinemia; IgA deficiency	Any age	Watery; sometimes steatorrhea.	Recurrent cutaneous and respiratory infection.
Combined immunodeficiency, AIDS, cellular defect	< 1 m Any age < 2 yr	Severe; watery; steatorrhea.	Stomatitis, skin rash, recurrent infection, opportunistic infection.
Genetic–Metabolic:			
Chloride losing diarrhea	< 1 m	Watery.	Alkalosis; growth failure.
Hypobetalipoproteinemia and a-betalipoproteinemia	< 3 m	Profuse; steatorrhea.	Progressive neurologic symptoms: low serum cholesterol; acanthocytosis.
Wolman's disease	< 1 m	Profuse; steatorrhea.	Emesis; severe growth failure; adrenal calcification; hypercholesterolemia.
Folate malabsorption	< 1 m	Watery.	Anemia; stomatitis, seizures, retardation.
Anatomic:			
Blind (stagnant) loop/ bacterial overgrowth	Any age	Watery; fat and carbohydrate malabsorption.	Caused by surgical adhesions, intestinal duplication, abnormal GI motility, partial obstruction.

682

Short bowel	Any age	Watery; malabsorption of all nutrients.	Rarely congenital, usually secondary to surgical resection.
Intestinal pseudoobstruction	Any age	Watery; malabsorption of all nutrients.	Distention; may be acquired or congenital; diarrhea secondary to bacterial overgrowth.
Inflammatory Bowel Disease:			
Crohn's disease		See Table 22–6.	
Ulcerative colitis		See Table 22–7.	
Eosinophilic gastroenteritis	Any age	Watery or bloody depending upon site of disease.	Intestinal or gastric obstruction, eczema, asthma, increased blood eosinophiles.
Hirschsprung's disease with enterocolitis	< 1 yr	Foul, liquid with WBC and a RBC.	Abdominal distention, fever, history of constipation.
Malnutrition	< 1 yr	Loose, steatorrhea, sometimes with carbohydrate malabsorption.	Becomes temporarily worse with refeeding.
Endocrine:			
Hyperthyroidism	Any age	Frequent, loose stool without malabsorption.	Other signs of hyperthyroidism.

683

Treatment

A. Parenteral Fluid Therapy: Parenteral fluid therapy is indicated in the following circumstances: (1) if vomiting or weakness prevents oral therapy; (2) in the presence of shock because of severe dehydration and acidosis; or (3) if surgical procedures are contemplated (see Chapter 4).

B. Oral Rehydration:

1. Replacement of fluid deficit–Commercially available oral solutions for replacement of fluid deficits resulting from viral gastroenteritis usually contain 75 meq Na/L, 20 meq K/L, 65 meq C1/L, 30 meq citrate or bicarbonate/L, and 25 g dextrose/L. Fluid deficit should be calculated by comparing weights or by physical signs. The desired volume should be administered by mouth over 12–24 hours.

2. Ongoing fluid needs–Commercially available oral solutions for maintenance during acute viral enteritis contain slightly less sodium (45 meq/L) and chloride (35 meq/L) than replacement solutions. As the calorie content of these solutions is only 100 kcal/L, they should not be used as the sole fluid intake for more than 48 hours.

3. Return to normal caloric intake–This should be fairly rapid in uncomplicated viral gastroenteritis. Intestinal lactase levels may be depressed for 7–14 days after acute gastroenteritis, and a lactose-free formula is advisable. Gastric retention and diminished bile salt secretion may temporarily decrease fatty food tolerance. High-fat solids should be reintroduced into the diet only after the child has demonstrated tolerance for carbohydrates.

4. Symptomatic therapy–Symptomatic treatment of acute gastroenteritis is rarely indicated and may seriously complicate fluid management. Diphenoxylate with atropine (Lomotil) should not be used in any infant under 3 years. Kaolin and pectin preparations are usually ineffective in acute gastroenteritis.

5. Specific therapy for infectious gastroenteritis—See Table 22–2.

CONSTIPATION

Normal frequency of defecation in children ranges from 3 per day to 1 per week. In healthy infants, stooling frequency is generally higher, but some normally defecate only 2–3 times per week. If stools are unusually hard or large, if pain or excessive straining is associated with defecation, if stooling frequency is less than once per week, if impaction of the rectum with fecal leakage occurs (this is a common manifestation of retentive constipation in school children) or if abdominal distention, emesis, or failure to thrive accompany infrequent stooling, symptomatic treatment and a careful assessment of possible organic causes should be undertaken.

Etiology (See Table 22–4.)

Table 22–4. Constipation.

	Agents
Infancy:	
Mechanical obstruction	Imperforate anus, anal stenosis. Intestinal obstruction.
Abnormal intestinal motility	Hirschsprung's disease: Lack of ganglion cells in the colon wall causes failure of peristalsis through affected areas. Intestinal pseudoobstruction. Hypothyroidism, congenital or acquired. Hypokalemia, hypercalcemia, hypermagnesemia.
Somatic weakness or incoordination	Hypotonia, acquired or congenital; cerebral palsy; sacral agenesis; spina bifida.
Pain on defecation	Anal fissure, perianal skin disease, or abscess.
Drugs	Narcotics, antihistamines, calcium salts, aluminum hydroxide antacids, vincristine.
Dehydrating conditions	Diabetes mellitus, diabetes insipidus, following acute gastroenteritis.
Childhood:†	
Retentive constipation	This is the most likely cause of constipation in healthy toddlers or school-age children. Boys are more commonly affected. Fecal leakage around an impaction is present in 60%. Urinary tract infection or obstruction may be associated, especially in females.

†All of the above conditions may present in childhood.

Treatment

A. Disimpaction:

1. If the impacted stool is soft or puttylike–disimpaction can be accomplished with oral laxatives such as Senokot or Milk of Magnesia given 2–3 days in a row.

2. If the impacted stool is very large or firm–enemas may be required. Rectal instillation of mineral oil (30–90 mL) will lubricate the impaction and a subsequent hypertonic phosphate enema (Fleet) or normal saline enema (20–40 mL per kg) will stimulate evacuation. It is rarely necessary to use more than 1000 mL of normal saline. Tap water enemas or soapy water enemas are not recommended because of the risk of water intoxication and colitis, respectively.

3. Rectal suppositories–glycerine or bisacodyl (Dulcolax) are useful occasionally.

B. Long-term therapy:

1. Increased fluid and fiber intake.

2. Addition of nonabsorbable carbohydrate to formula–Karo syrup.

3. Stool softeners–Mineral oil (2–3 mL/kg/d) may be used in ambulatory patients. The risk of aspiration and lipid pneumonia must be considered in infants and in recumbent patients, particularly those with psychomotor retardation. Detergent agents (Colace) may also function to soften stools.

4. Fiber supplements

5. Stimulant or osmotic laxatives–Laxatives such as Senokot, Dulcolax, or Milk of Magnesia may be used for short periods of time to prevent reimpaction while retraining of habit constipation is taking place.

COLIC

Colic in small infants is characterized by lengthy bouts of crying and apparent discomfort. It usually occurs in the firstborn infant, starting at around 10 days of age and lasting through the third month. It is a source of great anxiety for the parents whose ineffective attempts to calm the infant may exacerbate the condition.

The causes of colic are poorly understood. Some of the following factors may be of importance.

A. Gastrointestinal Distention with Air: Prolonged crying may fill the stomach and intestines with air. This may lead to crampy pain and the expulsion of gas per rectum. Continuous sucking on a pacifier or frequent breast or bottle feeding may do the same. A vicious cycle of crying, air swallowing, and more crying may be established.

B. Food: Overfeeding with large volumes of formula in an effort to quiet the infant may cause gastric distention and discomfort. Paradoxically, genuine hunger may initiate this cycle.

C. Emotional Factors: Colic occurs most often in a first-born infant during the first weeks at home. The hyperactive, tense infant is likely to have colic. Family tension and parental anxiety may be aggravating factors.

D. Allergy: Intestinal allergy to cow's milk protein, especially in families with a history of allergy in other members, may be associated with colic, emesis, and diarrhea.

Treatment

Treatment of colic is difficult. The most important first step is a careful physical examination and history to look for organic causes of fussiness such as otitis media, urinary infection, central nervous system disorders (tumors, seizures, infections), intestinal disease (ulcer, esophagitis, gastritis, infection, or obstruction), and other problems such as osteomyelitis or traumatic injury secondary to child abuse.

If careful evaluation indicates no cause for fussiness, the following conservative measures are sometimes helpful:

(1) Supportive, sympathetic instruction of parents regarding colic and its benign nature.

(2) Regular schedule for feedings and naps to avoid chaotic routines, overfeeding, or underfeeding.

(3) Low-level sound in the infant's sleeping area such as a radio or vacuum cleaner may be soothing.

(4) Gentle movement in a swing or rides in the automobile. There are even crib vibrators that simulate the sound and movement of an automobile.

(5) Trial of milk-free diet may help an infant with true protein allergy. Avoid frequent formula changes.

(6) Rest and assistance for the infant's caretakers is essential to prevent exhaustion.

(7) Medications are only occasionally useful and include antihistamines, antispasmodics, and antacids. Bentyl has been shown effective, but there is a risk of respiratory depression. The use of beer, wine, or other alcoholic beverages for sedation is not recommended.

Table 22–5. Peptic ulcer—primary vs. secondary.

	Primary	Secondary
Location	Duodenal > gastric.	Gastric = duodenal.
Age	More common > 5 yr.	Any age.
Cause	Hypersecretion; *Helicobacter pylori* infections; genetic factors (+ family history in 30%).	Burn, CNS trauma, local irritants, shock, decreased mucosal defenses.
Symptoms	Pain, emesis, irritability, bleeding.	Emesis, bleeding.
Diagnosis	Endoscopy.	Endoscopy.
Treatment	Histamine receptor antagonist; antibiotics for *H pylori*; antacids; local mucosal protective agents (sucralfate).	Remove primary stress; all other modalities noted for primary ulcer.

PEPTIC ULCER DISEASE
(See Table 22–5.)

INFLAMMATORY BOWEL DISEASE
(See Table 22–6.)

The two major inflammatory bowel diseases in children are Crohn's disease (regional enteritis) and ulcerative colitis. A comparison of the two conditions is found in Table 22–6. The etiology of both is unknown, but autoimmune factors are suspected. A family history of inflammatory bowel disease is obtained in 25% of cases. Ulcerative colitis and Crohn's disease may occur in the same family, suggesting some common etiology for the two conditions.

DISEASES OF THE LIVER
(See Tables 22–7 and 22–8.)

Cholestasis
Many newborns have elevated total serum bilirubin levels. This is secondary to physiologic jaundice or hemolytic disease for the most part. If the direct reacting fraction of bilirubin (conjugated fraction) is greater than 15% of the total, cholestatic liver disease should be suspected and thoroughly evaluated. Conjugated hyperbilirubinemia is *never* physiologic.

Table 22–6. Features of Crohn's disease and ulcerative colitis.

	Crohn's Disease	Ulcerative Colitis
Age at onset	10–20 yr	10–20 yr
Incidence (general population)	4–5/100,000	3–15/100,000
Relative incidence in children	2	1
Area of bowel affected	Oropharynx, esophagus, and stomach—rare Small bowel only, 25–30% Colon and anus only, 15% Ileocolitis, 40% Diffuse disease, 5%	Total colon, 90% Proctitis, 10%
Distribution	Segmental; disease-free skip areas common.	Continuous.
Pathology	Full thickness, acute and chronic inflammation; noncaseating granulomas (50%); fistulas, abscesses, strictures, and fibrosis may be present.	Superficial acute inflammation of mucosa with microscopic crypt abscess.
X-ray	Segmental lesions; thickened circular folds; cobblestone appearance of bowel wall secondary to longitudinal ulcers and transverse fissures; fixation and separation of loops; narrowed lumen "string sign"; fistulae.	Superficial colitis; loss of haustra; shortened colon and pseudopolyps (islands of normal tissue surrounded by denuded mucosa) are late findings.
Intestinal symptoms	Abdominal pain, diarrhea, perianal disease; enteroenteric/enterocutaneous fistula, abscess, anorexia.	Abdominal pain, bloody diarrhea, urgency, and tenesmus.

(Continued)

	Crohn's Disease	Ulcerative Colitis
Extraintestinal Symptoms:		
Arthritis/arthralgia	15%	9%
Fever	40–50%	40–50%
Stomatitis	9%	2%
Weight loss	90% (mean 5.7 kg)	68% (mean 4.1 kg)
Delayed growth and sexual development	30%	5–10%
Uveitis/conjunctivitis	15% (in Crohn's colitis)	4%
Sclerosing cholangitis	rare	4%
Renal stones	6% (oxalate)	6% (urate)
Pyoderma gangrenosum	1.3%	5%
Erythema nodosum	8–15%	4%
Laboratory findings	High ESR; microcytic anemia; low serum iron and total iron binding capacity; increased fecal protein loss; low serum albumin.	High ESR; microcytic anemia, high WBC with "left shift."
Treatment	Corticosteroids, azulfidine, metronidizole (especially for perianal disease); surgical resection as last resort.	Corticosteroids, azulfidine, azathioprine, or 6-mercaptopurine, colectomy for toxic megacolon, resistant symptoms, intractable pain or bleeding.

Table 22–7. Causes of neonatal cholestasis.

	Associated Findings
Infection:	
Bacterial (UTI, sepsis, meningitis)	+ Bacterial cultures.
Viral-intrauterine (rubella, CMV, herpes, toxoplasmosis)	+ Cultures; infant often SGA with DIC and other abnormalities secondary to infection.
Viral-acquired (HAV, HBV, HCV, EBV, herpes, Enterovirus)	+ serologic tests; enterovirus associated with encephalitis; cutaneous lesions in herpes.
Idiopathic (giant cell) hepatitis	Negative cultures; giant cells on liver biopsy.
Metabolic:	
Cystic fibrosis	+ Sweat test; pale, fatty stools, large gallbladder with viscid bile.
Galactosemia	Emesis, acidosis; reducing substances in urine while taking lactose; decreased RBC gal-1-PO_4-uridyl transferase.
Alpha-1-antitrypsin deficiency	Baby may be SGA; variable degrees of hepatitis and cirrhosis at presentation; serum α-1-antitrypsin $<$ 70 mg%.
Tyrosinemia	Hypoalbuminemia, coagulopathy, and hepatitis, increased urinary succinyl acetone.
Parenteral nutrition	Gradual onset; jaundice a late finding occurring after several weeks of IV nurition.
Extrahepatic biliary atresia, choledochal cyst	Alcoholic stools, firm large liver, generally healthy appearance.
Paucity of intrahepatic bile ducts:	
Alagille syndrome	Odd facies, growth failure. Hypogonadism. Peripheral pulmonic stenosis. Vertebral anomalies.
Other nonsyndromatic paucity	More rapidly progressive liver disease.

Table 22-8. Liver disease of older children.

	Agents
Acute infection (usually viral)	Cytomegalic inclusion virus
	Epstein-Barr virus
	Hepatitis A, hepatitis B,
	Non-A, non-B hepatitis (hepatitis C)
	Other systemic viral infections
	Bacterial agents include *N gonorrhea* (causes peri hepatitis)
Fatty liver	Malnutrition
	Storage (Wolman's disease)
	Reye's syndrome
	Mitochondrial dysfunction (eg, carnitine deficiency)
Tumors	Hepatoblastoma
	Hemangiomatosis
	Metastatic Wilms' tumor
	Neuroblastoma
	Gonadal tumor
	Leukemic infiltration
	Histiocytosis
Parasitic disease	*E histolytica*
	Visceral larva migrans
	Shistosoma mansoni
	S japonicum
Metabolic/genetic/ storage diseases	Cystic fibrosis—fatty liver/biliary cirrhosis
	Glycogen storage disease
	Galactosemia
	Tyrosinemia
	Alpha-1-antitrypsin deficiency
	Neiman–Pick disease
	Gaucher's disease
	Amyloidosis
	Congenital hepatic fibrosis
	Wilson's disease
Chronic inflammatory disease	Autoimmune chronic active hepatitis
	Chronic active Hepatitis B or C
	Sclerosing cholangitis, or chronic active hepatitis associated with inflammatory bowel disease

PANCREATIC DISEASE
(See Table 22–3.)

Cystic Fibrosis

In pediatrics, the most common cause of exocrine pancreatic insufficiency is cystic fibrosis (CF). Malabsorption, present from birth in 85% of persons with CF, is a result of obstruction of the ductular system and progressive destruction of the exocrine pancreas. Exogenous pancreatic enzymes must be provided with meals to improve digestion of complex carbohydrate, protein, and fat. Other gastrointestinal problems associated with CF include peptic ulcer, pancreatitis, cholecystitis, cholelithiasis, biliary cirrhosis, meconium ileus (in the newborn), meconium ileus equivalent (in older cystics, a result of large-volume fatty stool obstructing the distal small bowel or proximal colon), and rectal prolapse.

Shwachman Syndrome

This is a rare condition of unknown etiology (probably genetic) characterized by exocrine pancreatic insufficiency (because of fatty replacement of acinar tissue), neutropenia (either cyclic or continuous), growth failure, and metaphyseal dysostosis. Recurrent severe bacterial infections occur in some patients. Diarrhea and malnutrition are common. Sweat test is normal.

Pancreatitis

Pancreatitis is usually an acute viral infection is childhood. It is sometimes associated with overwhelming infection, connective tissue diseases, Reye's syndrome, drug toxicity, and rarely (in pediatrics) alcohol. Forty percent of cases are idiopathic. Trauma may cause pancreatitis and/or pancreatic pseudocyst. Abdominal tenderness, high serum amylase, and enlarged pancreas on abdominal ultrasound with ascites are diagnostic findings. Hemorrhagic pancreatitis carries a very high mortality.

GLUTEN ENTEROPATHY-CELIAC DISEASE

In celiac disease, malabsorption of all nutrients occurs owing to the diminished absorbing surface in the small intestine. Villous atrophy occurs in response to gluten present in wheat, rye, barley, and oats. It is thought that gliadin is bound by absorbing enterocytes in the intestine and that a local immune reaction ensues, which destroys the absorbing cells. Diarrhea and malabsorption usually appear in the second year of life, often after an acute viral illness. Weight loss, fatty stools, anorexia, and irritability are common. Occasionally, severe diarrhea, dehydration, electrolyte deficiency, and prostration occur (celiac crisis).

Diagnosis rests on typical villous atrophy and plasma cell infiltrate in small intestinal biopsies. Antigliadin antibodies are present. Diagnosis by trial of gluten-free diet is not recommended. Treatment is by gluten-free diet. Lactose tolerance is poor until intestinal recovery occurs. Vitamin and iron supplements may be necessary if diarrhea has been long-standing.

Full recovery is expected. The sensitivity to gluten is lifelong. Ten percent of first-degree relatives will be affected in this genetically determined disease.

DISACCHARIDASE DEFICIENCIES

Diminished levels of disaccharidase enzymes on the microvillous surface of the small intestine cause malabsorption of disaccharides and watery, acid, osmotic diarrhea upon ingestion of the offending sugar. Stools contain undigested disaccharide and their fermentation by-products. Symptoms also include nausea, vomiting, and flatulence. Disaccharidase deficiency may be primary (genetic) or secondary to bowel injury. Disaccharide tolerance tests or breath hydrogen assay after an oral disaccharide test meal may be diagnostic. Direct measurement of enzyme levels in intestinal biopsies can be performed (see Table 22–3). Treatment of deficiency is by avoidance of the offending sugars. Tolerance in genetic forms sometimes improves with age.

COW'S MILK ALLERGY

Cow's milk protein allergy is often suspected but rarely proved. The onset is usually in patients under 3 months of age, and the symptoms are diarrhea, vomiting, and, in older children, a malabsorption syndrome compatible with small bowel injury. Early introduction of milk into the diet, especially following gastrointestinal infection, may predispose to this condition. Laboratory findings include eosinophilia demonstrated in a smear of rectal mucus, eosinophilic mucosal infiltrate, proctitis at sigmoidoscopy, and occasionally an atrophic small bowel lesion.

Diagnosis must be confirmed by a response to elimination of cow's milk followed by recurrence of symptoms after reintroduction of milk.

Treatment depends upon the elimination of cow's milk and cow's milk products from the diet for 6 months to 1 year. Soy-based or protein hydrolysate formulas may be substituted. Concomitant soy protein allergy is up to 30% seen in these infants.

Cow's milk protein allergy usually resolves after 6–12 months.

ESOPHAGEAL ATRESIA WITH OR WITHOUT TRACHEOESOPHAGEAL FISTULA

In 90% of these cases, the upper esophagus ends blindly, and the lower esophagus communicates with the back of the trachea. In about 10% of cases, there is esophageal atresia without an associated tracheal fistula. Thirty percent have associated anomalies, usually cardiac or gastrointestinal. Imperforate anus is common.

Infants with esophageal atresia present early with cough and emesis during feedings and apparently excessive salivation. Aspiration pneumonia may occur either from reflux of gastric secretions into the lungs via the distal fistula or from aspiration of oral contents. Diagnosis is made by careful imaging using a small volume of barium instilled via a radio-opaque tube under fluoroscopy.

Immediate surgical repair is necessary. Aspiration pneumonia requires antibiotics. Gastrostomy placement is often necessary. Stricture and fistula formation at the site of esophageal anastomosis may occur, especially with high atresias. Gastroesophageal reflux is common postoperatively.

H-type tracheoesophageal fistula accounts for only 5% of cases. It is often diagnosed late, after repeated bouts of aspiration pneumonia and choking with feedings. Barium X-rays may not demonstrate the tiny fistula, which is usually located in the lower cervical esophagus. Endoscopy or bronchoscopy may demonstrate the fistula.

Early diagnosis, absence of lung disease and a short distance between the proximal and distal esophageal segments all improve the child's chances of a successful outcome. Prematurity and associated congenital anomalies add to the risk. Postoperative esophageal dilatation of stricture is often necessary.

ESOPHAGEAL OBSTRUCTION

Partial obstructions of the esophagus cause a variety of feeding problems during infancy or childhood including vomiting, aspiration, and malnutrition. Vascular ring may cause external compression, especially double aortic arch. Esophageal strictures develop after correction of tracheoesophageal fistula, ingestion of corrosive chemicals (eg, lye), or as a result of chronic peptic esophagitis from gastroesophageal reflux. Congenital strictures are rare, as is congenital achalasia. Globus hystericus, or a sensation of esophageal obstruction in the absence of obstructing lesions, may be seen even in preschool children. These children often refuse food but usually have no difficulty swallowing their own secretions.

Diagnosis

The upper GI series is the most informative study when symptoms suggest esophageal obstruction. Vascular ring causes characteristic external compression of the esophageal outline. Location and length of stricture, esophageal dysmotility, and hiatus hernia are easily seen. Endoscopy adds more information regarding esophagitis.

INGUINAL HERNIA & HYDROCELE

The testis forms cephalad to the kidney and descends into the scrotum during the last trimester of pregnancy. As it descends, the peritoneum descends with it to form the tunica vaginalis. The peritoneal connection between the abdominal cavity and the scrotum (the processus vaginalis) is normally obliterated. All hernias, hydroceles, and ectopic testes relate to abnormalities in this process.

Hernia

A hernia is seen as an intermittent bulge lateral to the pubic tubercle; the bulge appears when the patient is crying, straining, or standing and usually reduces spontaneously when the patient is relaxed or supine. Treatment in children usually consists of elective surgery performed when the child is in good health.

The incidence of hernia in the general population is 1%, and in premature infants, 5%. Males are affected most commonly (85% of cases). One half of cases of inguinal hernia during childhood occur in infants under 6 months of age. Right-sided hernias are more frequent than are those on the left (2:1). Irrespective of side, about 25% of patients have contralateral hernias. In females, hernias are often bilateral. For this reason, repair of the asymptomatic side is often performed in children less than 2 years of age, especially in females.

Incarceration (failure to reduce) occurs in about 10% of cases, most often in children under 1 year of age. Strangulation follows incarceration, and the hernia becomes tender and erythematous. The abdomen becomes distended, with vomiting and signs of bowel obstruction. Pressure on testicular vessels in the inguinal canal by an incarcerated hernia can cause testicular infarction.

Incarcerated hernia can often be reduced by gently squeezing the bowel back into the abdomen along the axis of the inguinal canal. Sedation (pentobarbital, 4 mg/kg, and meperidine, 1 mg/kg) is necessary in most cases.

Strangulation is managed by nasogastric suction, rehydration, correction of electrolyte deficiencies, and surgery when the patient's condition is stable. Attempted reduction may rupture ischemic bowel or return necrotic bowel into the abdomen.

The ovary is often incarcerated in females. Strangulation is rare, and hernias may usually be repaired on a relatively elective basis.

Hydrocele

Hydrocele is very common in newborns. Spontaneous regression by age 6 months is the rule. Frequent and rapid change in size of the hydrocele indicates a patent processus vaginalis with communication to the peritoneal cavity. Since hernia may develop, communicating hydroceles should be repaired.

Acute hydrocele may develop about the testis or in the spermatic cord and may be difficult to differentiate from incarcerated hernia. Examination at the internal ring level, with one finger in the upper rectum and another feeling the abdomen from the outside, may aid in differentiation. Acute hydrocele in the canal of Nuck presents as an oblong, firm swelling in the groin of a female infant and may be confused with a groin node. Exploration is required in doubtful cases.

GASTROESOPHAGEAL REFLUX
(Chalasia)

Gastroesophageal reflux occurs in 40% of healthy infants less than 6 months. Postprandial spitting and vomiting are the most common symptoms. Infants usually remain healthy, but aspiration pneumonia, esophagitis, esophageal stricture, and malnutrition may occur if vomiting is severe. Reflux is common in physically and neurologically handicapped children, in those with severe scoliosis, and after tracheoesophageal fistula repair.

Diagnosis is based upon characteristic history, upper GI series, sometimes esophageal scintiscan, and esophageal pH monitoring in atypical cases.

Conservative measures often suffice in healthy infants as the condition is usually self-limited. Infants are given small-volume, frequent feedings thickened with cereal and are kept in the prone position with the head elevated 60 degrees as much as possible to reduce reflux. Medication includes antacids, H_2 receptor antagonists, and smooth muscle stimulants such as bethanechol. In more resistant cases, gastric fundoplication may be necessary.

CONGENITAL HERNIA OF THE DIAPHRAGM

The most common area of herniation is in the left posterolateral portion, the foramen of Bochdalek. Foramen of Morgagni hernias rarely present during the newborn period and rarely cause significant respiratory symptoms.

Clinical Findings

A. Symptoms and Signs: Cyanosis and dyspnea is a newborn infant suggest the diagnosis. Respiratory distress is usually constant and severe. Chest movements are asymmetric with dullness on the affected side. Breath sounds may be absent. The abdomen is scaphoid and feels less full on palpation than usual. The mediastinum shifts away from the affected side. There is usually hypoplasia of the lung on the affected side with persistent pulmonary hypertension, which makes ventilatory management difficult.

B. Imaging: Chest x-ray (required for all infants with respiratory distress) usually shows a portion of the gastrointestinal tract in the thorax and displacement of the mediastinum. Avoid introducing contrast medium into the gastrointestinal tract.

Treatment

Diaphragmatic hernia is a surgical emergency. The viscera are reduced from the thorax through a subcostal incision. The diaphragm is closed and a chest tube left in place to water-seal drainage. The infant must be kept warm. If abdominal closure requires tension, close only the skin to prevent undue pressure on the diaphragm or inferior vena cava.

An endotracheal tube is left in place for ventilation. Persistent fetal circulation and pulmonary hypoplasia are the commonest cause of mortality. Pulmonary vasodilators are sometimes helpful. Recently, extracorporeal membrane oxygenation has been used with success in some of these infants.

Course & Prognosis

Survival depends on the degree of pulmonary hypoplasia; survival rate is about 50%. Lung weights of infants who do not survive are about half those of normal infants of the same gestational age and birth weight. The morphology of the lung on the side of the hernia is that of a 28- to 30-week-old fetus. Long-term survivors have normal lung weights, although they may have some degree of emphysema and decreased blood flow.

PYLORIC STENOSIS
(Congenital Hypertrophic Pyloric Stenosis)

Pyloric stenosis is more apt to occur in firstborn infants and is more common in males than in females (4:1 ratio). In most cases, the diagnosis is made between 3 and 12 weeks of age.

There is a marked increase in the size of the circular musculature of the pylorus, causing obstruction of the lumen. In the average case, the enlargement is the size and shape of an olive.

Clinical Findings

A. Symptoms and Signs: Vomiting begins in most cases after the 14th day of life. It is usually mild at first but becomes progressively more forceful and eventually projectile over 3–7 days. Vomiting occurs within one-half hour of feeding and does not contain bile. The infant is hungry and will refeed immediately. The child passes small, loose starvation stools. Weight loss, dehydration, and hypochloremic alkalosis may be severe. Jaundice develops in 2–5% of cases. Gastric stasis results in gastritis and hematemesis in some cases. On examination, the infant is alert, irritable, dehydrated, and hungry. The epigastrium may be distended and the gastric outline obvious. Gastric peristalsis passing from left to right during feeding can be seen on the abdomen. An olive shaped mass is palpable in the right upper quadrant, especially directly after vomiting, in 75–95% of cases. Inguinal hernias develop in 10% of cases secondary to forceful emesis. Tetany as a result of alkalosis and reduction of free serum calcium may occur.

B. Laboratory Findings: Findings include metabolic alkalosis, kypokalemia, and variable hyponatremia. Urinalysis usually reveals a markedly alkaline urine of high specific gravity. If potassium depletion is present, the infant may have an acid urine but still suffer from alkalosis. Hemoconcentration may be manifested by increased hemoglobin and hematocrit values. The indirect bilirubin fraction (unconjugated) may be elevated.

C. Imaging: If the typical mass in the right upper quadrant is not palpable, the pyloric muscle may be demonstrated by ultrasonography. The upper gastrointestinal series shows an enlarged stomach with a narrow, elongated pyloric channel and prolonged gastric retention of barium. The impression of the pyloric muscle on the antrum can be seen.

Treatment

A. Preoperative Care:

1. Rehydration–Rehydration by the intravenous route is preferred. The rate of infusion will depend on the severity of dehydration. Rarely, the patient will be cachectic and will require total parenteral nutrition.

2. Nasogastric intubation–Before operation, a No. 8 French nasogastric tube may be inserted to preclude regurgitation and aspiration of stomach contents during anesthesia.

B. Surgical Measures: Ramstedt pyloromyotomy divides the hypertrophied muscle bundles that obstruct the pylorus. Surgery should not be performed until rehydration and correction of alkalosis are complete.

Prognosis

Complete relief is to be expected following adequate surgical repair. Mortality rate is low.

MECONIUM ILEUS

Meconium ileus is the presenting sign in 15% of newborn infants with CF. Lack of pancreatic trypsin causes unusually thick meconium, which obstructs the lower 10–20 cm of ileum. The ileocecal valve and the entire colon are normal albeit small. There may be associated atresia of small bowel.

Clinical Findings

A. Symptoms and Signs: Intestinal obstruction in the newborn is characterized by progressively more severe vomiting, beginning within the first day or two of life. The vomitus contains bile.

The abdomen is distended, and loops of bowel may be seen through the abdominal wall. Firm masses within the loops strongly suggest meconium ileus. In most cases, no meconium will have been passed.

B. Laboratory Findings: If meconium appears in stools, it can be shown to contain no trypsin. The sweat test shows an increase in the chloride concentration of sweat (> 60 meq/L). Serum immunoreactive trypsinogen (a screening test for CF in the newborn) may be falsely normal in CF patients with meconium ileus, probably because of the severe reduction in exocrine pancreatic secretion.

C. Imaging: Marked intestinal dilatation may be seen, with characteristically few or no air-fluid levels in the loops of bowel (owing to the presence of inspissated meconium). A granular, mottled appearance within a loop because of bubbles of gas and meconium should suggest the presence of meconium ileus. Microcolon may be seen on barium enema. Free air seen in the peritoneal cavity or the presence of fluid between the loops of bowel indicates perforation. Calcification of the peritoneum, when present, represents antenatal perforation and meconium peritonitis.

Treatment

A. Preoperative Care: Provide continuous gastric suction through a nasogastric tube. Administer diatrizoate (Gastrografin) enemas but only when the infant is adequately hydrated. The hypertonic contrast medium draws water into the bowel and "floats out" the inspissated meconium. This procedure, which is often successful, must be done under fluoroscopy by a radiologist familiar with newborn infants. It will not relieve associated atresia, volvulus, or peritonitis.

B. Surgical Measures: Several choices are available. The portion of the distal ileum that contains the greatest amount of meconium may be resected. The ends are brought out and sutured to the skin. Postoperatively, the terminal ileum and colon are cleansed with pancreatic enzyme suspension. Closure of the enterostomy is performed 2–3 weeks later.

C. Postoperative Care: After the immediate obstruction is relieved, therapy for the prevention of pulmonary and nutritional disturbance of CF becomes necessary.

Prognosis

There is no relationship between meconium ileus and the severity of the respiratory symptoms of CF.

CONGENITAL ATRESIA OR STENOSIS OF INTESTINES & COLON

Congenital atresia and stenosis probably result from vascular obstruction in the mesenteric vessels during fetal development. Atresia designates a complete block, while stenosis indicates narrowing of the intestinal lumen. Atresia or stenosis of the duodenum is frequently associated with Down's syndrome.

Meconium ileus must be considered in any child with intestinal atresia (see above).

Clinical Findings

A. Symptoms and Signs: Atresia of the intestinal tract or colon causes vomiting on the first day of life. Intestinal stenosis may not come to the physician's attention for weeks or months. The vomitus contains bile. Depending on the level of involvement, abdominal distention is often present and becomes progressively worse. Peristaltic waves are often seen. Intestinal loops may be outlined on the abdominal wall. Dehydration is common because of persistent vomiting. Meconium may be dry and gray-green rather than black and viscous.

B. Imaging: Upright abdominal x-ray shows air and fluid levels with dilatation of the duodenum and the proximal loops of small bowel. The distal loops will be free of gas if the obstruction is complete. In partial obstruction, there may be gas without distention distal to the point of obstruction. Presence of free air in the abdominal cavity means that perforation has occurred. A granular, mottled appearance in the small bowel as a result of gas and meconium suggests meconium ileus.

Barium enema is an important part of the preoperative x-ray study. In low-intestinal atresia, it will often demonstrate the markedly decreased caliber characteristic of the unused portion of the gastrointestinal tract—the so-called microcolon. The chief indication for barium enema is to rule out Hirschsprung's disease and malrotation with volvulus, which can present with symptoms identical to those of intestinal atresia.

Treatment

For decompression, institute constant gastric sump suction. Give parenteral fluids and electrolytes.

Resection of the dilated, hypertrophic intestine proximal to the atresia and end-to-end anastomosis, where possible, are usually preferred for the surgical correction of atresia or stenosis. In all cases of atresia and marked stenosis, early intervention is essential to prevent perforation. If the infant is debilitated or if perforation has occurred, intestinal contents proximal to the stenosis may be diverted via an intestinal enterostomy and delayed ressection with anastomosis.

Course & Prognosis

The mortality rate in infants with atresia or marked stenosis is increased by delay in diagnosis. Postoperative hypomotility of the dilated proximal bowel may compromise enteral feedings, necessitating parenteral nutrition.

MALROTATION OF INTESTINES & COLON

Malrotation is the result of incomplete rotation of the gut and lack of attachment of the mesentery of the small intestine during intrauterine development. It may result in a volvulus of the midgut or obstruction of the second part of the duodenum by peritoneal bands. It may be associated with no symptoms.

Clinical Findings

A. Symptoms and Signs: If malrotation is accompanied by an intrinsic obstruction of the second portion of the duodenum (eg, atresia, stenosis), vomiting occurs within 48 hours of birth. In the early stages of midgut volvulus, the general condition is good; failure to diagnose and treat at this point will lead to rapid clinical deterioration indicative of widespread intestinal gangrene. Bilious emesis is the significant symptom. In older infants and children, there may be intermittent attacks of vomiting without significant abdominal distention. The presence of blood in the stools indicates ischemic mucosal changes and constitutes a surgical emergency.

B. Laboratory Findings: Hematocrit and red blood cell counts are elevated owing to dehydration. Slight leukocytosis is usually present. Marked leukocytosis suggests impending or actual gangrene of the bowel.

C. Imaging: Plain films of the abdomen may or may not show dilatation of the stomach and duodenum. Barium examination may show that the cecum and ascending colon are displaced to the left. Upper gastrointestinal barium studies are preferred by some pediatric radiologists for diagnosing malrotation.

Treatment

The goal of surgery is to relieve extrinsic compression in the duodenum by dividing the bands that bind the second and third portions to the retroperitoneum and by straightening the duodenojejunal junction. The midgut always twists in a clockwise fashion in North America; thus, the mass of bowel loops must be unwound in a counterclockwise direction. The small bowel is then placed in the right side of the abdomen and the colon to the left.

Course & Prognosis
Recurrences after surgical correction are uncommon.

MECKEL'S DIVERTICULUM

Meckel's diverticulum may be asymptomatic throughout life or may be associated with any of the following: hemorrhage; Meckel's diverticulitis, with symptoms identical to those of acute appendicitis; perforation; intussusception, with the diverticulum as the leading point; patent omphalomesenteric duct, with a diverticulum opening at the umbilicus; and intestinal obstruction from a vestigial band connecting the diverticulum to the umbilicus. It is found in 2% of the population and is usually located in the distal ileum.

Clinical Findings
Symptoms and signs depend upon the nature of the complication caused by Meckel's diverticulum. X-ray examinations are generally of no value in Meckel's diverticulum. Radioactive technetium perchlorate has been used to demonstrate ectopic gastric mucosa in the diverticulum.

Bleeding is usually massive and painless. The child passes tarry or bright-red blood through the rectum. The bleeding is from ulceration in the diverticulum or from the normal ileum adjacent to it. Bleeding, perforation, and diverticulitis occur only in the diverticuli that contain ectopic gastric mucosa and therefore secrete acid. Foreign bodies lodged in the diverticulum can cause any of these symptoms. Table 22–9 lists the differential diagnosis of rectal bleeding in infants and small children.

Treatment
Treatment consists of operative excision as soon as the diagnosis is made. In cases of gastrointestinal hemorrhage in which Meckel's diverticulum is suspected but unproved, operation may be deferred until the diagnosis is established or until bleeding occurs a second time. In the asymptomatic patient, elective excision or removal incidental to another surgical procedure is not indicated unless gastric mucosa is palpated in the diverticulum.

Table 22–9. Differential diagnosis of rectal bleeding in infants and children.

Cause	Usual Age Group	Additional Chief Complaints	Amount of Blood	Type of Blood	Treatment
Allergy	Colon	Colicky abdominal pain.	Moderate to large	Dark or bright	Eliminate allergen.
Anal fissure	< 2 yr	Pain.	Small	Bright	Soften stool; anal dilatation. See Table 22–2.
Bacterial enteritis	All ages	Diarrhea, cramps.	Small	Usually bright with diarrhea	Surgery.
Duplication of bowel	All ages	Variable.	Usually small	Usually dark	
Esophageal varices	> 4 yr	Bloody emesis; signs of portal hypertension; signs of chronic liver disease.	Variable	Usually dark	Reduce portal hypertension; sclerose varices.
Hemangioma or telangiectasia	All ages	Usually none.	Variable	Dark or bright	None.
Hemorrhagic disease of the newborn	Newborns	Other evidence of bleeding.	Variable	Dark or bright	Vitamin K, transfusion.
Inserted foreign body	Children	Pain.	Small	Bright	Removal.

(Continued)

Table 22–9 (cont'd). Differential diagnosis of rectal bleeding in infants and children.

Cause	Usual Age Group	Additional Chief Complaints	Amount of Blood	Type of Blood	Treatment
Intussusception	< 18 m	Abdominal pain; mass; bilious emesis.	Small to large	Red jelly-like	Barium enema or surgery.
Meckel's diverticulum	Young children	None or anemia.	Small to large	Dark or bright	Surgery.
Peptic ulcer	All ages	Abdominal pain, emesis, hematemesis.	Usually small	Dark	Antacid.
Swallowed maternal blood	Newborns	None.	Variable	Dark	None.
Volvulus	Infants or young children	Abdominal pain, intestinal obstruction.	Small to large	Dark	Surgery.
Ulcerative colitis; Crohn's colitis	> 3 yr	Pain, fever.	Small to large	Bright, with diarrhea	See Table 22–6.
Juvenile polyps	> 3 yr	None.	Small	Bright	May be removed endoscopically.

706

Course & Prognosis

The prognosis is excellent following surgery. If perforation through a gangrenous diverticulum has occurred, massive peritonitis may follow and is a serious threat to life.

DUPLICATIONS OF THE GASTROINTESTINAL TRACT

Cysts of enteric origin are associated with and often communicate with various levels of the gastrointestinal tract. They may occur anywhere from the upper esophagus to the anus and are often intimately associated with the adjacent areas of the gastrointestinal tract, usually sharing a common muscular wall. The nature of the mucosal lining varies considerably and may not necessarily correspond with the level of the gastrointestinal tract to which the cyst is adjacent. There is considerable variation in the size and shape of these cysts.

A duplication may present as an asymptomatic mass with gastrointestinal bleeding, as an intestinal obstruction resulting from volvulus or intussusception, or with evidence of localized peritonitis. Special types of duplications include neurenteric cysts and hindgut duplications. Neurenteric cysts usually arise from the proximal small bowel and extend toward the vertebral column; they are associated with a bony defect in the vertebral column and extension through the diaphragm and into the chest. Hindgut duplications actually represent a double colon and are often associated with doubling of the anus and the perineal structures.

Diagnosis can sometimes be made by use of radioactive technetium perchlorate to demonstrate ectopic gastric mucosa in the duplication.

Treatment consists of resection of the duplication and, in most cases, of the adjacent bowel also. The prognosis is good.

BILIARY ATRESIA

Biliary atresia is a progressive extrahepatic biliary obstruction in the newborn. If untreated, it eventually compromises the intrahepatic biliary system and results in cirrhosis, portal hypertension, ascites, and liver insufficiency.

Clinical Findings

Symptoms and signs include progressive jaundice, most often becoming apparent after the second week of life. Failure to thrive, hepatomegaly, and splenomegaly occur later.

Neonatal hepatitis is the condition most often confused with biliary atresia. This and other causes of jaundice (see table 22–7 & 22–8) must be ruled out.

Treatment

In infants with biliary atresia, bilioenteric drainage (portojejunostomy) procedures are performed preferably between the first and second months of life. The condition cannot be surgically palliated after 12–16 weeks, and death from liver failure or complications of portal hypertension usually occurs between 2 and 3 years.

Laparotomy and operative cholangiogram should be performed to confirm the diagnosis. The liver biopsy gives an indication of long-term prognosis, based upon the degree of hepatic cirrhosis.

Several modifications of the original hepatic portojejunostomy (Kasai procedure) have been developed in an effort to prevent postoperative intrahepatic cholangitis. If distal extrahepatic ducts of the gallbladder are patent, cholecystoenterostomy (Kasai gallbladder procedure) is the procedure of choice. Liver transplantation is increasingly used if the Kasai operation fails.

Course & Prognosis

The average survival of patients with untreated biliary atresia is 18 months. Progression of hepatic fibrosis is common even after surgical palliation, although 30–50% of patients may remain anicteric. The short-term transplant survival rate is about 75%.

CHOLEDOCHAL CYST

Choledochal cyst is less common than biliary atresia. The manifestations consist of intermittent jaundice, fever and chills (when infection is present), and a mass in the right upper quadrant. X-ray examination may show a mass on a plain film and indentation of the duodenum on an upper gastrointestinal series. Ultrasonography is the preferred method to confirm the diagnosis. The cyst should be excised rather than simply drained into the gastrointestinal tract. The overall prognosis is excellent if operative excision is done early. Newborns with symptomatic choledochal cysts have a poorer prognosis, with a course similar to that of extrahepatic biliary atresia.

INTUSSUSCEPTION

Intussusception is one of the most dangerous surgical emergencies in early childhood. It is characterized by the telescoping of a proximal portion of the intestine into a more distal portion, resulting in impairment of the blood supply and necrosis of the involved segment of bowel. In 95% of cases, no cause of intussusception can be found, but viral infections have been implicated. The condition is most common in infants between the ages of 5 months and 1 year. Telescoping occasionally occurs from a Meckel's diverticulum.

Intussusception most commonly involves the telescoping of the ileum into the colon (ileocolic type). Gangrene of the intussusception occurs if the incarcerated bowel loses its blood supply.

Clinical Findings

A. Symptoms and Signs: A sudden onset of recurrent, paroxysmal, sharp abdominal pain in a healthy child suggests intussusception. The child perspires and draws up the legs to ease the pain. The child may appear well or merely lethargic in the pain-free intervals. Vomiting frequently occurs after the onset of the abdominal pain but is not universally present. Fifteen percent of patients do not have pain.

After 1 or 2 hours of recurrent pain, there is pallor, sweating, and lassitude with each attack of pain. After 5 or more hours, dehydration and listlessness are noted, and the eyes are sunken and soft. A low-grade fever is usually present as a result of dehydration and obstruction.

Careful palpation usually reveals a nontender, firm, sausage-shaped mass in the abdomen. Its location varies, but it frequently is in the upper midabdomen. The right lower quadrant is characteristically less full than usual. If the leading point of the intussusception has reached the rectum, it may be possible to palpate a mass by rectal examination. Blood frequently is found on rectal examination. A "currant jelly" stool (blood and mucus clot) may be evacuated in a bowel movement.

B. Laboratory Findings: Depending on the duration of symptoms, dehydration may be found, requiring replacement fluid and electrolyte therapy.

C. Imaging: A plain film of the abdomen will frequently show absence of bowel gas in the right lower quadrant. Dilated loops of small bowel, when present, suggest partial or complete obstruction of the small intestine. When barium enema examination is performed, the intussusception is outlined as an inverted cap, and an obstruction to the further progression of the barium is noted. Barium enema may also be used to reduce the intussusception (see Treatment, below).

Treatment

A. General Measures: After intravenous fluids are given, nonoperative reduction by barium enema administered by a skilled radiologist under fluoroscopic control will safely reduce intussusception in two thirds of cases. The enema must reflux through the ileocecal valve, and unless the ileum is filled, it may be impossible to tell whether complete reduction has occurred. Subsequent laparotomy is necessary if reduction is not accomplished. If too much hydrostatic pressure is employed or if the bowel wall has been weakened owing to impairment of its vascular supply, perforation can occur. Hydrostatic reduction (barium enema) should *not* be attempted if there are physical findings of peritonitis.

B. Preoperative Care: One to 2 hours of intensive fluid and electrolyte therapy are usually necessary before the child can be considered a good risk for surgery. Parenteral fluids should be started, the blood should be typed and cross-matched before the patient is sent to x-ray for hydrostatic reduction. Deflation of the stomach by constant gastric suction is essential before, during, and after surgery.

C. Surgical Measures: Surgical reduction is possible in most cases of early diagnosis. The bowel is usually found to be viable. If not, resection and anastomosis should be done.

D. Postoperative Care: Parenteral feedings and nasogastric suction should be continued until the infant passes feces normally, since postoperative ileus may be prolonged. Fever may persist for 2 or 3 days. Antibiotics are rarely indicated unless the bowel has perforated preoperatively.

Course & Prognosis

With early diagnosis and treatment, the mortality rate is low. The longer the delay before treatment, the higher the mortality rate.

With adequate early treatment, the prognosis is excellent and recurrences are uncommon. For this reason, no attempt is made to do anything more than reduce the intussusception unless some condition that caused the obstruction such as a polyp or Meckel's diverticulum is discovered at surgery.

Children more than 4 years of age who have intussusception

frequently have a small bowel lymphosarcoma, polyp, or other leading point for the intussusception.

POLYPS OF THE INTESTINAL TRACT
(See Table 22–10.)

Juvenile Polyps

Most juvenile polyps are located in the colon (60% in the recto-sigmoid), but they may be found anywhere in the intestine. They may be single or multiple. They are usually soft, and they may show ulceration of the surface. Intussusception may occur with the polyp acting as the leading point.

In most cases, colonoscopic removal of juvenile polyps from the colon is possible. Single juvenile polyps have no malignant potential. Occasionally, adenomatous changes develop in patients with multiple juvenile polyps. Laparotomy is never indicated unless massive bleeding or intussusception develops. Most juvenile polyps will slough in time without complication.

Multiple polyps in the older child suggest the possibility of Peutz–Jegher's syndrome, Gardner's syndrome, or familial adenomatous polyposis. Family history, excisional biopsy of the lowest polyp, and examination for cutaneous manifestations will rule out these rare causes of polyps. A colectomy with ileorectal pull-through operation is usually the procedure of choice for children with Gardner's syndrome or adenomatous polyposis because of the high cancer risk.

HIRSCHSPRUNG'S DISEASE

Infants with Hirschsprung's disease lack normal development of Meissner's and Auerbach's plexuses in the distal bowel. The defect always begins at the anorectal junction and may involve all or most of the large bowel. In most cases, only the rectosigmoid is involved. The disease is 5 times more common in males and usually causes symptoms soon after birth.

Clinical Findings

A. Symptoms and Signs: Obstipation, abdominal distention, and vomiting may begin in the first days of life. Ninety percent of patients with aganglionosis fail to pass meconium during the first 24 hours of life. Obstipation may alternate with watery diarrhea. Complete obstruction, perforation, or acute

Table 22-10. GI polyposis syndromes.

	Location*	Number	Histology	Associated Findings	Malignant Potential
Juvenile polyps	Colon.	Usually single; rarely multiple.	Hyperplastic, hamartomatous.	None.	None in single polyps; rare in multiple polyps.
Familial polyposis	Colon (stomach and small bowel).	Multiple.	Adenomatous.	None.	Very common.
Peutz–Jegher syndrome	Small bowel, stomach, colon.	Multiple.	Hamartomatous.	Pigmented cutaneous and oral macules; ovarian cysts and tumors; bony exostoses.	2–3%.
Gardner syndrome	Colon (stomach, small bowel).	Multiple.	Adenomatous.	Cysts, tumors, and desmoids of skin and bone; other tumors.	Very common.
Cronkhite–Canada syndrome	Stomach, colon (esophagus, small bowel).	Multiple.	Hamartomatous.	Alopecia, onychodystrophy, hyperpigmentation.	Rare.
Turcot syndrome	Colon.	Multiple.	Adenomatous.	Thyroid and brain tumors.	Possible.

*Parentheses indicate less common locations.

enterocolitis may develop at any time. Poor weight gain is common.

The abdomen is distended, often with palpable loops of bowel. Rectal examination shows no stool in the ampulla. There may be an explosive release of feces and flatus when the examining finger is withdrawn. Signs of malnutrition are present.

B. Imaging: An upright abdominal x-ray may show massive distention of the colon with gas and feces. In advanced cases, there may be air-fluid levels. Look carefully for air in the wall of the bowel, which is occasionally a sign of enterocolitis.

Barium enema should be performed *without* the usual bowel preparation. Use only sufficient barium to study the colon up to the junction of the aganglionic and the stool-filled ganglionic segment. The transitional segment is spastic, with an irregular, saw-toothed outline. This may be best seen on a lateral view. In the newborn, this may not be striking, and the only positive finding may be retention of barium in the proximal bowel for more than 24 hours after the examination.

C. Rectal Biopsy: This should be performed after the barium enema has been completed if there is doubt in the diagnosis. A biopsy specimen shows absence of ganglion cells in both Meissner's and Auerbach's plexuses. Marked hypertrophy of nerve trunks may be seen.

D. Rectal Manometry: Rectal manometry demonstrates loss of the normal reflex relaxation of the internal anal sphincter upon rectal distention.

Treatment

Colostomy is usually performed early and must be done as an emergency procedure if perforation or enterocolitis is suspected. Resection of the aganglionic segment, with reestablishment of continuity (Swenson, Duhamel, or Soave procedure), may be performed when the patient is 6 months or older. Waiting allows the patient to resume normal growth and allows the distended proximal colon to resume its normal size.

ANORECTAL MALFORMATIONS
(Imperforate Anus)

Most males with an anorectal malformation have a fistula to the membranous urethra and no connection between the hindgut and the perineal skin. Most females have a fistula to the perineum at the posterior junction of the labia (posterior fourchette). In the female, communication between the rectum and the urinary tract is rare.

Clinical Findings

A. Males: There is no opening where the anus should be. The intergluteal fold may be well developed, with good sphincter response to perineal stimulation. Look for a fistula along the median raphe. Watch for meconium in urine. There is a significant incidence of associated tracheoesophageal fistula. Absence of a perineal fistula means that the patient probably has a communication to the urethra and requires a colostomy. In doubtful cases, this communication (fistula) can sometimes be seen on urethrogram.

B. Females: Look for a fistula in the posterior fourchette and perineum. Gentle dilation of the fistula with a sound will often relieve obstipation temporarily. A high vaginal fistula cannot be handled by dilation; the patient should have a colostomy.

C. General Findings: Since there is a high incidence of absence of kidneys and strictures of the ureteropelvic and ureterovesical structures, all infants with imperforate anus require thorough study of the urinary tract.

Treatment

A. Conservative Measures: Pass a nasogastric tube if no fistula is found or if the abdomen is distended. Perforation can occur if the bowel is allowed to become massively distended. Time should not be wasted waiting for air to distend the rectum for x-ray confirmation.

B. Surgical Measures: Perineal fistulas in males and females require only dilation during the newborn period; anoplasty can be done later. Pull-through operations for patients with a high imperforate anus should be done after the age of 6 months. The best results are reported when a transcoccygeal approach is used. The results are poor if the child has myelomeningocele or a significant malformation of the lumbosacral spine.

Prognosis

All infants with perineal fistulas should be continent since bowel passes normally through the levators. Infants with a high pouch have only a fair chance for complete rectal continence.

APPENDICITIS

Appendicitis is the most common pathologic lesion of the intestinal tract requiring surgery in childhood. Most cases are seen in children between the ages of 4 and 12 years and may be associated with other illnesses, especially measles. The cause is not clear, although some cases seem to result from impaction of a fecalith in the lumen of the appendix with resultant congestion of the distal appendix and bacterial invasion by organisms residing in the intestinal tract. Pinworms may occasionally cause appendicitis.

Clinical Findings

A. Symptoms: Acute periumbilical or generalized abdominal pain is usually constant. After 1–5 hours, the pain becomes localized in the right lower quadrant. Urinary pain or frequency may be present if the appendix lies near the bladder or ureters. When vomiting occurs, it is usually only after prolonged pain. Constipation occurs frequently, but diarrhea is only occasionally seen.

B. Signs: Fever is low-grade, varying from 37.8 to 38.4 °C (100 to 101.6 °F), or may be absent early in the course. Very high fevers are suggestive of appendiceal perforation, with peritonitis, or of the simultaneous presence of bacterial enteritis, especially if accompanied by diarrhea. **Note:** Appendicitis may complicate enteritis.

The child usually is anxious and may be "doubled up" (with hips flexed) or walk bent over, often holding the right side.

Palpation may reveal a difference in muscular tension between the 2 sides of the abdomen. The hand should be warm and palpation gentle. Localization of tenderness may be difficult, but an opinion about whether the pain is greater on the right or left side may be formed by observing the child's expression while palpating each area and noting the involuntary spasm of the abdominal musculature. Most children tend to flex the right thigh in an effort to decrease the spasm of the psoas muscle. However, the elicitation of a positive psoas sign on hyperextension of the leg, revealing spasm and pain, is generally of doubtful value in small children.

There may be rectal tenderness, a mass consisting of peritoneal fluid, or an indurated omentum wrapped around an inflamed appendix.

C. Laboratory Findings: Two or 3 consecutive determinations of white blood cells will frequently show a rise in the total white blood cell count, with an accompanying shift to the left in the neutrophilic series. It is imperative that a careful urinalysis be made in order to rule out inflammation of the kidney or bladder. **Note:** Irritation of the ureter may occur, and a few white or red blood cells may appear in the urine. A neglected abscess behind the bladder may lead to hematuria and urgency.

D. Imaging: In uncomplicated appendicitis, plain films of the abdomen may show a fecalith, scoliosis, or an abnormal gas pattern. When exudate has formed, evidence of peritoneal inflammation may be established by noting disappearance of the peritoneal line and preperitoneal fat line along the right wall of the abdomen or by noting obliteration of the psoas shadow.

The judicious use of a barium enema may be of value if the diagnosis is not clear. Normal filling of the appendix tends to exclude the diagnosis of appendicitis. In well-established cases of appendicitis, persistent pressure defects and other abnormalities of the cecum may be noted.

In the presence of perforation, fluid may accumulate between loops of the bowel. However, free intra-abdominal air is rare except in children under 2 years of age. With abscess formation, there may be evidence of a soft tissue mass in the region of the perforation. In atypical cases, a plain film of the chest is of value to rule out reflex pain and abdominal spasm of an undiagnosed pneumonitis.

Differential Diagnosis

Differential diagnosis includes mesenteric adenitis, pyelitis, cystitis, pneumonitis (especially pneumococcal), gastroenteritis, peritonitis, constipation, Meckel's diverticulitis, and acute onset of inflammatory bowel disease (especially Crohn's ileitis/ileocolitis).

Treatment

A. Surgical Measures: Appendectomy should be done as soon as the child has been prepared by adequate fluid and electrolyte administration. If there is doubt as to diagnosis, an exploratory laparotomy, with removal of the appendix and culture of peritoneal fluid, should be performed. Intravenous antibiotic therapy may be indicated if peritoneal contamination has occurred. Penrose drains are indicated for localized abscesses.

B. Postoperative Care: Patients with simple appendectomy do not require a nasogastric tube. Intravenous fluids are usually required for 24 hours.

For patients with ruptured appendix, continuous gastric suction should be employed until intestinal peristalsis is normal. Fowler's position (semi-sitting) should be maintained in order to permit drainage into the pelvic region. Parenteral fluid therapy is administered as indicated (see Chapter 4). Antibiotics (see Chapter 8) are given as determined by peritoneal culture data.

FOREIGN BODIES IN THE GASTROINTESTINAL TRACT

The incidence of foreign bodies in the gastrointestinal tract is highest in children 1–3 years of age. Coins, toys, and marbles may lodge in the esophagus and should be removed by esophagoscopy. If passed into the stomach, they usually pass through the entire gastrointestinal tract without incident. If x-rays are taken for presumed ingestion, be sure to include the esophagus and pharynx if the foreign body is not in the abdomen.

Pointed foreign bodies (eg, pins, nails, screws) usually pass without incident. Remove endoscopically if the patient has pain, fever, vomiting, or local tenderness. Only 2–4% of such cases require surgery. X-ray examination is required only if the foreign body has not passed in 4 or 5 days. If a pin or other sharp object remains in the same location for 4 or 5 days, the point may have penetrated the bowel, and endoscopic removal or surgery is then indicated.

23 | Blood

Taru Hays, MD

CHILDHOOD ANEMIAS

Anemia is a common blood disorder in children and differs from that in adults in that the anemia may be more pronounced. This is due in part to the fact that growth in childhood is associated with an increased need for blood-building substances. Furthermore, infections, which are so common in childhood, have a more profound effect on blood formation in early life than in adulthood. A classification of childhood anemia based on mean corpuscular volume (MCV) is presented in Table 23–1.

PHYSIOLOGIC "ANEMIA" OF THE NEWBORN

A gradual drop in red cells and hemoglobin occurs normally during the first 10–12 weeks of life, owing to shortened red cell survival time, expanded intravascular volume, and improved oxygenation. The red blood count is reduced to 3.5–4.5 million/μL, and the hemoglobin level may reach a low of 10–12 g/dL in full-term infants and 7 g/dL in premature infants. This is followed by a gradual increase in the number of red cells, with a correspondingly slower rise in hemoglobin level.

ANEMIA OF PREMATURITY

Although at birth the red cell count and hemoglobin levels of a premature infant are only slightly lower than those of a full-term one, the subsequent reduction that occurs is greater in premature infants. The magnitude of the drop of red cell count and hemoglobin level is inversely proportionate to the size of the infant. In very small infants (< 1 kg at birth), a reduction of hemoglobin to 7–8 g/dL and a reduction of red cells to 2.5–

Table 23–1. Classification of anemias based on mean corpuscular volume (MCV).

Microcytic	Normocytic	Macrocytic
Iron deficiency	Hemolytic anemias	Folate deficiency
Thalassemia	Chronic disease anemia	Vitamin B_{12} deficiency
Lead poisoning	Acute blood loss	Congenital hypoplastic anemia (Diamond–Blackfan)
Pyridoxine deficiency	Anemia of infection	Fanconi's anemia
Copper deficiency	Anemia of inflammation	Preleukemia
Hemoglobin E	Infiltrative process	Other bone marrow failure states
	Aplastic process	

3 million/μL may occur. Lowest levels are reached at about the end of the second month of life. More severe anemia occurs in premature infants than in full-term infants, because premature infants undergo a greater growth in body size and a correspondingly greater increase in blood volume. Furthermore, the total iron stores are smaller in the premature infant, since most of a newborn's iron is acquired during the last 3 months of gestation and erythropoietin production in response to anemia is less than in the term infant.

Pallor is the principal manifestation. The anemia generally is normochromic and normocytic early in the course of the disease and relatively hypochromic and microcytic late in the course.

The initial drop in hemoglobin level or red blood cell count cannot be prevented by early treatment with iron. After the second month of life, supplemental iron should be given.

IRON DEFICIENCY ANEMIA

Because expansion of blood volume is part of the growth process, the need for iron in children is greater than that in adults. In the average full-term infant, the stores of iron available at birth are adequate for 3–6 months. In the premature infant, twin, or child born of a mother with severe iron deficiency, the iron reserves will be expended earlier, placing these children at increased risk of developing iron deficiency anemia.

Iron deficiency anemia may result from inadequate storage, deficient intake, chronic blood loss, poor absorption and utilization of iron, or milk protein sensitivity. Iron deficiency anemia is uncommon in breast-fed infants.

Clinical Findings

A. Symptoms and Signs: Pallor may be the only early finding. Weakness, listlessness, and irritability appear later. Interference with growth may occur in long-standing cases, and delayed development (reversible) may occur in anemia of short duration. Congestive heart failure occurs occasionally; generalized edema, rarely.

B. Laboratory Findings: In hypochromic microcytic anemia, hemoglobin values are decreased, and there is relatively less reduction in red cells. Anisocytosis and poikilocytosis may be marked. The reticulocyte count may be low, normal, or slightly elevated. The serum ferritin concentration is reduced; serum iron level is low; iron-binding capacity is increased; transferrin saturation is reduced; and the level of free erythrocyte protoporphyrin is elevated. Blood may be present in stools. Histologic abnormalities of the bowel may be present. Severe iron deficiency may be associated with copper deficiency, a decreased serum albumin level, and thrombocytosis.

Treatment

Iron is specific therapy. Other blood-building elements are not necessary.

A. Medicinal Iron: Iron should be given as the ferrous salt. Elemental iron, 5–6 mg/kg/d in 3 divided doses, should be given before meals. Therapy should be continued for several months after the concentration of hemoglobin returns to normal in order to build reserves of iron.

Intramuscular iron (iron dextran injection [Imferon]) should be used only when treatment with oral iron is not feasible.

B. Dietary Iron: Food contains insufficient iron for effective therapy of iron deficiency anemia. Absorption of iron from most foods is generally good; phytates (oatmeal, brown bread) may inhibit absorption. Good sources of iron include red meats; liver; dried fruits such as apricots, prunes, and raisins; and pinto beans. Fair food sources of iron include carrots, beans, spinach, peas, sweet potatoes, and peaches.

C. Transfusions: Transfusions of packed red cells are reserved for patients with severe symptomatic anemia in whom a rapid rise in hemoglobin concentration is desired. If evidence of heart failure is present, transfuse very slowly. Parenteral diuretics and partial exchange transfusion may be of value.

Course & Prognosis

Progressive anemia will result unless medicinal or dietary therapy is instituted and the underlying abnormality, if any, corrected. Improvement is then prompt, with a significant rise in the reticulocyte count appearing in 4–7 days and a rise in the hemoglobin concentration of approximately 0.1–0.2 g/dL/d. Simple iron deficiency anemia due to a low intake of iron should clear rapidly, but the presence of other deficiencies, congenital malformation, infection, or poor compliance with therapy may alter this favorable outcome.

Administration of iron, 2 mg/kg/d for full-term infants and 4 mg/kg/d for premature infants at high risk for developing iron deficiency during the first year, either in infant formulas or in a medicinal form, has been recommended to prevent iron deficiency.

ANEMIA OF CHRONIC INFECTION & INFLAMMATION

Chronic infection or inflammation is often accompanied by anemia. These chronic conditions may inhibit iron exchange by blocking the release of catabolized iron from the red cells to the reticuloendothelial system. This form of anemia is often confused with iron deficiency anemia because the red cells may be slightly hypochromic (although they are often normal) and the reticulocyte count is low. However, in anemia of chronic infection, serum ferritin and serum iron levels are normal but total iron binding capacity is low, and the anemia does not respond to iron therapy. Anemia may be an important clue to an underlying inflammatory condition; it resolves when the primary disease process is controlled or resolves.

HYPOPLASTIC & APLASTIC ANEMIAS

Congenital hypoplastic anemia (Diamond-Blackfan anemia, aregenerative pure red blood cell anemia) is associated with decreased hemoglobin concentration and reticulocyte counts and increased MCV. Erythroid precursors are decreased or absent from the marrow. Patients usually respond well to corticosteroids; transfusions may be necessary. They are short children with some skeletal malformations.

Children may develop transient erythroblastopenia, with a temporary halt in red cell production manifested by normochromic normocytic anemia, reticulocytopenia, and the absence of red cell precursors in otherwise normal bone marrow. Erythroblastopenia is usually preceded by viral or bacterial infection and can be differentiated from congenital hypoplastic anemia by the presence of normal MCV. Recovery is spontaneous without treatment, often within a few weeks.

Fanconi's anemia (hypoplastic anemia, often with pancytopenia) presenting after the age of 2 years may occur as an autosomal recessive disorder in association with abnormal pigmentation, skeletal anomalies (eg, absent, hypoplastic, or supernumerary thumb; hypoplastic or absent radius), retarded growth, hypogonadism, small head, renal anomalies, microphthalmos, strabismus, and abnormalities of the reproductive tract (Fanconi's syndrome). The anemia usually responds to testosterone. Bone-marrow transplantation, using a nonrelated HLA donor, may be considered.

Acquired aplastic anemia, characterized by pancytopenia

and hypoplasia of the bone marrow, is rare in childhood. The peak incidence is 3–5 years of age. Acquired aplastic anemia may occur as a toxic reaction to drugs or chemicals (chloramphenicol, phenylbutazone, sulfonamides, solvents, insecticides), as a complication of infection, or in association with early manifestations of leukemia. Although anemia appears to be acquired in most cases, no causative agent can be identified in as many as 50% of patients (idiopathic aplastic anemia). Children with aplastic anemia present with pallor, fatigue, fever, and an increased tendency to bleed. Hepatosplenomegaly and adenopathy do not result. The prognosis of aplastic anemia without treatment is extremely poor; fewer than 10% of patients recover fully within 5 years, and 50% of patients die from hemorrhage or infection within the first 6 months. Bone marrow transplant from a sibling with HLA-compatible marrow may increase survival to 50–70% and is presently the treatment of choice. When bone marrow transplant is not feasible, the use of immunosuppressive therapy with high-dose corticosteroids and antithymocyte globulin (ATG) may be of value in up to 50% of patients.

HEMOLYTIC ANEMIAS

GENERAL CONSIDERATIONS

Anemias associated with shortened red cell survival are known as **hemolytic anemias.** Symptoms and signs may include pallor, jaundice, and splenomegaly. Gallstones may develop after many episodes of hemolysis.

Anemia, reticulocytosis, hyperbilirubinemia, and haptoglobinemia are the hallmarks of hemolytic anemia. The urine and feces contain increased amounts of urobilinogen. With severe chronic hemolysis, erythroid hyperplasia of the bone marrow often results in widening of the marrow spaces, and hemosiderosis may occur.

Classification of Congenital Hemolytic Anemia

A. Membrane Defects: Congenital spherocytosis, congenital elliptocytosis, congenital stomatocytosis, pyropoikilocytosis.

B. Hemoglobinopathies: Sickle cell anemia, sickle syndromes (S-thalassemia, SC hemoglobinopathy), thalassemias, unstable hemoglobins.

C. Enzyme Defects: Glucose-6-phosphate dehydrogenase (G6PD) deficiency, pyruvate kinase deficiency, hexokinase deficiency.

Classification of Acquired Hemolytic Anemia

(1) Autoimmune process.
(2) Infections.
(3) Toxins and drugs.
(4) Thermal injury.
(5) Disseminated intravascular coagulation (DIC).
(6) Hemolytic-uremic syndrome.
(7) Transfusion reactions.

AUTOIMMUNE HEMOLYTIC ANEMIA

In autoimmune hemolytic anemia, hemolysis occurs when IgG or IgM antibodies are directed against and cause damage to the red cell membranes. IgG-mediated disease is primarily an extravascular process, with hemolysis occurring in the spleen or other reticuloendothelial organs, while IgM-mediated disease is generally intravascular. The cause of anemia cannot be identified in about half of affected patients (idiopathic autoimmune hemolytic anemia). Anemia in other patients may be associated with immunoproliferative disorders (lupus erythematosus, Hodgkin's disease, and other malignant diseases), infection (especially Epstein-Barr virus, cytomegalovirus, other viral infections, and *Mycoplasma*), and chronic inflammatory conditions (ulcerative colitis).

The clinical presentation may be indolent (IgG-mediated) or fulminant (complement and IgM-mediated), with symptoms of anemia (pallor, malaise, and congestive heart failure); jaundice (common), with increased amounts of urobilinogen in the urine; and splenomegaly, which is more common with the IgG-mediated form of the disease. Laboratory findings include reticulocytosis and the presence of microspherocytes. Results of direct Coomb's tests are positive for IgG antibody in sera from patients with IgG-mediated anemia; negative for IgG antibody in sera from those with IgM-mediated anemia; and positive for complement fixation with IgM and, occasionally, with IgG.

If hemolysis is mild, treatment may not be necessary. Most patients respond to prednisone administered for 7–10 days; an initial larger dose is decreased over the next few days. Splenectomy is reserved for patients with severe hemolysis that is unresponsive to an adequate trial of corticosteroids. Other immunosuppressive therapy may be used in refractory cases. Transfusions are given if signs of congestive heart failure are present.

ISOIMMUNE HEMOLYTIC ANEMIA

Isoimmune hemolytic anemia is seen primarily in the newborn and is due to incompatibility with maternal Rh, ABO, or other antibodies. It may also occur with transfusion reactions in patients of all ages. Findings are similar to those of autoimmune hemolytic anemia. After the source of exogenous antibody has been discontinued, the anemia is usually self-limited. However, exchange transfusion may be required, especially in infants with Rh incompatibility.

CONGENITAL (HEREDITARY) SPHEROCYTOSIS

Congenital spherocytosis is a hereditary (dominant) disease caused by excessive destruction of abnormally shaped cells (spherocytes). The disease may be discovered during a "hypoplastic" crisis, when the reticulocyte count may be very low and the degree of anemia more profound than usual. Crises may occur at periodic intervals.

Other members of the family may have overt or subclinical disease with slight spherocytosis and increased osmotic fragility of red blood cells (demonstrated in hypotonic saline solution). In a small percentage of cases, no family involvement can be determined.

Findings include spherocytosis, increased osmotic fragility, and reticulocytosis. The osmotic fragility test will show abnormal findings if the blood is incubated (at 37 °C for 24 hours) prior to testing. The autohemolysis test results are also abnormal. Maturation arrest of all elements in the marrow may be present at times of aplastic crises. Neonates may show early and exaggerated jaundice. Cholelithiasis may develop in the second or third decade.

Treatment is by splenectomy, ideally performed in patients after the age of 5 years. Until the time of splenectomy, folic acid, 1 mg/d, should be given. Pneumococcal vaccine provides additional protection.

Following removal of the spleen, the underlying defect of the red cells persists, but most patients will have a complete remission of hemolysis and anemia.

HEREDITARY ELLIPTOCYTOSIS

Hereditary elliptocytosis (ovalocytosis) is a congenital disease characterized by numerous elongated or oval cells. It is usually asymptomatic, but some patients may have mild to severe hemolysis. In the latter, splenectomy may be of value.

NONSPHEROCYTIC HEMOLYTIC ANEMIA ASSOCIATED WITH DEFICIENCIES OF VARIOUS ENZYMES

Glucose-6-phosphate dehydrogenase (G6PD) deficiency is the most common red cell enzyme deficiency. It is inherited as an X-linked recessive trait and primarily affects males. It occurs in high frequency in Africa, the Mediterranean region, the Arabian peninsula, the Middle East, and Southeast Asia. Approximately 15% of black males in the USA are affected. Chronic anemia usually is not present, but acute episodes of severe hemolysis occur with exposure to certain drugs and foods, including primaquine, sulfonamides, aspirin, acetanilide, phenacetin, nitrofurans, synthetic vitamin K, compounds containing naphthalene, and fava beans. Tbe deficiency is less severe in blacks, and hemolysis usually occurs only with use of antimalarials and nitrofurans. Hemolysis is occasionally precipitated by infections. A screening test and assay are available, although the results may be normal if the reticulocyte count is high. With drug exposure, there is a rapid development of hemolytic anemia with hemoglobinuria and subsequent reticulocytosis. Blood transfusion may be required for treatment.

A number of other red cell enzyme deficiencies have been reported as causes of chronic nonspherocytic hemolytic anemia. They are usually autosomal recessive disorders and hence symptomatic only in the homozygous state. These disorders are very rare except for pyruvate kinase deficiency. Specific diagnosis is made by red cell enzyme assays. Patients with pyruvate kinase deficiency show a partial response to splenectomy. Transfusions may be needed for hemolytic or aplastic crises.

HEMOLYTIC-UREMIC SYNDROME

Hemolytic-uremic syndrome (HUS), occurring mainly in children between the ages of 6 months and 6 years, is characterized by (1) a sudden onset of Coomb's negative hemolytic anemia; (2) thrombocytopenic purpura; and (3) nephropathy (with renal insufficiency, azotemia, and acute renal necrosis). Occasionally, there is central nervous system involvement, with drowsiness and convulsions. Clinical manifestations of the syndrome are frequently preceded by diarrhea (commonly due to enterovirus infection or *Escherichia coli*) or, less often, by an upper respiratory tract infection, with an intervening symptom-free period of 1–10 days. Other findings may include hepato-splenomegaly, severe abdominal pain, hypertension, and cardiac failure. Helmet-shaped and fragmented red cells are the hallmark of HUS. Fibrinogen and platelet deposition in the arterioles may play a very significant role in the pathophysiology of HUS.

Packed red blood cell transfusions and peritoneal dialysis are often required as supportive measures. Heparin, inhibitors of platelet function, or activators of fibrinolysin have been used in treatment, with very little effect on the course of the renal disease. Complete recovery from hematologic manifestations usually occurs, but permanent impairment of renal function is not uncommon.

Partial forms of the disease may occur. The patient's siblings may also be affected.

HEREDITARY HEMOGLOBINOPATHIES

BETA-THALASSEMIA

Beta-thalassemia is a relatively common anemia that is due to an inherited defect in the synthesis of the beta chains of hemoglobin. It may occur in a severe homozygous form, characterized by pronounced changes in the blood and in various organ systems; or it may occur as the "trait," with little or no anemia and no systemic changes. It is most common in Italians, Greeks, and Southeast Asians and occurs occasionally in other persons of non-Mediterranean background. A mild beta-thalassemia gene (β^+) also occurs in blacks of African descent and may be seen in association with the sickle gene.

Beta-Thalassemia Major (Homozygous Form; Mediterranean Anemia, Cooley's Anemia)

The homozygous form is a severe hypochromic microcytic anemia with hemolysis in the bone marrow that starts in the first year of life. Both parents will be carriers of the "trait." Symptoms are secondary to the anemia and include pallor, characteristic facies due to widening of the tabular bones of the skull, jaundice of varying degrees, and hepatosplenomegaly. Laboratory findings (Table 23–2) include hypochromic microcytic anemia, anisocytosis, poikilocytosis, basophilic stippling, and decreased fragility of the red cells, with the presence of target cells, nucleated erythrocytes, and an increased number of reticulocytes in the peripheral blood. Levels of hemoglobin F and A_2 are elevated; hemoglobin A is usually absent. Findings on x-ray include changes in the bones due to extreme marrow hyperplasia. These changes include widening of the medulla, thinning of the cortex, and coarsening of trabeculation (the so-called hair-on-end appearance).

Beta-Thalassemia Minor (Heterozygous Form; Thalassemia Trait, Cooley's Carrier State)

In the heterozygous form, evidence of mild anemia and splenomegaly may be present. Blood smears show hypochromic microcytosis, target cells, anisocytosis, and poikilocytosis. The diagnosis may be confirmed by finding elevated levels of F or A_2 hemoglobin on hemoglobin electrophoresis.

Treatment

Transfusions are the only effective means of temporarily overcoming the anemia in severe cases, but they do not alter the underlying disease. Other hematopoietic agents are entirely ineffective and should not be used. Iron chelation with deferoxamine and vitamin C combined with hypertransfusion (maintaining hemoglobin at levels greater than 11 g/dL) are very beneficial. Chronic hypoxia and iron loading are the significant factors in the production of myocardial and hepatic damage.

Splenectomy may be necessary when the spleen is so large as to produce discomfort or if an acquired hemolytic component is superimposed on the primary disease. However, the risk of infection is splenectomized children with thalassemia is great, and prophylactic penicillin and pneumococcal vaccine should be given.

Course & Prognosis

In the past, in spite of repeated transfusions, children with thalassemia major generally died within the first 2 decades of life from intercurrent infections or from hemochromatosis. However, with hypertransfusion and iron chelation, the outlook is greatly improved. Gallbladder stones frequently develop in patients surviving to the early teens. Thalassemia trait is associated with a normal life span.

Table 23–2. Summary of findings in abnormal hemoglobin diseases and thalassemia.

	Hemoglobin Type	Anemia	Spleno- megaly	Pain Crises	Increased Blood Destruction	Target Cells	Sickling (Solubility) Test	Microcytosis	Hypochromia
Normal adult and child	AA (A_2* F*)	0	0	0	No	0	0	0	0
Normal newborn	AF†	0	0	0	No	0	0	0	0
Iron deficiency anemia	AA (A_2* F*)	+ to ++++	±	0	No	±	0	+ to ++++	+ to ++++
β^0-Thalassemia major	F† A_2†	++++	++++	0	Yes	++	0	++++	++++
β^0-Thalassemia minor	A (A_2† F†)	±	0 to +	0	±	+	0	++	++
β^+-Thalassemia– hemoglobin C disease	CA (F*)	+	0	0	Yes	+++	0	+	+
β^0-Thalassemia– hemoglobin E disease	EF†	+++	+++	0	Yes	++	0	+++	+++
Sickle cell trait	AS (A_2* F*)	0	0	0	No	0	+	0	0
Sickle cell anemia	SS (A_2* F†)	+++	±	+++	Yes	++	+	0	0 to +
Sickle-β^+-thalassemia	SA (A_2† F†)	+	±	+	Yes	++	+	++	++
Sickle-β^0-thalassemia	S (A_2† F†)	+++	+++	+++	Yes	++	+	++	++
Sickle-hemoglobin C disease	SC (F†)	+	++	++	Yes	+++	+	0	0

(Continued)

Table 23-2. (cont'd). Summary of findings in abnormal hemoglobin diseases and thalassemia.

	Hemoglobin Type	Anemia	Spleno-megaly	Pain Crises	Increased Blood Destruction	Target Cells	Sickling (Solubility) Test	Microcytosis	Hypochromia
Sickle-hemoglobin D disease	SD (A₂* F†)	++	++	++	Yes	+	+	+	+
Hemoglobin C trait	AC (F*)	0	0	0	No	+++	0	0	0
Homozygous hemoglobin C disease	CC (F*)	+	0 to ++	0	Yes	++++	0	0	0
Hemoglobin D trait	AD (A₂* F*)	0	0	0	No	0	0	0	0
Hemoglobin E trait	AE (F*)	0	0	0	No	±	0	0	0
Homozygous hemoglobin E disease	EE (F†)	+	±	0	Yes	+++	0	++	0
α-Thalassemia "carrier"	A (A₂* F*)‡	±	0	0	0	+	0	++	+
α-Thalassemia-hemoglobin H disease	AH (A₂* F*)‡	++	++	0	++	+++	0	+++	+++
α-Thalassemia-fetal hydrops	Bart's	++++	++++	0	++	+++	0	++++	++++

*A₂ is usually < 4% and F < 2% of the total hemoglobin.
†Elevated levels.
‡Hemoglobin Bart's is also present at birth.

ALPHA-THALASSEMIA

Alpha chains of the hemoglobin molecule are genetically determined by 4 genes, and thus gene deletions can result in 4 degrees of alpha-thalassemia.

Type 2 is always mild, and its incidence is high in Africa, Arabia, the Middle East, and Southeast Asia. The heterozygote with one gene deletion ($-\alpha/\alpha\alpha$) is called the "silent carrier" and is clinically and hematologically normal, while the homozygote with 2 deletions ($-\alpha/-\alpha$) is called the "carrier" and has microcytosis, hypochromia, and mild or borderline anemia.

Type 1 alpha-thalassemia occurs primarily in Southeast Asians. The heterozygote, or "carrier," with 2 gene deletions ($-/\alpha\alpha$) also shows microcytosis, hypochromia, and mild anemia, while the homozygous state ($-/-$) results in fetal hydrops and is incompatible with life.

In the double heterozygous state for type 1 and type 2 alpha-thalassemia, genes are deleted ($-/-\alpha$); this is known as hemoglobin H disease and occurs in people of Southeast Asia. It is characterized by splenomegaly and a moderate hemolytic anemia with microcytosis, hypochromia, and elevated reticulocyte count.

Diagnosis is made in the mild forms by ruling out iron deficiency (by documenting a normal serum iron or ferritin level) and beta-thalassemia minor (A_2 and F hemoglobin levels are normal in alpha-thalassemia). Hemoglobin Bart's (4 gamma globins) is present in varying degrees in all forms in the newborn infant, while hemoglobin H (4 beta globins) is present in the older child with the 3-gene deletion disease.

Treatment is not needed in the mild forms. Hemoglobin H disease may require transfusions, but most patients maintain hemoglobin levels of 9–10 g/dL.

SICKLE CELL ANEMIA

Sickle cell anemia is an inherited abnormality of hemoglobin (hemoglobin S). It has a high incidence in blacks but is also common in people of the Arabian peninsula, Sicily, and certain parts of Greece, Turkey, and India. In hemoglobin S, the amino acid valine replaces the normally occurring glutamic acid in the beta chain. Although the sickle trait occurs in about 8% of the black population in the USA, the disease with anemia occurs in only fewer than 1% of blacks.

Clinical Findings

A. Symptoms and Signs: Onset of clinical manifestations may be at any time in the first decade. Findings include fever, headache, "pain crises" in the long bones, osteopathy (particularly of metacarpals and phalanges), abdominal pain and tenderness, pallor, jaundice, splenomegaly (in the very young), hepatomegaly, cardiomegaly, and hemic heart murmurs. The spleen ceases to function normally early in childhood, and "autosplenectomy" occurs as a result of repeated infarctions. Patients with sickle cell anemia have an increased resistance to malarial infection; an increased susceptibility to bacterial sepsis, osteomyelitis, pneumonia, and meningitis [in particular with encapsulated organisms (eg, pneumococcus)]; and an increased risk of anesthetic complications. Enuresis and nocturia may be present. Strokes are commonly seen in young teens. In the severe form, the general picture is of poor health, development, and nutrition. Folic acid deficiency is common. During a pain crisis, the disease may mimic acute surgical abdomen or osteomyelitis. Aplastic crises may occur, with diminished red cell production superimposed on rapid destruction. In young infants, acute anemia and hypovolemia can be seen with splenic sequestration.

B. Laboratory Findings: Sickle-shaped red blood cells are seen in peripheral blood smears. Other findings include normochromic anemia, reticulocytosis, nucleated red blood cells in the peripheral blood, leukocytosis, hyperbilirubinemia, increased excretion of urobilinogen, increased lactate dehydrogenase levels, and an abnormal electrophoretic pattern, with 75–100% hemoglobin S and increased amounts of fetal hemoglobin. There is excretion of excessive quantities of urine of low specific gravity. Severe hyponatremia may occur during a crisis. Zinc deficiency has been described and may contribute to short stature and delayed onset of puberty.

Heterozygotes (carriers of sickle trait) may be identified by use of a screening test (Sickledex Test; sodium metabisulfite test) and hemoglobin electrophoresis. Characteristically, 25–45% hemoglobin S is found. Heterozygotes are not anemic and—except for conditions with extreme hypoxia—are asymptomatic. Hematuria has rarely been associated with sickle trait.

Treatment

Parenteral fluid therapy, analgesics, and transfusion for severe anemia and crises are the only consistently effective methods of treatment. Placing the patient in oxygen during the crisis and giving bicarbonate have been recommended.

Adequate hydration of the patient at the onset of a crisis sometimes obviates the need for transfusions. Because infection exacerbates sickling of the patient's red blood cells, all infections should be treated promptly and vigorously. Sepsis and meningitis should be suspected in the febrile infant.

Folic acid, 1 mg/d, should be given. The routine administration of prophylactic penicillin has been advocated, and pneumococcal vaccine should be given at 2 years of age.

Course & Prognosis

The course is determined by the severity of the sickling tendency and resulting hemolysis, the frequency and duration of crises, and the age of the patient. Interference with growth, nutrition, and general activity is common, although many patients lead active lives with persistent hemoglobin levels of 7–9 g/dL.

Repeated transfusions in conjunction with iron chelation using deferoxamine, designed to maintain hemoglobin levels above 11 g/dL and thus decrease bone marrow production of S hemoglobin, is recommended for patients with strokes and heart failure.

SICKLE-HEMOGLOBIN C DISEASE

Sickle-hemoglobin C disease is caused by the inheritance of hemoglobin S from one parent and hemoglobin C from the other. It occurs almost exclusively in the black population.

The clinical manifestations are similar to those of sickle cell anemia but tend to be less severe. Splenomegaly may be present and acute enlargement may occur with splenic sequestration crises. Proliferative retinopathy is common after the age of 15 years. Diagnosis is suspected by the presence of mild to moderate anemia, elevated reticulocyte counts, many target cells on blood smear, and positive results in the sickling (solubility) test. It is confirmed by hemoglobin electrophoresis.

Treatment is similar to that for sickle cell anemia and is primarily symptomatic. Patients should receive annual retinal examinations and be treated with laser therapy if retinopathy is detected.

BLEEDING DISEASES IN CHILDHOOD

GENERAL CONSIDERATIONS

Family History

A family history of easy bruising and excessive bleeding is valuable in the following disorders: (1) hemophilia (males only), (2) von Willebrand's disease (both sexes), (3) congenital thrombocytopenia or platelet dysfunction syndromes, (4) hereditary hemorrhagic telangiectasia, and (5) deficiencies of factor II, V, VII, X, or XI (Table 23–3), which may be hereditary and not X-linked.

Table 23–3. Blood clotting factors and hemorrhagic disorders.

	Clotting Factor*	Deficiency Disease
I	Fibrinogen	Afibrinogenemia
II	Prothrombin	Prothrombin deficiency disease
III	Tissue thromboplastin	None
IV	Calcium (Ca^{2+})	None
V	Proaccelerin; labile factor	Factor V deficiency disease
VII	Proconvertin; stable factor	Factor VII deficiency disease
VIII	Antihemophilic factor (AHF)	Hemophilia A, AHF deficiency disease, factor VIII deficiency disease
IX	Plasmin thromboplastin component (PTC); Christmas factor	Hemophilia B, PTC deficiency disease, Christmas disease, factor IX deficiency disease
X	Stuart factor; Stuart–Prower factor	Stuart–Prower factor deficiency disease, factor X deficiency disease
XI	Plasma thromboplastin antecedent (PTA)	Hemophilia C, PTA deficiency disease, factor XI deficiency disease
XII	Hageman factor	None
XIII	Fibrin-stabilizing factor	Fibrin-stabilizing factor deficiency disease, factor XIII deficiency disease
	α_2-Antiplasmin	α_2-Antiplasmin deficiency disease

*Factor VI is not considered a separate entity.

Physical Examination

Bleeding disorder should be considered in patients with abrupt changes in the pattern or severity of bruising and bleeding, unexplained bleeding from a circumcision, or excessive bleeding at the site of surgery.

Bruises on the extremities are found in many normal children following trauma and usually have no clinical significance. In infants and young children, petechiae can occur in the head and neck areas in association with crying, vomiting, or coughing without an underlying bleeding disorder. Mucocutaneous bleeding usually signifies an abnormality in the number or function of the platelets or a defect of the blood vessels. Hemarthrosis is uncommon except in patients with hemophilia.

Laboratory Examination

Recommended basic screening tests include bleeding time, platelet count, partial thromboplastin time (PTT), prothrombin time (PT), thrombin time, and fibrinogen level.

HEMOPHILIA

Hemophilia is an X-linked bleeding disorder transmitted by females to their male offspring. Hemophilia A (factor VIII deficiency, or classic hemophilia) accounts for 75% of cases of hemophilia. It occurs with an incidence of 1 per 10,000 population. Affected family members generally have equally severe disease. Hemophilia B (factor IX deficiency, or Christmas disease) is much less common. It may demonstrate the same levels of severity.

Clinical Findings

A. Symptoms and Signs: Symptoms vary greatly in severity; many cases are mild. Severely affected patients are usually identified at circumcision or in the first year of life and show signs of increased bruising and hemarthrosis (most commonly of the knees, ankles, or hips) as they begin to walk. In older patients, bleeding may occur in the large muscle groups, the genitourinary tract, or the skin. Mucous membrane bleeding, usually of the mouth, is also a problem after even a minor laceration or contusion. Mildly affected patients rarely have bleeding into the joints and may present with hemophilia only at the time of a surgical procedure.

B. Laboratory Findings: See Table 23–4. The PTT should be determined and other screening tests performed in any sus-

Table 23–4. Differentiation by laboratory findings of coagulation defects.

Disease*	Bleeding Time	Platelet Count	One-Stage Prothrombin Time	Partial Thromboplastin Time	Thrombin Time
Afibrinogenemia	N or ↑		↑	↑	↑
Factor II deficiency disease	V†	N	↑	N or ↑	N
Factor V deficiency disease	N	N	↑	↑	N
Factor VII deficiency disease	N	N	↑	N	N
Factor VIII deficiency disease	N	N	N	↑	N
Factor IX deficiency disease	N	N	N	↑	N
Factor X deficiency disease	N	N	↑	↑	N
Factor XI deficiency disease	N	N	N	↑	N
Factor XIII deficiency disease	N	N	N	N‡	N
Thrombasthenia (Glanzmann's syndrome)	↑	N	N	N	N
Thrombocytopenia	↑	↓	N	N	N
Von Willebrand's disease	↑	N	N	↑	N

*See Table 23–3 for synonyms of factor deficiency diseases.
†Variable.
‡Diagnosis should be suspected in a congenital bleeding state when results of all screening tests are normal. Diagnosis is confirmed by showing instability of fibrin clot in urea.
§Associated with factor VIII deficiency in most cases.

pected case of hemophilia. If the PTT is prolonged, a specific-factor assay should be carried out to confirm the diagnosis.

Treatment

A. Specific Measures: The specific treatment of hemophilia consists of replacing missing clotting factors. In hemophilia A, only fresh frozen plasma, factor VIII concentrates, or cryoprecipitates of fresh plasma should be used. In younger children, this can be achieved with cryoprecipitates (100 units of factor VIII per plastic pack); for dosage, see Therapeutic Blood Fraction Products, below. Older children with hemophilia A may be given factor VIII concentrates (250 units per vial). The use of concentrates carries a higher risk of hepatitis and HIV than does use of cryoprecipitates. In hemophilia B, use of stored or fresh blood, fresh frozen plasma (200–250 units per plastic pack), or a concentrate of factor IX (Konyne; 550 units of factor IX per vial) is effective; for dosage, see Therapeutic Blood Fraction Products, below. In mild cases, because of the danger of hepatitis and other infections, frozen plasma should be used instead of pooled plasma when possible. Dosage is determined by the severity of the bleeding to be treated. Hypervolemia may be avoided by the use of antihemophilic factor (AHF) or factor VIII concentrates. Adjuncts to transfusion therapy include (1) aminocaproic acid (Amicar), 100 mg/kg every 6 hours, for oral mucosal bleeding; and (2) desmopressin acetate (DDAVP, Stimate), 0.3 μg/kg given intravenously in 20 mL of saline over a 20-minute period, in mild cases of hemophilia A.

B. Special Problems:

1. Head injuries–Head injuries can be life-threatening in severe hemophiliacs. Raise the factor VIII level to over 50% as soon as possible. Patients with head injuries often require repeated factor replacement initially and, if intracranial hemorrhage is documented, for several weeks.

2. Hemarthroses–In patients with bleeding into the joints or muscles, raise the factor VIII levels to 20–40% every day until the pain becomes less severe. Bed rest and a short period of immobilization (usually for no longer than 24 hours) are indicated. This is followed by a slow increase in the level of physical therapy, with an active range of motion to regain full use of the joint. Acetaminophen is usually sufficient for analgesia if the patient receives transfusion early. Aspirin should not be used. Subsequent therapy includes exercises (passive and then active) and prevention of ankylosis in the unphysiologic position. Repeated episodes of joint effusion as well as hematuria may be treated by corticosteroids.

3. Sutures–If suturing is necessary, raise the factor VIII levels to 20–40% every other day until the sutures are removed, including the day of removal.

4. Hematuria–Patients with hematuria may be treated with a short course of corticosteroids.

5. Open wounds–In patients with bleeding from open wounds (skin, tooth socket), follow the measures outlined above, as indicated. Do *not* cauterize the wounds. Use sutures as necessary. Use pressure bandage and application of cold to accessible areas.

Prognosis

The prognosis has been much improved since the institution of home care programs of prophylactic therapy. Many of the problems of chronic joint disease have been avoided. Major problems of repeated administration of blood products include the increased risk of hepatitis, HIV infection, and the development of inhibitors (IgG antibody) to factor VIII in 10–15% of patients. With home transfusion programs, most patients are successful in leading independent and nearly normal lifestyles.

VON WILLEBRAND'S DISEASE

Von Willebrand's disease is a mild to severe familial bleeding disorder characterized by abnormalities of the factor VIII molecule. In severe classic von Willebrand's disease, the factor VIII procoagulant activity (VIIIc), the portion of the molecule that corrects the bleeding time defect and supports ristocetin-induced aggregation of platelets (VIIIvWd), and the factor VIII measured by heterologous antibodies (VIII antigen) are reduced. Variants of the disorder are seen in which combinations of the above portions of the factor VIII molecule are defective.

Patients with von Willebrand's disease show skin and mucous membrane bleeding (epistaxis, menorrhagia). The disorder is usually inherited as an autosomal dominant trait. The bleeding time is usually prolonged, as is the PTT, although in mild cases measurements of VIIIc, VIII antigen, and VIIIvWd must be made to establish the diagnosis.

Treatment consists of infusions of fresh frozen plasma, 10–15 mL/kg; cryoprecipitate, one plastic pack per 5 kg; or desmopressin acetate (DDAVP, Stimate), 0.3 μg/kg in 20 mL of saline, given intravenously over a 20-minute period.

DISSEMINATED INTRAVASCULAR COAGULATION

Disseminated intravascular coagulation (DIC) is characterized by intravascular consumption of plasma clotting factors (factors I, II, V, and VIII) and platelets; fibrinolysis, with production of fibrin split products; widespread deposition of fibrin thrombi that produce tissue ischemia and necrosis in various organs (principally the lungs, kidneys, gastrointestinal tract, adrenals, brain, liver, pancreas, and skin); generalized hemorrhagic diathesis; microangiopathic hemolytic anemia, with fragmented, burred, and helmet-shaped erythrocytes; and shock and death. The disorder has been found in association with infections, surgical procedures, burns, neonatal conditions (especially sepsis and respiratory distress syndrome), neoplastic diseases, severe hypoxia and acidosis, other metabolic disorders, and a variety of miscellaneous causes (eg, hemangioma, transfusion reactions, drugs, hemolytic-uremic syndrome). The clinical manifestations depend on the systems involved. Laboratory findings include prolonged PT and PTT, elevated levels of monomers and fibrin split products, decreased levels of fibrinogen, and decreased platelet counts.

Therapy consists of treating the underlying cause (sepsis, acidosis, hypoxia) and replacing clotting factors with fresh frozen plasma, 10 mL/kg, or platelet transfusions. In the newborn with severe DIC, exchange transfusion may be of value. Indications for use of heparin include severe meningococcemia, associated large vessel thrombosis, purpura fulminans, and promyelocytic or monocytic leukemia.

THERAPEUTIC BLOOD FRACTION PRODUCTS

When therapeutic blood fractions are given, there is a risk of transmitting the virus of serum hepatitis; this risk is greater when pooled blood fraction products are given than when single donor products are used. There appears to be an increased risk of acquired immune deficiency syndrome (AIDS) with the use of factor VIII concentrates or other blood components; however, this risk is decreased by use of heat-treated concentrates and screening of donors.

AHF or Factor VIII Concentrates (Cryoprecipitates)

Cryoprecipitates are a blood bank product made from fresh frozen plasma. One pack of cryoprecipitate contains 100 units.*

*A unit of clotting factor is the amount contained in the equivalent of 1 mL of fresh plasma with 100% clotting activity.

A. Indications: For therapy of factor VIII deficiency (hemophilia A or von Willebrand's disease).

B. Dosage and Administration: Reconstitute lyophilized material (stored at 4° C) and inject by intravenous push. Dose is calculated as follows:

Units* of factor VIII = Desired in vivo level in percent × 0.5 × Weight (kg)

A dosage of one pack per 5 kg usually gives a factor VIII level of 40%. The usual level desired is 40%; however, 20% is the minimal hemostatic level.

Factor IX Complex

Factor IX complex (Konyne, Profilnine, Proplex) is a lyophilized product containing factors IX, II, VII, and X in vials of 500 units.*

A. Indications: For therapy of congenital factor IX deficiency (hemophilia B, or Christmas disease) or severe liver disease.

B. Dosage and Administration: Dosage is calculated as for factor VIII (see above) except that twice the calculated dose is given initially (for tissue diffusion).

PURPURAS

Purpuras are bleeding diseases that may be due to a reduced number or abnormal function of platelets or to a defect in or abnormality of the vascular system.

Classification of Purpuras

Purpuras are differentiated by the clinical picture, the number and type of platelets in the peripheral blood, and the number and type of megakaryocytes in the bone marrow.

A. Purpuras with Low Platelet Counts and Normal or Increased Numbers of Megakaryocytes:

1. Immunologic purpura, including (a) postinfectious purpura; (b) drug-induced purpura; (c) certain collagen diseases (eg, lupus erythematosus); and (d) congenital purpura due to isoim-

---

*A unit of a clotting factor is the amount contained in the equivalent of 1 mL of fresh plasma with 100% clotting activity.

munization resulting from maternal sensitization to some drugs, with passive transfer of maternal antiplatelet antibody.

2. Hypersplenic states (eg, Banti's syndrome, Gaucher's disease, postinfectious states, cirrhosis).

3. Thrombotic thrombocytopenia.

4. Hemolytic-uremic syndrome.

5. Purpura associated with large hemangiomas.

6. Wiskott-Aldrich syndrome.

B. Purpuras with Normal Platelet Counts and Abnormalities of the Vascular System:

1. Anaphylactoid or "vascular" (Henoch-Schönlein) purpura.

2. Scurvy.

3. Nonthrombocytopenic purpura associated with infection (eg, meningococcemia, subacute infective endocarditis) or chemical agents (eg, penicillin).

4. Hereditary hemorrhagic telangiectasia.

5. Traumatic or mechanical purpuras, including those associated with certain skin diseases (eg, Ehlers-Danlos syndrome, telangiectatic purpura).

6. Purpura associated with chronic disease (eg, hypertension, cardiac disease, Cushing's syndrome).

7. Psychogenic purpura.

8. Toxic purpura.

C. Purpuras with Normal Platelet Counts, Normal Megakaryocytes, and Defective Function of Platelets:

1. Thrombasthenia (Glanzman's).

2. Storage pool disease.

3. Bernard-Soulier syndrome.

4. Liver disease.

5. Von Willebrand's disease.

6. Purpura following drug ingestion (aspirin, penicillins).

7. Uremia.

D. Purpuras with Low Platelet Counts and Decreased Numbers of Megakaryocytes:

1. Purpura due to severe infections.

2. Purpura associated with hypoplastic and aplastic anemias.

3. Leukemia and other malignant neoplastic diseases.

4. Purpura resulting from ionizing irradiation.

5. Uremia.

6. Congenital purpura, which may be associated with absence of the radius.

IDIOPATHIC THROMBOCYTOPENIC PURPURA

Idiopathic thrombocytopenic purpura (ITP) of childhood is a relatively common bleeding disorder most likely mediated by antiplatelet antibodies. It usually occurs in patients between 2 and 10 years of age and commonly follows an infection by 2–3 weeks. In the neonatal period, ITP may follow infection or exchange transfusion or may be due to material isoantibodies to the infant's platelets.

Clinical Findings

A. Symptoms and Signs: Bleeding into the skin or from the nose, gums, and urinary tract is the most common symptom. Bleeding into joints or from the bowel is uncommon. Central nervous system bleeding occurs rarely but may be fatal. Petechiae are usually present. Splenomegaly is rare.

B. Laboratory Findings: The platelet count is low, and the bleeding time is prolonged. Large immature platelets are occasionally seen. Red and white blood cell counts are normal unless severe hemorrhage has occurred. Megakaryocytes in the bone marrow are normal or increased in number. Antiplatelet antibodies may be demonstrated. Results of other hematologic tests are normal.

Treatment

A. Specific Measures: There is no specific treatment for ITP. Corticosteroids are useful in 60–70% of children. Indications include patients with severe thrombocytopenia with bleeding and patients at increased risk for central nervous system bleeding. More recently, intravenous gamma globulin has been useful in acute bleeding episodes and also in steroid-refractory thrombocytopenia.

B. General Measures: Eradicate infection, if present. In the presence of active infection, antibiotics and chemotherapeutic agents are not contraindicated unless the thrombocytopenia is the result of the administration of these drugs, in which case therapy with other agents is indicated. All medications should be given either orally or intravenously.

Other measures include transfusions to maintain hemoglobin levels, prevention of trauma, institution or maintenance of regular diet with vitamins, and avoidance of aspirin. Watchful waiting for 6–8 months is appropriate for many cases.

C. Surgical Measures: Splenectomy is indicated (preferably after age 5 years) if conservative therapy has been carried out for 6–12 months without improvement, if the disease process is very severe, if the patient is becoming steadily worse in spite of other therapy, if the patient develops a sudden intracranial hemorrhage, or if the patient is having recurrent bouts of severe ITP for which no definite cause can be determined. Splenectomy is also indicated in an adolescent girl with severe menorrhagia. Splenectomy should be avoided, if possible, in children under 5 years of age, and the procedure is contraindicated if the number of megakaryocytes in the bone marrow is decreased.

Course & Prognosis

Clinical activity may continue to be evident for 2 weeks to several months, but significant improvement usually occurs within 4–6 weeks. Eighty-five percent of children who have ITP with normal or elevated numbers of megakaryocytes in the bone marrow will have a spontaneous and complete recovery within 6 months even without therapy, but spontaneous recovery may occur after a period of as long as 3½ years. A few will need splenectomy.

Adolescents tend to have a more chronic course, often associated with the presence of other antibodies, proteinuria, or abnormal renal function. ITP during adolescence may be associated with subsequent development of subacute lupus erythematosus.

ANAPHYLACTOID OR "VASCULAR" PURPURA

Anaphylactoid purpura (Henoch-Schönlein purpura) is a disease of unknown cause. Many patients have a history of allergic manifestations. Some cases of anaphylactoid purpura follow infections; a causal relationship with group A streptococcal infections has been suspected. The disease tends to recur, and it may persist over a span of many years.

Clinical Findings

A. Symptoms and Signs: Abdominal and joint pains are present in most children, but the pain may occur only in the abdomen (Henoch type) or only at the joints (Schönlein type). The pain may precede the development of skin lesions. Either small or large joints may be involved. The joints are painful and swollen. Ecchymoses, petechiae, or bullous hematomas may be present. The initial lesions may resemble urticaria, but these soon become hemorrhagic. They often appear first around the elbows and ankles and over the buttocks. Gastrointestinal hemorrhage is common in children. Nephritis may occur early or after the acute phase in over one-third of cases. Intussusception may develop. Associated group A beta-hemolytic streptococcal infections are frequent.

B. Laboratory Findings: Platelet counts and most hematologic test results are normal. Eosinophilia may be present in some cases. Serum IgA levels may be elevated.

Treatment

In many cases, treatment is either unnecessary or ineffective.

A. Specific Measures: Therapy includes eradication of infection, using appropriate antibiotics, and elimination of allergens (if known). Antihistamines may be given if allergy is suspected.

B. General Measures: Corticosteroids may relieve joint and abdominal symptoms. They do not appear to benefit patients with renal complications.

C. Prevention of Recurrences: Give prophylactic penicillin if a streptococcal cause can be established. Remove other known allergens.

Course & Prognosis

The disease may vary in degree from mild to quite severe. Complete recovery eventually occurs in most cases, but recurrences are not infrequent and nephritis occasionally persists and may become chronic. Death during the acute phase of the disease is rare.

HYPERCOAGULABILITY

Hypercoagulability describes an increased tendency toward thrombosis in patients with certain underlying conditions. Patients at risk include those with a deficiency of antithrombin III, protein C, protein S, or plasminogen; newborns and older children with central plastic catheters or prosthetic heart valves; postsurgical patients who required prolonged periods of bed rest and thus are susceptible to venous stasis; and patients with vasculitic processes (eg, systemic lupus erythematosus, nephritis, hemolytic-uremic syndrome) in which damaged endothelium provides a nidus for clot formation and occasionally for progression to a more generalized disease process.

The patient may present with pain and swelling of the involved extremity or with symptoms of a stroke. Homozygous protein C deficiency can present as purpura fulminans in neonates. The diagnosis of thrombosis is made by physical examination. Supporting laboratory findings may include decreased levels of fibrinogen, antithrombin III, protein S, or protein C; decreased platelet counts; or elevated levels of fibrin split products or monomers. However, laboratory findings may be normal even in the face of significant thrombosis.

Treatment involves interruption of the triggering process. Heparinization should be instituted at once, with the goal of increasing the PTT to 1½ times that of normal. Give a loading dose of heparin, 100 units/kg, followed by a continuous intravenous infusion of 15–20 units/kg/h. Newborn infants may require an increased dosage. Prolonged anticoagulation for 4–6 months with warfarin (Coumadin) may be indicated once the initial thrombosis is controlled. Antiplatelet agents (aspirin, sulfinpyrazone, dipyridamole) may be indicated in cases in which a prosthetic heart valve or arterial malformation is the inciting agent for thrombosis. The use of fibrinolytic agents (streptokinase, urokinase) in children is reserved for extensive and life-threatening thrombus. Local urokinase therapy is very useful in catheter-induced thrombosis.

ABSENCE OF THE SPLEEN

Absence of the spleen, whether the absence is congenital, postsurgical, or functional (secondary to an underlying disease such as sickle cell anemia), places the child at significant risk for infection with encapsulated bacteria. The overall incidence of infection is 5–10%, with the fatality rate 30–50%. Those at greatest risk are children under 2 years of age and children with recent splenectomy (ie, for the first 2 years following splenectomy). The classic hematologic finding is the presence of Howell-Jolly bodies on the peripheral blood smear.

The tendency to develop life-threatening infections is markedly decreased in older children when the spleen is removed for trauma, ITP, portal vein thrombosis, local tumors, or hereditary spherocytosis. The risk is significant in those with histiocytosis, inborn errors of metabolism, hepatitis with portal hypertension, thalassemia, and Wiskott-Aldrich syndrome.

The use of prophylactic antibiotics remains controversial. Some physicians use continuous penicillin prophylaxis in the younger child, while others treat at the first sign of fever. Polyvalent pneumococcal vaccine (Pneumovax 23), which protects against infection with many of the common pneumococci, may be given to all splenectomized children and repeated in early childhood if given to infants under 2 years of age. Prompt therapy with antibiotics in any child with fever has been recommended.

SPLENOMEGALY

Splenomegaly is generally an indicator of systemic disease. The tip of the spleen may normally be felt in 30% of newborn infants and 5% of young children. Splenomegaly may be associated with other signs of systemic disease, particularly adenopathy, hepatomegaly, petechiae, ecchymoses, and jaundice. Less common causes of splenomegaly include acute viral infections (particularly infectious mononucleosis and cytomegalovirus), hematologic disorders (eg, congenital or acquired hemolytic anemias, red cell membrane defects, disorders of hemoglobin synthesis), metabolic diseases (eg, Gaucher's disease, Niemann-Pick disease), vascular abnormalities (eg, portal hypertension), and, rarely, cysts (eg, splenic cysts). When leukemia or other malignant neoplastic disease presents with splenomegaly, it is usually accompanied by adenopathy, pallor, and other signs of systemic illness.

Evaluation of patients with splenomegaly should include an assessment of the complete blood count, platelet count, peripheral blood smear, and reticulocyte count. Other studies may include tests for viral infection, liver-spleen scan, work-up for hemolytic anemias, and bone marrow examination for evaluation of storage diseases.

NEUTROPENIA

Neutropenia, a total granulocyte count below $1500/\mu L$, may result from poor release of granulocytes from the bone marrow, decreased survival of granulocytes in the circulation, or abnormalities of granulocyte production and development. The congenital forms of neutropenia include (1) cyclic neutropenia, occurring at 2- to 4-week intervals in association with mucous membrane ulcers, cervical lymphadenopathy, and stomatitis; (2) benign chronic neutropenia, which may be genetically transmitted (as a dominant or recessive trait), with manifestations of mild infection; (3) severe congenital neutropenia, transmitted as a recessive trait, with life-threatening infection in early infancy; (4) Shwachman-Diamond syndrome, with metaphyseal chondrodysplasia, dwarfism, pancreatic exocrine insufficiency, anemia, and thrombocytopenia; (5) cartilage-hair hypoplasia, with short limb dwarfism, abnormally fine hair, and T cell deficiencies; and (6) Chédiak-Higashi syndrome. Acquired neutropenias are the most common forms of childhood neutropenia and are induced by an autoimmune mechanism. Viral infections are the commonest reason for neutrophil antibodies causing both leukopenia and neutropenia. Atypical lymphocytosis and monocytosis are common associated findings. Drugs and toxins may cause neutropenia.

Benign forms of neutropenia may not require therapy. In other forms, infections should be treated with appropriate antibiotics. Patients with neutropenia associated with acute suppression of the bone marrow from cytotoxic drugs should be treated with broad-spectrum antibiotics; leukocyte transfusions may be of value.

IMMUNOLOGIC DEFICIENCY SYNDROMES
(Antibody Deficiency Syndromes, Hypogammaglobulinemias)

Immunologic deficiency diseases are characterized by (1) increased susceptibility to bacterial, viral, fungal, and protozoal infections; (2) a generalized or selective deficiency in the serum immunoglobulins; (3) a diminished capacity (in varying degrees) to form circulating antibodies or to develop cellular immunity (delayed hypersensitivity) after an appropriate antigenic stimulus; and (4) clinical and immunologic variability. Several broad categories are definable based upon whether the defect originates with a disturbance of antibody-producing lymphoid cells (B cells) or with thymus-derived cells that mediate cellular immunity (T cells).

Classification of Immunologic Disorders
   A. Immunoglobulin Deficiencies:
   1. Infantile X-linked agammaglobulinemia (IgG, IgA, or IgM deficiency).
   2. Selective immunoglobulin deficiency (dysgammaglobulinemia).
   3. Acquired hypogammaglobulinemia.
   4. Transient hypogammaglobulinemia of infancy.
   B. Cellular Immune Deficiency with "Normal" Immunoglobulins:
   1. Thymic dysplasia (Nezelof type).
   2. DiGeorge's syndrome (congenital absence of thymus and parathyroids; third and fourth pharyngeal pouch syndrome).
   C. Combined Immunoglobulin and Cellular Immune Deficiencies:
   1. Congenital–
   a. Severe combined immunodeficiency (Swiss type agammaglobulinemia, thymic dysplasia).

b. Wiskott-Aldrich syndrome (dysgammaglobulinemia and progressive cellular immunity deficiency).

2. Acquired–

a. Hodgkin's disease.

b. Iatrogenic conditions (steroid or antimetabolite therapy).

c. Acquired immune deficiency syndrome (AIDS).

Clinical Findings

A. Signs and Symptoms: In patients with immunoglobulin deficiency disease, recurrent pyogenic bacterial infections predominate, and chronic otitis media, sinusitis, and bronchiectasis are especially common. In agammaglobulinemia, viral infections (such as measles, varicella, and mumps) are weathered without incident. In individuals with cellular immunity defects, progressive vaccinia has been a frequent complication, and vaccination should be avoided. Candidal infections are not uncommon in such patients, and unusually severe infections with cytomegalovirus, herpesvirus, and *Pneumocystis* occur as well. In the acquired forms, malignant disorders of the lymphoreticular system occur with increased frequency. AIDS, which has been reported in children with hemophilia and in infants born to infected mothers (eg, IV drug abusers), is often difficult to distinguish from congenital deficiency disease.

Laboratory Findings

Diagnosis is based on results of the following.

(1) Quantitative immunochemical determination of the serum levels of IgG, IgM, and IgA.

(2) Isohemagglutinin determination. These antibodies to the blood group substance belong for the most part to the IgM class. They are normally present after about 1 year of age in all individuals of blood groups A, B, and O. Therefore, their absence is presumptive evidence of IgM deficiency.

(3) Absolute lymphocyte count. The count is 4000–6000/μL in normal children but reduced in patients with cellular immunity deficiency (especially in patients with severe combined immunodeficiency).

(4) Examination of bone marrow for plasma cells.

Confirmatory tests include the following:

(1) Results of immunization with well-characterized antigens (eg, diphtheria toxoid, tetanus toxoid) in terms of specific antibody production and plasma cell development.

(2) Presence of germinal center formation, plasma cells, and small lymphocytes in a biopsy of the regional lymph node taken 1 week after antigenic stimulation.

(3) Reaction to *Candida* and mumps skin tests.

(4) Induction of contact dermal hypersensitivity with dinitrochlorobenzene.

(5) Results of in vitro tests of lymphocyte function [phytohemagglutinin (PHA), concanavalin A (ConA), pokeweed mitogen, antigens, and allogeneic cells].

Treatment

Treatment for patients with immunoglobulin deficiency consists of replacement therapy with immune globulin, which is chiefly IgG. Give 200 mg/kg intravenously and then 100 mg/kg every 3 or 4 weeks. Preparations consisting solely of IgM and IgA are not yet available. Preparations suitable for intravenous use (Gamimune, Sandoglobulin) are now available.

Each individual has genetically determined differences in gamma globulins, and isoimmunization can occur as a result of giving genetically foreign gamma globulin. Since isoimmunization may have some deleterious effects, injudicious administration of immune globulin should be avoided.

Therapy of cellular immune deficiencies with bone marrow transplant is still experimental, but results are improving.

24 | Kidney & Urinary Tract

Gary M. Lum, MD

CLINICAL FINDINGS

Clinical manifestations of diseases of the kidneys or urinary tract include those symptoms that suggest (1) infection (eg, urgency; frequency; dysuria; and abdominal, suprapubic, or costovertebral angle pain); (2) urolithiasis (abdominal pain, colic); (3) voiding problems (frequency, straining, incontinence); and (4) chronic renal failure (CRF) from abnormal renal development (polyuria, enuresis, failure to thrive). The inability of the kidneys to elaborate a concentrated urine is one of the first signs of inadequate renal development (if urinary concentrating ability is the *only* renal abnormality noted, the diagnosis of diabetes insipidus must be entertained as well).

Renal inflammation, such as glomerulonephritis, is often asymptomatic unless it produces an immediate, severe compromise in renal function. Subsequent disease progression can produce symptoms of CRF, including anorexia, nausea and vomiting, malaise and easy fatigability, and bone pain.

Renal compromise should be suspected in newborns with congenital absence of the abdominal musculature; presence of a single umbilical artery; abdominal masses; or abnormalities of the spinal cord, sacrum, perineum, or external genitalia. Renal anomalies may also be seen in association with ear deformities, aniridia, hemihypertrophy, chromosomal disorders, hepatic cysts or fibrosis, pulmonary hypoplasia, and congenital ascites. The presence of oligohydramnios and spontaneous pneumothorax should also raise the question of renal disease. With the application of prenatal ultrasonography, abnormalities of the urinary tract may be demonstrated early in pregnancy.

Findings such as hypertension; edema; skeletal deformity; pallor or anemia; hematuria; proteinuria; bacteriuria; crystalluria; acidosis; and elevations in BUN, creatinine, potassium, and serum phosphate may be encountered in various renal disease states.

DIAGNOSTIC STUDIES

Laboratory assessment of renal function begins with a carefully performed urinalysis. The urinary dipstick is a helpful screening tool. The detection of hematuria, leukocyturia, and/or bacteruria, however, should be followed by microscopic inspection of the urinary sediment. Abnormal amounts of urinary protein should be quantitatively measured. If infection is suspected, the urine is sent for culture and sensitivity. A reliably performed mid-stream, clean-catch urinary specimen is adequate for culture. If this cannot be obtained with confidence a bladder catheterization or suprapubic bladder tap may be performed. Bacterial colony counts of less than 10,000/mL, or multiple flora, are usually considered contaminants unless obtained by catheterization or bladder tap (provided proper technique is followed). Appropriate diagnostic work-up should follow to exclude genitourinary abnormalities or conditions predisposing to infection (eg, obstruction, reflux, foreign body, trauma, hygiene, infestations such as pinworms).

Abnormalities or disease resulting in functional renal disturbance is demonstrated and monitored by the serum BUN and creatinine (Cr). Serum creatinine is a reflection of muscle metabolism and therefore is related to total body muscle mass. In general in pediatrics the normal range is from 0.3–0.8 mg%. Since normal renal function maintains the serum level in a "steady-state," a doubling of the serum creatinine reflects approximately a 50% reduction in renal function. Thus, even a level of 0.8 mg% is of concern, if normal serum creatinine for a given-sized child is 0.4 mg%. Calculation of the renal creatinine clearance (CrCl) can be useful in estimating renal function; however, it requires the reliable collection of a timed (12–24 h) urinary specimen. The calculation is as follows:

$$\frac{\text{Urine Cr mg\%} \times \text{Volume mL/min}}{\text{Serum Cr mg\%}}$$

Verification of reliability can be demonstrated by determination of the creatinine index (24-h creatinine excretion in mg/kg body wt = 12–20). The difficulties encountered in obtaining such a specimen are avoided by estimating glomerular filtration rate with the serum creatinine. The following formula derives creatinine clearance:

$$\frac{0.55 \times \text{height (length) cm}}{\text{Serum Cr mg\%}}$$

BUN also reflects renal function, but it may be altered in other ways (eg, increased catabolism, low urinary flow rate). For example, although the usual BUN:creatinine ratio is 1:10, urinary obstruction typically produces a disproportionate rise in BUN.

Other biochemical markers of renal disease include acidosis, hyperkalemia, hypocalcemia, hyperphosphatemia, and, as a result of disturbed calcium and phosphate homeostasis, elevated alkaline phosphatase. Serologic data, such as immunoglobulins, serum complement, or antinuclear antibodies (ANA) are useful in the work-up of glomerulonephritis and should be obtained when clinically indicated. A normocytic, normochromic anemia is found later in renal failure, as are rickets or long-bone deformity secondary to renal osteodystrophy.

SPECIAL DIAGNOSTIC STUDIES

Renal ultrasonography and nucleotide scans can provide important information regarding renal size, blood flow, and architecture. Excretory urography (intravenous pyelography) may also be used to demonstrate renal excretion of iodinated contrast material. Voiding cystourethrography will demonstrate reflux and bladder dysfunction. Cystoscopy permits direct visualization of ureteral ostia and bladder mucosa and outlet. Cystometrics can further delineate proper bladder function. Renal arteriography is most helpful in demonstrating renovascular abnormalities. Renal biopsy readily provides histologic verification of suspected renal parenchymal disease.

NONOBSTRUCTIVE CONGENITAL MALFORMATIONS

1. CYSTIC KIDNEYS

Classification
    A. Polycystic Kidneys (Infantile Type; Autosomal Recessive): The renal tissue is filled with multiple small cysts. The kidneys are generally very enlarged. Polycystic disease is often present in the liver, pancreas, or lungs.
    B. Polycystic Kidneys (Adult Type; Autosomal Dominant): Numerous cysts involve all portions of both kidneys and, occasionally, other organs.
    C. Multicystic Kidneys: Multicystic disease usually affects only one kidney, which is moderately enlarged with large cysts;

the renal parenchyma is hypoplastic or absent. The calices and pelvis are malformed, hypoplastic, or absent, and the ureter is atretic. The other kidney is often dysplastic.

D. Other Cystic Kidneys: Other varieties of cystic kidneys include medullary cystic disease (juvenile nephronophthisis), microcystic disease, dysplastic kidney, solitary renal cyst, and hamartomatous cystic or multilocular kidney.

Clinical Findings

A. Symptoms and Signs: Clinical findings depend on the type of cystic disease. A multicystic kidney or solitary cyst, for example, is commonly a static abnormality, and given the presence of another normally functioning kidney may be of little clinical consequence. Microcystic disease (congenital nephrosis) leads to early renal failure with initial symptoms related to the nephrotic syndrome. Polycystic kidney disease (PKD) or tuberous sclerosis (depending on the degree and rate of progression of renal parenchymal compromise) may present little symptomatology early in the course. The autosomal recessive form of PKD (infantile) tends to enlarge rapidly, so increasing abdominal girth may be noticeable, especially in the infant or small child. Cystic disease of the liver is associated with infantile PKD. Lastly, another cystic lesion to consider in childhood is juvenile nephronophthisis (medullary cystic disease). Renal tubular dysfunction (eg, Fanconi syndrome)—develops early in the course, and CRF will likely follow.

Hypertension is an early problem with cystic disease and should be strictly controlled as it can hasten progression of renal failure. Microhematuria is expected. Symptoms of CRF, of course, will vary with the development of significant functional compromise.

B. Laboratory Findings: Again, depending on the type of cystic abnormality as described above, laboratory findings may include hematuria, proteinuria, renal tubular acidosis, glycosuria, and phosphaturia. In any of the cystic lesions (excluding a multicystic kidney) increases in BUN, creatinine, serum phosphate, and other abnormalities associated with CRF will develop as renal insufficiency progresses.

Treatment

Microcystic disease requires early intervention with vigorous nutritional support, given the massive protein loss, and will usually progress to end-stage renal disease (ESRD) within the first few years of life. Treatment is directed at the complications of protein wasting and early CRF.

Since the major manifestation of functional renal disturbance in juvenile nephronophthisis is renal tubular dysfunction, supplementation of bicarbonate, phosphate, sodium, and potassium losses are the initial treatment, followed by management of ensuing CRF.

In polycystic disease, CRF management becomes an issue at varying times depending on the type, severity, and rate of progression to ESRD. An early concern is hypertension control; otherwise, the condition has no specific therapy. The angiotensin-converting enzyme class of antihypertensive drugs are particularly helpful.

2. MALFORMATIONS OF THE URINARY TRACT

Conditions in the newborn resulting from abnormal development of the kidneys and urinary tract that lead to compromise of renal function include total renal aplasia, dysplasia, or hypoplasia. The cystic dysplasias and their clinical relevance have been previously discussed. Abnormalities of the collecting system (ie, renal pelves, ureters, bladder, and urethra) can result in renal maldevelopment and functional compromise. Thus, postnatal renal function will be affected by the degree of interference with in utero renal development, as well as the effect upon residual renal tissue of timely diagnosis and the success of surgical intervention, if feasible.

Such abnormalities of genitourinary development may be detected in utero through the application of ultrasonography. The demonstration of oligohydramnios or poor pulmonary development may reflect abnormal renal development. In the immediate postnatal period poor urinary stream, abdominal mass (kidney or bladder), or alternating periods of anuria and polyuria are suggestive of obstruction at various levels of the urinary tract (eg, ureteropelvic junction, ureterovesical junction, or posterior urethral valves in males).

Appropriate and rapid surgical intervention in an effort to relieve and prevent further damage to renal tissue, as well as medical management of any significant reduction in renal function and the clinical consequences of CRF, are the most important aspects of the treatment approach to these conditions.

URINARY TRACT INFECTION

Acute urinary tract infection may be limited to the lower urinary tract, but persistent or recurrent cases often result in reflux nephropathy, and at times one may observe acute pyelonephritis. Newborns of both sexes and females of all ages seem at highest risk of developing urinary tract infections.

Infection may be caused by a variety of organisms, particularly *Escherichia coli* and other organisms commonly found in the intestinal tract. Kidney involvement often results from ascending infection. Congenital abnormalities associated with obstruction and ureterovesical reflux may be important predisposing factors.

Clinical Findings

A. Symptoms and Signs: Symptoms may be mild or absent. Common symptoms, however, are fever and chills, urinary urgency and frequency, incontinence, dysuria, and abdominal pain. Occasionally, there may be complaints of anorexia and nausea or vomiting. With acute pyelonephritis, these symptoms may be more obvious. Any of the findings listed on p 750 may be present. Asymptomatic bacteriuria occurs in 1% of schoolgirls.

Signs include dull or sharp pain and tenderness in the kidney area or abdomen. Hypertension and evidence of chronic renal failure may be present. Jaundice may occur, particularly during early infancy.

B. Laboratory Findings: Pyuria is characteristic, but it may be absent in the majority of patients during some phase of the disease. Slight or moderate hematuria occasionally occurs. There may be slight proteinuria. Pathogenic organisms and casts of all types may be present in the urine, but the urine may be normal for long periods of time. Anemia is found in cases of long-standing infection. Leukocytosis is usually in the range of $15,000-35,000/\mu L$. The diagnosis of urinary tract infection should be suspect if it is based on examination of a single voided urine specimen. A reliably performed mid-stream, clean-catch urine specimen is suitable for culture. If that cannot be obtained with confidence, suprapubic bladder tap or catheterization may be performed.

C. Urologic Studies: Intravenous urography and voiding cystourethrography are recommended by many investigators for all children after the initial infection. Others feel that these procedures should be performed after the first urinary tract infection only for newborn infants, boys of all ages, and girls with symptoms suggestive of pyelonephritis; otherwise, they should be performed after second infections. The need for further urologic evaluation depends on the nature and severity of any abnormalities noted.

Treatment

A. Specific Measures: Eradicate infection with appropriate chemotherapeutic or antibiotic therapy (see Chapter 8), usually for at least 10 days and particularly with drugs to which the patient has not recently been exposed. A prolonged course of urinary tract antisepsis (2–6 months or longer) may be indicated, especially for repeated infections. Repeat urinalyses at intervals of 1 or 2 months for at least a year is recommended.

B. General Measures: Force fluids during the acute stage. If possible, have the patient shower instead of bathing. Discontinue "bubble baths." Avoid constipation. Look for evidence of pinworms, which are often associated with repeated episodes of cystitis.

C. Surgical Measures: There is no clear evidence that routine surgical correction—by either bladder neck revision, dilation, urethrotomy, or meatotomy—alters the course of recurrent urinary tract infections to any significant degree, but repair of clearly obstructive lesions is indicated.

D. Prophylactic Measures: After control of the infection, a prophylactic regimen using nitrofurantoin, sulfisoxazole, or methenamine mandelate may be of value depending on the organism; if methenamine is used, the urine should be kept acid. Nalidixic acid may be an effective substitute for methenamine. The dipstick nitrite test is a useful adjunct to home screening for infection. Urine cultures should be repeated as clinically indicated or suggested by urinalysis.

In some cases, it is not sufficient to institute treatment only for clinical exacerbations, since subclinical infection may persist and be associated with progressive severe renal damage.

Reinfection in children, regardless of the absence of obstruction or reflux, is not uncommon. However, recurrences are most likely in cases in which there is an underlying urologic abnormality, especially when reflux nephropathy exists. In such cases, the patient should be checked periodically for at least 5 years.

ASYMPTOMATIC HEMATURIA

The finding of abnormal numbers of red blood cells (RBCs) in the urine, especially if asymptomatic, suggests the possible presence of glomerular disease. Other "nonrenal," and largely symptomatic, problems (eg, trauma, bleeding diathesis, infection, lithiasis, hypercalciuria, history of sickle cell disease, renal tumors, cystic diseases, as well as factitious causes) should be excluded.

Clinical Findings

A. Symptoms and Signs: Hematuria of glomerular etiology is generally asymptomatic unless the cause is acute glomerulonephritis (AGN) with symptoms arising from severe disturbances in renal function. Associated signs include hypertension and other signs of systemic vascular disease (eg, dermatologic).

B. Laboratory Findings: Asymptomatic hematuria is detected by urine dipstick. Microscopic urinalysis should verify the presence of RBCs as well as the presence of RBC casts, which would support the diagnosis of glomerulonephritis [GN]. Significant proteinuria suggests more concerning glomerular pathology. Associated pyuria may indicate infection, but severe renal inflammation can also produce pyuria. Serum analysis may be unrevealing or may show findings supportive of GN (eg, elevations in BUN and creatinine, hypocomplementemia, positive ANA). If significant glomerular disease can be excluded, familial hematuria or benign persistent hematuria may be the cause. If GN is clinically suspected, renal biopsy is indicated, especially if chronic GN is the major consideration. Chronic hereditary glomerulonephritis (Alport syndrome) may be considered on the basis of a strong family history and compatible renal histologic findings.

Treatment

The treatment of asymptomatic hematuria depends on the etiology. Discussion of those treatable entities follow in the section on Glomerulonephritis. Benign hematuria, by definition, requires no treatment.

GLOMERULONEPHRITIS

Inflammation of the renal glomerulus—glomerulonephritis—produces characteristic glomerular morphologic changes. In presentations of acute GN, a typical clinical picture is manifested by gross hematuria (tea-colored or a "smokey-red-brown" urine), edema (generally mild, eg, periorbital), and hypertension. The most common form of acute GN in childhood is the "postinfectious" variety. The condition presents approximately 2 weeks after the initial infection (usually streptococcal but other bacterial and viral processes have been shown to produce subsequent glomerular reaction) and will display varying degrees of clinical severity, depending on the reduction in glomerular filtration rate (GFR), degree of hypertension, and/or associated protein loss (eg, nephrotic syndrome).

Other glomerulonephritides may also present with the acute GN syndrome, as well as with asymptomatic hematuria. These include the GN of systemic lupus erythematosus (SLE), Henoch-Schönlein purpura (HSP), IgA nephropathy, and membranoproliferative GN (histologic types I, II, and III). Occurring rarely in children are the entities of antiglomerular basement membrane (anti-GBM) disease (eg, Goodpasture's syndrome) and idiopathic, rapidly progressive GN.

Clinical Findings

A. Symptoms and Signs: Unless the GN is part of a systemic vasculitic entity such as HSP or SLE, the clinical findings will vary primarily with the degree of renal inflammation, disturbance in GFR, hypertension, and proteinuria. In the former cases other systemic signs and symptoms would be expected (rashes, arthralgias, or gastrointestinal disturbances).

In typical presentations of acute poststreptococcal GN, signs are few and symptoms are usually mild. However, depending on the severity of renal insufficiency, symptoms can range from mild (malaise, anorexia) to severe (nausea, vomiting, uremic CNS depression, hypertensive encephalopathy). The presence and degree of edema will not only depend on the reduction in GFR (sodium and water retention), but will also be influenced by the degree of urinary protein loss and its effect on plasma oncotic pressure. Proteinuria of the magnitude resulting in the nephrotic syndrome suggests the presence of a severe form of poststreptococcal GN or one of the other more serious forms of GN.

B. Laboratory Findings: Since urine color (evidence of gross hematuria) is often the first sign noted in the presentation of acute GN, urinalysis will confirm the presence and numbers of RBCs. The demonstration of RBC casts in the urine supports the clinical impression of GN, but their absence does not exclude it. Severe glomerular and renal interstitial inflammation can also produce pyuria. Proteinuria, especially the degree resulting in nephrotic syndrome, can be seen in more severe cases.

Serum BUN and creatinine will reflect the degree of renal functional disturbance. If the GFR is reduced significantly, expect alterations in serum bicarbonate, potassium, calcium, and phosphate as well. As mentioned, severe proteinuria will result in hypoalbuminemia, and associated hyperlipidemia may also be demonstrated.

Since preceding streptococcal disease is most frequently the cause of acute, postinfectious forms of GN, the search for evidence of recent exposure may reveal elevations in antistreptolysin O titer and/or streptozyme. Such data are of little relevance in "nonacute" GN or purely nephrotic syndrome presentations.

Other helpful laboratory data in evaluating GN include the serum complement. Complement may be found to be depressed in postinfectious GN, membranoproliferative GN, and SLE-GN. Normalization of serum complement is expected rapidly (1–30 days) in typical poststreptococcal GN. Intermittent or persistent depression suggests chronic GN (eg, membranoproliferative GN varieties), or SLE, where complement depression and antinative DNA elevations, hallmarks of disease activity, can be used to guide therapy.

Treatment

There is no specific therapy for poststreptococcal GN. Treatment is aimed at controlling hypertension and following the effect of disease on GFR. Depending on the degree of associated renal failure, measures can be taken to reduce protein, salt, and potassium intake; phosphate binders can be used to reduce dietary phosphate; and dialysis can be used as indicated in severe renal failure until (and if) renal recovery occurs. Such extreme measures would be instituted earlier in the more severe forms of GN, in which acute renal failure (ARF) progresses at a more rapid rate.

There are, of course, specific therapeutic measures that can be taken in the more severe or chronic forms of GN. Corticosteroids are useful in membranoproliferative GN and SLE. High dose, intravenous corticosteroids, cytotoxic agents, anticoagulation, and plasmapheresis have been used alone and in combination with variable results in these and other GNs (eg, anti-GBM disease, rapidly progressive GN). Some cases of HSP GN and IgA nephropathy, when severe (usually with excessive proteinuria and/or marked reduction in renal function) have also prompted attempts at treatment intervention, although there is no universally accepted therapy for these clinical entities. The likelihood of ARF or CRF progressing toward ESRD requiring chronic dialysis treatment and/or transplant is of considerable concern in all such cases.

PROTEINURIA

Like hematuria, the presence of abnormal amounts of protein in the urine suggests renal or urinary tract abnormalities.

Excretion of more than 250 mg of protein in 24 hours should raise the suspicion of significant proteinuria. Urinary dipstick can estimate the amount of protein in a given specimen, but total 24-hour quantitation should be undertaken (apply creatinine index to verify collection). The albumin:creatinine ratio in a spot urine specimen provides a practical screening tool. Although there is some variation with age, it is convenient to think of a ratio of less than 0.1 as normal, 0.1–1.0 as slight, 1.0–10 as moderate, and greater than 10 as heavy proteinuria. Some children will excrete abnormal amounts of protein only while maintaining an upright posture (orthostatic or postural proteinuria). This phenomenon can be documented by measuring the protein content of urine produced during the day (upright) and comparing it with the urine formed overnight (recumbent). In such cases more than 80% of the protein lost in the urine will be demonstrated in the upright specimen. The total quantity should not exceed 1.5 g in 24 hours.

Further pursuit of the etiology of proteinuria is undertaken if there is no orthostatic component, or if the quantity exceeds 1.5 g or produces the nephrotic syndrome (NS). The NS is produced when proteinuria results in hypoproteinemia with subsequent edema formation (degree varies with sodium intake) secondary to the loss of plasma oncotic pressure. Hyperlipidemia is also described as part of this syndrome.

Slight to moderate amounts of proteinuria can also be found in conditions where there are abnormalities of the collecting system (reflux, obstruction) or with infection. Benign persistent proteinuria (eg, exercise-induced) is a diagnosis of exclusion.

Moderate to heavy proteinuria is more suggestive of true glomerular histopathology, but massive proteinuria producing NS in children (especially ages 2–6 years) is likely to represent the idiopathic nephrotic syndrome of childhood (INSC), which has no, as yet, demonstrable glomerular morphologic abnormality ("nil lesion," "minimal change," lipoid nephrosis). However, distinct glomerular lesions that can produce NS include focal glomerular sclerosis, mesangial nephropathy, and membranous nephropathy (more common in teenagers and adults.)

Clinical Findings

A. Symptoms and Signs: Mild to moderate proteinuria is generally asymptomatic. Most often its detection is fortuitously part of routine screening. In NS, symptomatology, if any, will generally be related to the degree and location of edema. Its degree will vary with the level of serum albumin and sodium intake. Periorbital edema may not permit satisfactory opening of the eyelids (this location has prompted many a mistaken pursuit of allergy). Severe ascites may interfere with appetite and/or respiration. Symptomatic scrotal or vulvar edema may be of concern. Irritability or lethargy may be present.

The most numerous and clinically significant signs are generally only observed in cases of NS. Hypertension should raise the suspicion of the presence of significant renal pathology. Signs of volume depletion and circulatory compromise will likewise vary. Oliguria (concentrated urine) is expected. Fever suggests infection, especially spontaneous pneumococcal peritonitis if acute abdominal signs are present.

B. Laboratory Findings: Urinalysis is expected to be otherwise unrevealing in cases of isolated proteinuria (although the presence of significant quantities of RBCs would suggest glomerular disease). However, as many as 20 RBCs per high-power field (no RBC casts) can be seen in the urine of children with INSC where no glomerular lesion is expected. If NS is present, lipid droplets (maltese crosses) can be seen in the urine with the use of Polaroid filters.

Glomerular lesions can also produce reductions in GFR; thus, serum BUN and creatinine may be elevated. However, keep in mind that in NS, whether or not glomerular injury is responsible, circulatory volume contraction can lead to renal underperfusion ("prerenal" insufficiency) also resulting in elevations of BUN (primarily) and creatinine.

Furthermore, in NS, serum albumin will be decreased (as will measured total calcium) and serum lipids will be increased. Hyponatremia may be present. Although total body sodium is high owing to renal affinity for sodium in this state, the kidney is also avidly reabsorbing water (vasopressin) in defense of circulating volume. Factitious hyponatremia is also created by measurement of serum sodium in lipemic sera.

Treatment

There is no treatment per se for proteinuria, but therapy is directed at the various causes. For example, there is no treatment for postural or excercise-induced proteinuria.

The complications of NS may require immediate attention while awaiting the response, if any, to therapy directed at reducing or eliminating proteinuria. Restoration of life-threatening volume depletion should be accomplished with the administration of albumin. Care must be taken if hypertension is also paradoxically present. Administration of diuretics can lead to further circulating volume contraction, but can aid in mobilization of problematic edema and urine production, if administered while replenishing serum albumin. Infections should be promptly treated. The tendency to increased intravascular thrombosis can also be a threat.

Therapy directed against specific renal lesions will first demand documentation by renal biopsy. If the clinical presentation strongly supports the diagnosis of INSC, corticosteroids are the treatment of choice. Approximately 85% of children with this disease respond to prednisone. A dose of 2 mg/kg of body weight (maximum 60 mg) is given as a single daily dose until the urine is protein-free (negative to trace by dipstick) for a maximum of 6 weeks. After remission has been maintained for 3–5 days, the same dose is administered every other day for 6–8 weeks and then is slowly tapered over another 4–6 weeks and discontinued. Of patients who do not respond to this treatment, a few will still reveal no significant histopathology on renal biopsy, but the rest will likely have either focal glomerular sclerosis (most prevalent), mesangial nephropathy, or membranous lesions. Even some of initial responders may prove "steroid-dependent" (frequent relapses, more than 2 months between episodes) or "steroid-resistant" with time.

When prolonged steroid exposure poses the risks associated with steroid toxicity, cytotoxic drugs such as chlorambucil and cyclophosphamide can induce longer, if not permanent, remission. They must be administered judiciously as they are not without significant side effects. Diagnostic confirmation of renal morphology with steroid resistance is again needed.

Course & Prognosis

INSC, despite multiple relapses and the use of cytotoxic agents, is expected to resolve without sequelae. The most concerning aspects of the entity relate to the complications of the nephrotic condition, which have been previously addressed. Complications of NS are likewise of considerable concern in the

Table 24–1. Causes of acute renal failure in children.

Prerenal:	Dehydration, congestive heart failure, renal arterial thrombosis, nephrotic syndrome.
Postrenal:	Urinary tract obstruction (eg, ureteropelvic and ureterovesical junctional stenoses and posterior urethral valves), urolithiasis, clot, foreign body.
Renal:	Glomerulonephritis, hemolytic uremic syndrome, systemic vasculitis, acute tubular necrosis (asphyxia, hypotension, ischemia), drugs, interstitial disease.

other glomerular lesions capable of producing it. Of these, mesangial nephropathy has a guarded prognosis relative to progressive renal failure, whereas as many as 15–20% of children with focal glomerular sclerosis develop CRF, although improved results with attempts at various treatment regimens have been reported. Corticosteroid therapy is reported to improve the prognosis of membranous nephropathy.

ACUTE RENAL FAILURE

Renal insufficiency, or acute renal failure (ARF)—"the clinical appearance of the inability of the kidneys to maintain their role in body homeostasis"—may be practically divided into causes resulting from compromise in renal perfusion (prerenal), obstruction to urinary flow (postrenal), or renal parenchymal disease (renal). Examples of each of these entities are listed in Table 24–1.

Clinical Findings

A. Symptoms and Signs: Depending on the degree of reduction in GFR and urine production, symptoms will range from those associated with fluid overload (eg, shortness of breath) to those of uremia (anorexia, nausea and vomiting, lethargy, etc).

Clinical signs vary from mild to severe edema, hypertension, congestive heart failure, pulmonary edema, anemia, and encephalopathy.

B. Laboratory Findings: Serum BUN and creatinine are increased and must be monitored. Serum analysis will reveal disturbances in electrolytes, most importantly potassium and bicarbonate (acidosis). Serum calcium generally decreases while phosphate increases. Anemia may be noted.

Treatment

All immediately correctable causes (usually prerenal or postrenal) should be addressed. Renal glomerular or interstitial diseases, once identified, are treated accordingly. The complications of ARF should be carefully monitored and controlled. Timely intervention with dialysis is important in reducing morbidity. Recovery is largely dependent on the nature of the renal lesion and its response to therapy.

The Hemolytic Uremic Syndrome (HUS) (see Chapter 23) is responsible for many cases of ARF in children. Management is directed at the consequences of the renal failure (dialysis in severe cases), although there have been reported improvements seen with plasma infusion or plasmapheresis in isolated cases.

Acute tubular necrosis (ATN)—or vasomotor nephropathy—is the disturbance in renal function usually suspected in clinical settings where renal ischemia or nephrotoxicity (hemoglobin, myoglobin, drugs, etc) is implicated and no other immediately identifiable cause is elucidated. Precipitating factors should be quickly identified and eliminated. The urinary indices (Table 24–2) are helpful in assessing oliguria when a distinction must be made between diminished renal perfusion and ATN. Rapid restoration of renal perfusion and induction of diuresis (furosemide, up to 5 mg/kg IV) may avert ATN or at least establish nonoliguric ATN, which by virtue of reasonable urinary output is considerably easier to manage. The treatment for this entity is otherwise largely supportive, including dialysis as indicated. Renal recovery is expected unless renal ischemia is of the degree producing cortical necrosis, or unless metabolic toxins have caused irreversible injury. Recovery from oligoanuric ATN generally includes a nonoliguric or "diuretic" phase, and thus careful attention is directed toward preventing severe volume depletion during this period.

Overall management of prolonged ARF with oliguria includes careful attention to fluid balance. Measurement of input and output as well as daily weight is advised. Central venous pressure monitoring may be indicated. Urinary bladder catheterization may be helpful in assessing the clinical situation early in ARF, but if oliguria is established the presence of a foreign body in the bladder invites infection.

Hypertension should be controlled with appropriate antihypertensive medications and normalization of intravascular volume. Intake of water, sodium, potassium, and phosphate should be restricted. Dietary phosphate binders, eg, calcium carbonate, should be administered as well. Reduced protein intake and adequate calories to decrease catabolism will minimize

Table 24–2. Urinary findings in oliguria–prerenal vs ATN.

Test	Prerenal	ATN
Sodium (meq/L)	<20	>20
Fractional Na excretion*	<1	>1
Urine/serum creatinine	>40	<40
Osmolality (mosm/L)	>400	<400

*$FENa = \dfrac{U/P\ Na}{U/P\ Cr} \times 100.$

the rate of rise in serum BUN. On the other hand, such restrictions can be greatly modified or eliminated with the use of dialysis.

Metabolic acidosis may be treated with bicarbonate, intravascular volume permitting. Likewise, correction of pH will aid in the intracellular movement of serum potassium.

Other temporizing measures to combat hyperkalemia include the infusion of dextrose and insulin. Calcium administration is "cardioprotective" in this situation; moreover, hypocalcemia itself may be a problem, and may be clinically manifest in tetany with correction of acidosis—alkalinization increases protein-bound calcium. Such temporizing treatment of life-threatening hyperkalemia must be followed by the removal of excess potassium with either Na–K^+ exchange resins (Kayexalate) or dialysis. Again, most, if not all, of the complexities of management and consequences of uremia may be easily handled with the institution of dialysis.

RENAL TUBULAR DEFECTS

As previously mentioned in the discussion concerning juvenile nephronophthisis, there are renal disorders that are expressed primarily, if not solely, by abnormal function of the renal tubule. The most commonly encountered abnormality of this type is isolated renal tubular acidosis (RTA). Although this is a "renal" acidosis, it is to be distinguished from the acidosis seen in CRF, which is primarily the result of decreasing renal mass. The De Toni-Fanconi-Debré syndrome describes the more extensively malfunctioning nephron that produces not only renal bicarbonate losses but also phosphaturia, glycosuria, and aminoaciduria. This abnormality is most frequently encountered in metabolic diseases such as cystinosis, renal developmental conditions such as juvenile nephronophthisis, and acquired conditions of either unknown etiology or renal toxin exposure. Some of the acquired conditions may resolve but the usual course in untreated cystinosis, for example, is progressive CRF to end-stage disease.

Depending on the type of isolated RTA, however, the prognosis varies. Type 1 RTA (distal tubule—hydrogen ion gradient defect/bicarbonate loss) is generally associated with more complex metabolic disorders and nephrocalcinosis. Type 2 RTA (proximal tubule—lowered "threshold" for bicarbonate reabsorption-bicarbonate wasting) is most frequently encountered as a transient form in infancy (suggesting delayed renal development of normal proximal bicarbonate reclamation). If this type is an isolated tubular problem it is expected to spontaneously resolve by age 2–4 years. Type 3 can be said to be a combination of types 1 and 2, and type 4 (deficiency in the renal physiologic effect of aldosterone) is primarily seen in adults with renal tubulo-interstitial disease.

1. RENAL TUBULAR ACIDOSIS

Clinical Findings

A. Symptoms and Signs: Failure to thrive is the most common presenting symptom. Polydypsia and polyuria may be noted. Anorexia, vomiting, constipation, and general listlessness may also be prominent features depending on the severity of systemic acidosis and extent of urinary losses. Skeletal pain associated with rickets (usually in more severe forms of type 1 and Fanconi syndrome) can also occur. There may be associated hypokalemia, producing symptomatic muscle weakness.

Poor gains in length and weight or skeletal deformity may be the only signs. Hematuria may be noted as a consequence of nephrocalcinosis (more commonly seen in type 1).

B. Laboratory Findings: Non–anion gap acidosis (hyperchloremic) is demonstrated with inappropriate urine pH (nonacidified). Hypokalemia may be present, or may come about with the administration of alkali therapy. Glycosuria, phosphaturia, and aminoaciduria are noted in Fanconi syndrome. Normal urinalysis should help exclude tubulo-interstitial disease. Demonstration of normal renal architecture with ultrasonography is advisable.

Treatment

Administration of alkali is the mainstay of treating the metabolic abnormality. Sodium citrate solution (Bicitra, 1 meq each Na and HCO_3 per mL, or Polycitra, 1 meq each Na and K and 2 meq HCO_3 per mL) is commonly used. Type 1 RTA will require 1–3 meq/kg body wt/d in 3 divided doses. Type 2, owing to the magnitude of proximal tubular bicarbonate losses, will generally require 5–15 meq/kg/d.

Course & Prognosis

Genetically transmitted or sporadic type 1 (with or without associated systemic disease) disorders resulting in nephrocalcinosis, or autoimmune diseases associated with type 1, are likely to be permanent defects. Drug-induced type 1 may resolve with discontinuation of the offending agent, as should RTA secondary to reflux nephropathy or obstruction if there is satisfactory recovery with correction of the urinary tract abnormality. Transient forms of type 2 are expected to resolve, as are those associated with drugs. Familial type 2 or that associated with the Fanconi syndrome are permanent defects, or are at least a significant management problem until CRF occurs in those entities with progressive renal interstitial and glomerular deterioration.

2. NEPHROGENIC DIABETES INSIPIDUS

Another tubular disorder less frequently encountered is this inherited (primarily X-linked) disorder, in which there is impaired or absent renal response to antidiuretic hormone.

Clinical Findings
A. Symptoms and Signs: Nephrogenic diabetes insipidus occurs early in infancy with irritability, failure to thrive, and poor feeding. Polyuria, polydipsia, dehydration, and rapid weight loss are remarkable, and fever may be noted.

B. Laboratory Findings: Urine output is increased and the osmolality is low, but urinalysis is otherwise unremarkable. Urinary concentration does not respond to vasopressin administration. Hypernatremia is marked (serum osmolality high) and metabolic acidosis develops with severe dehydration.

Treatment
Intake should be reduced in solutes (which obligate urinary water excretion) but appropriate in caloric content. However, care must be taken to assure adequate protein intake for growth, and to avoid hyponatremia. Thiazide diuretics are useful as they decrease sodium reabsorption in the cortical diluting segment of the renal tubule, resulting in increased sodium loss, while the resulting volume contraction leads to enhanced proximal tubule absorption of fluid. A dose of 30 mg/kg of chlorthiazide per day in 3 divided doses is helpful in treating this abnormality.

25 | Eye

Philip P. Ellis, MD

Eye examination should be a part of every general physical examination. Testing of visual acuity is the singly most important test of visual function. In children 3 years or older, visual acuity can usually be tested with standard test charts. In infants, it can be evaluated by observing whether the eyes focus on and follow a light or attractive toy. By the age of 2 years vision is normally about 20/60; at 4–5 years it should be almost 20/20.

Ocular alignment is evaluated by observing the corneal light reflection, which should come from corresponding central positions if the eyes are straight. Extraocular muscle function may be tested by having the subject follow a light or toy in different directions of gaze. Ophthalmoscopy is an essential part of the eye examination and usually requires dilatation of the pupils. In infants, the pupils can be dilated by use of (1) drops containing a combination of 1% tropicamide (Mydriacyl) and 2.5% phenylephrine or (2) drops containing 0.2% cyclopentolate and 1% phenylephrine (Cyclomydril). Either of these should be instilled 2 or 3 times at 10- to 15-minute intervals. In children 2 years or older, 1% cyclopentolate (Cyclogyl) or 5% homatropine instilled once or instilled twice at 5- to 10-minute intervals provides good pupillary dilatation, usually within 30–45 minutes. The 10% solution of phenylephrine should not be used in infants and should be avoided in small children, because of possible absorption into the bloodstream and systemic toxicity. When the ophthalmoscope is placed 10–15 inches (25–40 cm) in front of the eye and a +10 or +15 dioptric lens is used, a uniform red reflex should be observed in the pupil. An irregular red reflex or unequal reflexes in the 2 pupils suggests the possibility of opacities in the ocular media or a major difference in refractive error between the 2 eyes.

DISORDERS OF THE EYELIDS

EPICANTHUS

Epicanthus is a concave bilateral lidfold at the inner angle of the lids. It is normal in Orientals, is found in children with Down's syndrome, and may be observed also in otherwise normal children, usually as a family trait.

If epicanthus is marked, it may give the appearance of a convergent squint, since the pupil is closer to the lidfold at the inner angle than at the outer angle. No therapy is indicated.

STY
(Hordeolum)

A sty is a purulent infection of a sebaceous gland in the lid, usually caused by *Staphylococcus aureus*. There is localized edema, swelling, redness near the lid edge, and pain, with the point of maximum tenderness over the affected gland. Internal hordeolum is an infection of a meibomian gland or duct. It is an acute form of chalazion (see below).

Treatment
A. Local Measures: Hot moist compresses constitute the most effective treatment. Topical antibiotics may prevent complicating conjunctivitis, hasten resolution, and prevent recurrences and involvement of other glands. Use sodium sulfacetamide (10% ointment) or an antibiotic ophthalmic ointment. Never squeeze the sty.

B. Systemic Antibiotics: Systemic antibiotics should be given in severe cases, especially if there is a surrounding cellulitis.

Prognosis
The acute inflammation usually resolves in 4–10 days, but recurrences are frequent. Continued therapy at night with an antibiotic ointment may prevent recurrence.

CHALAZION

Chalazion is a relatively painless mass that may result from obstruction, retention, and granulomatous inflammation of one of the meibomian glands in the upper or lower lid.

The irregularity of the lid may be cosmetically disturbing. A slight feeling of irritation of the eye may also be present.

Treatment

A. Local Measures: In the acute phase warm, moist compresses may be applied. Topical antibacterial ointments may be used for treatment of the acute form and for recurrences.

B. Surgical Measures: Give local anesthesia, and open the chalazion by conjunctival incision and curettage. Incision is made at a right angle to the lid margin. Avoid the lid margin. Do not perform surgery during the acute phase. Intralesional injection of 1 to 2 mg of triamcinolone acetonide suspension is an effective alternative to surgery.

Complete excision for biopsy is suggested in recurrent or unusual cases.

Prognosis

The prognosis for eradication is good with incision and curettage or corticosteroid injection. Without such definitive treatment, recurrences are common. In the absence of repeated infections, chalazion produces irritation and is a cosmetic problem, which may make surgery desirable. A large chalazion can produce astigmatism through pressure on the globe.

BLEPHARITIS
(Granulated Lids)

Chronic inflammation of the lid margins is caused by infection with pyogenic bacteria (usually *S aureus*). *Pityrosporum ovale* is associated with the seborrheic type of blepharitis in adolescents. Seborrheic dermatitis and dandruff are often associated.

Blepharitis is characterized by chronic reddening and thickening of the lid margins and frequent rubbing and irritation of the eye. Fine scales and granulations may be seen along the base of the eyelashes, and ulceration and bleeding occur at the base of the lash in the staphylococcal type of blepharitis.

Treatment

Depending on the causative agent, local antibiotic or chemotherapeutic medication is indicated, together with warm water soaks of the lid margins. The lid margins should be cleansed with a cotton applicator moistened with a diluted baby shampoo. Treat dandruff and seborrheic dermatitis.

Examine and treat siblings and parents.

Prognosis

There is a marked tendency to chronicity. Treatment usually controls the condition, but complete cures are difficult to obtain. Spontaneous cures are common in staphylococcal infections. Permanent loss of the eyelashes may result from severe staphylococcal blepharitis.

PTOSIS
(Drooping of the Upper Eyelids)

Ptosis is characterized by drooping lids and backward tilting of the head in an attempt to see below the upper lids. It is due to paresis or paralysis of the levator muscle of the upper lid, which is supplied by a branch of the oculomotor nerve. There may be associated weakness of the superior rectus muscle.

Practical note: When ptosis is acquired, myasthenia gravis should be suspected and ruled out by specific tests.

Ptosis may be congenital (sometimes accompanied by a marked epicanthus) or acquired. It is generally bilateral but frequently asymmetric. Acquired ptosis is seen less often in children than in adults and suggests neurologic disease. Slight ptosis results from interruption of cervical sympathetics (Horner's syndrome).

Treatment

To prevent visual loss, early plastic surgery is indicated when ptosis is severe and interferes with vision. In patients with milder forms of ptosis, no surgical treatment is required except for cosmetic reasons and can be delayed until the age of 4–5 years.

Prognosis

Prognosis is excellent for surgical cure when levator paralysis is partial. Good results are usually obtained when the paralysis is complete.

TICS OF THE EYELIDS
(Blepharospasm)

Frequent blinking may be due to refractive errors, chronic blepharitis, or conjunctivitis, but it usually suggests emotional tension. Correction of the physical cause may lead to rapid improvement. Blepharospasm due to tension states may disappear spontaneously or with psychotherapy or use of tranquilizers. The patient's parents should be reassured of the good prognosis and urged to adopt a more permissive attitude toward the child. Not infrequently, however, signs of blepharospasm give way to other signs of tension states during the postadolescent period.

OBSTRUCTION OF THE LACRIMAL APPARATUS
(Dacryostenosis)

Dacryostenosis is one of the most common congenital abnormalities of the eye and usually results from incomplete canalization of the nasolacrimal duct. It may also be acquired. Trauma and chronic conjunctivitis may predispose to the development of this disorder.

Tearing and conjunctivitis may be noted. Mucopurulent discharge is often present or may be expressed from the lacrimal sac. The condition may be unilateral or bilateral.

Treatment & Prognosis
A. Local Measures: The lacrimal sac should be gently massaged, using a pumping action with a small finger in the lacrimal fossa. If infection is present, local chemotherapy with sodium sulfacetamide ophthalmic drops is advised. In 95% of cases, correction occurs spontaneously or following massage.

B. Surgical Measures: Probing is easily and safely performed in patients after 6–9 months of age. It is seldom performed earlier, because the condition usually resolves spontaneously. Probing is successful in most cases; if it fails, however, dacryocystorhinostomy may be indicated.

CONJUNCTIVITIS OF THE NEWBORN
(Ophthalmia Neonatorum)

Etiology
There are 4 main causes of conjunctivitis in the newborn:

A. Silver Nitrate: This is by far the most common cause. Onset is in the first 2 days of life, usually the first.

B. Gonococci or Staphylococci: The onset is at any time after birth, usually between the second and fifth days.

C. Chlamydiae: The onset of inclusion blennorrhea is between the third and 14th days.

D. Herpes simplex: The onset is within the first 2 weeks of life.

Clinical Findings

   A. Symptoms and Signs:

   1. Silver nitrate conjunctivitis–The mucoid discharge may become purulent if secondary infection occurs.

   2. Gonococcal or staphylococcal conjunctivitis–The discharge is frankly purulent and very profuse.

   3. Inclusion blennorrhea–The discharge is moderately profuse. Characteristically, the conjunctiva in the lower fornix is hypertrophied.

   4. Herpes simplex conjunctivitis–The discharge is thin and watery. Dendritic or geographic corneal ulceration may follow the conjunctivitis.

   B. Laboratory Findings:

   1. Silver nitrate conjunctivitis–Smears of pus reveal cellular debris but few, if any, bacteria. Bacteriologic cultures yield negative results early in the course.

   2. Gonococcal or staphylococcal conjunctivitis–Gram-stained smears of discharge will reveal gram-negative intracellular diplococci (gonococci) or gram-positive cocci in clusters (staphylococci). Cultures should be obtained and plated on the appropriate media.

   3. Inclusion blennorrhea–Staining epithelial cells obtained by conjunctival scraping will demonstrate paranuclear inclusion bodies using Giemsa or hematoxylin-eosin stains. *Chlamydia trachomatis* infection can be definitively diagnosed by isolating the organism in tissue culture or by utilizing a rapid antigen detection test: (1) direct fluorescent staining for elementary bodies or (2) enzyme-linked immunoassay.

   4. Herpes simplex conjunctivitis–Conjunctival smears and scrapings reveal lymphocytes, plasma cells, and multinucleated giant cells. Cultures for herpes simplex are usually positive.

Treatment

   Silver nitrate conjunctivitis is usually self-limited and no treatment is required. Saline irrigations may be used. Bacterial conjunctivitis requires prompt therapy with chemotherapeutic agents such as sodium sulfacetamide, bacitracin, tetracycline, gentamicin, or tobramycin ointment every 4 hours for 7 days. The treatment of gonococcal conjunctivitis is penicillin 100,000 U/kg/d intravenously in 4 divided doses. Penicillinase-producing strains should be treated with intravenous or intramuscular ceftriaxone, 25–50 mg/kg daily for 7 days or gentamicin 5 mg/kg/d intramuscularly in 2 divided doses for 7 days. Topical antibiotic therapy is unnecessary when systemic antibiotic treatment is given. Inclusion blennorrhea should be treated with systemic antibiotics because pneumonitis, otitis media, and vulvo-vaginitis often accompany the conjunctivitis. Erythromycin syrup, 50 mg/kg/d orally in 4 divided doses for 14 days should be employed. Herpes simplex infections should be treated with 1% trifluridine drops every 2 hours for 7 days.

Prophylaxis

Replacement of silver nitrate with an antibiotic ophthalmic ointment has been advocated to prevent silver nitrate conjunctivitis.

Prepartum therapy of gonorrhea-infected mothers may prevent gonococcal conjunctivitis, but instillation of silver nitrate or an antibiotic affords an additional safeguard.

Inclusion blennorrhea originates from an asymptomatic subclinical infection of the mother's cervix with *C trachomatis*. Screening and treating the mother before delivery for chlamydial cervicitis can prevent inclusion conjunctivitis.

The advisability of topical and/or systemic antiviral prophylactic treatment for newborns of mothers with active genital herpetic lesions has not been determined.

Prognosis

The prognosis with treatment is generally very good, and cure should result within 2–4 days. If bacterial conjunctivitis is untreated, permanent scarring of the cornea and partial or complete loss of vision may result, depending on the severity and duration of the untreated condition.

CONJUNCTIVITIS

Etiology

Conjunctivitis is most often caused by local bacterial, viral, or fungal infections (secondary to other mycotic infections) or by systemic diseases.

A. Bacterial Conjunctivitis: *S aureus, Streptococcus pneumoniae*, beta-hemolytic streptococci, *Neiserria gonorrhoeae, N meningitidis*, and *Haemophilus influenzae* are the agents usually responsible for "pinkeye." Inclusion blennorrhea and trachoma are due to chlamydial infection.

B. Viral Conjunctivitis: Viruses of epidemic keratoconjunctivitis (usually adenovirus type 8 or 19), pharyngoconjunctival fever (usually adenovirus type 3 or 7), and herpes simplex may occur.

C. Fungal Conjunctivitis: A variety of fungal organisms (often secondary to other mycotic infections) may rarely produce conjunctivitis.

D. Allergic Conjunctivitis:–Conjunctivitis may be due to seasonal allergy (eg, vernal conjunctivitis), and may progress to phlyctenular keratoconjunctivitis.

E. Systemic Disease: Systemic diseases may cause conjunctivitis, eg, vitamin A deficiency (xerophthalmia), measles, and erythema multiforme (Stevens-Johnson disease).

Clinical Findings
See Table 25–1.

Treatment
A. Specific Measures:

1. Bacterial conjunctivitis–Local instillation of ophthalmic sulfacetamide eyedrops or ointment is indicated. Because most organisms are gram-positive, erythromycin may be used. Other choices include gentamicin or tobramycin. For trachoma and inclusion conjunctivitis, apply tetracycline antibiotic ointment locally 4 times daily.

2. Viral conjunctivitis–There is no specific treatment. Warm compresses often provide relief of symptoms. Secondary bacterial infections should be treated with topical antibiotics or sulfacetamide.

3. Fungal conjunctivitis–Local instillation of natamycin (Natacyn) drops, 5% suspension, 1% micanazole, or amphotericin B suspension, 0.05–1.5%, is indicated.

4. Allergic conjunctivitis–Instillation of a weak ophthalmic vasoconstrictor (eg, 0.05% naphazoline, 0.05% tetrahydrozoline, or 0.12% phenylephrine) and the systemic use of antihistaminic drugs may provide relief. Topical instillation of a weak corticosteroid solution such as 0.125% prednisolone (or equivalent) every 2 hours is also effective. Observe closely for complications. Topical 4% cromolyn sodium (Opticrom) every 6 hours is useful and may avoid the need for corticosteroid drops.

5. Systemic disease–The treatment or recovery from systemic disease usually results in improvement of the eye lesion.

B. General Measures: Measures include use of cool compresses (not ice) for allergic conjunctivitis and hot compresses for bacterial conjunctivitis. Never use eye patches.

Prognosis
The prognosis in all types of conjunctivitis is generally excellent if proper treatment is instituted. In untreated cases, cor-

Table 25–1. Clinical and laboratory features of conjunctivitis.[*]

	Viral	Bacterial	Chlamydial	Allergic
Itching	Minimal	Minimal	Minimal	Severe
Hyperemia	Generalized	Generalized	Generalized	Generalized
Tearing	Profuse	Moderate	Moderate	Moderate
Exudation	Minimal, mucoid	Profuse, purulent	Profuse, mucoid or mucopurulent	Minimal, slightly mucous
Preauricular adenopathy	Common	Uncommon	Common only in inclusion conjunctivitis	None
Stained conjunctival smears and scrapings	Lymphocytes, plasma cells, multinucleated giant cells, eosinophilic intranuclear inclusions	Neutrophils, bacteria	Neutrophils, plasma cells, basophilic intracytoplasmic inclusions	Eosinophils
Associated sore throat and fever	Occasionally	Occasionally	Never in inclusion conjunctivitis; often present in neonatal conjunctivitis	Never

[*]Modified, with permission, from Vaughn D, Asbury T, Tabbara KF: *General Ophthalmology*, 12th ed. Appleton & Lange, 1989.

neal infection, ulceration, and scarring with visual loss may occur.

REFRACTIVE ERRORS

MYOPIA
(Nearsightedness)

In myopia, the focus of distant objects lies anterior to the retina, resulting in poor vision for distant objects. The focus of near objects lies closer to the retina (ie, nearsighted). Myopia is often hereditary and is frequently associated with prematurity.

Myopia should be suspected when the condition exists in either parent. It usually results from excessive length of the eyeball but may be caused by increased refractive power in the cornea or lens. Myopia tends to become gradually more severe during the growing period.

Clinical Findings

Myopia is manifested by poor vision for distant objects, squinting, and difficulty in reading the blackboard at school. Routinely, when the patient is 3 years of age, a fundus examination should be done after instillation of a cycloplegic agent (see p 768).

Holding reading matter close up is not necessarily a sign of myopia, since children have much greater powers of accommodation than do adults.

The refractive error in either myopia or hyperopia may be estimated by use of the direct ophthalmoscope. Use of a cycloplegic agent is necessary in children. If the examiner is emmetropic or wearing corrective lenses, the subject's approximate refractive error can be read in diopters as the most plus (black numbers) in the ophthalmoscope with which retinal detail can be seen clearly. (With less plus, the examiner will accommodate to maintain a clear view.) This technique of examination has definite limitations and should not be relied on completely for the diagnosis of refractive errors.

Treatment & Prognosis

Except for patients with mild cases, proper lenses for full correction of the refractive error should be worn at all times. In general, it is the parents' distaste for eyeglasses rather than the child's lack of cooperation that interferes with early treatment. Children as young as 2 years of age usually can wear eyeglasses comfortably. Contact lenses may be prescribed for adolescents who can assume responsibility for the lenses and care of their eyes.

HYPEROPIA
(Farsightedness)

An emmetrope has perfect vision for distance without focusing (accommodating). The hyperope usually has good distance vision but must accommodate to see clearly. Hyperopia usually results from shortness of the eyeball but may be caused by reduced refractive power of the cornea or lens. Some degree of hyperopia is normal before puberty. The condition is largely familial and should be suspected if either of the parents suffers from it.

The condition may be asymptomatic. Headache and eyestrain may be present in older children during close work. Internal strabismus (esotropia) is often related to moderate or severe hyperopia.

For diagnosis by direct ophthalmoscope, see the discussion in the section on myopia (above).

Treatment & Prognosis

Only in children with marked degrees of hyperopia or strabismus is optical correction required, since some improvement can be expected as the child grows.

ASTIGMATISM

Astigmatism is characterized by a difference in refractive power of one meridian of the cornea as compared with the meridian at right angles to it. The difference between the 2 is the degree of astigmatism, and the meridian in which a corrective cylinder is placed is the axis of the astigmatism. Optically, this causes the horizontal component to be out of focus with the vertical component (or vice versa, depending upon the meridian of astigmatism).

Astigmatism is largely familial and is usually caused by developmental variations in the curvature of the cornea. Lenticular astigmatism is much less common than corneal astigmatism.

Clinical Findings

Astigmatism is usually seen in children who also have either myopia or hyperopia. Common findings are headache, fatigue, eye pain, reading difficulties, and a tendency to frown.

Treatment & Prognosis

Eyeglasses or contact lenses may be required, at least for reading and for watching television or movies. The degree of farsightedness or nearsightedness determines whether eyeglasses must be worn constantly. No spontaneous improvement may be expected. Corneal astigmatism is not corrected by most soft contact lenses but is corrected with either hard or semisoft gas-permeable lenses. However, special soft contact lenses may be made to correct corneal astigmatism.

CONTACT LENSES

Contact lenses can be fitted satisfactorily on any patient who is sufficiently motivated to undergo the discomforts of adaptation, but the child should be old enough to remove and insert the lenses without help. Contact lenses may be useful in infants who have undergone unilateral cataract surgery, provided that the parents are understanding and cooperative and learn the techniques of contact lens care. Since corneal damage may result from improper fitting or handling, contact lenses should be prescribed and fitted only by persons qualified to give crucial follow-up care and to treat injury or infection early.

Soft contact lenses may be used for optical purposes and also for therapeutic purposes—protection of the cornea, bandaging of corneal injury, and treatment of corneal edema. Many patients who cannot wear the conventional hard lenses may tolerate the soft lenses.

AMBLYOPIA

Amblyopia is a unilateral or bilateral reduction in vision, uncorrectable with glasses, that occurs in an eye that is normal on ophthalmoscopy. It is found in 2–4% of the general pediatric population. In children the most common cause of amblyopia is strabismus and results from long, continuous deviation of one eye with suppression of the retinal image in this eye to avoid diplopia. Amblyopia also may occur when there is a large difference in the refractive error between the 2 eyes (anisometropia).

Generally the eye with the greatest refractive error does not develop a clear retinal image and as a result vision fails to develop normally.

STRABISMUS
(Squint)

Strabismus is characterized by ocular deviations or failure of the eyes to maintain parallelism. It occurs in up to 5% of children. Intermittent squinting in infants under 6 months of age may not be true strabismus. Persistent deviations or deviations after 6 months are true strabismus, and require treatment.

Because the eyes fail to maintain parallelism, the image of the deviating eye is suppressed, with consequent progressive diminution of vision on that side leading to loss of sight (amblyopia), which may be permanent if not recognized and treated. All patients with strabismus should be examined by an ophthalmologist.

Etiology

The exact cause of strabismus cannot be determined in most cases. Congenital or hereditary strabismus is more common than the acquired form.

A. Paralytic Strabismus: Paralytic strabismus is due to a congenital or acquired anomaly of a particular extraocular muscle or paresis of its nerve supply.

B. Comitant (Nonparalytic) Strabismus: There are 3 types of comitant strabismus.

1. The accommodative type is due to hyperopia and has its onset in patients at 2–4 years of age.

2. The congenital (muscular, innervational) form has its onset at or near birth.

3. In the visual form of comitant strabismus, there is poor vision in one eye, due to a developmental anomaly or malignant tumor of the retina, or there are opacities of the media, interfering with fixation and fusion.

Clinical Findings

A. Symptoms: Eso (internal) deviations are most common in children; older children and adults tend to develop exo (external) deviations. Vision may be decreased on the affected side. With alternating squint, good vision is maintained in both eyes. Personality disorders may occur and may be reflected in social maladjustment and poor schoolwork.

B. Signs: Deviation of the eye may be in any direction and may be intermittent or constant, alternating or monocular. If strabismus is paralytic and the lesion is neurologic in nature, the angle of deviation varies with the direction of the gaze, increasing in the direction of action of the paretic muscle. If strabismus is comitant, the angle of deviation remains unaffected by the direction of the gaze.

Treatment

Diagnosis of the usual congenital types should be possible in a patient by 6 months of age, and early therapy should be instituted. In many cases of accommodative strabismus, visual problems become apparent with increasing use of near vision in the preschool and school years, eg, when attention is focused on books. Ocular disease must be ruled out by ophthalmoscopic examination.

A. General Measures: If the squint is constantly monocular, a patch must be placed over the unaffected eye to force the child to use the deviated eye and prevent amblyopia. This patch must be worn all day and should cover the entire eye. The use of a patch may be required for many months. Patching is generally of little value in patients after the age of 7 years.

Correction by glasses is imperative if marked refractive errors are found on cycloplegic refraction.

Orthoptic exercises have been recommended in an attempt to avoid surgery, but children under 5–7 years of age are rarely able to cooperate satisfactorily. Injudicious use of orthoptics often merely postpones definitive therapy unnecessarily.

If nonoperative procedures result in improvement, surgery may be postponed.

B. Surgical Measures: Surgery is indicated when vision is equal in both eyes and the deviation cannot be corrected by glasses; it is also indicated for cosmetic reasons when vision cannot be equalized. Surgery may be performed in a child as early as 6–12 months of age. Early correction is desirable if there is a good potential for fusion. Cosmetic surgery is usually done in children closer to the school years.

Prognosis

Good results are usually obtained in the treatment for strabismus associated with refractive errors. Good cosmetic results usually follow surgical treatment. Normal binocular vision, which is dependent upon sensory mechanisms, does not usually develop after surgery for congenital esotropia.

MISCELLANEOUS EYE DISORDERS

INFLAMMATION OF THE CORNEA
(Keratitis)

The healthy cornea possesses no blood vessels and is clear. Any blood vessels or opacities seen in it are pathologic.

Etiology

A. Xerophthalmia: Keratitis may be due to vitamin A deficiency occurring in malnourished children, in allergic children on restricted diets, and in children with biliary tract anomalies that interfere with absorption of vitamin A. (See also Chapter 4.)

B. Bacterial Ulcers: Bacterial ulcers usually follow trauma by a foreign body or injuries infected by bacteria, including *S pneumoniae,* hemolytic streptococci, *Klebsiella pneumoniae, Pseudomonas aeruginosa,* and *M liquefaciens.* These ulcers lead to hypopyon (pus in the anterior chamber), great corneal destruction, and loss of the eye if not treated intensively. Gonococcal conjunctivitis also frequently leads to corneal ulceration, hypopyon, and, ultimately, perforation.

C. Phlyctenular Keratitis: This may be due to an allergic reaction to tuberculoprotein but may also result from sensitivity to other proteins (bacterial or fungal). Tuberculosis can also cause a deep form of keratitis.

D. Interstitial Keratitis: Interstitial keratitis is associated with congenital or acquired syphilis (90% of cases) or may follow infectious diseases such as herpes zoster, mumps, and tuberculosis.

E. Viral Keratitis: Lesions are most often due to herpes simplex.

F. Mycotic Ulcers: These lesions are usually associated with penetration of the cornea with vegetable material, eg, a stick.

Clinical Findings

A. Symptoms and Signs: Regardless of the course, keratitis is usually characterized by pain, redness, photophobia, tearing, and blurred vision. Defects in the epithelium will stain with fluorescein. This green stain can be seen with an ordinary flashlight but is fluorescent with a blue-filtered light. Iritis is usually associated with keratitis and is characterized by a ciliary flush (limbal injection) and by aqueous flare and cells (seen only with a slit lamp).

1. Xerophthalmia–Xerophthalmia is characterized by a cornea that has lost luster and appears cloudy and dry (xerosis). Typically, there is little vascular reaction. Epithelial defects and secondary infection occur. As the condition progresses, these dry areas become keratinized and the cornea softens. The end stage is keratomalacia and obscured vision. Bitot's spots are triangular, grayish-white, foamy lesions, usually on the temporal conjunctiva, with the base adjacent to the limbus. They are associated with poor nutritional states but are not always accompanied by vitamin A deficiency.

2. Bacterial ulcers–In the early stages, there is a gray area of infiltration of the cornea associated with a dilatation of the circumcorneal blood vessels, producing the characteristic ciliary flush. There is more pain than is expected from such a small lesion, and the corneal epithelium is markedly hazy. The area enlarges, and ulceration develops; a level of pus often appears in the anterior chamber (hypopyon).

3. Phlyctenular keratitis–The limbus is usually first affected, with the appearance of a small, vascularized, elevated nodule. Gray infiltrates with secondary vascularization may occur in the superficial layers of the corneal stroma and may progress to shallow ulcers. The ulcer extends toward the center of the cornea and results in extensive scar formation. Photophobia is most marked in phlyctenulosis.

4. Interstitial keratitis–Marked, insidious, early congestion is present, with coincident iridocyclitis and clouding of the cornea. The cornea may become so cloudy that the iris cannot be seen. Photophobia may be severe. Fine, deep stromal vessels are present.

5. Viral keratitis–The dendrite is suggestive of herpes simplex, which may also present as stippling or as a geographic corneal ulcer. Corneal hypesthesia is usually present.

6. Mycotic ulcers–The corneal surface typically appears gray and rough and is sometimes elevated. The margins of the ulcer are irregular; "feathery" opacities often extend into the stroma beyond the ulcer margins. Hypopyon (pus in the anterior chamber) and a ring infiltration surrounding the primary lesion may be present.

B. Laboratory Findings: Bacteriologic cultures of ulcers usually reveal the presence of pathogenic bacteria; direct scrapings for Gram's stain often can give more prompt specific diagnosis. Serologic tests for syphilis and tuberculin testing with very dilute ($\geq$1:100,000) tuberculin material should be done in suspected cases. Vitamin A levels and tolerance test results are abnormal in patients with vitamin A deficiency.

Complications

Corneal involvement may give rise to iritis and glaucoma. Clouding of the central area can occur with severe visual loss. Purulent endophthalmitis may lead to loss of the eye.

Treatment

   A. Specific Measures:

   1. Xerophthalmia–Vitamin A therapy is specific. Parenteral therapy may be required in some cases.

   2. Bacterial ulcers–Intensive, early specific topical antibiotic therapy is imperative and must be based on findings obtained from scrapings and cultures from the ulcer itself. Systemic treatment is usually not required except for gonococcal infections (see Ophthalmia Neonatorum, above). Bacitracin-neomycin-polymyxin, tobramycin, or gentamicin ophthalmic ointment or solution may be used pending bacterial diagnosis. These drugs are effective against *Pseudomonas* ulcers and will also combat common cocci or rods. The pupil should be kept dilated with 1% atropine or 5% homatropine. Combination corticosteroid–antibiotic drops or ointment should not be used. Corticosteroids are detrimental for use in some patients with viral infections, especially those with herpes simplex.

   3. Phlyctenular keratitis–Use of topical corticosteroids, 1 drop every 2 hours, results in dramatic improvement. **Note:** Children with phlyctenular keratitis may be hypersensitive to tuberculin, and skin testing should be done with the greatest of caution at dilutions of 1:100,000 or greater.

   4. Interstitial keratitis–Specific therapy for syphilis and tuberculosis may improve the eye lesion. Topical cortisone probably minimizes scarring. Local use of cycloplegics is important in relieving photophobia and ciliary spasm.

   5. Viral keratitis–For treatment of patients with herpes simplex and vaccinia keratitis, use 0.1% idoxuridine (Herplex, Stoxil) topically, 1 drop each hour during the day and every 2 hours at night for 4–7 days. Idoxuridine ointment, 0.5%, instilled 5 times a day, may be equally effective. Topical application of vidarabine (Vira-A), 3% ointment, or trifluridine (Viroptic), 1% solution applied every 2 hours, is often effective in controlling herpes simplex keratitis when topical idoxuridine is unsuccessful. Corticosteroids should never be used in viral types of keratitis. They may enhance invasiveness of the virus and lead to serious complications, including corneal perforation in patients with herpetic keratitis.

6. Mycotic ulcers–Treat with natamycin (Natacyn), 5% suspension, or topical amphotericin B, 1.5 mg/mL. A 1% solution of miconazole is often effective.

B. General Measures: Sedation and analgesia are most important in symptomatic care. Topical anesthetics are contraindicated because they impair corneal healing. A cycloplegic, such as 1% atropine or 5% homatropine, should be instilled, 1 drop 2–3 times a day. Hot compresses applied for 15 minutes 3 or 4 times a day may decrease pain. Dark glasses will relieve photophobia.

The routine use of systemic broad-spectrum antibiotics should be discouraged. Specific bacteriologic diagnosis should guide therapy when possible. All patients with corneal ulcers should be managed by an ophthalmologist.

Course & Prognosis

A. Xerophthalmia: Even when marked clouding of the cornea has interfered with vision, complete regression frequently will occur after adequate vitamin A therapy.

B. Bacterial Ulcers: With early specific antibiotic therapy, prognosis is good. Prognosis is guarded in *Pseudomonas,* gonococcal, and hemolytic streptococcal ulcers.

C. Phlyctenular Keratitis: Recurrences are frequent and in many cases are of unknown cause. The ultimate prognosis depends on the frequency and severity of these recurrences. Prognosis for vision is much better now that attacks can be controlled with corticosteroids.

D. Interstitial Keratitis: Corneal scars may interfere with vision. In many of these, however, visual acuity is eventually excellent. Corneal transplants may be of value in selected cases.

E. Viral Keratitis: Complaints of photophobia and pain usually persist for a long time, frequently for several months, until healing has occurred. Secondary iritis may occur. Recurrences of herpes simplex keratitis are common. The ulcers rarely perforate spontaneously but may give rise to considerable scarring. (Perforation has occurred when corticosteroids have been used topically.)

F. Mycotic Ulcers: Depending upon the depth and area of involvement, dense corneal scarring may occur. Keratoplasty may be indicated in cases not responding to medical treatment and for improvement of vision after the active infection has resolved.

ORBITAL & PERIORBITAL CELLULITIS

Cellulitis is often secondary to sinusitis and may also occur as a complication of trauma and septicemia. The most common organisms are streptococci, staphylococci, and *H influenzae*.

Periorbital cellulitis is characterized by erythema and swelling of the eyelids. The conjunctiva and orbital tissues are not involved. Preauricular lymphadenopathy may be present.

Orbital cellulitis is marked by erythema and swelling of the eyelids, conjunctival chemosis, proptosis, limitation of ocular movements, fever, and leukocytosis. In cases of *H influenzae* infection, the skin of the eyelids has a distinct magenta discoloration.

Complications include meningitis and cavernous sinus thrombosis.

Treatment consists of use of hot packs and specific systemic antibiotic drugs. Drainage of loculated abscesses is occasionally necessary.

CATARACT

Cataract is an opacity of the lens or of its capsule and may be present at birth or may develop in childhood. Cataracts are often bilateral and symmetric.

Etiology
A. Congenital Cataract: Maternal rubella occurring during the first or early in the second trimester of pregnancy may result in congenital cataracts. It is probable that other viral and systemic diseases may result in congenital cataracts. These causes, however, have been less well explored.

B. Cataracts of Childhood:

1. Trauma–Traumatic cataract results from penetrating wounds or blunt trauma to the eyeball. The cataract may develop in a short time and progress rapidly; it frequently is followed by secondary glaucoma.

2. Systemic disease–Diabetes, hypoparathyroidism, galactosemia, Down's syndrome, and Lowe's syndrome may cause cataracts.

3. Poisoning–Cataracts may result from poisoning, chiefly from ingestion or inhalation of naphthalene or diphenyl.

4. Other eye disease–Cataracts may result as a complication of other diseases of the eye, including retinitis pigmentosa, glaucoma, uveitis, and iridocyclitis; cataracts may be a late stage of retrolental fibroplasia.

5. Corticosteroids–Cataracts may be due to long-term use of systemic or topical corticosteroids in high doses.

Clinical Findings

A. Symptoms: Visual acuity is diminished. There is no pain if the cataract is uncomplicated by other diseases of the eye.

B. Signs: The lens nucleus and cortex both may be opaque. If no clear lens remains, the cataract is termed "mature." Strabismus may be the first indication of cataract. Nystagmus (searching or pendular type) develops if visual acuity is impaired to 20/100 (6/30) or worse.

On dilation of the pupil, the opaque areas are seen to be white by direct light (leukocoria). The red reflex of the retina is not seen if the cataract is dense.

Treatment

A. General Measures: In the unusual case of dense central cataract, it is worthwhile to try to improve vision with 1% tropicamide (Mydriacyl), 1 drop in the involved eye twice during the day. If this is successful, surgery may be postponed until the visual status can be evaluated more completely.

B. Surgical Measures: In cases of dense complete cataracts or in those that cannot be managed temporarily with mydriatic eye drops, surgical removal should be done early (ie, within the first few weeks of life).

Prognosis

The extent of the cataract and the presence or absence of complicating ocular disease will determine whether or not useful vision can be expected. If nystagmus has developed, vision will rarely be better than 20/200 (6/60), even after successful surgery. If monocular cataract surgery is performed, correction of the refractive error with a contact lens or a surgically placed corneal button (epikeratophakia) is necessary. Intraocular lens implants in children are controversial. They should not be used below age 6–7 years.

GLAUCOMA

Glaucoma is increased intraocular pressure involving one or both eyes, giving rise to optic nerve damage and visual field loss. Infantile congenital glaucoma (in children under 3 years of age) is an autosomal recessive trait. Most cases of congenital glaucoma are sporadic; some show a hereditary pattern. Glaucoma may also follow injury or disease of the eye. It can occur as a complication of topical corticosteroid therapy. A juvenile form of glaucoma (in persons 6 years and older) may also occur.

Clinical Findings

A. Congenital Glaucoma: Photophobia is often the earliest symptom. The eyes may water. Persistent pain may be present, but more often there is none. Vision gradually deteriorates. Peripheral vision is affected first.

The eye may enlarge, and the corneal diameter may increase. Corneal edema may be present. The pupil is often dilated, and the sclera may be thin and bluish. The eyeball is large and firm to pressure. The optic nerve shows increased cupping. The difference between the normal and the affected eye in unilateral glaucoma is marked.

B. Juvenile Glaucoma: The signs and symptoms are similar to those in congenital glaucoma but less pronounced.

Treatment

A. General Measures: Antiglaucoma drugs (eg, pilocarpine and timolol) will control intraocular pressure in some cases of juvenile glaucoma but have little effect on congenital glaucoma. Acetazolamide given orally may be of value in the treatment of juvenile glaucoma; it is of little or no value in the treatment of infantile congenital glaucoma.

B. Surgical Measures: Surgery generally is required to relieve intraocular pressure. In congenital glaucoma, goniotomy or trabeculotomy may improve the function of the filtration angle. If these procedures fail to control the intraocular pressure, filtering surgical procedures or ciliary body destruction with cryotherapy or ultrasound should be tried. Enucleation is indicated if the eye continues to be painful and if vision has been lost.

Course & Prognosis

Generally, glaucoma is slowly progressive. Without treatment, blindness usually occurs eventually, although impairment of vision may progress gradually over a period of many months. With surgical treatment, vision frequently is saved. Prognosis is always guarded.

RETINOPATHY OF PREMATURITY
(Retrolental Fibroplasia)

Retinopathy of prematurity is a disease of the retina that occurs almost exclusively in premature infants of low birth weight (< 1500 g) and gestational age (< 32 weeks). It is invariably bilateral—sometimes unequally so—and leads, in its severe form, to wildly disorganized retinal vascular overgrowth and permanent blindness. In the past, it was the most common cause of blindness in children in the USA. The incidence has declined with awareness of the toxic effects of oxygen on the retina. Recently, therapy employing high concentrations of oxygen to treat respiratory distress syndrome in premature infants has again been used, and retrolental fibroplasia has occurred with increasing frequency.

High oxygen tension in the bloodstream for a prolonged period is the main precipitating factor. The disease is quite rare when supplemental oxygen therapy is not used and is uncommon when oxygen concentrations in incubators are kept below 40%. If oxygen therapy is necessary, the concentration in the incubator should be controlled by direct measurement with an oximeter rather than by monitoring the rate of flow from the tank; this has recently assumed considerable medicolegal importance. Monitoring of arterial O_2 is the best method of determining oxygen tension in the bloodstream.

All premature infants should have a careful ophthalmoscopic examination, including detailed inspection of the peripheral retina through a dilated pupil, by a skilled ophthalmologist by the sixth week of life, by which time severe forms of the disease are most common. Mild forms of the disease regress spontaneously. Refractive errors (myopia) are common sequelae and are recognizable in early childhood. Cryotherapy of the peripheral retina may be of benefit in halting progression in the severe forms of the disease.

UVEITIS

Inflammation of the uveal tissues (iris, ciliary body, and choroid) may be granulomatous or nongranulomatous and acute or chronic. Uveitis occasionally is due to specific infection with bacteria, viruses, fungi, or parasites; more commonly it is due to a nonspecific inflammatory reaction, probably as a hypersensitivity or autoimmune process. Anterior uveitis (iritis and cyclitis) in children and adolescents is often associated with juvenile rheumatoid arthritis.

Anterior involvement (iridocyclitis) is characterized by an inflamed eye, photophobia, blurred vision, ciliary injection, pupillary constriction, inflammatory cells in the anterior chamber, and keratic precipitates on the back of the cornea. Posterior involvement (choroiditis) is characterized by blurred vision and vitreous floaters. The vitreous is hazy on ophthalmoscopic examination. Acute choroid lesions appear as white indistinct masses; old lesions are seen as pigmented, disorganized scar tissue of the choroid and retina.

Complications consist of glaucoma, cataracts, and retinal detachment. Optic neuritis may be associated.

Patients with nonspecific anterior uveitis should be treated with topical administration of 1% atropine twice a day and topical corticosteroids (1% prednisolone or equivalent) 4–8 times a day. Patients with posterior involvement require systemic corticosteroids. Subconjunctival injection of repository corticosteroids may be beneficial in the treatment of cyclitis.

OPTIC NEURITIS

Two types of optic neuritis are seen in childhood: (1) papillitis (anterior involvement with papilledema) and (2) retrobulbar neuritis (disks appear normal). Most cases follow viral infections or represent localized encephalomyelitis. Optic neuritis may also be due to drug toxicity or associated with neurologic disease.

The symptoms consist of loss of visual acuity, field defects (usually central scotomas), and, occasionally, pain on movement of the eye. Papilledema is present in the anterior form only.

Treatment is nonspecific. Systemic corticosteroids are of questionable value. The prognosis is good.

RETINOBLASTOMA

Retinoblastoma is a rare, malignant tumor of children, affecting approximately 1 infant in 20,000 live births. A family history is found in less than 10% of cases, but about 30% may have a hereditary predisposition to tumor formation. Approximately 25% of cases are bilateral. Patients who survive bilateral retinoblastoma or have a family history of retinoblastoma have about a 50% chance of transmitting the disease to their offspring.

Genetic counseling is advisable for survivors of retinoblastoma as well as for parents of children with retinoblastoma.

The presenting symptom is usually a white spot in the pupil. Strabismus may be present. Glaucoma may occur. Diagnosis is usually made by ophthalmoscopy after wide pupillary dilatation. With unilateral disease treatment consists of enucleation of the eye, although small tumors may be treated with irradiation or cryotherapy. All patients with retinoblastoma should be referred to an ophthalmologist with expertise in management of this difficult problem.

26 | Bones & Joints

Robert E. Eilert, MD

Orthopaedic surgery is the medical discipline that deals with disorders of neuromuscular and skeletal systems. Patients with bone & joint problems usually present with pain, loss of function, or deformity. As is true of most medical and surgical disorders, the diagnosis of musculoskeletal disorders can often by made on the basis of a carefully taken history. The physical examination is the most important feature of diagnosis and depends upon an intimate knowledge of extremity & spinal anatomy.

DISTURBANCES OF PRENATAL ORIGIN

CONGENITAL AMPUTATIONS

Congenital amputations may be due to teratogens (eg, drugs or viruses), amniotic bands, or metabolic diseases (eg, diabetes in the mother) or, in rare cases, may be hereditary defects. Most are spontaneous and not genetically determined. The history of the pregnancy must be carefully reviewed in a search for possible teratogenic factors. According to the currently accepted international classification, amputations are either terminal or longitudinal. In terminal amputation, all parts are missing distal to the level of involvement—eg, absence of the forearm, wrist, and hand in the case of a terminal below-the-elbow amputation. A longitudinal amputation consists of partial absence of structures in the extremity along one side or the other. In radial clubhand, the entire radius is absent, but the thumb may be either hypoplastic or completely absent—ie, the effect on structures distal to the amputation may vary. Complex tissue defects are nearly always associated with longitudinal amputations in that the associated nerves and muscles are usually not completely represented when a bone is absent. Bones within the axial skeleton likewise may be absent. Congenital absence of the sacrum is often associated with diabetes in the mother.

Terminal amputations are treated by means of a prosthesis, eg, to compensate for shortness of one leg. With longitudinal deficiences, constructive surgery may be feasible with the objective of reducing deformity and stabilizing joints.

Lower extremity prostheses are best fitted at about the time of normal walking (12–15 months of age). Lower extremity prostheses are consistently well accepted, as they are necessary for balancing and walking. Upper extremity prostheses are not as well accepted. Fitting the child with a dummy type prosthesis as early as 6 months of age has the advantage of instilling an accustomed pattern of proper length and bimanual manipulation. Children fitted later than age 2 years nearly always reject upper extremity prostheses.

Children quickly learn how to function with their prostheses and can lead active lives, participating in sports with peers.

DEFORMITIES OF THE EXTREMITIES

1. METATARSUS VARUS

Metatarsus varus is characterized by adduction of the forefoot on the hindfoot, with the heel in normal position or slightly valgus. The longitudinal arch is often creased vertically when the deformity is more rigid. The lateral border of the foot demonstrates sharp angulation at the level of the base of the fifth metatarsal, and this bone will be especially prominent. The deformity varies from flexible to rigid. Most flexible deformities are secondary to intrauterine posture and usually resolve spontaneously.

If the deformity is rigid and cannot be manipulated past the midline, splinting is appropriate to ensure the resolution of the deformity. The prognosis for this common deformity of the foot is excellent in that 85% correct by age 3–4 yrs with the remainder having mild problems fitting shoes.

2. CLUBFOOT
(Talipes Equinovarus)

When foot deformity consists of the following 3 elements, the diagnosis of classic talipes equinovarus, or clubfoot, is made: (1) equinus or plantar flexion of the foot at the ankle joint, (2) varus or inversion deformity of the heel, and (3) forefoot varus. The incidence of talipes equinovarus is approximately

1:1000 live births. Any infant with a clubfoot should be examined carefully for associated anomalies, especially of the spine. Clubfoot tends to follow a hereditary pattern in some families or may be part of a generalized neuromuscular syndrome such as arthrogryposis or myelodysplasia.

Treatment consists of massage and manipulation of the foot to stretch the contracted tissues on the medial and posterior aspects, followed by splinting to hold the correction. When this is instituted in the nursery shortly after birth, correction is achieved much more rapidly. When treatment is delayed, the foot tends to become more rigid within a matter of days.

About half of children with clubfoot eventually need an operative procedure to lengthen the tightened structures about the foot.

A supple foot that is easily corrected by strapping and casting has a more favorable prognosis. If the foot is rigid operative correction is indicated for normal function in walking.

3. CONGENITAL DYSPLASIA OF THE HIP JOINT
(Congenital Hip Dislocation)

In a child with congenital dysplasia of the hip, the femoral head and the acetabulum may be in partial contact at birth. This condition is termed subluxation of the hip. A more severe defect is complete loss of contact between the femoral head and acetabulum, in which case there is frank dislocation of the hip, with the femoral head nearly always displaced laterally and superiorly due to muscle pull. At birth, there is lack of the development of both the acetabulum and the femur in cases of congenital hip dysplasia. The dysplasia becomes progressive with growth unless the dislocation is corrected. If the dislocation is corrected in the first few days or weeks of life, the dysplasia is completely reversible and a normal hip will develop. As the child becomes older and the dislocation or subluxation persists, the deformity will worsen to the point where it will not be completely reversible, especially after the walking age. For this reason, it is important to diagnose the deformity in the nursery or, at the latest, the 6-week checkup.

Clinical Findings

The diagnosis of congenital hip dislocation in the newborn depends upon demonstrating instability of the joint by placing the infant on its back and obtaining complete relaxation by feeding with a bottle if necessary. The examiner's long finger is then placed over the greater trochanter and the thumb over the inner side of the thigh. Both hips are flexed 90 degrees and then slowly abducted from the midline. With gentle pressure, an attempt is made to lift the greater trochanter forward. A feeling of slipping as the head goes into the acetabulum is a sign of instability. In other infants, the joint is more stable, and the deformity must be provoked by applying slight pressure with the thumb on the medial side of the thigh as the thigh is adducted, thus slipping the hip posteriorly and eliciting a jerk as the hip dislocates. The signs of instability are the most reliable criteria for diagnosing congenital dislocation of the hip in the newborn. X-rays of the pelvis are notoriously unreliable until about 6 weeks of age.

After the first month of life, the signs of instability become less evident. Contractures begin to develop about the hip joint, causing limitation of abduction. Normally, the hip should abduct fully to 90 degrees on either side during the first few months of life. It is important that the pelvis be held level to detect asymmetry of abduction. When the hips and knees are flexed, the knees are at unequal heights, with the dislocated side lower. After the first few weeks of life, x-ray examination becomes more valuable, with lateral displacement of the femoral head being the most reliable finding. In mild cases, the only abnormality may be increased steepness of acetabular alignment, so that the acetabular angle is greater than 35 degrees.

If congenital dislocation of the hip has not been diagnosed during the first year of life and the child begins to walk, there will be a painless limp and a lurch to the affected side. When the child stands on the affected leg, there is a dip of the pelvis on the opposite side owing to weakness of the gluteus medius muscle. In children with bilateral dislocations, the loss of abduction is almost symmetric and may be deceiving. Abduction, however, is never complete, and x-ray of the pelvis is indicated in children with incomplete abduction in the first few months of life. As a child with bilateral dislocation of the hips begins to walk, the gait is waddling. The perineum is widened as a result of lateral displacement of the hips, and there is flexion contracture as a result of posterior displacement of the hips. This flexion contracture contributes to marked lordosis, and the greater trochanters are easily palpable in their elevated position. Treatment is still possible in the first 2 years of life, but the results are not nearly as effective as in children treated in the nursery.

Treatment

Dislocation or dysplasia diagnosed in the first few weeks or months of life can easily be treated by splinting, with the hip maintained in flexion and abduction. Forced abduction is contraindicated, as this often leads to avascular necrosis of the femoral head. The use of double or triple diapers is never indicated for medical reasons, since diapers are not adequate to obtain proper positioning of the hip. In cases of joint laxity without true dislocation, improvement will be spontaneous and diapers are excessive treatment.

Various splints to maintain flexion and abduction of the hip, such as the ones designed by Pavlik, Ilfeld, or von Rosen, are available. Treatment of children requiring splints is best supervised by an orthopedic surgeon with a special interest in the problem.

In the first 4 months of life, reduction can be obtained by simply flexing and abducting the hip; no other manipulation is usually necessary. If force is used to reduce the hip, the excessive pressure may cause avascular necrosis. In such cases, preoperative traction for 2–3 weeks is important to relax soft tissues about the hip. Following traction in which the femur is brought down opposite the acetabulum, reduction can be easily achieved without force under general anesthesia. It is then necessary to place the child in a plaster cast, which is used for approximately 6 months. If the reduction is not stable within a reasonable range following closed reduction, open reduction may be necessary combined with plication of the lax capsule in order to maintain reduction.

If reduction is done at an older age, operations to correct the deformities of the acetabulum and femur may be necessary during growth.

4. TORTICOLLIS

Wryneck deformities in infancy may be due either to injury to the sternocleidomastoid muscle during delivery or to disease affecting the cervical spine. In the case of muscular deformity, the chin is rotated to the side opposite to the affected sternocleidomastoid muscle contracture, and the head is tilted toward the side of the contracture. A mass felt in the midportion of the sternocleidomastoid muscle does not represent a true tumor but fibrous transformation within the muscle.

In mild cases, passive stretching is usually effective. If the deformity has not been corrected by passive stretching within the first year of life, surgical division of the muscle will correct it. It is not necessary to excise the "tumor" of the sternocleidomastoid muscle, since this tends to resolve spontaneously. If the deformity is left untreated, an unsightly facial asymmetry will result.

Torticollis is occasionally associated with congenital deformities of the cervical spine, and x-rays of the spine are indicated in all cases.

Acute torticollis may follow upper respiratory infection or mild trauma in children. Rotatory subluxation of the upper cervical spine should be sought by appropriate x-ray views. Traction or a cervical collar usually results in resolution of the symptoms within 1 or 2 days.

GENERALIZED AFFECTIONS OF SKELETON OR MESODERMAL TISSUES

1. ARTHROGRYPOSIS MULTIPLEX CONGENITA
(Amyoplasia Congenita)

Arthrogryposis multiplex congenita consists of incomplete fibrous ankylosis (usually symmetric) of many or all of the joints of the body. There may be contractures either in flexion or extension. Upper extremity deformities usually consist of adduction of the shoulders, extension of the elbows, flexion of the wrists, and stiff, straight fingers with poor muscle control of the thumbs. In the lower extremities, common deformities are dislocation of the hips, extension of the knees, and severe clubfoot. The joints are fusiform and the joint capsules decreased in volume, producing contractures. Various investigations have attributed the basic defect to an abnormality of muscle or of the lower motor neuron. Muscular development is poor, and muscles may be represented only by fibrous bands. The joint deformities appear to be secondary to a lack of active motion during intrauterine development.

2. MARFAN'S SYNDROME

Marfan's syndrome is characterized by unusually long fingers and toes (arachnodactyly); hypermobility of the joints; subluxation of the ocular lenses; other eye abnormalities including cataract, coloboma, megalocornea, strabismus, and nystagmus; a high-arched palate; a strong tendency to scoliosis; pectus carinatum; and thoracic aneurysms due to weakness of the media of the vessels. Serum mucoproteins may be decreased and urinary excretion of hydroxyproline increased. The condition is easily confused with homocystinuria, as the phenotypic presentation is identical. The 2 diseases may be differentiated by the presence of homocystine in the urine in homocystinuria.

Treatment is usually supportive for associated problems such as flatfeet. Scoliosis may involve more vigorous treatment by bracing or spine fusion. The long-term prognosis has improved for patients as better treatment for their aortic aneurysms has been devised.

3. CRANIOFACIAL DYSOSTOSIS
(Crouzon's Disease)

Craniofacial dysostosis is a syndrome consisting of acrocephaly, hypoplastic maxilla, beaked nose, protrusion of the lower lip, exophthalmos, exotropia, and hypertelorism. It is usually familial. No orthopedic treatment is necessary. Heroic efforts have been made by neurosurgeons and plastic surgeons to correct the grotesque deformity of patients, who generally have normal intelligence. These operative procedures are complicated and hazardous, involving multiple osteotomies of the skull and facial bones.

4. KLIPPEL-FEIL SYNDROME

Klippel-Feil syndrome is characterized by fusion of some or all of the cervical vertebrae. Multiple spinal anomalies may be present, with hemivertebrae and scoliosis. The neck is short and stiff, the hairline is low, and the ears are often low-set. Common associated defects include congenital scoliosis, cervical rib, spina bifida, torticollis, web neck, high scapula, renal anomalies, and deafness. Examination of the urinary tract by urinalysis, blood urea nitrogen, and intravenous urograms is indicated as well as a hearing test.

Scoliotic deformities, if progressive, may require treatment. Occasionally, it is necessary to correct the high scapula, also called Sprengel's deformity.

5. OSTEOGENESIS IMPERFECTA

Osteogenesis imperfecta is a rare, mainly dominantly inherited connective tissue disease. The severe fetal type (osteogenesis imperfecta congenita) is characterized by multiple intrauterine or perinatal fractures. Affected children continue to have fractures and are dwarfed as a result of bony deformities and growth retardation. Intelligence is not affected. The shafts of the long bones are reduced in cortical thickness, and wormian bones are present in the skull. Other features include blue scleras, thin skin, hyperextensibility of ligaments, "otosclerosis" with significant hearing loss, and hypoplastic and deformed teeth. Recurrent epistaxis, easy bruisability, mild hyperpyrexia (which may increase significantly during anesthesia), and excessive diaphoresis are common. In the tarda type, fractures begin to occur at variable times after the perinatal period, resulting in relatively fewer fractures and deformities in these cases. The patients are sometimes suspected of having suffered induced fractures, and the condition should be ruled out in any case of nonaccidental trauma.

Metabolic defects include elevated serum pyrophosphate, decreased platelet aggregation, and decreased incorporation of sulfate into acid mucopolysaccharides by skin fibroblasts. Normal parents can be counseled that the likelihood of a second affected child is negligible.

There is no effective treatment by medication. Surgical treatment involves correction of deformity of the long bones. Multiple intramedullary rods have been used to prevent deformity from poor healing of fractures.

The overall prognosis is poor, and patients are often confined to wheelchairs during adulthood.

6. ACHONDROPLASIA
(Classic Chondrodystrophy)

In achondroplasia, the arms and legs are short, with the upper arms and thighs proportionately shorter than the forearms and legs. Findings frequently include bowing of the extremities, a waddling gait, limitation of motion of major joints, relaxation of the ligaments, short stubby fingers of almost equal length, a prominent forehead, moderate hydrocephalus, depressed nasal bridge, and lumbar lordosis. Mentality and sexual function are normal. A family history is often present. X-rays demonstrate short, thick tubular bones and irregular epiphyseal plates. The ends of the bones are thick, with broadening and cupping. Epiphyseal ossification may be delayed. The medullary canal is narrowed, so that herniated disk in adulthood may lead to acute paraplegia.

7. OSTEOCHONDRODYSTROPHY
(Morquio's Disease)

Osteochondrodystrophy is characterized by shortening of the spine, kyphosis, scoliosis, moderate shortening of the extremities, pectus carinatum, protuberant abdomen, hepatosplenomegaly, and a waddling gait resulting from instability of the hips and laxity of the knee joints. The skull is minimally involved. The child may appear normal at birth but begins to develop deformities between 1 and 4 years of age as a result of abnormal deposition of mucopolysaccharides. The disorder is commonly familial. Inheritance appears to be on an autosomal recessive basis.

X-rays demonstrate wedge-shaped flattened vertebrae and irregular, malformed epiphyses. The ribs are broad and have been likened to canoe paddles. The lower extremities are more severely involved than the upper ones.

There is no treatment, and the prognosis is poor. Death may occur in childhood or adolescence. Progressive clouding of the cornea leads to increasing visual impairment.

8. CHONDROECTODERMAL DYSPLASIA
(Ellis-van Creveld Syndrome)

Manifestations include ectodermal dysplasia, congenital heart disease, polydactyly, syndactyly, poorly formed teeth, and mental retardation. The disease is familial and inbred in certain ethnic groups such as the Amish people of Pennsylvania.

X-ray changes include chondrodystrophy; shortening and bowing of the tibias and fibulas; hyperplastic, eccentric proximal tibial metaphyses; and fusion of the carpal bones.

No treatment is available. The long-term prognosis depends on the severity of heart involvement.

GROWTH DISTURBANCES
OF THE MUSCULOSKELETAL SYSTEM

SCOLIOSIS

The term *scoliosis* denotes lateral curvature of the spine, which is always associated with some rotation of the involved vertebrae. Scoliosis is classified by its anatomic location, in either the thoracic or lumbar spine, with rare involvement of the cervical spine. The apex of the curve is designated right or left. Thus, a left thoracic scoliosis would denote a convex leftward curve in the thoracic region, and this is the most common type of idiopathic curve. Posterior curvature of the spine (kyphosis) is normal in the thoracic area, though excessive curvature may become pathologic. Anterior curvature is called lordosis and is normal in the lumbar spine. Idiopathic scoliosis generally begins at about 8 or 10 years of age and progresses during growth. In rare instances, infantile scoliosis may be seen in children 2 years of age or less.

Idiopathic scoliosis is about 4–5 times more common in girls than in boys. The disorder is usually asymptomatic in the adolescent years, but severe curvature may lead to impairment of pulmonary function or low back pain in later years. It is important to examine the back of any adolescent coming in for a physical examination. The examination is performed by having the patient bend forward 90 degrees with the hands joined in the midline. An abnormal finding consists of asymmetry of the height of the ribs or paravertebral muscles on one side, indicating rotation of the trunk associated with lateral curvature.

Diseases that may be associated with scoliosis include neurofibromatosis, Marfan's syndrome, cerebral palsy, muscular dystrophy, and poliomyelitis. Neurologic examination should be performed in all children with scoliosis to determine whether these disorders are present.

Five to 7% of cases of scoliosis are due to congenital vertebral anomalies such as a hemivertebral or unilateral vertebral bridge. These curves are more rigid than the more common idiopathic curve and will often increase with growth, especially during the rapid growth spurt during adolescence.

The most common type of scoliosis is so-called idiopathic scoliosis, which may be due to asymmetry of neuromuscular development. In 30% of cases, other family members are affected.

Postural compensation of the spine may lead to lateral curvature from such causes as unequal length of the lower extremities. Antalgic scoliosis may result from pressure on the spinal cord or roots by infectious processes or herniation of the nucleus pulposus; the underlying cause must be sought. The curvature will resolve as the primary problem is treated.

Clinical Findings

A. Symptoms and Signs: Scoliosis in adolescents is classically asymptomatic. It is imperative to seek the underlying cause in any case where there is pain, since in these instances the scoliosis is almost always secondary to some other disorder such as a bone or spinal cord tumor. Deformity of the rib cage and asymmetry of the waistline are evident with curvatures of 30 degrees or more. A lesser curvature may be detected by the forward bending test as described above, which is designed to detect early abnormalities of rotation that are not apparent when the patient is standing erect.

B. Imaging: The most valuable x-rays are those taken of the entire spine in the standing position in both the anteroposterior and lateral planes. Usually, there is one primary curvature with a compensatory curvature that develops to balance the body. At times there may be 2 primary curvatures, usually in the left thoracic and right lumbar regions. Any right thoracic curvature should be suspected of being secondary to neurologic or muscular disease, prompting a more meticulous neurologic examination.

Treatment

Curvatures of less than 20 degrees usually do not require treatment unless they show progression. Bracing is indicated for curvature of 20–40 degrees in a skeletally immature child. Treatment is indicated for any curvature that demonstrates progression on serial x-ray examination. Curvatures greater than 40 degrees are resistant to treatment by bracing. Thoracic curvatures greater than 60 degrees have been correlated with a poor pulmonary prognosis in adult life. Curvatures of such severity are an indication for surgical correction of the deformity and posterior spinal fusion to maintain the correction. Curvatures between 40 and 60 degrees may also require spinal fusion if they appear to be progressive, are causing decompensation of the spine, or are cosmetically unacceptable.

Prognosis

Compensated small curvatures that do not progress may be well tolerated throughout life, with very little cosmetic concern. The patients should be counseled regarding the genetic transmission of scoliosis and cautioned that their children should be examined at regular intervals during growth. Large thoracic curvatures greater than 60 degrees are associated with shortened life span and may progress even during adult life. Large lumbar curvatures may lead to subluxation of the vertebrae and premature arthritic degeneration of the spine, producing disabling pain in adulthood. Early detection allows for simple brace treatment or surface electrical stimulation. In patients so treated, the long-term prognosis is excellent and surgery is not necessary. For this reason, school screening programs for scoliosis have gained popular support in many sections of the country.

EPIPHYSIOLYSIS
(Slipped Capital Femoral Epiphysis)

Epiphysiolysis is the separation of the proximal femoral epiphysis through the growth plate. The head of the femur is usually displaced medially and posteriorly relative to the neck of the femur. The condition occurs in adolescence and is more common in overweight children. Slightly over 40% of the children so affected are of the obese, hypogenital body type.

Occasionally, the condition occurs as an acute episode resulting from a fall or direct trauma to the hip. This is called a fracture and must be differentiated. Commonly, there are vague symptoms over a protracted period of time in an otherwise healthy child who presents with pain and limp. The pain is often referred into the thigh or the medial side of the knee. It is important to examine the hip joint in any child complaining of knee pain, particularly in adolescents. The consistent finding on physical examination is limitation of internal rotation of the hip. There usually is also an associated hip flexion contracture as well as local tenderness about the hip. X-rays should be taken in both the anteroposterior and lateral planes. These must be carefully examined in early cases in order to show an abnormality where displacement of the femoral head occurs posteriorly, which is usually most easily seen on the lateral view.

Treatment is based on the same principles that govern treatment of fracture of the femoral neck in adults in that the head of the femur is fixed to the neck of the femur and the fracture line allowed to heal. Unfortunately, the severe complication of avascular necrosis occurs in 30% of these patients.

The long-term prognosis is guarded because most of these patients continue to be overweight and overstress their hip joints. Follow-up studies have shown a high incidence of premature degenerative arthritis in this group of patients—even those who do not develop avascular necrosis. The development of avascular necrosis almost guarantees a poor prognosis, since new bone does not replace the femoral head at this late stage of skeletal growth.

About 30% of patients have bilateral involvement, and patients should be followed for slipping of the opposite side, which may occur as long as 1 or 2 years after the primary episode.

GENU VARUM & GENU VALGUM

Genu varum (bowleg) is normal from infancy through 2 years of life. The alignment then changes to genu valgum (knock-knee) until about 8 years of age, at which time adult alignment is attained. Criteria for referral to an orthopedist include persistent bowing beyond age 2, bowing that is increasing rather than decreasing, bowing of one leg only, and knock-knee associated with short stature.

Bracing may be appropriate, or, rarely, an osteotomy is necessary for a severe problem such as Blount's disease (proximal tibial epiphyseal dysplasia).

TIBIAL TORSION

The physician is often asked about "toeing in" in small children. The disorder is routinely asymptomatic. Tibial torsion is rotation of the leg between the knee and the ankle. Internal rotation amounts to about 20 degrees at birth but decreases to neutral rotation by 1 year of age. The deformity is sometimes accentuated by laxity of the knee ligaments, allowing excessive internal rotation of the leg in small children. In children who have a persistent internal rotation of the tibia beyond 1 year of age, it is often due to sleeping with feet turned in and can be reversed with an external rotation splint worn only at night.

FEMORAL ANTEVERSION

"Toeing in" beyond 2 or 3 years of age is usually based on femoral anteversion, which produces excessive internal rotation of the femur as compared with external rotation. This femoral alignment follows a natural history of progressive decrease toward neutral up to 8 years of age, with slower change to 16 years of age. Studies comparing the results of treatment with shoes or braces to the natural history have shown that little is gained by active treatment. Active external rotation exercises such as ballet, skating, or bicycle riding may be worthwhile. Osteotomy for rotational correction is rarely required. Refer those who have no external rotation of hip in extension.

COMMON FOOT PROBLEMS

When a child begins to stand and walk, the long arch of the foot is flat with a medial bulge over the inner border of the foot. The forefeet are mildly pronated or rotated inward, with a slight valgus alignment of the knees. As the child grows and muscle power improves, the long arch is better supported and more normal relationships occur in the lower extremities. (See also Metatarsus Varus and Talipes Equinovarus.)

1. FLATFOOT

Flatfoot is a normal condition in infants. Children presenting for examinations should be checked to determine that the heel cord is of normal length when the heel is aligned in the neutral position, allowing complete dorsiflexion and plantar flexion. As long as the foot is supple and the presence of a longitudinal arch is noted when the child is sitting in a non–weight-bearing position, the parents can be assured that a normal arch will probably develop. There is usually a familial incidence of relaxed flatfeet in children who have prolonged malalignment of the foot. In any child with a shortened heel cord or stiffness of the foot, other causes of flatfoot such as tarsal coalition or vertical talus should be ruled out by a complete orthopedic examination and x-ray.

In the child with an ordinary relaxed flatfoot, no active treatment is indicated unless there is calf or leg pain. In children who have leg pains attributable to flatfeet, an orthopedic shoe with Thomas heel may relieve discomfort. An arch insert should not be prescribed unless passive correction of the arch is easily accomplished; otherwise, there will be irritation of the skin over the medial side of the foot.

2. TALIPES CALCANEOVALGUS

Talipes calcaneovalgus is characterized by excessive dorsiflexion at the ankle and eversion of the foot. It is often present at birth and almost always corrects spontaneously. The deformity is the reverse of classic clubfoot (talipes equinovarus) and is due to intrauterine position.

Treatment consists of passive exercises by the parents, stretching the foot into plantar flexion. In rare instances, it may be necessary to use plaster casts to help with manipulation and positioning.

Complete correction is the rule.

3. CAVUS FOOT

In cavus foot, the deformity consists of an unusually high longitudinal arch of the foot. It may be hereditary or associated with neurologic conditions such as poliomyelitis, Charcot-Marie-Tooth disease, Friedreich's ataxia, or diastematomyelia. There is usually an associated contracture of the toe extensor, producing a claw toe deformity in which the metatarsal phalangeal joints are hyperextended and the interphalangeal joints acutely flexed. Any child presenting with cavus feet should have a careful neurologic examination including x-rays of the spine.

In resistant cases that do not respond to shoe adjustments (metatarsal bars and supports), operation may be necessary to lengthen the contracted extensor and flexor tendons. Arthrodesis of the foot may be necessary later. If these feet are left untreated, they are often painful and limit walking.

The overall prognosis is much poorer than with low arch or pes planus.

4. CLAW TOES

In patients with claw toes, there is a flexion deformity of either or both interphalangeal joints, which results in the "claw." The condition is usually congenital and may be seen in association with disorders of motor weakness, such as Charcot-Marie-Tooth disease or pes cavus. Surgical correction can alleviate symptoms if the toes are painful.

5. BUNIONS
(Hallux Valgus)

Girls may present in adolescence with lateral deviation of the great toe associated with a prominence over the head of first metatarsal. This deformity is painful only with shoe wear and almost always can be relieved by fitting shoes that are wide enough. Surgery should be avoided in the adolescent age group, as the results are much less successful than in adult patients with the same condition.

DEGENERATIVE PROBLEMS
(Arthritis, Bursitis, & Tenosynovitis)

Degenerative arthritis may follow childhood skeletal problems such as infection, slipped capital femoral epiphysis, avascular necrosis, or trauma or may occur in association with hemophilia. Early effective treatment of these disorders will prevent arthritis. Late treatment is often unsatisfactory.

Degenerative changes in the soft tissues around joints may occur as a result of overuse syndrome in adolescent athletes. Young boys throwing excessive numbers of pitches, especially curve balls, may develop "little leaguer's elbow," consisting of degenerative changes around the humeral condyles associated with pain, swelling, and limitation of motion. In order to enforce the rest necessary for healing, a plaster cast may be necessary. A more reasonable preventive measure is to limit the number of pitches thrown by children.

Acute bursitis is quite uncommon in childhood, and other causes should be ruled out before this diagnosis is accepted.

Tenosynovitis is most common in the region of the knees and feet. Children taking dancing lessons, particularly toe dancing, may have pain around the flexor tendon sheaths in the toes or ankles. Rest is effective treatment. At the knee level, there may be irritation of the patellar ligament, with associated swelling in the infrapatellar fat pad. Synovitis in this area is usually due to overuse and is also treated by rest. Corticosteroid injections are contraindicated.

TRAUMA

SOFT TISSUE TRAUMA
(Sprains, Strains, & Contusions)

A sprain is the stretching of a ligament, and a strain is a stretch of a muscle or tendon. In either of these injuries, there may be some degree of tissue tearing. Contusions are generally due to tissue compression, with damage to blood vessels within the tissue and the formation of hematoma.

A severe sprain is one in which the ligament is completely divided, resulting in instability of the joint. A mild or moderate sprain is one in which incomplete tearing of the ligament occurs, but in which there is associated local pain and swelling.

If there is more severe trauma resulting in tearing of a ligament, instability of the joint may be demonstrated by gross examination or by stress testing with x-ray documentation. Such deformity of the joint may cause persistent instability resulting from inaccurate apposition of the ligament ends during healing. If instability is evident, surgical repair of the torn ligament is indicated. If a muscle is torn, usually at its end, it should be repaired.

The initial treatment of any sprain consists of ice, compression, and elevation. The purpose of the treatment is to decrease local edema and residual stiffness resulting from gelling of blood proteins in the interstitial space. Splinting of the affected joint protects against further injury and relieves swelling and pain.

1. ANKLE SPRAINS

The history will indicate that the injury was by either forceful inversion or eversion. The more common inversion injury results in tearing or injury to the lateral ligaments, whereas an eversion injury will injure the medial ligaments of the ankle. The injured ligaments may be identified by means of careful palpation for point tenderness around the ankle. The joint should be supported or immobilized at a right angle, which is the functional position. Prolonged use of a plaster cast is usually not necessary, but the sprained ankle should be rested sufficiently to allow complete healing. This may take 3–6 weeks. Because fractures usually receive more attention and adequate follow-up, the results are often better. A properly treated ankle sprain should not be the source of prolonged and repeated disability.

2. KNEE SPRAINS

Sprains of the collateral and cruciate ligaments are uncommon in children. These ligaments are so strong that it is more common to injure the epiphyseal growth plates, which are the weakest structures in the region of the knees of children. In adolescence, however, the joints and growth plates attain adult growth, and a rupture of the anterior cruciate ligament can result from a twisting injury that may avulse the anterior tibial spine. In such instances, the injury is apparent on physical examination and x-ray and requires anatomic reduction and immobilization for 6 weeks. In most instances, this means open operative correction.

3. BACK SPRAINS

Sprains of the ligaments and muscles of the back are unusual in children but may occur as a result of violent trauma from automobile accidents or athletic injuries. A child with back pain should not be presumed to have had trauma to the spine unless the history warrants that conclusion. The reason for back pain should be carefully sought by x-ray and physical examination. Inflammation, infection, and tumors are more common causes of back pain in children than sprains.

4. CONTUSIONS

Contusion of muscle with hematoma formation produces the familiar "charley horse" injury. Treatment of such injuries is by application of ice, compression, and rest. Exercise should be avoided for 5–7 days. Local heat may hasten once the acute phase of tenderness and swelling is past.

5. MYOSITIS OSSIFICANS

Ossification within muscle occurs when there is sufficient trauma to cause a hematoma that later heals in the manner of a fracture. The injury is usually a contusion and occurs most commonly in the quadriceps of the thigh or the triceps of the arm. When such a severe injury with hematoma is recognized, it is important to splint the extremity and avoid activity. If further activity is allowed, ossification may reach spectacular proportions and resemble an osteosarcoma.

Disability is great, with local swelling and heat and extreme pain upon the slightest motion of the adjacent joint. The limb should be rested, with the knee in extension or the elbow in 90 degrees of flexion, until the local reaction has subsided. Once local heat and tenderness have decreased, gentle active exercises may be initiated. Passive stretching exercises are not indicated, because they may stimulate the ossification reaction. It is occasionally necessary to excise excessive bony tissue if it interferes with muscle function once the reaction is mature. Surgery should not be attempted before 9 months to a year after injury, because it may restart the process and lead to an even more severe reaction.

TRAUMATIC SUBLUXATIONS & DISLOCATIONS

Dislocation of a joint is always associated with severe damage to the ligaments and joint capsule. In contrast to fracture treatment, which may be safely postponed, dislocations must be reduced immediately. Dislocations can usually be reduced by gentle sustained traction. It often happens that no anesthetic is necessary for several hours after the injury, because of the protective anesthesia produced by the injury. Following reduction, the joint should be splinted for transportation of the patient.

The dislocated joint should be treated by immobilization for at least 3 weeks, followed by graduated active exercises through a full range of motion. Physical therapy is usually not indicated for children with injuries. As a matter of fact, vigorous manipulation of the joint by a therapist may be harmful. The child should be permitted to perform therapy alone. No stretching should be permitted.

1. SUBLUXATION OF THE RADIAL HEAD
(Nursemaid's Elbow)

Infants frequently sustain subluxation of the radial head as a result of being lifted or pulled by the hand. The child appears with the elbow fully pronated and painful. The usual complaint is that the child's elbow will not bend. X-rays are normal, but there is point tenderness over the radial head. When the elbow is placed in full supination and slowly moved from full flexion to full extension, a click may be palpated at the level of the radial head. The relief of pain is remarkable, as the child usually stops crying immediately. The elbow may be immobilized in a sling for comfort for a day.

Pulled elbow may be a clue to battering. This should be remembered during examination, especially if the problem is recurrent.

2. RECURRENT DISLOCATION OF THE PATELLA

Recurrent dislocation of the patella is more common in loose-jointed individuals, especially adolescent girls. If the patella completely dislocates, it nearly always goes laterally. Pain is severe, and the patient is brought to the doctor with the knee slightly flexed and an obvious bony mass lateral to the knee joint and a flat area over the usual location of the patella anteriorly.

X-rays confirm the diagnosis. The patella may be reduced by extending the knee and placing slight pressure on the patella while gentle traction is exerted on the leg. In subluxation of the patella, the symptoms may be more subtle, and the patient may say that the knee "gives out" or "jumps out of place."

In the case of complete dislocation, the knee should be immobilized for 3–4 weeks, followed by a physical therapy program for strengthening the quadriceps muscle. Operation may be necessary to tighten the knee joint capsule if dislocation or subluxation is recurrent. In such instances, if the patella is not stabilized, repeated dislocation produces damage to the articular cartilage of the patellofemoral joint and premature degenerative arthritis.

EPIPHYSEAL SEPARATIONS

In children, epiphyseal separations and fractures are more common than ligamentous injuries. This finding is based on the fact that the ligaments of the joints are generally stronger than the associated growth plates. In instances where dislocation is suspected, an x-ray should be taken in order to rule out epiphyseal fracture. Films of the opposite extremity, especially around the elbow, may be valuable for comparison. Reduction of a fractured epiphysis should be done under anesthesia in order to align the growth plate with the least amount of force necessary. Fractures across the growth plate may produce bony bridges that will cause premature cessation of growth or angular deformities in the growth plate. Epiphyseal fractures around the shoulder, wrist, and fingers can usually be treated by closed reduction, but fractures of the epiphyses around the elbow often require open reduction. In the lower extremity, accurate reduction of the epiphyseal plate is necessary to prevent joint deformity if a joint surface is involved. Unfortunately, some of the most severe injuries to the epiphyseal plate occur from compression injuries, where the amount of force is not immediately apparent. If angular deformities result, corrective osteotomy should be necessary.

TORUS FRACTURES

Torus fractures consist of "buckling" of the cortex as a result of minimal angular trauma. They usually occur in the distal radius or ulna. Alignment is satisfactory, and simple immobilization for 3–5 weeks is sufficient.

GREENSTICK FRACTURES

With greenstick fractures there is frank disruption of the cortex on one side of the bone but no discernible cleavage plane on the opposite side. These fractures are angulated but not displaced, as the bone ends are not separated. Reduction is achieved by straightening the arm into normal alignment, and reduction is maintained by a snugly fitting plaster cast. It is necessary to x-ray children with greenstick fractures again in a week to 10 days to make certain that the reduction has been maintained in plaster. A slight angular deformity will be corrected by remodeling of the bone. The farther the fracture is from the growing end of the bone, the longer the time required for healing. The fracture can be considered healed when there are no findings of tenderness and local swelling or heat and when adequate bony callus is seen on x-ray.

FRACTURE OF THE CLAVICLE

Clavicular fractures are very common injuries in infants and children. They can be immobilized by a figure-of-8 dressing that retracts the shoulders and brings the clavicle to normal length. The healing callus will be apparent when the fracture has consolidated, but this unsightly lump will generally resolve over a period of months to a year.

SUPRACONDYLAR FRACTURES OF THE HUMERUS

Supracondylar fractures tend to occur in the age group from 3 to 6 years and are potentially dangerous because of the proximity to the brachial artery in the distal arm. They are usually associated with a significant amount of trauma, so that swelling may be severe. Volkmann's ischemic contracture of muscle may occur as a result of vascular embarrassment. When severe swelling is present, the safest course is to place the arm in traction and carefully observe nerve function and the vascular supply to the hand. In these cases, the children should be hospitalized. If the blood supply is compromised, exposure of the brachial artery may be necessary, although this is rarely needed when satisfactory reduction and traction are employed. Complications associated with supracondylar fractures also include a resultant cubitus valgus secondary to poor reduction. It is often difficult to ascertain adequacy of the reduction because a flexed position is necessary to maintain normal alignment. Such a "gun-stock" deformity of the elbow may be somewhat unsightly but does not usually interfere with joint function.

GENERAL COMMENTS ON OTHER FRACTURES IN CHILDREN

Reduction of fractures in children is usually accomplished by simple traction and manipulation; open reduction is not commonly indicated. Remodeling of the fracture callus will usually produce an almost normal appearance of the bone over a matter of months. The younger the child, the more remodeling is possible. Angular deformities remodel with ease. Rotatory deformities do not remodel, and this produces the cubitus valgus deformity sometimes seen after supracondylar fractures.

The physician should be suspicious of child battering whenever the age of a fracture does not match the history given or when the severity of the injury is more than the alleged accident would have produced. In suspected cases of battering where no fracture is present on the initial x-ray, a repeat film 10 days later is in order. Bleeding beneath the periosteum will be calcified by 7–10 days, and the x-ray appearance is almost diagnostic of severe closed trauma characteristic of a battered child.

INFECTIONS OF THE BONES & JOINTS

OSTEOMYELITIS

Osteomyelitis is an infectious process that usually starts in the spongy or medullary bone and then extends to involve compact or cortical bone. It is more common in boys than in girls or in adults of either sex. The lower extremities are most often affected, and there is commonly a history of trauma. Osteomyelitis may occur as a result of direct invasion from the outside through a penetrating wound (nail) or open fracture, but hematogenous spread of infection (eg, pyoderma or upper respiratory tract infection) from other infected areas is more common. The most common infecting organism is *Staphylococcus aureus*, which seems to have a special tendency to infect the metaphyses of growing bones. Anatomically, circulation in the long bones is such that the arterial supply to the metaphysis just below the growth plate is by end arteries, which turn sharply to end in venous sinusoids, causing a relative stasis. In the infant under 1 year of age, there is direct vascular communication with the epiphysis across the growth plate, so that direct spread may occur from the metaphysis to the epiphysis and subsequently into the joint. In the older child, the growth plate provides an effective barrier and the epiphysis is usually not involved, although the infection spreads retrograde from the metaphysis into the diaphysis and, by rupture through the cortical bone, down along the diaphysis beneath the periosteum.

1. EXOGENOUS OSTEOMYELITIS

In order to avoid osteomyelitis by direct extension, all wounds must be carefully examined and cleansed. Puncture wounds are especially liable to lead to osteomyelitis if not carefully debrided. Cultures of the wound made at the time of exploration and debridement may be useful if signs of inflammation and infection develop subsequently. In extensive or contaminated wounds, antibiotic coverage is indicated. Contaminated wounds should be left open and secondary closure performed 3–5 days later. If at the time of delayed closure further necrotic tissue is present, it should be excised.

Parenteral administration of antibiotics is satisfactory, and local irrigation is not needed. If the wound is acquired outside the hospital, penicillin is adequate for most wounds. After cultures have been read, an appropriate alternative antibiotic can be chosen if there is lingering inflammation. A tetanus toxoid booster is indicated for any questionable wound.

Once exogenous osteomyelitis has become established, treatment becomes more complicated, requiring extensive surgical debridement and drainage followed by careful antibiotic management. These cases require hospitalization and the use of intravenous antibiotics.

2. HEMATOGENOUS OSTEOMYELITIS

Hematogenous osteomyelitis is usually caused by pyrogenic bacteria; 85% of cases are due to staphylococci. Streptococci are rare causes of osteomyelitis today, but *Pseudomonas* organisms have often been documented in cases of nail puncture wounds. Children with sickle cell anemia are especially prone to osteomyelitis caused by salmonellae.

Clinical Findings

A. Symptoms and Signs: In infants, the manifestations of osteomyelitis may be quite subtle, presenting as irritability, diarrhea, or failure to feed properly; the temperature may be normal or slightly low; and the white blood count may be normal or only slightly elevated. In older children, the manifestations are more striking, with severe local tenderness and pain, high fever, rapid pulse, and elevated white blood cell count and sedimentation rate. Osteomyelitis of a lower extremity often presents around the knee in a child 7–10 years of age. Tenderness is most marked over the metaphysis of the bone where the process has its origin.

B. Laboratory Findings: Blood cultures are often positive early. The most significant test in infancy is the aspiration of pus when suspicion arises because of lack of movement in a painful extremity. It is useful to insert a needle to the bone in the area of suspected infection and aspirate any fluid present. This fluid can be smeared and stained for organisms as well as cultured. Even edema fluid may be useful for determining the causative organism. The white blood cell count is usually elevated, as is the sedimentation rate.

C. Imaging: The first manifestations to appear on x-ray is nonspecific local swelling. This is followed by elevation of the periosteum, with formation of new bone from the cambium layer of the periosteum occurring after 3–6 days. As the infection becomes chronic, areas of cortical bone are isolated by pus spreading down the medullary canal, causing rarefaction and demineralization of the bone. Such isolated pieces of cortex become ischemic and form sequestra (dead bone fragments). These x-ray findings are late, and osteomyelitis should be diagnosed clinically before significant x-ray findings are present. Bone scan is valuable in suspected cases before x-rays become positive.

Treatment

A. Specific Measures: Antibiotics should be started intravenously as soon as the diagnosis of osteomyelitis is made. Use of methicillin, another semisynthetic penicillin, or a cephalosporin that covers penicillinase-producing *S aureus* is recommended. Gentamicin can also be given to combat gram-negative organisms until the results of cultures are available. Antibiotics should be continued until swelling, tenderness, and local discharge have ceased and the white blood cell count and erythrocyte sedimentation rate are normal. Serial x-rays can also be used to follow bone healing. Antibiotic therapy by the intravenous route should be continued until all clinical signs are improved, including sedimentation rate. For a reliable family, oral medication may be started at that time (about 10 days), adjusting dosage by serum killing power and continued monitoring of erythrocyte sedimentation rate for at least 1 month after the rate has returned to normal.

B. General Measures: Splinting of the limb minimizes pain and decreases spread of the infection by lymphatic channels through the soft tissue. The splint should be removed periodically to allow active use of adjacent joints and prevent stiffening and muscle atrophy. In chronic osteomyelitis, splinting may be necessary to guard against fracture of the weakened bone.

C. Surgical Measures: Aspiration of the metaphysis is a useful diagnostic measure in any case of suspected osteomyelitis. Osteomyelitis represents a collection of pus under pressure within the body. In the first 24–72 hours, it may be possible to abort osteomyelitis by the use of antibiotics alone. However, if frank pus is aspirated from the bone, surgical drainage is indicated. If the infection has not shown a dramatic response to antibiotics within 24 hours in questionable cases, surgical drainage is also indicated. It is important that all devitalized soft tissue be removed and adequate exposure of the bone obtained in order to permit free drainage. Excessive amounts of bone should not be removed when draining acute osteomyelitis, since they may not be completely replaced by the normal healing process.

In questionable cases, little damage has been done by surgical drainage, but failure to drain the pus in acute cases may lead to more severe damage.

Prognosis

When osteomyelitis is diagnosed in the early clinical stages and prompt antibiotic therapy is begun, the prognosis is excellent. If the process has been unattended for a week to 10 days, there is almost always some permanent loss of bone structure, as well as the possibility of growth abnormality.

PYOGENIC ARTHRITIS

The source of pyogenic arthritis varies according to the age of the child. In the infant, pyogenic arthritis often develops by spread from adjacent osteomyelitis. In the older child, it presents as an isolated infection, usually without bony involvement. In teenagers with pyogenic arthritis, an underlying systemic disease is usually the cause, eg, an obvious generalized infection or an organism that has an affinity for joints, such as the gonococcus.

In infants, the most common cause of pyogenic arthritis is *S aureus,* although gram-negative organisms may be seen. In children between 4 months and 4 years of age, *Haemophilus influenzae* is a common causative organism.

The initial effusion of the joint rapidly becomes purulent. An effusion of the joint may accompany osteomyelitis in the adjacent bone. A white blood cell count exceeding $100,000/\mu L$ in the joint fluid indicates a definite purulent infection. Generally, spread of infection is from the bone into the joint, but unattended pyogenic arthritis may also affect adjacent bone. The sedimentation rate is elevated.

Clinical Findings

A. Symptoms and Signs: In older children, the signs are striking, with fever, malaise, vomiting, and restriction of motion. In infants, paralysis of the limb due to inflammatory neuritis may be evident. Infection of the hip joint in infants can be diagnosed if suspicion is aroused by decreased abduction of the hip in an infant who is irritable or feeding poorly. A history of umbilical catheter treatment in the newborn nursery should alert the physician to the possibility of pyogenic arthritis of the hip.

B. Imaging: Early distention of the joint capsule is nonspecific and difficult to measure by x-ray. In the infant with unrecognized pyogenic arthritis, dislocation of the joint may follow within a few days as a result of distention of the capsule by pus. Later changes include destruction of the joint space, resorption of epiphyseal cartilage, and erosion of the adjacent bone of the metaphysis.

Treatment

Diagnosis may be made by aspiration of the joint. In the hip joint, pyogenic arthritis is most easily treated by surgical drainage because the joint is deep and difficult to aspirate as well as being inaccessible to thorough cleaning through needle aspiration. In more superficial joints, such as the knee, aspiration of the joint at least twice daily may maintain adequate drainage. If fever and clinical symptoms do not subside within 24 hours after treatment is begun, open surgical drainage is indicated. Antibiotics can be specifically selected based on cultures of the aspirated pus. Before the results of cultures are available, treatment by methicillin and gentamicin will cover the usual etiologic organisms. It is not necessary to give intra-articular antibiotics, since good levels are achieved in the synovial fluid.

Prognosis

The prognosis is excellent if the joint is drained early, before damage to the articular cartilage has occurred. If infection is present for more than 24 hours, there is dissolution of the proteoglycans in the articular cartilage, with subsequent arthrosis and fibrosis of the joint. Damage to the growth plate may also occur, especially within the hip joint, where the epiphyseal plate is intracapsular.

TRANSIENT ("TOXIC") SYNOVITIS OF THE HIP

The most common cause of limping and pain in the hip of children in the USA is transitory synovitis, an acute inflammatory reaction that often follows an upper respiratory infection and is generally self-limited. In questionable cases, aspiration of the hip yields only yellowish fluid, ruling out pyogenic arthritis. Generally, however, toxic synovitis of the hip is not associated with elevation of the white blood cell count or a temperature above 38.3°C (101°F). It classically affects children 3–10 years of age and is more common in boys. There is limitation of motion of the hip joint, particularly internal rotation, and x-ray changes are nonspecific, with some swelling apparent in the soft tissues around the joint.

Treatment consists of bed rest and the use of traction with slight flexion of the hip. Aspirin may shorten the course of the disease, although even with no treatment the disease usually is self-limited to a matter of days. It is important to maintain x-ray follow-up, since transient synovitis may be the precursor of avascular necrosis of the femoral head (see next section) in a small percentage of patients. X-rays can be obtained at 1 month and 3 months, or earlier if there is persistent limp or pain.

VASCULAR LESIONS & AVASCULAR NECROSIS

AVASCULAR NECROSIS OF THE PROXIMAL FEMUR
(Legg-Calvé-Perthes Disease)

The vascular supply of bone is generally precarious, and when it is interrupted, necrosis results. In contrast to other body tissues that undergo infarction, bone removes necrotic tissue and replaces it with living bone in a process called "creeping substitution." This replacement of necrotic bone may be so complete and so perfect that a completely normal bone results. Adequacy of replacement depends upon the age of the patient, the presence or absence of associated infection, congruity of the involved joint, and other physiologic and mechanical factors.

Because of their rapid growth in relation to their blood supply, the secondary ossification centers in the epiphyses are subject to avascular necrosis. Even though the pathologic and radiologic features of avascular necrosis of the epiphyses are well known, the cause is not generally agreed upon. Necrosis may follow known causes such as trauma or infection, but idiopathic lesions usually develop during periods of rapid growth of the epiphyses. Thus, the highest incidence of Legg-Calvé-Perthes disease is between 4 and 8 years of age.

Clinical Findings

A. Symptoms and Signs: Persistent pain is the most common symptom, and the patient may present with limp or limitation of motion.

B. Laboratory Findings: Laboratory findings, including studies of joint aspirates, are normal.

C. Imaging: X-ray findings correlate with the progression of the process and the extent of necrosis. The early finding is effusion of the joint associated with slight widening of the joint space and periarticular swelling. Decreased bone density in and around the joint is apparent after a few weeks. The necrotic ossification center appears more dense than the surrounding viable structures, and there is collapse or narrowing of the femoral head.

As replacement of the necrotic ossification center occurs, there is rarefaction of the bone in a patchwork fashion, producing alternating areas of rarefaction and relative density or "fragmentation" of the epiphysis.

In the hip, there may be widening of the femoral head associated with flattening, giving rise to the term coxa plana. If infarction has extended across the growth plate, there will be a radiolucent lesion within the metaphysis. If the growth center of the femoral head has been damaged so that normal growth does not occur, varus deformity of the femoral neck will occur as a result of overgrowth of the greater trochanteric apophysis.

Eventually, complete replacement of the epiphysis will become apparent as new bone replaces necrotic bone. The final shape of the head will depend upon the extent of the necrosis and collapse that has been allowed to occur.

Differential Diagnosis

Differential diagnosis must include inflammatory and infectious lesions of the joints or apophyses. Transient synovitis of the hip may be distinguished from Legg-Calvé-Perthes disease by serial x-rays.

Treatment

Treatment consists simply of protection of the joint. If the joint is deeply seated within the acetabulum and normal joint motion is maintained, a reasonably good result can be expected. The hip is held in abduction and internal rotation in order to fulfill this purpose. Braces are generally used. Surgery may be necessary for an uncooperative patient or one whose social or geographic circumstances do not allow use of a brace.

Prognosis

The prognosis for complete replacement of the necrotic femoral head in a child is excellent, but the functional result will depend upon the amount of deformity that develops during the time the softened structure exists. In Legg-Calvé-Perthes disease, the prognosis depends upon the completeness of involvement of the epiphyseal center. In general, patients with metaphyseal defects, those in whom the disease develops late in childhood, and those who have more complete involvement of the femoral head have a poorer prognosis.

OSTEOCHONDRITIS DISSECANS

In osteochondritis dissecans, there is a pie-shaped necrotic area of bone and cartilage adjacent to the articular surface. The fragment of bone may be broken off from the host bone and displaced into the joint as a loose body. If it remains attached, the necrotic fragment may be completely replaced by creeping substitution.

The pathologic process is precisely the same as that described above for avascular necrosing lesions of ossification centers. However, since these lesions are adjacent to articular cartilage, there may be joint damage.

The most common sites of these lesions are the knee (medial femoral condyle), the elbow joint (capitellum), and the talus (superior lateral dome).

Joint pain is the usual presenting complaint. However, local swelling or locking may be present, particularly if there is a fragment free in the joint. Laboratory studies are normal.

Treatment consists of protection of the involved area from mechanical damage. If there is a fragment free within the joint as a loose body, it must be surgically removed. For some marginal lesions, it may be worthwhile to drill the necrotic fragment in order to encourage more rapid vascular ingrowth and replacement. If large areas of a weight-bearing joint are involved, secondary degenerative arthritis may result.

MISCELLANEOUS DISEASES OF BONE

FIBROUS DYSPLASIA

Dysplastic fibrous tissue replacement of the medullary canal is accompanied by the formation of metaplastic bone in fibrous dysplasia. Three forms of the disease are recognized: monostotic, polyostotic, and polyostotic with endocrine disturbances (precocious puberty in females, hyperthyroidism, and hyperadrenalism, ie, Albright's syndrome).

Clinical Findings
A. Symptoms and Signs: The lesion or lesions may be asymptomatic. Pain, if present, is probably due to pathologic fractures. In females, endocrine disturbances may be present in the polyostotic variety and associated with café au lait spots.

B. Laboratory Findings: Laboratory findings are normal unless endocrine disturbances are present, in which case there may be increased secretion of gonadotropic, thyroid, or adrenal hormones.

C. Imaging: The lesion begins centrally within the medullary canal, usually of a long bone, and expands slowly. Pathologic fracture may occur. If metaplastic bone predominates, the contents of the lesion will be of the density of bone. Marked deformity of the bone may result, and a shepherd's crook deformity of the upper femur is a classic feature of the disease. The disease is often asymmetric, and limb length disturbances may occur as a result of stimulation of epiphyseal cartilage growth.

Differential Diagnosis
The differential diagnosis may include other fibrous lesions of bone as well as destructive lesions such as bone cyst, eosinophilic granuloma, aneurysmal bone cyst, nonossifying fibroma, enchondroma, and chondromyxoid fibroma.

Treatment

If the lesion is small and asymptomatic, no treatment is needed. If the lesion is large and produces or threatens pathologic fracture, curettage and bone grafting are indicated.

Prognosis

Unless the lesions impair epiphyseal growth, the prognosis is good. Lesions tend to enlarge during the growth period but are stable during adult life. Malignant transformation has not been recorded.

UNICAMERAL BONE CYST

Unicameral bone cyst appears in the metaphysis of a long bone, usually in the femur or humerus. It begins within the medullary canal adjacent to the epiphyseal cartilage. It probably results from some fault in enchondral ossification. The cyst is "active" when it abuts onto the metaphyseal side of the epiphyseal cartilage and "inactive" when a border of normal bone exists between the cyst and the epiphyseal cartilage. The lesion is usually identified when a pathologic fracture occurs, producing pain. Laboratory findings are normal. On x-rays, the cyst is identified centrally within the medullary canal, producing expansion of the cortex and thinning over the widest portion of the cyst.

Treatment consists of curettage of the cyst if it is producing pain. The cyst may heal after a fracture and not require treatment. Curettage should be delayed if surgery would risk damage to the adjacent growth plate. In such cases, methylprednisolone injection may be curative.

The prognosis is excellent. Some cysts will heal following pathologic fracture.

ANEURYSMAL BONE CYST

Aneurysmal bone cyst is similar to unicameral bone cyst, but it contains blood rather than clear fluid. It usually occurs in a slightly eccentric position in the long bone, expanding the cortex of the bone but not breaking the cortex, although some extraosseous mass may be produced. On x-rays, the lesion appears somewhat larger than the width of the epiphyseal cartilage, and this feature distinguishes it from unicameral bone cyst.

The aneurysmal bone cyst is filled by large vascular lakes, and the stoma of the cyst contains fibrous tissue and areas of metaplastic ossification.

The lesion may appear quite aggressive histologically, and it is important to differentiate it from osteosarcoma or hemangioma. Treatment is by curettage and bone grafting, and the prognosis is excellent.

GANGLION

A ganglion is a smooth, small cystic mass connected by a pedicle to the joint capsule, usually on the dorsum of the wrist. It may also be seen in the tendon sheath over the flexor surfaces of the fingers. These ganglions can be excised if they interfere with function or cause persistent pain.

BAKER'S CYST

Baker's cyst is a herniation of the synovium in the knee joint into the popliteal region. In children, the diagnosis may be made by aspiration of mucinous fluid, but the cyst nearly always disappears with time. Whereas Baker's cysts may be indicative of intraarticular disease in the adult, they usually are of no clinical significance in children and rarely require excision, usually resolving spontaneously by age 5 years.

27 | Neuromuscular Disorders

W. Davis Parker, Jr MD, Paul G. Moe,
Alan Seay, MD

ABNORMAL HEAD SIZE

General Considerations:
Head size reflects brain growth. The average head circumference in males is about 1 cm larger than in females from term birth on, except during girls' earlier pubertal spurt. Generally, taller and heavier people have larger heads; parental head sizes do influence the child's head size. Head circumference should be measured at each well-child visit (oftener if indicated) and plotted on a graph of standard head circumference based on sex.

MICROCEPHALY

A head circumference 3 SD or more below the mean for age and sex, or a head circumference increasing too slowly or not at all denotes microcephaly. A head circumference of near 2 SD below the mean and falling off is equally significant.

Etiology
The causes of microcephaly with irreparable interference to brain development are provided in Table 27–1.

A head size *small at birth* proves intrauterine onset; a baby suffering asphyxia *at birth* will have normal newborn head size, which may later slow down in growth.

Family history of small heads and measurement of close relatives may aid in diagnosing (rare) autosomal dominant microcephaly.

Clinical Findings
A. Symptoms and Signs: Microcephaly may be discovered when the child is examined because of delayed developmental milestones or neurologic problems. There may be a marked backward slope of the forehead, as in familial microcephaly, with

824

Table 27–1. Causes and examples of irreparable microcephaly.

Cause	Examples
Prenatal chromosomal	Trisomy 13, 18, 21
Malformation	Lissenencephaly, schizencephaly
Syndromes	Rubenstein-Taybi, Cornelia de Lange
Toxins	Alcohol, anticonvulsants (?), maternal PKU*
Infections (intrauterine)	TORCHES†
Radiation	Maternal pelvis, 1st and 2nd trimester
Placenta insufficiency	Toxemia, infection
Familial	AD, AR (autosomal dominant, recessive)
Perinatal hypoxia, trauma	Birth asphyxia, injury
Infections (perinatal)	Bacterial meningitis (especially Group B Strep) Viral encephalitis (Coxsackie B, Herpes II)
Metabolic	Hypoglycemia, PKU,* MSUD‡
Postnatal sequela from earlier insult	As above
Degenerative Disease	Tay Sachs, Krabbe's

*Phenylketonuria.
†Toxoplasmosis, Rubella, Cytomegalovirus, Herpes Simplex, Syphilis.
‡Maple syrup urine disease.

narrowing of the bitemporal diameter; and there may be occipital flattening that is not positional. The fontanel may be closed earlier than expected; sutures may be unexpectedly prominent.

B. Laboratory Findings: These vary with the cause. If clinical factors warrant, TORCH titers must be assessed. Elevated IgM titer, if available at birth, is most helpful; comparison to maternal titers, passive transfer to the infant, and rising titer postnatally are all important factors to analyze. Amino and organic acid screens on the baby are occasionally diagnostic. The mother may need to be screened for PKU. Karyotyping should be considered.

C. Imaging: Skull films are indicated if there is suspicion of craniosynostosis. Sometimes microcephaly causes secondary acquired craniosynostosis. CT or MRI brain imaging may aid in diagnosis (eg, of intracranial calcification, malformations, atrophy) and prognosis.

Treatment & Prognosis

Treatment is usually supportive and directed at the multiple neurologic and sensory deficits and any endocrine disturbances (eg, diabetes insipidus) encountered. Catch-up growth after correction of an underlying metabolic disturbance may rarely occur. Many children with head circumferences more than 2 SD below the mean show variable degrees of mental retardation.

ELECTROENCEPHALOGRAPHY

EEG has its most distinct clinical applicability in the study of seizure disorders. "Activation" techniques (photic stimulation, well-sustained hyperventilation for 3 minutes, and depriving the patient of sleep) may accentuate abnormalities or disclose latent abnormalities. The EEG has a role in assessing brain maturation, for example in sleep ontogeny in the newborn.

EEG is also used in the evaluation of tumors, cerebrovascular accidents, neurodegenerative diseases, and other neurologic disorders causing brain dysfunction. However, with some notable exceptions, it is nonspecific. Recordings over a 24-hour period or all-night recordings are invaluable in the diagnosis of sleep disturbances such as sleep apnea and narcolepsy. The electroencephalogram can be helpful in determining a possible cause or mechanism of coma and is frequently used to determine whether the coma is irreversible and brain death has occurred.

The limitations of EEG are considerable, and results are often misinterpreted. In most cases, the duration of the actual tracing is only about 45 minutes, and records only a very small fraction of the brain's overall activity. About 15% of normal (nonepileptic) individuals, especially children, may show some paroxysmal activity on EEG. Electroencephalographic findings such as those seen in migraine, learning disabilities, or behavior disorders may not reflect permanent "brain damage."

Evoked Potentials

Cortical auditory, visual, or somatosensory evoked potentials (evoked responses) may be recorded from the scalp surface over the temporal, occipital, or frontoparietal cortex after repetitive stimulation of the retina by light flashes, of the cochlea by sounds, or of the skin by galvanic stimuli of varying frequency and intensity, respectively. Computer averaging is used to recognize and enhance these responses while subtracting or suppressing the asynchronous background electroencephalographic activity. The presence or absence of evoked potential waves and their latencies (time from stimulus to wave peak or time between peaks) figure in the clinical interpretation. While results of these tests alone are usually not diagnostic, the tests are noninvasive, sensitive, objective, and relatively inexpensive extensions of the clinical neurologic examination. Since the auditory and somato-sensory tests and one type of visual test are totally passive, requiring only that the patient remain still, they are particularly useful in the evaluation of functions in neonates and small children as well as in patients unable to cooperate (eg, due to mental retardation, degenerative disorder, anesthesia, or coma).

Brainstem Auditory Evoked Potentials

A brief auditory stimulus (click) of varying intensity and frequency is delivered to the ear to activate the auditory nerve (nerve VIII) and sequentially activate the cochlear nucleus, tracts and nuclei of the lateral lemniscus, and inferior colliculus. Thus, this technique assesses hearing and function of the brainstem auditory tracts.

Pattern-Shift Visual Evoked Potentials

The preferred stimulus is a shift (reversal) of a checkerboard pattern, and the response is a single wave (called P100) generated in the striate and parastriate visual cortex. The absolute latency of P100 (time from stimulus to wave peak) and the difference in latency between the 2 eyes are sensitive indicators of disease. The amplitude of response is affected by any process resulting in poor fixation on the stimulus screen or affecting visual acuity. Ability to focus on a checkerboard pattern is thus necessary to evaluate visual acuity. (A bright flash evoked potential can be used in younger and uncooperative children, but the norms are less standardized.) Evoked potentials suggest that visual acuity may be 20/20 in infants by 6–7 months of age.

Short-Latency Somatosensory Evoked Potentials

Responses are commonly produced by electric stimulation of peripheral sensory nerves, as this evokes potentials of greatest amplitude and clarity; finger tapping and muscle stretching may also be used. The function of this test is similar to that of the auditory test in closely correlating wave forms with function of the sensory pathways and permitting localization of conduction deficits. Short-latency somatosensory evoked potentials are used in the assessment of a wide variety of lesions of the peripheral nerve, root, spinal cord, and central nervous system following trauma, neuropathies (eg, in diabetes mellitus or Landry-Guillain-Barré syndrome), myelodysplasias, cerebral palsy, and many other disorders.

PEDIATRIC NEURORADIOLOGIC PROCEDURES

Sedation for Procedures

Radiologic procedures in infants and children are usually performed by pediatric radiologists, but sedation for these procedures remains largely the responsibility of the physician caring for the child. The choice of sedation must take into account the patient's age and physical condition, the type of neurologic disorder, the effect and duration of the procedure, and whether immediate neurosurgery is anticipated.

Oral or rectal chloral hydrate may be used, 30–60 mg/kg/dose. However, many radiology departments use only nonoral methods of adminstration because of fears of vomiting and aspiration. An alternative is pentobarbital, 6 mg/kg for children weighing less than 15 kg and 5 mg/kg for larger children (up to a maximum of 200 mg) given intramuscularly, rectally (at least 20 minutes before a procedure), or intravenously 2–4 mg/kg. Training and equipment to support blood pressure and respirations must be available. Pentobarbital usually achieves sedation for up to 2 hours. However, if sedation is inadequate 30 minutes after injection, and depending on the condition of the child, a second dose of pentobarbital, 2 mg/kg, is given. General anesthesia may be indicated, especially if the child is to undergo surgery immediately on completion of a radiologic procedure.

Computerized Tomography

Computerized tomography (CT) scanning consists of a series of cross-sectional ("axial") roentgenograms. The procedure is almost risk free and can be performed on an outpatient basis. Radiation exposure is approximately the same as that from a skull roentgenogram series; shielded gonads receive less than 0.1 mrad. The CT scan is often repeated after intravenous injection of iodized contrast medium for "enhancement," which reflects the vascularity of a lesion or its surrounding tissues. Precautions should be taken to ensure that the patient is not hypersensitive to iodinated dyes and that allergic reactions can be managed promptly. Sufficient information is often obtained from a nonenhanced scan, reducing both cost and risk.

Magnetic Resonance Imaging

Magnetic, or nuclear magnetic, resonance imaging (MRI) is a noninvasive technique that uses the magnetic properties of certain nuclei to produce signals that are translated into an image. MRI can provide information about the histologic, physiologic, and biochemical status of tissues, in addition to gross anatomic data.

Clinically, MRI has been applied chiefly to the study of lesions in the head, but it can be used in examinations of the spine, body organs, and tissues such as muscles and nerves. It has been used to delineate brain tumors, edema, ischemic and hemorrhagic lesions, hydrocephalus, vascular disorders, inflammatory and infectious lesions, and degenerative processes. MRI can be used to study myelination and demyelination and, through the demonstration of changes in relaxation time, metabolic disorders of the brain, muscles, and glands. Since bone causes no artifact in the images, the posterior fossa and its contents can be studied far better than with CT scans; even blood vessels and the cranial nerves can be imaged. On the other hand, the inability to detect calcification limits the detection of calcified lesions. It is believed that the strong magnetic fields used in this procedure do not cause molecular or cellular damage.

The cost is 2–3 times that of a contrast-enhanced CT scan. The procedure can be frightening, and complete immobility of the child is necessary: this necessitates sedation or light anesthesia.

Ultrasonography

Ultrasonography offers a pictorial display (eg, echoencephalogram, echocardiogram) of the varying density of tissues in a given anatomic region or structure by recording the echoes of ultrasonic waves reflected from it. The many advantages of ultrasonography include the ability to make quick assessment of a structure and its positioning by means of portable equipment, without ionizing radiation and at about one-fourth the cost of CT scanning. Sedation is usually not necessary, and ultrasonography can be repeated as often as indicated. In brain imaging, B mode and real-time sector scanners are usually employed, permitting excellent detail to be obtained in the coronal and sagittal planes.

Ultrasonography has been used for in utero diagnosis of hydrocephalus and other anomalies. In neonates, the thin skull and the open anterior fontanelle have facilitated imaging of the brain, and ultrasonography is now used in many nurseries to screen and follow all infants of less than 32 weeks' gestation or under 1500 g for intracranial hemorrhage. Other uses in neonates include detection of hydrocephalus, major brain and spine malformations, and even calcifications from intrauterine infection with cytomegalovirus or *Toxoplasma*.

Cerebral Angiography

Arteriography remains a very useful procedure in the diagnosis of many cerebrovascular disorders, particularly vascular malformations, and is sometimes used when a potentially operable lesion is suspected. In some instances of brain tumor, arteriography may be necessary to define the precise location or vascular bed, to differentiate among tumors, or to distinguish tumor from abscess or infarction. Noninvasive CT scanning and MRI scans are often satisfactory for static or flowing blood pathology (eg, sinus thromboses). Thus, use of (invasive) arteriography is often being replaced by these less dangerous procedures.

Myelography

X-ray examination of the spine following injection of a dye, water-soluble contrast medium, or air into the subarachnoid space via the lumbar or, rarely, the cervical route may be indicated in cases of spinal cord tumors or various forms of spinal dysraphism and in rare instances of herniated discs in children. However, in most institutions, spine scanning MRI or CT metrizamide myelography is now employed instead.

FEBRILE SEIZURES

Febrile seizures are very common, occuring in 2–3% of children. Most (> 90%) are generalized, brief (less than 5 minutes), and occur early with an "OMPA" (otitis media, pharyngitis, adenitis) illness. These seizures probably reflect a lowered seizure threshold in some children who convulse in response to the stress of fever. While some children with febrile seizures may subsequently have recurrent nonfebrile seizures in later childhood and adult life, this probably reflects a continued lowered seizure threshold. Febrile seizures themselves probably do not cause nonfebrile seizures. The chance of later epilepsy is higher if the febrile seizures have complex features (eg, duration greater than 15 minutes, more than one seizure in the same day, or focal features). Other adverse factors are an abnormal neurologic status preceding the seizures (eg, cerebral palsy or mental retardation), early onset of febrile seizure (before 1 year of age), and positive family history for epilepsy. Even with adverse factors the risk of epilepsy in later life is low—in the 15–20% range. Febrile seizures may recurr in 20–40%, but, in general, recurrent febrile seizures don't worsen the long-term outlook.

Management

The child with a febrile seizure must be examined. Routine studies (eg, electrolytes, glucose, calcium, skull x-rays, or brain imaging studies) are seldom helpful and the laboratory evaluation must be tailored to the specifics of each child. CNS INFECTION MUST BE RULED OUT either by clinical observation or by spinal fluid examination. Bacterial meningitis can present with a fever and seizure. Signs of meningitis, (eg, bulging fontanel, stiff neck, stupor, irritability) may all be absent, especially in a child under 18 months. The fact that the child has had a previous febrile seizure does not rule out meningitis as the cause of the current episode. The younger the child, the more important the tap as the less reliable are physical findings in diagnosing meningitis. Although the yield will be low, a tap should probably be done in a child under age 2, if recovery is slow, if no other cause for the fever is found, and if close follow-up is not going to be possible. Sometimes observation in the emergency room for several hours will obviate the need for a tap. A negative tap does not rule out the emergence of meningitis during the same febrile illness; sometimes a second tap needs to be done.

Treatment after the seizure is over is problematic. Many clinicians choose to treat the child with a maintenance anticonvulsant during the course of that febrile illness. However, the relatively benign nature of febrile seizures must be balanced against the potential side effects of anticonvulsants. Phenobarbital and valproate are possible choices, although the somnolence from the phenobarbital load (5–10/kg) often discomforts both the doctor and parent and sometimes confuses follow-up assessments. Valproic acid has more dangers and should be avoided in the acute situation with vomiting and/or acidosis.

Most clinicians chose to follow the youngster without anticonvulsant medication. Fever control measures with sponging and antipyretics, and appropriate antibiotics if a bacterial illness is suspected or confirmed will be the major treatment. The family can be reassured that simple febrile seizures are not thought to have any long-term adverse consequences. An electroencephalogram should be ordered if the febrile seizure is complicated or unusual; in the uncomplicated febrile seizure, the EEG is most often normal. About 10% will have slowing or other occipital abnormalities. Ideally, the study should be done at least a week after the illness to avoid transient findings due to the fever or seizure itself. In older children, 3/second spike wave discharge, suggestive of a genetic propensity to epilepsy, may occur. In the young infant EEG findings seldom aid in predicting the chance of recurrence of febrile or nonfebrile seizures.

Prophylactic anticonvulsants are not indicated in the uncomplicated febrile seizure patient. If febrile seizures are complicated, for example very prolonged, or if family anxiety is unrequited by information, anticonvulsant prophylaxis may be indicated to reduce the incidence of recurrent febrile or afebrile seizures. Phenobarbital 3–5 mg/kg/d as a single bedtime dose is an option. Often increasing the dose gradually, for example starting with 2 mg/kg/d the first week, 3 mg/kg/d the second week, etc, will decrease side effects and noncompliance. A phenobarbital level in the 15–40 μg/mL range is desirable.

Sodium valproate is the other medication that has been successful, but has more hazards. In the infant age group, liquid suspension is often necessary; it has a short half-life and causes more GI upset than the coated capsules useful in older age groups. The dose is 15–60 mg/kg/d divided into 3 or 4 daily doses. Precautionary laboratory studies are necessary. Diphenylhydantoin and carbamazepine have not shown effectiveness in febrile seizure prophylaxis.

SEIZURE DISORDERS
(See Table 27–2.)

General Considerations
A seizure is a sudden, transient disturbance of brain function, manifested by involuntary motor, sensory, autonomic, or psychic phenomena, alone or in any combination, often accompanied by alteration or loss of consciousness.

Repeated seizures without evident time-limited cause justify the label of epilepsy. Seizures and epilepsy occur most commonly at the extremes of life. The incidence is highest in the newborn, and higher in childhood than in later life. Epilepsy in childhood often remits. Factors adversely influencing recurrence include difficulty in getting the seizures under control (that is, the number of seizures occurring before control is achieved), neurologic dysfunction or mental retardation, age of onset under 2 years, and abnormal EEG at the time of discontinuing medication. The type of seizures also often determines prognosis.

Seizures are caused by any factor that can disturb brain function. The causes of seizures and epilepsy are often divided into symptomatic (when a cause is strongly identified or presumed) and idiopathic (the cause is unknown or genetic influences are strongly etiologic). The younger the infant or child, the more likely the cause can be identified. Idiopathic or genetic epilepsy most often appears between ages 4 and 16. A seizure disorder or epilepsy should not be considered idiopathic unless a thorough history, examination, and appropriate laboratory tests have turned up no apparent cause.

Clinical Findings

A. Symptoms and Signs: The key to making the diagnosis of epilepsy is, of course, the history. A seizure may be preceded by an aura—transient symptoms such as a feeling of fear, numbness or tingling in the fingers, or bright lights in one visual field are examples of an aura, really the onset of the seizure. Sometimes the patient recalls nothing. Occasionally there is a more distant prodrome to the seizure; for example, a feeling of unwellness, or a feeling of something about to happen, or a recurrent thought that occurred over minutes or hours prior to the aura and seizure itself.

Minute details of the seizure can help determine proper classification. Did the patient become extremely pale before she fell? Was she able to respond to queries during the episode? Did she go completely "out" or become unconscious? Did she fall stiffly or gradually slump to the floor? Did she injure herself? How long did the stiffening or jerking last? Where were the sites of jerking?

Events occurring after the seizure also can be helpful in diagnosis. Was there loss of speech? Was the patient able to respond accurately prior to going to sleep?

All these prior-to, during, and after-the-seizure events can help to classify the seizure, and indeed may help to decide if the event actually was a probable epileptic seizure or a pseudo-seizure—that is, a nonepileptic phenomenon mimicking a seizure. As alluded to above, classifying the seizure type may aid in diagnosis and prognosis and suggest desirable or necessary laboratory tests and medication choices.

B. Differential Diagnosis: It is terribly important not to label a nonepileptic condition as epileptic. The label "epilepsy" often has connotations to the layperson of brain damage and limitation of activity; diagnosis may prevent or preclude certain occupations in later life. It is often very difficult to change an inaccurate diagnosis many years later.

1. Breath-holding Attacks–Age 6 months to 3 years (0–6 years), always precipitated by trauma and fright. Cyanosis; sometimes stiffening, tonic (or jerking-clonic), convulsion (anoxic seizure); may sleep after. Family history positive in 30%. EEG is normal. Treatment is interpretation and reassurance.

Table 27-2. Seizure disorders.

Age Group and Seizure Type	Age at Onset	Clinical Manifestations	Causative Factors	Electro-encephalographic Pattern	Other Diagnostic Studies	Treatment and Comments (Anticonvulsants by Order of Choice)
Neonatal seizures	Birth to 2 weeks	Often "atypical"; sudden limpness or tonic posturing, brief apnea and cyanosis; odd cry, eyes "rolling up," blinking or mouthing or chewing movements, nystagmus, twitchiness or clonic movements, focal, multifocal, or generalized.	Neurologic insults (hypoxia/ischemia, intracranial hemorrhage) present more in first 3 days or after 8th day; metabolic disturbances alone between third and eighth days; hypoglycemia, hypocalcemia, hyper- and hyponatremia. Drug withdrawal. Pyridoxine deficiency and other metabolic	May correlate poorly with clinical seizures. Focal spikes or slow rhythms; multifocal discharges.	Lumbar puncture, serum Ca^{2+}, PO_4^{-}, glucose, Mg^{2+}; BUN, amino acid screen, blood ammonia, organic acid screen, TORCHES screen. Ultrasound and/or CT scan for suspected intracranial hemorrhage and structural abnormalities.	Phenobarbital, IV or IM, if seizures not controlled, add phenytoin IV (loading dose 20 mg/kg each). Diazepam, approximately 0.2 mg/kg. Treat underlying disorder. Seizures due to brain damage often resistant to anticonvulsants. When cause in doubt, stop protein feedings until enzyme deficiencies of urea cycle or

Name	Age at onset	Clinical features	Cause	EEG	Diagnosis	Treatment
West's syndrome: "infantile spasms." (See also Lennox-Gastaut syndrome below.)	3–18 months; occasionally up to 4 years	Sudden, usually symmetric adduction and flexion of limbs with concomitant flexion of head and trunk; also abduction and extensor movements like Moro reflex. Tendency for spasms to occur in clusters, on waking or falling asleep, or when fatigued, or may be noted particularly when the infant is being handled, is ill, or is otherwise	causes. CNS infections and structural abnormalities. Pre- or perinatal brain damage or malformation in approximately ⅓, biochemical, infectious, degenerative causes in approximately ⅓, unknown in approximately ⅓. With early onset, pyridoxine deficiency, amino- or organic aciduria. Tuberous sclerosis in 5–10%. Chronic inflammatory disease and toxoplasmosis.	Hypsarrhythmia; chaotic high-voltage slow waves, random spikes, all leads (90%); other abnormalities in rest. Rarely "normal." EEG normalization usually correlates with reduction of seizures; not helpful prognostically regarding mental development.	Funduscopic and skin examination, trial of pyridoxine. Amino- and organic acid screen. Chronic inflammatory disease. TORCHES screen. CT or MRI scan should be done to (1) establish definite diagnosis and (2) aid in genetic counseling.	amino metabolism ruled out. Corticotropin preferred (2–4 units/kg/d IM Acthar gel 1/day, then slow withdrawal). Some prefer oral corticosteroids. Diazepam, clonazepam, valproic acid. In resistant cases, ketogenic or medium-chain triglyceride (MCT) diet. Retardation of varying degree in approximately 90% of cases.

(Continued)

835

Table 27–2 (cont'd). Seizure disorders.

Age Group and Seizure Type	Age at Onset	Clinical Manifestations	Causative Factors	Electro-encephalographic Pattern	Other Diagnostic Studies	Treatment and Comments (Anticonvulsants by Order of Choice)
		irritable. Tendency for each patient to have own stereotyped pattern.	Aicardi syndrome (females with mental retardation agenesis of corpus callosum, ocular and vertebral anomalies).			
Febrile convulsions	3 months to 5 years	Usually generalized seizures, less than 15 minutes; rarely focal in onset. May lead to status epilepticus.	Nonneurologic febrile illness (temperature rise to 102.5°F or higher); family history frequently positive for febrile convulsions.	Normal interictal EEG, especially when obtained 8–10 days after seizure. In older infants 3/s spikes often seen.	In infants or whenever suspicion of meningitis exists, perform lumbar puncture.	Treat underlying illness, fever. Diazepam po 0.3–0.5 mg/kg q8h during illness. Prophylaxis with phenobarbital (valproic acid if phenobarbital not tolerated), with neurologic

						deficits, prolonged seizure, family history of epilepsy.
Myoclonic astatic (akinetic, atonic) seizures, formerly atypical absence. With mental retardation, Lennox–Gastaut syndrome	Any time in childhood; normally 2–7 years	Shocklike violent contractions of one or more muscle groups, singly or irregularly repetitive; may fling patient suddenly to side, forward, or backward. Usually no or only brief loss of consciousness. Half or more of patients also have generalized grand mal seizures.	Multiple causes, usually resulting in diffuse neuronal damage. History of West's syndrome; pre- or perinatal brain damage; viral meningo-encephalitides; subacute sclerosing panencephalitis, CNS degenerative disorders; lead or other encephalopathies; structural cerebral abnormalities, eg. porencephaly.	Atypical slow (1–2.5 Hz) spike-wave complexes ("petit mal variant") and bursts of high voltage generalized spikes, often with diffusely slow background frequencies.	As dictated by index of suspicion. Lumbar puncture with measles antibody titre and CSF IgG index. Nerve conduction studies. Urine for lead, arylsulfatase A, etc. Skin biopsy for electron microscopy and enzyme studies. CT scan and brain biopsy may be justified.	Difficult to treat. Valproic acid, clonazepam, or ethosuximide. Imipramine as adjunct. Diazepam. Ketogenic or medium-chain triglyceride (MCT) diet. ACTH or corticosteroids as in West's syndrome. Protect head with helmet and chin padding.

(Continued)

837

Table 27–2 (cont'd). Seizure disorders.

Age Group and Seizure Type	Age at Onset	Clinical Manifestations	Causative Factors	Electro-encephalographic Pattern	Other Diagnostic Studies	Treatment and Comments (Anticonvulsants by Order of Choice)
Absence ("petit mal"). Also juvenile and myoclonic absence	3–15 years	Lapses of consciousness or vacant stares, lasting about 10 seconds; often in "clusters." Automatisms of face and hands; clonic activity in 30–45%. Often confused with complex partial seizures but no aura or postictal confusion.	Unknown. Genetic component: probably an autosomal dominant gene.	Three-second bilaterally synchronous, symmetric, high-voltage spikes and waves. EEG "normalization" correlates closely with control of seizures.	Hyperventilation when patient on inadequate or no medication often provokes attacks. CT scan is rarely of value.	Valproic acid or ethosuximide; with latter, add phenobarbital if EEG suggests other abnormalities (grand mal). In resistant cases, ketogenic or MCT diet. Also, in resistant cases, valproic acid and ethosuximide together.
Simple partial or focal seizures (motor/sensory/ jacksonian). (Complex partial or psychomotor	Any age	Seizure may involve any part of body; may spread in fixed pattern (jacksonian	Often secondary to birth trauma, inflammatory process, vascular accidents, meningo-	Focal spikes or slow waves in appropriate cortical region; sometimes diffusely	If seizures are difficult to control or progressive deficits occur, neuroradiodi-agnostic studies,	Carbamazepine, phenytoin, phenobarbital, or primidone. Valproic acid useful adjunct.

					particularly CT
seizures, below.)		march), becoming generalized. In children, epileptogenic focus often "shifts" and epileptic manifestations may change concomitantly.	encephalitis, etc. If seizures are coupled with new or progressive neurologic deficits, a structural lesion (eg, brain tumor) is likely.	abnormal or even normal.	brain scan, imperative.	
Complex partial seizures (psychomotor, temporal lobe, or limbic seizures)	Any age	Aura may be a sensation of fear, epigastric discomfort, odd smell or taste (usually unpleasant), visual or auditory hallucination (either vague and "unformed" or well-formed image, words, music). Aura and seizure stereotyped for each patient. Seizure may	As above. Temporal lobes especially sensitive to hypoxia; thus, this seizure type may be sequela of birth trauma, febrile convulsions, etc. Also especially vulnerable to certain viral infections, especially herpes simplex. Remediable other causes are small	As above, but occurring in temporal lobe and its connections, eg, frontotemporal, temporoparietal, temporooccipital regions.	CT scan when structural lesions suspected. Temporal lobe biopsy when herpes simplex encephalitis suspected. Carotid amobarbital injection when lateralization of speech dominance in question.	Carbamazepine, phenytoin, phenobarbital, or primidone. More than one drug may be necessary. Valproic acid may be useful. Phenacemide in difficult-to-control seizures uncontrolled by drugs and where a primary epileptogenic focus is identifiable,

(Continued)

839

Table 27-2 (cont'd). Seizure disorders.

Age Group and Seizure Type	Age at Onset	Clinical Manifestations	Causative Factors	Electro-encephalo-graphic Pattern	Other Diagnostic Studies	Treatment and Comments (Anticonvulsants by Order of Choice)
		consist of vague stare; facial, tongue, or swallowing movements and throaty sounds; or various complex automatisms. Unlike absences, complex partial seizures tend not to occur in clusters but singly and to last longer (1 minute or more) followed by confusion. History of aura (or child running to adult from "vague	cryptic tumors or vascular malformations.			excision of anterior third of temporal lobe. Adjunctive psychotherapy required frequently.

	Age	Clinical features	Genetics	EEG	Laboratory	Treatment
		fear") and of automatisms involving more than face and hands establishes diagnosis. About 60% also develop generalized grand mal seizures.				Carbamazepine or phenytoin. Primidone or phenobarbital.
"Benign epilepsy of childhood" (with "centrotemporal" or "rolandic" foci)	5–16 years	Partial motor or generalized seizures. Similar seizure patterns may be observed in patients with focal cortical lesions.	Seizure history or abnormal EEG findings in 40% of relatives of affected probands and 18–20% of parents and siblings, suggesting transmission by a single autosomal dominant gene, possibly with age-dependent penetrance.	Centrotemporal spikes or sharp waves ("rolandic discharges") appearing paroxysmally against a normal EEG background.	Serum Ca^{2+} and glucose, BUN, urinalysis. Seldom need CT scan.	

(Continued)

Table 27-2 (cont'd). Seizure disorders.

Age Group and Seizure Type	Age at Onset	Clinical Manifestations	Causative Factors	Electroencephalographic Pattern	Other Diagnostic Studies	Treatment and Comments (Anticonvulsants by Order of Choice)
Juvenile myoclonic epilepsy (of Janz)	Late childhood and adolescence, peaking at 13 years	Mild myoclonic jerks of neck and shoulder flexor muscles after waking up ("awakening" grand mal seizures). Intelligence usually normal.	40% of relatives have myoclonias, especially in females; 15% have the abnormal EEG pattern without clinical attacks.	Interictal EEG shows fast variety of spike-and-wave sequences or 4 to 6 Hz multi-spike-and-wave complexes.	Differentiate from progressive myoclonic encephalopathy of Unverricht-Lafora and other degenerative disorders by appropriate biopsies (muscle, liver, etc).	Valproic acid.
Generalized tonic-clonic seizures (grand mal)	Any age	Loss of consciousness; tonic-clonic movements often preceded by vague aura or cry.	Often unknown. Genetic component. May be seen with metabolic disturbances,	Bilaterally synchronous, symmetric multiple high-voltage spikes, spikes and waves,	As above.	Phenobarbital in first 12 months; carbamazepine or valproic acid; phenytoin; primidone.

Bladder and bowel incontinence in approximately 15%. Postictal confusion; sleep. Often mixed with or masking other seizure patterns.	trauma, infection, intoxication, degenerative disorders, brain tumors, etc.	mixed patterns. Often normal under age 4.	Combinations may be necessary.

2. Infantile Syncope *(Pallid Breath-Holding)*–No external precipitant (internal pain, cramp, or fear the precipitant?), pallor, then may have seizure (anoxic/ischemic). Vagally (heart-slowing) mediated, like adult syncope. EEG normal; may get cardiac slowing with vagal stimulation (eyeball pressure, cold cloth on face) during EEG.

3. Tics or Tourette's Syndrome–Simple or complex stereotyped. (The same, time after time.) Jerks or movements, coughs, grunts, sniffs. Worse at repose or with stress. May be suppressed during MD visit. Family history often positive. EEG negative. Nonanticonvulsant drugs may benefit.

4. Night Terrors; Sleep Talking, Walking, "Sit-Ups"–Three to 10 year olds. Usually occur in first sleep cycle (30–90 minutes after going to sleep) with crying, screaming, and "autonomic discharge" (pupils dilated, perspiring, etc). Lasts minutes. Child goes back to sleep and has no recall of event the next day. Sleep studies (polysomnogram and EEG) are normal. Disappears with maturation. Sleep talking and walking and short "sit-ups" in bed are fragmentary arousals. If a spell is recorded, EEG shows arousal from deep sleep, but the behavior seems wakeful. The youngster needs to be protected from injury and gradually settled down and taken back to bed.

5. Nightmares–Vivid dreams occur in subsequent cycles of sleep, often in the early morning hours and generally are partially recalled the next day. The bizarre and frightening behavior may sometimes be confused with complex partial seizures. These occur during REM (rapid eye movement) sleep; epilepsy usually doesn't occur during that phase of sleep. In extreme or difficult cases, an all night sleep EEG may help to differentiate seizures from nightmares.

6. Migraine–One variant of migraine can be associated with an acute confusional state. There may be the usual migraine prodrome with spots before the eyes, dizziness, visual field defects, and then agitated confusion. If the patient has had other more typical migraine with severe headache and vomiting without confusion, that may aid in the diagnosis. The severe headache with vomiting as the youngster comes out of the migraine may aid in distinguishing the attack from epilepsy. Other seizure manifestations are practically never seen. The EEG in migraine is usually normal and seldom shows epileptiform abnormalities as are often seen in patients with epilepsy.

7. Syncope–Syncope often has a precipitant. The patient usually remembers feeling dizzy, lightheaded, the room going dark, beginning to fall, feeling nauseated or "ill," etc. Observers may notice extreme pallor at the onset. Often the fall is gradual but not always. If the heart rate is taken it is often very slow. When the patient awakens, he may remember beginning to fall. Occasionally a very brief tonic or tonic-clonic seizure may occur due to anoxia. Incontinence is rare. An EEG will invariably be normal. The family history is often positive for syncope.

8. Shuddering–Shuddering or shivering attacks can occur in infancy and be a forerunner of essential tremor in later life. Often the family history is positive for tremor. The shivering may be very frequent. EEG will be normal. There is no clouding or loss of consciousness.

9. Gastroesophageal Reflux–Reflux of acid gastric contents may lead to discomfort and produce unusual posturings of the head and neck or trunk. Appropriate circumstances and upper GI series, cineangiogram of swallowing, sometimes even an EEG (which will always be normal), may be necessary to distinguish this condition from seizures.

10. Conversion Reaction/Pseudoseizures–Many patients with clear-cut pseudoseizures also have genuine seizures. The episodes may be writhing, intercourse-like movements, tonic episodes, bizarre jerkings and thrashing around or even seeming sudden unresponsiveness. Often there is ongoing psychological trauma.

The spells must often be seen or recorded on video in a controlled situation to distinguish them from epilepsy. A normal EEG during a spell is a key diagnostic feature. Often the spells are so bizarre as to be easily distinguished. Sometimes pseudoseizures can be precipitated by suggestion with injection of normal saline in a controlled situation. Combativeness is common, self-injury and incontinence rare.

11. Staring Spells–School teachers often make referral for absence or petit mal seizures in youngsters who stare or seem preoccupied at school. Helpful in the history is the lack of these spells at home, for example, in the early morning hours prior to breakfast as might be seen with absence seizures. A lack of other epilepsy in the child and/or family history often is helpful. Sometimes these children have difficulties with school, and have cognitive or learning disability. The child can generally be brought out of this spell by a firm command. An EEG is sometimes necessary to reassure all that absence seizures aren't occurring. A 24-hour ambulatory EEG to record attacks during the child's everyday school activities occasionally is necessary.

Status Epilepticus

Status epilepticus is a clinical or electric seizure and is somewhat arbitrarily defined as a single seizure lasting at least 30 minutes, or a series of seizures without complete recovery over the same period of time. Eventually, high fever, hypotension, respiratory depression, and even death may occur. Thus, status epilepticus is a relative medical emergency.

A child with status epilepticus often has a high fever with or without intracranial infection such as viral encephalitis or bacterial meningitis. Status epilepticus may be the youngster's initial seizure; various studies show that in one- to three-quarters of children status epilepticus is the initial seizure. Often the status is a reflection of a remote insult, for example anoxia or trauma. Tumor, vascular disease ("strokes"), or head trauma are common causes of status epilepticus in adults but are uncommon causes in childhood. One-half are symptomatic of acute (25%) or chronic (25%) CNS disorders. Infection or metabolic disorders are the most common symptomatic causes in children. The cause is unknown in half, but many of these will be febrile. Status is more common under one year with 37% occurring under that age and 85% under the age of 5. Thus the pediatrician is going to see status epilepticus most commonly in infants and preschoolers.

Treatment of status is first directed toward basic life support of the patient and correction of any identifiable metabolic abnormalities or other serious stressors. Glucose should be given both because hypoglycemia itself can cause status and to meet the metabolic requirements of the patient. Drugs used for treatment of status include lorazepam, phenobarbital, and phenytoin. The intravenous route of administration is usually preferred because of faster onset of action. Intravenous anticonvulsants can produce apnea, hypotension, and arrhythmias; the clinician should be prepared in advance to deal with these eventualities.

CONGENITAL MALFORMATIONS OF THE NERVOUS SYSTEM

Malformations of the nervous system occur in 1–3% of living neonates and are present in 40% of infants who die. Developmental anomalies of the central nervous system (CNS) may result from a variety of causes, including infectious, toxic, metabolic, and vascular insults that affect the fetus. The specific type of malformation that results from such insults, however, may be more dependent upon the time during gestation when the insult occurs than on the specific etiology. The period of induction, 0–28 days' gestation, is the period during which the neural plate appears and the neural tube forms and closes. Insults during this phase can result in a major absence of neural structures, such as anencephaly, or in a defect of neural tube closure, such as spina bifida, meningomyelocele, or encephalocele. Cellular proliferation and migration characterize neural development that occurs after 28 days of gestation. Lissencephaly, pachygyria, agyria, and agenesis of the corpus callosum represent disorders caused by insults that occur during the period of cellular proliferation and migration.

Abnormalities of Neural Tube Closure

Defects of neural tube closure constitute some of the commonest forms of congenital malformations affecting the nervous system. Spina bifida with associated meningomyelocele or meningocele are commonly found in the lumbosacral region. Depending on the extent and severity of spinal cord and peripheral nerve involvement, clinical findings include lower extremity weakness, bowel and bladder dysfunction, and hip dislocation. Surgical intervention is usually indicated to close meningoceles and meningomyeloceles. Additional treatment is necessary to manage chronic urinary tract abnormalities, orthopedic abnormalities such as kyphosis and scoliosis, and lower extremity paresis. Hydrocephalus commonly associated with meningomyelocele usually requires ventriculoperitoneal shunting.

Arnold-Chiari malformations occur as 2 distinct types. Arnold-Chiari malformation type I consists of elongation and displacement of the caudal end of the brainstem into the spinal canal with protrusion of the cerebellar tonsils through the foramen magnum. In association with this hindbrain malformation, there is often minor-to-moderate abnormalities of the base of the skull, including basilar impression, platybasia, and small foramen magnum. Arnold-Chiari malformation type I may remain asymptomatic for years, but in older children and young adults it may cause progressive ataxia, lower cranial nerve paresis, and progressive vertigo. This malformation is often associated with a lumbosacral meningomyelocele and is termed Arnold-Chiari type II. Hydrocephalus is present in approximately 90% of children with Arnold-Chiari type II. These patients may also have aqueductal stenosis, hydromyelia, or syringomyelia. The clinical manifestations of Arnold-Chiari type II malformation are most commonly caused by the associated hydrocephalus and meningomyelocele.

In general, the diagnosis of neural tube defects is obvious at the time of birth. Prenatal diagnosis may be strongly suspected based on ultrasonographic findings and the presence of elevated levels of alpha fetoprotein in the amniotic fluid.

Disorders of Cellular Proliferation and Migration

A. Lissencephaly: Lissencephaly is a severe malformation of the brain characterized by an extremely smooth cortical surface with minimal sulcal and gyral development and often, a primitive cytoarchitectural construction of the cerebral mantle. Pachygyria and agyria are closely associated with lissencephaly but represent more restricted forms of migrational abnormalities. Patients with lissencephaly usually suffer from severe neurodevelopmental delay, microcephaly, and seizures, including infantile spasms. Patients with lissencephaly frequently have additional associated malformations and dysmorphic features (eg, Walker-Warburg syndrome or Miller-Dieker syndrome, or metabolic disorders such as Zellweger syndrome). It is particularly important to identify these syndromes because of their genetic importance.

B. Agenesis of the Corpus Callosum: Agenesis of the corpus callosum, once thought to be a relatively rare cerebral malformation, has been seen frequently with modern neuroimaging techniques. Occasionally agenesis of the corpus callosum appears to be inherited in an autosomal dominant or autosomal recessive pattern. X-linked recessive patterns have also been described. Agenesis of the corpus callosum may be found in conjunction with metabolic defects (pyruvate dehydrogenase deficiency, nonketotic hyperglycinemia). Most cases, however, are sporadic. Maldevelopment of the corpus callosum may be partial or complete. Many patients with agenesis of the corpus callosum have associated seizures, developmental delay, microcephaly, or mental retardation although this condition may be found incidentally in functionally normal individuals. A special form of agenesis of the corpus callosum occurs in Aicardi's syndrome. In this X-linked disorder, agenesis of the corpus callosum is associated with infantile spasms, mental retardation, lacunar choreoretinopathy, and vertebral body abnormalities.

C. Dandy-Walker Malformation: Dandy-Walker malformation is characterized by vermal aplasia, cystic enlargement of the fourth ventricle, rostral displacement of the tentorium, and absence or atresia of the foramina of Magendie and Luschka. Although hydrocephalus is usually not present congenitally, it often develops within the first few months of life, and in those patients who develop hydrocephalus, 90% have developed hydrocephalus by 1 year of age. On physical examination, there is often a rounded protuberance or exaggeration of the occiput of the cranium. In the absence of hydrocephalus and increased intracranial pressure, there may be few physical findings to suggest neurologic dysfunction. An ataxic syndrome, if it develops, usually appears late and occurs in fewer than 20% of patients. Many long-term neurologic deficits result directly from hydrocephalus. Diagnosis of Dandy-Walker malformation is confirmed by head CT or MRI scanning. Treatment is directed at the management of hydrocephalus.

Craniosynostosis

Craniosynostosis, or premature closure of cranial sutures, is usually sporadic and idiopathic. However, some patients have syndromes such as Apert's and Crouzon's that are inherited and that are associated with abnormalities of the digits, extremities, and heart. Very rarely, craniosynostosis may be associated with an underlying metabolic disturbance such as hyperthyroidism and hypophosphotasia. The most common form of craniosynostosis involves the sagittal suture and results in scaphocephaly, an elongation of the head in the anterior to posterior direction. Premature closure of the coronal sutures causes brachycephaly, an increase in cranial diameter from left to right. Unless many or all cranial sutures close prematurely, intracranial volume will not be compromised, and the brain's growth will not be impaired, nor will neurologic dysfunction result. Management of craniosynostosis is directed at preserving normal skull shape.

Hydrocephalus

Hydrocephalus is characterized by increased volume of cerebrospinal fluid in association with progressive ventricular dilatation and may result from failure of reabsorption of CSF (communicating hydrocephalus) or from an obstruction that blocks the flow of spinal fluid within the ventricular system or blocks the egress of spinal fluid from the ventricular system into the subarachnoid space (noncommunicating hydrocephalus). A wide variety of disorders, such as hemorrhage, infection, tumors, and congenital malformations may play an etiologic role in development of hydrocephalus.

Clinical features of hydrocephalus include macrocephaly, and/or excessive head growth rate. Increased intracranial pressure may cause irritability, vomiting, loss of appetite, impaired upward gaze, impaired extraocular movements, hypertonia of the lower extremities, and generalized hyperreflexia. Without treatment, optic atrophy may occur. In infants, papilledema may not be present, whereas in older children with closed cranial sutures, optic disc swelling may eventually develop.

Hydrocephalus can be diagnosed based upon the clinical course, physical examination findings, and CT scan or MRI findings. Treatment of hydrocephalus is directed at providing an alternative outlet for CSF from the intracranial compartment, usually by ventriculoperitoneal shunting. Other treatment should be directed, if possible, at the underlying etiology for the hydrocephalus.

FLACCID PARALYSIS

Flaccid paralysis evolving over hours or a few days suggests involvement of the lower motor neuron complex. *Anterior horn cells* (spinal cord) may be involved by viral infection (paralytic poliomyelitis) or para or post viral immunologically mediated disease (acute transverse myelitis). The *nerve trunks* (polyneuritis) may be diseased as in Landry-Guillian-Barre syndrome or affected by toxins (diphtheria, porphyria). The *neuromuscular junction* may be blocked by tick toxin or botulinum toxin.

The paralysis rarely will be due to metabolic (periodic paralysis) or inflammatory muscle disease (myositis). *A lesion compressing the spinal cord must be ruled out.* The features that aid in diagnosis are age, history of preceding or waning illness, presence (at the time of paralysis) of fever, rapidity of progression, cranial nerve findings, and sensory findings. Exam may show "long tract" findings (pyramidal tract), causing increased reflexes and a positive Babinski sign. There may be decreased sensation for pain and temperature. Back pain, even tenderness to percussion may occur. Bowel and bladder dysfunction (incontinence) may occur. Often the paralysis is ascending, symmetric, and painful (muscle tenderness or myalgia). Laboratory findings occasionally are diagnostic.

Differential Diagnosis

The child who is "well" and becomes paralyzed often has polyneuritis. Acute transverse myelitis (ATM) occurs in an afebrile child. The child who is ill and febrile at the time of paralysis often has ATM (or polio); *acute* epidural spinal cord abscess (or other compressive lesion) must be ruled out. Poliomyelitis is very rare in our immunized population. Tick bite paralysis occurs "in season" (spring-summer). Removal of the tick is curative.

Infantile botulism occurs under age 1 and has been associated with honey ingestion. Food-borne and wound botulism are very rare. Intravenous drug abuse can lead to myelitis and paralysis. Chronic myelopathy is emerging as a result of two HIV viruses, HTLV-I and HTLV-III.

HYPOKALEMIC PERIODIC PARALYSIS

This rare condition is inherited as a dominant trait, with decreased occurrence in females, but it may appear sporadically. Onset is during childhood. The proximal muscles are affected first. Cranial and respiratory muscles are spared. Attacks of weakness may be precipitated by rest after exercise, exposure to cold, emotional stress, and high dietary intake of carbohydrate and sodium. The serum potassium level is low during an attack. An attack may be provoked by exercising the patient. Acetazolamide 5–30 mg/kg/d orally is usually effective in preventing attacks.

HYPERKALEMIC PERIODIC PARALYSIS

This form of periodic paralysis has its onset in the first decade of life and is usually detected in infancy because of "staring" eyes (myotonic form of lid lag) or a very feeble cry (especially on waking). It is inherited as an autosomal dominant trait. Pseudohypertrophy of the calves is often present. There is an increased incidence of diabetes mellitus. The attacks are relatively short, lasting 30 minutes to 2 hours, and may be precipitated by rest after exercise, cold, and fatigue. Attacks usually occur in children of school age and then abate, though permanent muscle weakness may develop. The serum potassium level rises during attacks. Treatment is with hydrochlorothiazide 50 mg/d orally, or acetazolamide 250 mg/d orally. The disorder is consistent with a normal life span.

NORMOKALEMIC PERIODIC PARALYSIS

In this disorder, the onset is in the first decade of life. It is inherited as an autosomal dominant trait. Attacks come on during rest after exercise, with cold, following ingestion of foods high in potassium (eg, many fruit juices), and following ingestion of alcohol. The attacks may last days. In normokalemic paralysis, serum electrolyte levels do not change during attacks. Muscle biopsy may show vacuolar myopathy.

Treatment consists of increased salt intake; acetazolamide 250 mg/d orally, with dosage adjusted for each case; and fludrocortisone 0.1 mg/d orally. The prognosis is good.

MYASTHENIA GRAVIS

Myasthenia gravis is characterized by easy fatigability of muscles, particularly the extraocular muscles and those of mastication, swallowing, and respiration. However, in the neonatal period or early infancy, the weakness may be so constant and general that an affected infant may present nonspecifically as a "floppy infant." Girls are involved more frequently than boys. The age at onset is over 10 years in 75% of cases. If diagnosed before age 10, congenital myasthenia should be considered in retrospect. The disorder is thought to be immunologically mediated and a circulating antibody to the acetylcholine receptor protein has been identified.

Clinical Findings

A. Symptoms and Signs:

1. Neonatal (transient) myasthenia gravis–This occurs in 12% of infants born to myasthenic mothers. The condition is due to maternal factors transferred across the placenta; a thymic factor in the infant may also be involved.

2. Congenital (persistent) myasthenia gravis–In this form of the disease, the mothers of the affected infants rarely have myasthenia gravis but other relatives may. Sex distribution is equal. Symptoms are often subtle and not recognized initially. Differential diagnosis includes many other causes of the "floppy infant" syndrome, such as infant botulism, ocular myopathy, congenital ptosis, and Mobius syndrome (facial nuclear aplasia and other anomalies). This condition is probably not immunologic and often responds poorly to therapy.

3. Juvenile myasthenia gravis–In this autoimmune form, the symptoms and signs are like those in adults. Receptor antibodies are usually present. The more prominent signs are difficulty in chewing, dysphagia, a nasal voice, ptosis, and ophthalmoplegia. Pathologic fatigability of limbs, chiefly involving the proximal limb and neck muscles, may be more prominent than the bulbar signs. Weakness may be limited to ocular muscles only. Associated disorders include autoimmune conditions, especially thyroid disease.

The differential diagnosis includes Landry-Guillain-Barre syndrome and bulbar poliomyelitis. Administration of anticholinesterase agents helps with the diagnosis and may be lifesaving.

B. Laboratory Findings:

1. Neostigmine test–In newborns and very young infants, the neostigmine (Prostigmin) test may be preferable to the edrophonium (Tensilon) test because the longer duration of its response permits better observation, especially of sucking and swallowing movements. The test dose of neostigmine is 0.02 mg/kg subcutaneously, usually given with atropine, 0.01 mg/kg subcutaneously. There is a delay of about 10 minutes before the effect may be manifest. The physician should be prepared to suction secretions.

2. Edrophonium test–Testing with edrophonium is used in older children who are capable of cooperating in certain tasks, such as raising and lowering their eyelids and squeezing a sphygmomanometer bulb or the examiner's hands. The test dose is 0.1–1 mL intravenously, depending on the size of the child. Maximum improvement occurs within 2 minutes.

3. Other laboratory tests–Serum acetylcholine receptor antibodies are found in the neonatal and juvenile forms. In juveniles, thyroid studies are indicated.

C. Electrical Studies of Muscle: Repetitive stimulation of a motor nerve at slow rates (3/s) with recording over the appropriate muscle reveals a progressive fall in amplitude of the muscle potential in myasthenic patients. If this study is negative, single fiber electromyography may be employed.

D. Imaging: Chest x-ray and/or other imaging procedures should be done in cases of autoimmune myasthenia gravis to evaluate the thymus. Thymus tumors are rare in children.

Treatment

A. General and Supportive Care: Management of the airway is of overriding importance. Suctioning and/or respiratory assistance may be required. Treatment should be carried out by physicians with experience in this disorder.

B. Anticholinesterase Drug Therapy:

1. Pyridostigmine (Mestinon)–The dose must be adjusted for each patient. A frequent starting dose is 15–30 mg orally every 6 hours.

2. Neostigmine (Prostigmin)–Fifteen milligrams of neostigmine are roughly equivalent to 60 mg of pyridostigmine. Neostigmine often causes gastric hypermobility with diarrhea. It may be given parenterally.

3. Atropine–Atropine may be added on a maintenance basis to control mild cholinergic side effects such as hypersecretion, abdominal cramps, and nausea and vomiting.

4. Immunologic intervention–This is primarily by use of prednisone. Plasmapheresis is effective in some patients.

5. Myasthenic crisis–Relatively sudden difficulties in swallowing and respiration may be observed in myasthenic patients. Edrophonium will result in dramatic but brief improvement; this may make it difficult to evaluate the condition of the small child. Suctioning, respiratory assistance, and fluid and electrolyte maintenance may be required.

6. Cholinergic crisis–Cholinergic crisis may result from overdosage of anticholinesterase drugs. The resulting weakness may be similar to that of myasthenia, and the muscarinic effects (diarrhea, sweating, lacrimation, miosis, bradycardia, hypotension) are often absent or difficult to evaluate. The edrophonium test may help to determine whether the patient is receiving too little of the drug or is manifesting toxic symptoms due to overdosage. Improvement after the drugs are withdrawn suggests cholinergic crisis. Respirator facilities should be available.

C. Surgical Measures: Early thymectomy is beneficial in many patients; the effects are usually delayed. *Experienced surgical and postsurgical care are prerequisites.*

Prognosis

Neonatal (transient) myasthenia presents a great threat to life, primarily due to aspiration of secretions. With proper treatment, the symptoms usually begin to disappear within a few days to 2–3 weeks, after which the child usually requires no further treatment.

In the congenital (persistent) form, the symptoms may initially be as acute as in the transient variety; more commonly, however, they are relatively benign and constant, with gradual worsening as the child grows older. Fatal cases occur.

In the juvenile form, patients may become resistant or unresponsive to anticholinesterase compounds and require corticosteroids or treatment in a hospital, where respiratory assistance can be given as needed. The overall prognosis for survival, for remission, and for improvement after therapy with prednisone and thymectomy is favorable.

Endocrine & Metabolic Disorders | 28

Ronald W. Gotlin, MD

DISTURBANCES OF GROWTH & DEVELOPMENT

SHORT STATURE

Abnormally short stature in relation to age is a common finding in childhood. In most instances, it is due to a normal variation from the usual pattern of growth. The possible roles of such factors as sex, race, size of parents and other family members, intrauterine factors, nutrition, pubertal maturation, and emotional status must all be evaluated in the total assessment of the child (Table 28–1). The causes of unusually short stature can usually be differentiated on the basis of significant findings in the history, physical examination, and radiographic estimation of skeletal maturation ("bone age").

1. CONSTITUTIONAL DELAYED GROWTH & ADOLESCENCE

Many normal children have a delay in the onset of skeletal maturation that is considered to be "constitutional." Puberty progresses normally after a delayed onset. In other respects, they appear entirely normal. There is often a history of a similar pattern of growth in one of the parents or other members of the family. These children are usually short throughout childhood but reach normal adult height, although at an age later than average.

2. GROWTH HORMONE DEFICIENCY

The incidence of growth hormone (GH) deficiency is approximately 1:10,000. More than 75% of cases are the result of

Table 28–1. Causes of short stature.

Familial, racial, or genetic

Constitutional retarded growth and delayed adolescence

Endocrine disturbances
  Growth hormone deficiency
    Isolated somatotropin or somatotropin-releasing hormone
    deficiency
    Somatotropin deficiency with other pituitary hormone deficiencies
  Hypothyroidism
  Adrenal insufficiency
  Cushing's disease and Cushing's syndrome (including iatrogenic
  causes)
  Sexual precocity (androgen or estrogen excess)
  Diabetes mellitus (poorly controlled)
  Diabetes insipidus
  Hyperaldosteronism

Primordial short stature
  Intrauterine growth retardation
    Placental insufficiency
    Intrauterine infection
  Primordial dwarfism with premature aging
    Progeria (Hutchinson-Gilford syndrome)
    Progeroid syndrome
      Werner's syndrome
      Cachectic (Cockayne's syndrome)
  Short stature without associated anomalies
  Short stature with associated anomalies (eg, Seckel's bird-headed
  dwarfism, leprechaunism, Silver's syndrome, Bloom's syndrome,
  Cornelia de Lange syndrome, Hallerman-Streiff syndrome)

Inborn errors of metabolism
  Altered metabolism of calcium or phosphorus (eg, hypophosphatemic
  rickets, hypophosphatasia, infantile hypercalcemia,
  pseudohypoparathyroidism)
  Storage diseases
    Mucopolysaccharidoses (eg, Hurler's syndrome, Hunter's
    syndrome)
    Mucolipidoses (eg, generalized gangliosidosis, fucosidosis,
    mannosidosis)
    Sphingolipidoses (eg, Tay-Sachs disease, Niemann-Pick disease,
    Gaucher's disease)
    Miscellaneous (eg, cystinosis)
  Aminoacidemias and aminoacidurias
  Epithelial transport disorders (eg, renal tubular acidosis, cystic
  fibrosis, Bartter's syndrome, vasopressin-resistant diabetes insipidus,
  pseudohypoparathyroidism)
  Organic acidemias and acidurias (eg, methylmaionic aciduria, orotic
  aciduria, maple syrup urine disease, isovaleric acidemia)

Metabolic anemias (eg, sickle cell disease, thalassemia, pyruvate kinase deficiency)

Disorders of mineral metabolism (eg, Wilson's disease, magnesium malabsorption syndrome)

Body defense disorders (eg, Bruton's agammaglobulinemia, thymic aplasia, chronic granulomatous disease)

Constitutional (intrinsic) diseases of bone

Defects of growth of tubular bones or spine (eg, achondroplasia, metatropic dwarfism, diastrophic dwarfism, metaphyseal chondrodysplasia)

Disorganized development of cartilage and fibrous components of the skeleton (eg, multiple cartilaginous exostoses, fibrous dysplasia with skin pigmentation, precocious puberty of McCune-Albright)

Abnormalities of density of cortical diaphyseal structure or metaphyseal modeling (eg, osteogenesis imperfecta congenita, osteopetrosis, tubular stenosis)

Short stature associated with chromosomal defects

Autosomal (eg, Down's syndrome, cri du chat syndrome, trisomy 18)

Sex chromosomal (eg, Turner's syndrome-XO, penta X, XXXY)

Chronic systemic diseases, congenital defects, and cancers (eg, chronic infection and infestation, inflammatory bowel disease, hepatic disease, cardiovascular disease, hematologic disease, central nervous system disease, pulmonary disease, renal disease, malnutrition, cancers, collagen vascular disease)

Psychosocial dwarfism (deprivation dwarfism)

Miscellaneous syndromes (eg, arthrogryposis multiplex congenita, cerebrohepatorenal syndrome, Noonan's syndrome, Prader-Willi syndrome, Riley-Day syndrome)

hypothalamic releasing hormone deficiency. Approximately half of all cases involving the hypothalamus and pituitary are idiopathic (rarely familial), and the remainder are secondary to pituitary, central nervous system, or hypothalamic disease (empty sella syndrome, septooptic dysplasia, craniopharyngioma, infections, tuberculosis, sarcoidosis, toxoplasmosis, syphilis, trauma, reticuloendotheliosis, vascular anomalies, and other tumors such as gliomas). GH deficiency may be an isolated defect or may occur in combination with other pituitary hormone deficiencies.

At birth, affected infants may be small. Growth retardation is evident during infancy, and there may be infantile fat distribution, youthful facial features, small hands and feet, and delayed sexual maturation. Excessive wrinkling of the skin is present in older individuals. Hypoglycemia and microphallus may occur.

Dental development and epiphyseal maturation ("bone age") are delayed to an equal degree or more so than height age (median age for patient's height). Headaches, visual field defects, abnormal skull x-rays, and symptoms of posterior pituitary insufficiency (polyuria and polydipsia) may precede or accompany the GH deficiency in cases resulting from central nervous system disease.

GH deficiency is associated with low levels of somatomedin C and GH in the serum and a failure of the GH level to rise in response to arginine, oral levodopa, oral clonidine, exercise, or insulin-induced hypoglycemia or during normal physiologic sleep. Patients with hypothalamic deficiency may respond to growth hormone-releasing hormone. Laron type dwarfism is a rare condition in which there is an inability to generate somatomedin in response to GH. Other children may have an immunoreactive GH with reduced bioactivity.

Treatment is with synthetic human growth hormone (hGH) or growth hormone-releasing hormone, which is expected to be available soon. Protein anabolic agents (testosterone, fluoxymesterone, oxandrolone, etc) may be effective in promoting linear growth, but these drugs may cause acceleration of epiphyseal closure with decrease in eventual height.

Treatment trials employing hGH in conditions with non–hGH-dependent short stature are proceeding and in Turner's syndrome hGH treatment is efficacious. Use of hGH for *normal* short children is controversial.

3. HYPOTHYROIDISM
(See p 871.)

4. PRIMORDIAL SHORT STATURE
(Intrauterine Growth Retardation)

Primordial short stature may occur in a number of disorders, including craniofacial disproportion (see Table 28–1), or may occur in individuals with no accompanying significant physical abnormalities. Children with primordial short stature have birth weight and length below normal for gestational age. Head circumference may be normal or reduced. Thereafter, they grow parallel to but below the third percentile. Plasma GH levels are usually normal but may be elevated. In some instances, somatomedin levels are subnormal. There is an increased incidence of functional fasting hypoglycemia. In most instances, skeletal maturation ("bone age") corresponds to chronologic age or is only mildly delayed, in contrast to the more marked delay often present in children with GH and thyroid deficiency.

There is no satisfactory treatment for primordial short stature, although there may be an increase in growth rate in response to pharmacologic doses of human GH.

5. SHORT STATURE DUE TO EMOTIONAL FACTORS
(Psychosocial Short Stature, Deprivation Dwarfism)

Psychologic and emotional deprivation with disturbances in motor and personality development may be associated with short stature. Growth retardation in some of these children is the result of undernutrition; in others, undernutrition does not seem to be a factor. In some instances, in addition to being small, the child may have an increased (often voracious) appetite and a marked delay in skeletal maturation. Polydipsia and polyuria are sometimes present. These children are of normal size at birth and grow normally for a variable period before growth stops. A history of feeding problems during early infancy is common. Emotional disturbances in the family are the rule.

Placement in a foster home or a significant change in the psychologic and emotional environment at home usually results in significantly improved growth, a decrease of appetite and dietary intake to more normal levels, and personality improvement. Treatment with growth-promoting agents is not indicated.

DIFFERENTIAL DIAGNOSIS OF SHORT STATURE

Short stature may accompany or be caused by a large number of conditions (see Table 28–1). When the etiologic diagnosis is not apparent from the history and physical examination, the following laboratory studies, in addition to bone age, are useful in detecting or categorizing the common causes of short stature:

(1) Complete blood count (to detect chronic anemia, infection, cancer).

(2) Erythrocyte sedimentation rate (often elevated in collagen vascular disease, cancer, chronic infection, inflammatory bowel disease).

(3) Urinalysis and microscopic examination (occult pyelonephritis, glomerulonephritis, renal tubular disease, etc).

(4) Stool examination for occult blood, parasites, and parasite ova (inflammatory bowel disease, overwhelming parasitism).

(5) Serum electrolytes and phosphorus levels (mild adrenal insufficiency, renal tubular diseases, parathyroid disease, rickets, etc).

(6) Blood urea nitrogen and creatinine levels (occult renal insufficiency).

(7) Karyotyping (should be performed in all short girls with delayed sexual maturation with or without clinical features of Turner's syndrome).

(8) Thyroid function assessment: serum free thyroxin (FT_4) and thyroid-stimulating hormone (TSH) assay (short stature may be the only sign of hypothyroidism).

(9) GH evaluation. Blood samples for GH determination should be obtained following 20 minutes of exercise, during normal sleep, or after administration of one of the conventional provocative agents (arginine, glucagon, levodopa, clonidine, and insulin-induced hypoglycemia). Samples obtained during the first 90 minutes of sleep are preferable, since they demonstrate both the presence and the physiologic release of GH.

FAILURE TO THRIVE

Failure to thrive is present when there is a perceptible declination of growth from an established pattern or when the patient's height and weight plot consistently below the third percentile. (The term is usually reserved for infants who for various reasons fail to gain weight.) Linear growth and head circumference may also be affected; when this occurs, the underlying condition is generally more severe. There are many reasons for failure to thrive (see below and Table 28–1), although a specific cause often cannot be established. Nonaccidental trauma may be an important cause of failure to thrive.

Classification & Etiologic Diagnosis

The diagnosis of failure to thrive is usually apparent on the basis of the history and physical examination. In failure to thrive, it is useful to compare the patient's chronologic age with the height age (median age for the patient's height), weight age, and head circumference. On the basis of these measurements, 3 principal patterns can be defined and will provide a starting point in the diagnostic approach.

Group 1: This group is the most common type. The head circumference is normal, and the weight is reduced out of proportion to height. In the majority of cases of failure to thrive, undernutrition is present as a result of deficient caloric intake, malabsorption, or impaired caloric utilization.

Group 2: The head circumference is normal or enlarged for age, and the weight is only moderately reduced, usually in proportion to height. Failure to thrive is due to structural dystrophies, constitutional dwarfism, or endocrinopathies.

Group 3: Although the head circumference is normal, the weight is reduced in proportion to height, owing to a primary central nervous system deficit or intrauterine growth retardation (see Primordial Short Stature, above).

An initial period of observed nutritional rehabilitation, usually in a hospital setting, is often helpful in the diagnosis. The child should be placed on a regular diet for age, and the caloric intake and weight should be carefully plotted for 1–2 weeks. During this period, evidence of lactose intolerance is sought by checking pH and reducing substances in the stool. If stools are abnormal, the child should be placed on a lactose-free diet and further observed. Caloric intake should be increased if weight gain does not occur but intake is well tolerated. The following 3 patterns are often noted during the rehabilitation period. Pattern 1 is by far the most common.

Pattern 1: In this most common type, the intake is adequate and the weight gain is satisfactory, but the feeding technique is at fault. A disturbed infant-mother relationship leads to the decreased caloric intake.

Pattern 2: The intake is adequate, but there is no weight gain. If weight gain is unsatisfactory after increasing the calories to an adequate level (based on the infant's ideal weight for his or her height), malabsorption is a likely diagnosis. If malabsorption is present, it is usually necessary to differentiate pancreatic exocrine insufficiency (cystic fibrosis) from abnormalities of intestinal mucosa (celiac disease). In cystic fibrosis, growth velocity commonly declines from the time of birth, and appetite usually is voracious. In celiac disease, growth velocity is usually not reduced until 6–12 months of age, and inadequate caloric intake may be a prominent feature.

Pattern 3: The intake is inadequate, owing to the following: (1) Sucking or swallowing difficulties due to central nervous system or neuromuscular disease or to esophageal or oropharyngeal malformations may result in inadequate intake. (2) Inability to eat large amounts is common in patients with cardiopulmonary disease or in anorexic children suffering from chronic infections, inflammatory bowel disease, and endocrine problems (eg, hypothyroidism). Patients with celiac disease often have inadequate caloric intake in addition to malabsorption. (3) Inadequate intake may be due to vomiting, spitting up, or rumination in patients with upper intestinal tract obstruction (eg, pyloric stenosis, hiatal hernia, chalasia), chronic metabolic aberrations and acidosis (eg, renal insufficiency, diabetes mellitus or insipidus, methylmalonic acidemia), adrenogenital syndrome, increased intracranial pressure, or psychosocial abnormalities.

TALL STATURE

Although there are several conditions (Table 28–2) that may produce tall stature, by far the most common cause is a constitutional variation from normal. Tall stature is usually of concern only to adolescent and preadolescent girls.

On the basis of family history, previous pattern of growth, state of physiologic development, assessment of epiphyseal development ("bone age"), and standard growth data, the physician should make a tentative estimate of the patient's eventual height. Hormonal therapy with conjugated estrogenic substances (eg, Premarin), 5–10 mg/d orally (continuously or cyclically), has been recommended by some in cases in which the patient's predicted height is considered to be excessive and the physiologic age as determined by stage of sexual maturity and epiphyseal development has not reached the 12-year-old level. Because of known and unknown long-term effects of estrogen administration in children and variable effects of therapy, treatment with

Table 28–2. Causes of tall stature.

Constitutional (familial, genetic) factors	**Genetic causes**
	Kilinefelter's syndrome
	Syndromes of XYY, XXYY (tall as adults)
Endocrine causes	Testicular feminization
Androgen deficiency (normal height as children, tall as adults)	
Anorchidism (infection, trauma, idiopathic)	**Miscellaneous syndromes and entities**
Klinefelter's syndrome	Cerebral gigantism (Soto's syndrome)
Androgen excess (tall as children, short as adults)	Diencephalic syndrome
Pseudosexual precocity	Homocystinuria
True sexual precocity	Marfan's syndrome
Hyperthyroidism	Total lipodystrophy
Somatotropin excess (pituitary gigantism)	

estrogen seldom is recommended and should be used with caution.

Testosterone in high doses has been used to decrease height in excessively tall boys. The results are variable (average reduction in adult height is approximately 5 cm). Testicular function may be altered for a prolonged period after treatment.

DIABETES INSIPIDUS

Diabetes insipidus may result from deficient secretion of vasopressin (ADH), lack of response of the kidney to ADH, or failure of osmoreceptors to respond to elevations of osmolality. Hypofunction of the posterior lobe of the pituitary with ADH deficiency may be idiopathic or may be associated with lesions of the anterior pituitary or hypothalamus (trauma, infections, suprasellar cysts, tumors, reticuloendotheliosis, or some developmental abnormality). Congenital ADH deficiency may be transmitted as an autosomal dominant trait. In nephrogenic diabetes insipidus, a hereditary X-linked (dominant) disease affecting both sexes but more severe in males, the renal tubules fail to respond normally to ADH, and no lesion of the pituitary or hypothalamus can be demonstrated.

Clinical Findings

The onset is often sudden, with polyuria, intense thirst, constipation, and evidence of dehydration. High fever, circulatory collapse, and secondary brain damage may occur in young infants on an ordinary feeding regimen. Serum osmolality may be elevated (above 305 mosm/L), but urine osmolality remains below 280 mosm/L (specific gravity approximately 1.010) even after a 7-hour test period of thirsting. Rate of growth, sexual maturation, and general body metabolism may be impaired, and hydroureter and bladder distention may develop.

Diabetes insipidus may be differentiated from psychogenic polydipsia and polyuria by permitting the normal intake of fluid for several days and then withholding water for 7 hours or until weight loss (3% or more) demonstrates adequate dehydration. With neurogenic or nephrogenic diabetes insipidus, the urine osmolality does not increase above 300 mosm/L even after the period of dehydration. Normal children and those with psychogenic polydipsia will respond to the dehydration with a urinary osmolality above 450 mosm/L. Patients with long-standing psychogenic polydipsia may be unable to concentrate urine initially, and the test may have to be repeated on several successive days. Eventually, dehydration will increase urine osmolality well above plasma osmolality. The ADH and hypertonic saline tests may be employed to distinguish between the various forms of diabetes insipidus.

Treatment

The treatment of choice for central diabetes insipidus is intranasal desmopression acetate (1-desamino-8-D-arginine vasopressin; DDAVP).

The cautious use of chlorothiazide and ethacrynic acid may be of value in nephrogenic diabetes insipidus. (Check levels of serum electrolytes, uric acid, and blood glucose periodically.) For nephrogenic diabetes insipidus, also administer abundant quantities of water at short intervals and feedings containing limited electrolytes and minimal (but nutritionally adequate) amounts of protein.

SEXUAL PRECOCITY

In sexual precocity, the onset of secondary sexual development is earlier than anticipated by chronologic age, body mass, and family history. Sexual precocity is generally divided into 2 *major* types: Gonadotropin releasing hormone dependent (GnRH) true precocity, and GnRH independent pseudoprecocity. **True (complete) precocity** is the result of premature increases in gonadotropin either from stimulation of the hypothalamic-pituitary mechanism (eg, in children with no abnormality or in those with tumor, infection, trauma, etc) or rarely from gonadotropin-producing tumors (eg, hepatoma, choriocarcinoma). **Pseudoprecocity** is initiated by nongonadotropin-producing conditions (eg, adrenal, ovarian, and testicular tumors and other lesions) or by administration of sex steriods.

A third type, which resembles true sexual precocity but is not associated with premature elevation of gonadotropin concentrations, has been described and is termed **gonadotropin-independent true sexual precocity.** This condition is more common in males and is often familial.

In the past, true sexual precocity was considered to be idiopathic in approximately 80% of girls and 50% of boys. Currently, through the use of CT and MRI scans, small abnormalities in the region of the hypothalamus are most commonly recognized.

Sexual precocity has been arbitrarily defined as the development of secondary sex characteristics beginning before age 8 in girls and age 9½ in boys. Breast development is usually the first sign in girls, but the pattern of development is variable. Height may be normal initially, but it is often increased; osseous maturation ("bone age") may be even more advanced than height age, particularly in pseudoprecocious patients. Psychologic development tends to correspond to chronologic age. Ovarian luteal cysts may be present in response to gonadotropin stimulation. When sensitive assays are employed, urinary and serum gonadotropin levels are elevated for age, and adrenal androgen levels may be elevated to the pubertal range. Findings on EEG are frequently abnormal, particularly in boys.

Adrenal lesions (see Diseases of the Adrenal Cortex, below) are the most common causes of pseudoprecocity. Gonadal tumors are uncommon causes; the granulosa cell and theca-lutein cell tumors of the ovary are the most common, are generally unilateral and of low malignant potential, and produce excessive amounts of estrogen. In almost all instances, the tumor can be palpated transabdominally or rectally, but it is advisable to examine females with pelvic ultrasonography.

When possible, treatment is directed at the underlying cause. In the idiopathic variety the treatment of choice is a GnRH agonist. These agents result in gonadotropin suppression through endocrine "down regulation." Treatment with medroxyprogesterone acetate (Depo-Provera) and cyproterone is often unsatisfactory. Psychologic management of the patient and family is important. Children who initially have no definable causative lesion should be examined at periodic intervals for evidence of previously occult abdominal or central nervous system lesions.

Precocious Development of the Breast (Premature Thelarche)

Precocious development of one or both breasts may occur at any age. In most cases, the onset is in the first 2 years of life; in two-thirds of these cases, breast development is obvious in the first year. The condition is not associated with other evidence of sexual maturation. It may represent unusual sensitivity of the breasts to normal amounts of circulating estrogen or a temporarily increased secretion or ingestion of estrogen. Both breasts are usually involved, and enlargement may persist for months or years; the nipples generally do not enlarge. Rapid growth, advanced skeletal maturation, and menstruation do not occur in these patients, in contrast to patients with sexual precocity. Extensive diagnostic investigation is seldom warranted; no treatment is necessary. Puberty occurs at the normal time.

Premature Adrenarche (Premature Pubarche)

Premature development of sexual hair may occur at any age and in both sexes (more often in females than in males) and must be differentiated from adrenal hyperplasia. About a third of cases occur in organically brain-damaged children. It appears to result from a premature slight increase in production of adrenal androgens. (Serum dehydroepiandrosterone concentrations are elevated.) Pubic hair usually develops first, but axillary hair is present in about half of cases when these patients are first seen. True virilization does not develop; children are of normal stature, and osseous development is not advanced. Urinary 17-ketosteroid and testosterone excretions are normal. Premature adrenarche requires no treatment.

Menstruation

The age at menarche ranges from 9 to 16 years; menarche is considered delayed if it has not occurred by age 17 years or within 5 years after development of the breasts. Primary amenorrhea is the result of gonadal lesions (ie, gonadal dysgenesis) in about 60% of patients, and in such cases serum and urine gonadotropin levels are elevated. In the remaining cases of primary amenorrhea, extragonadal abnormalities are present (eg, pituitary-hypothalamic hypogonadotropinism; congenital anomalies of the tubes, uterus, or vagina; androgen excess or other endocrine imbalance; and chronic systemic disease or pelvic inflammatory disease).

Once regular periods are established, amenorrhea (ie, secondary amenorrhea; see Table 28–3) during adolescence is often the result of pregnancy, strenuous physical activity, or chronic systemic disease. Secondary amenorrhea should therefore be viewed as a symptom requiring prompt evaluation and, when possible, treatment.

GONADAL DISORDERS

Deficiency of gonadal tissue or function may result from a genetic or embryologic defect; from hormone excess affecting the fetus in utero; from inflammation and destruction following infection (eg, mumps, syphilis, tuberculosis); from trauma, irradiation, autoimmune disease, or tumor; or as a consequence of surgical castration. Secondary hypogonadism may result from pituitary insufficiency (eg, destructive lesions in or about the

Table 28–3. Causes of secondary amenorrhea.

I. Pregnancy.
II. Decreased ovarian function.
  A. Decreased gonadotropin level (secondary ovarian insufficiency).
    1. Due to organic and idiopathic hypothalamic disease, pituitary disease, or both.*
    2. Due to "functional abnormalities of the hypothalamic-pituitary axis" ("psychogenic").
    3. Due to hypothalamic-pituitary disease secondary to chronic systemic illness.
      a. Nutritional disorder (eg, anorexia nervosa).
      b. Chronic infection or systemic disease (eg, cancer, collagen vascular disease, inflammatory bowel disease).
    4. Secondary to endogenous hormones (eg, androgen excess, feminizing or masculinizing ovarian tumor).
    5. Secondary to exogenous drugs (eg, long-term contraceptive drugs, androgens, estrogens, tranquilizers).
    6. Associated with strenuous and prolonged physical activity (eg, ballet dancing, marathon running).
  B. Increased gonadotropin level (primary ovarian insufficiency).
    1. Due to acquired diseases (destruction of ovaries by infection or tumor, "premature menopause," radiation castration, surgical removal of ovaries).
    2. Due to ovarian agenesis and dysgenesis* (eg, Turner's syndrome).
III. Congenital and acquired lesions of the uterine tubes and uterus, including cases of chromosomal intersex (eg, adhesions, congenital absence of the uterus, cryptomenorrhea, hysterectomy, synechia of the uterus, testicular feminization syndrome).

*Usually or often associated with primary amenorrhea.

anterior pituitary, irradiation of the pituitary, starvation), diabetes mellitus, androgen excess (eg, adrenogenital syndrome), or insufficiency of either the thyroid or adrenals.

CRYPTORCHIDISM

Cryptorchidism (undescended testes) is a common disorder in children. It may be unilateral or bilateral and may be classified as ectopic, total, or incomplete. About 3% of term male infants and 20% of premature male infants have undescended testes at birth. In over half of these cases, the testes will descend by the second month; by age 1 year, 80% of all undescended testes are in the scrotum. If cryptorchidism persists into adult life, failure of spermatogenesis is the rule, but testicular androgen production usually remains intact. The incidence of cancer (usually seminoma) is appreciably greater in testes that remain in the abdomen after puberty.

Cryptorchidism may merely represent delayed descent of the testes or may be due to prevention of normal descent by some mechanical lesion such as adhesions, short spermatic cord, fibrous bands, or endocrine disorders (ie, decreased gonadotropins). It is probable that many undescended testes are congenitally abnormal and that this abnormality in itself prevents descent.

A causal relationship between failure of spermatogenesis and an abdominal location of testes after puberty is assumed. On occasion, the apparent abnormality of abdominal testes may be reversible (even if the testes are histologically abnormal at the time they are placed in the scrotum).

Clinical Findings

In palpating the scrotum for the testes, the cremasteric reflex may be elicited, with a resultant ascent of the testes into the abdomen (pseudocryptorchidism). To prevent this ascent, the fingers first should be placed across the upper portion of the inguinal canal. Examination in a warm bath is also helpful.

Treatment

The best age for medical or surgical treatment has not been determined, but early childhood is currently recommended. Some recommend surgery before age 5 years; others say during the first year. There appears to be a high incidence of azoospermia in testes operated on after age 10 years; recent evidence indicates that damage to germ and Leydig cells of intra-abdominal testes may occur by age 3–4 years, but the relationship of these changes to fertility is unproved. The risk of surgical injury to the testes must be weighed against the possible benefits. Surgical repair is indicated for cryptorchidism persisting beyond puberty, since the incidence of cancer is appreciably greater in glands that remain in the abdomen beyond the second decade of life.

A. Unilateral Cryptorchidism: Most cases are due to local mechanical lesions or a defective testis on the involved side. If pseudocryptorchidism has been ruled out and if descent has not occurred by age 5 years, many investigators recommend surgical exploration, with testicular biopsy and relocation by a surgeon skilled in this procedure.

B. Bilateral Cryptorchidism: The child with bilaterally undescended testes should be evaluated for sex chromosome abnormalities and genetic sex determined by chromosome analysis in the newborn period. Androgen treatment (testosterone enanthate) is indicated only as replacement therapy in the male beyond the normal age of puberty who has been shown to lack functional testes.

C. Pseudocryptorchidism: Retractile testes, ie, those that are sometimes in the scrotum but not at the time of examination, generally require no treatment.

Prognosis

Following surgery, the prognosis is guarded with respect to spermatogenesis in the involved testis.

KLINEFELTER'S SYNDROME

Klinefelter's syndrome is occasionally familial, presents at the time of puberty, and is characterized by atrophic sclerosis of the seminiferous tubules with normal Leydig cells and virilization. It is often accompanied by bilateral gynecomastia, relatively long extremities, abnormally small testes, and azoospermia or oligospermatogenesis. Gonadotropin levels (particularly luteinizing hormone levels) are usually elevated. Testosterone levels are normal or low. Many patients are mentally retarded. Some patients have histories of severe psychopathologic disorder. There is an extra X chromosome (most commonly an XXY chromosome pattern). Typical histopathologic changes may occur in men whose only complaint is sterility.

Klinefelter's syndrome must be differentiated from gonadotropin deficiency, the physiologic gynecomastia that occurs in some boys at puberty, and feminizing tumors of the adrenal cortex or testes.

There is no satisfactory treatment, but methyltestosterone, 20–40 mg/d orally, or testosterone enanthate, 200–400 mg intramuscularly every 3 weeks, continued for several months, may produce positive physical and behavioral changes and reduce gynecomastia. If it does not, surgical mastectomy for cosmetic purposes is indicated.

DISEASES OF THE THYROID

GOITER

Goiter is not uncommon in children and adolescents and is most commonly due to chronic lymphocytic thyroiditis (see Thyroiditis, p 877). It may also result from acute inflammation, iodine deficiency, infiltrative processes, neoplasms, ingestion of goitrogens, or an inborn error in thyroid metabolism (familial goiter). With the exception of hyperthyroidism (and possibly pregnancy), thyroid enlargement results from the stimulation of excess thyroid-stimulating hormone (TSH). Regardless of the cause, patients may be clinically and biochemically euthyroid, hypothyroid, or hyperthyroid.

Familial goiter results from enzymatic defects in hormonogenesis, eg, (1) iodide trapping, (2) iodide organification, (3) coupling, (4) deiodination, and (5) production of thyroglobulin and serum carrier protein. Patients with any of these defects display an autosomal recessive mode of inheritance; the organification defect may be associated with severe congenital deafness (Pendred's syndrome). The age at onset of symptoms of hypothyroidism is variable.

Substances implicated in the development of goiter include cabbage, soybeans, turnips, rutabagas, aminosalicylic acid (PAS), resorcinol, phenylbutazone, iodides (particularly in individuals who have also received corticosteroids), and drugs that interfere with iodide trapping (eg, thiocyanates).

Clinical Findings

The clinical features and physical characteristics of patients with goiters vary depending on the cause and are seldom diagnostic.

Nodular goiter may occur during childhood. The likelihood that a nodule is malignant increases when the nodule is single, hard, or associated with paratracheal lymph node enlargement or does not concentrate radioactive iodide (see Carcinoma of the Thyroid, below).

Treatment

Remove or avoid precipitating factors if possible. With the exception of hyperthyroidism and instances where specific causes can be eliminated or corrected (eg, iodide deficiency, goitrogens), treatment is with full replacement of thyroid hormone (see p 873). Surgery is necessary if cancer is a possibility.

Prophylaxis

Prophylaxis in endemic areas of iodine deficiency consists of the use of bread containing iodides or iodized salt (1 mg of iodine per 100 g of salt) or the administration of 1–2 drops of saturated solution of potassium iodide per week. Iodination of the water supply is also a satisfactory preventive measure.

NEONATAL GOITER

Neonatal goiter may result from the transplacental passage, from mother to infant, of iodides, goitrogens, antithyroid drugs, or human-specific thyroid-stimulating immunoglobulin (TSI). The latter may occur in pregnancies in which the mother has or once had Graves' disease. The offspring may temporarily be hyperthyroid, with exophthalmos. Regardless of the cause, the goiter is usually diffuse and relatively soft but may be large and firm enough to compress the trachea, esophagus, and adjacent blood vessels. Treatment varies with the cause; iodides, antithyroid drugs, or thyroid hormone (eg, levothyroxine, 0.05 mg/d) for a few weeks may be indicated. Occasionally, surgical division of the thyroid isthmus may be necessary.

HYPOTHYROIDISM

Hypothyroidism may be either congenital or acquired. Congenital hypothyroidism may be due to aplasia, hypoplasia, or maldescent of the thyroid, resulting from an embryonic defect of development; the administration of radioiodide to the mother; or, possibly, an autoimmune disease. It may be caused by defective synthesis of thyroid hormone (familial goiter; see Goiter, above). Other cases of congenital hypothyroidism may result from the maternal ingestion of medications (eg, goitrogens, propylthiouracil, methimazole, iodides), from iodide deficiency (endemic cretinism), or, rarely, from thyroid hormone unresponsiveness. Thyroid tissue in an aberrant location is present in most patients with sporadic "athyreotic" cretinism.

Acquired (juvenile) hypothyroidism is most commonly the result of chronic lymphocytic thyroiditis (see Thyroiditis, p 877) but may be idiopathic or the result of surgical removal, thyrotropin deficiency (usually associated with other pituitary tropic hormone deficiencies), the ingestion of medications (eg, iodides, cobalt), or a deficiency of iodides. An ectopic thyroid gland, a relatively common cause of hypothyroidism, may maintain normal function for variable periods postnatally. Breast-feeding may mitigate severe hypothyroidism and perhaps prevent impaired neurologic development in the hypothyroid patient.

Clinical Findings

The findings depend on age at onset and the degree of deficiency.

A. Symptoms and Signs:

1. Functional changes–Findings include decreased appetite; physical and mental sluggishness; pale, dry, coarse cool skin; decreased intestinal activity (constipation); large tongue; poor muscle tone (protuberant abdomen, umbilical hernia, lumbar lordosis); hypothermia; bradycardia; diminished sweating (variable); carotenemia; decreased pulse pressure; hoarse voice or cry; and slow relaxation on eliciting tendon reflexes. Prolonged gestation, large size at birth, nasal obstruction and discharge, large fontanelles, hypoactivity, and persistent jaundice may also be present during the neonatal period. Even with congenital deficiency of thyroid hormone, the first findings may not appear for several days or weeks.

2. Retardation of growth and development–Findings include decreased growth velocity with resultant shortness of stature; infantile skeletal proportions, with relatively short extremities; infantile naso-orbital configuration (bridge of nose flat, broad, and undeveloped; eyes seem to be widely spaced); retarded "bone age" and epiphyseal dysgenesis; retarded dental development and enamel hypoplasia; and large fontanelles in the neonate. Slowing of mental responsiveness and retardation of development of the brain may occur. In older children and adolescents, growth failure may be the only manifestation of hypothyroidism.

3. Sexual precocity–Rarely, isosexual precocity may occur, resulting from elevated gonadotropin levels. Galactorrhea may be present, and menometrorrhagia has been reported in older girls. Testicular enlargement occurs rarely in boys.

4. Other changes–Myxedema of tissues may occur. The skin may be dry, thick, scaly, and coarse, with a yellowish tinge from excessive deposition of carotene. The hair is dry, coarse, and brittle (variable) and may be excessive. The axillary and supraclavicular pads may be prominent. Muscular hypertrophy (Kocher, Debré-Sémélaigne syndromes) occasionally is present. Psychosis secondary to myxedema has been described. An ectopic thyroid gland may produce a mass at the base of the tongue or in the midline of the neck.

B. Laboratory Findings: Thyroxine (T$_4$) and thyroid-stimulating hormone (TSH) levels are the most helpful aids in diagnosing hypothyroidism. Levels of T$_4$ and free T$_4$ are reduced; TSH levels are increased in primary hypothyroidism. Serum carotene and cholesterol levels are usually elevated in hypothyroid children but may be normal in some hypothyroid infants; a rise to abnormally high levels occurs 6–8 weeks after cessation of therapy. The basal metabolic rate is low (unreliable in children). Serum alkaline phosphatase levels are reduced; BUN and creatinine levels may be increased. Erythrocyte glucose 6-phosphate dehydrogenase activity is decreased. Sweat electrolyte levels are often increased. Circulating autoantibodies to thyroid constituents may be found. Plasma GH levels and GH response to insulin-induced hypoglycemia and arginine stimulation may be subnormal.

C. Imaging: Epiphyseal development ("bone age") is delayed. The cardiac shadow may be increased. Epiphyseal dysgenesis, coxa vara, coxa plana, and vertebral anomalies may occur. The pituitary fossa may be enlarged.

Treatment

Levothyroxine sodium is a reliable synthetic agent for thyroid replacement therapy. The dose is 100 μg/m^2 (10–12 μg/kg in neonates). Older children, adolescents, and adults require 0.15–0.2 mg daily in one dose. In hypothyroid patients, particularly myxedematous infants, low doses (0.025–0.05 mg) should be used initially and increased weekly in small increments. The therapeutic range is evaluated by clinical response (appearance, growth, development), sleeping pulses, and thyroid function tests. (T$_4$ levels, when a euthyroid state has been reached, may be 25% higher than accepted "normal" levels in untreated individuals.) Improvement usually occurs in 1–3 weeks.

Course & Prognosis

In patients with congenital hypothyroidism, growth and motor development can be returned to normal with adequate replacement therapy. The prognosis for mental development is guarded if treatment is delayed beyond 3 months of life. In patients with acquired hypothyroidism, restoration of physical and mental function to the predisease level is variable following replacement therapy. Overtreatment with thyroid drugs may produce accelerated skeletal maturation and craniosynostosis.

HYPERTHYROIDISM

Hyperthyroidism appears to occur in individuals who demonstrate a reduced capacity to remove host-directed thyroid-stimulating immunoglobulins. In addition, psychic trauma, psychologic maladjustments, disturbances in pituitary function, infectious disease, heredity, and imbalance of the endocrine system all have been incriminated in the etiology and pathogenesis of hyperthyroidism. Congenital hyperthyroidism, sometimes persisting or recurring for months or years with or without exophthalmos, may occur in infants of thyrotoxic mothers and be associated with premature synostosis, minimal brain dysfunction, accelerated "bone age," and goiter.

Hyperthyroidism (with normal T_4 levels) may result from isolated hypersecretion of triiodothyronine (T_3 toxicosis) but is uncommon during childhood except in relapse.

Clinical Findings

A. Symptoms and Signs: The disease usually develops rapidly and is more common in girls, (5:1), with the highest incidence between ages 12 and 14 years. The manifestations may include the following in any combination: "nervousness" (ie, restlessness, mood swings, hand tremors); palpitations and tachycardia, even during sleep, and systolic hypertension with increased pulse pressure; warm and moist skin and flushed face; exophthalmos; diffuse goiter, usually firm, with or without bruit and thrill; weakness and loss of weight in spite of polyphagia; accelerated growth and development; and poor school performance. Amenorrhea is common in adolescent girls. Premature craniosynostosis may occur.

B. Laboratory Findings: Levels of T_4, free T_4, and T_3 resin uptake are elevated. T_3 levels may be elevated. Serum cholesterol and TSH levels are low. Circulating TSI levels are usually above normal. There is moderate leukopenia and glucosuria. Glycosuria may be present.

Treatment

Antithyroid drugs, radioactive iodide, and surgical methods are equally capable of eliminating the manifestations of hyperthyroidism and yield approximately equal numbers of "cured" patients.

A. General Measures:

1. Restricted physical activity–Activity should be restricted, especially in severe cases, in preparation for surgery or at the beginning of a medical regimen.

2. Diet–The diet should be high in calories, proteins, and vitamins.

3. Sedation–Large doses of barbiturates or tranquilizers may be necessary to control nervousness.

4. Sympatholytic drugs–These drugs (eg, propranolol) decrease the peripheral conversion of T_4 to T_3 and diminish cardiovascular and some neurologic symptoms. They are also helpful in preparation for thyroid surgery.

B. Specific Measures: With medical treatment, clinical response may be noted in about 2–3 weeks, and adequate control may be achieved in 2–3 months. The thyroid gland frequently increases in size after initiation of treatment, but it usually decreases in size after 3 months.

1. Propylthiouracil–This drug blocks the hormonogenesis and release of thyroid hormone as well as the peripheral conversion of T_4 to T_3. It may be used in the initial treatment of the patient with hyperthyroidism, but if the T_4 fails to return to a normal range, surgery may be necessary, although some patients may be controlled by long-continued (> 5 years) medical therapy. Relapses occur in 25–50% of patients, and severe cases may not respond. Therapy must usually be continued at least 2–3 years with the minimum drug dosage that will produce a euthyroid state.

a. Initial dosage–Give 100–800 mg/d in 3 or 4 divided doses 6 or 8 hours apart until results of thyroid function tests are normal and all signs and symptoms have subsided. Larger doses may be necessary.

b. Maintenance dosage–Give 100–150 mg/d in 1–3 divided doses. The drug may be continued at higher doses until hypothyroidism has resulted, and then a supplement of oral thyroid may be added. Thyroid hormone should also be given if the gland remains large after 1–2 months of control with propylthiouracil therapy.

2. Methimazole (Tapazole)–This may be used in $\frac{1}{15}$–$\frac{1}{10}$ the dosage of propylthiouracil. Toxic reactions are slightly more common with this drug than with the thiouracils.

3. Iodide–Iodide is generally not recommended.

4. Radioactive iodide–Radioiodide therapy is currently recommended by some either as initial treatment or if medical therapy fails. Regardless of the dose or type of radioactive iodide employed, hypothyroidism generally can be anticipated at variable periods after treatment.

5. Other drugs–Antithyroid drugs, antibiotics, sedation, propranolol, reserpine, and guanethidine may be of value for the treatment of thyroid storm.

C. Surgical Measures: Subtotal thyroidectomy is considered by some to be the treatment of choice for children, especially if close follow-up is difficult or impossible. The patient should be prepared first with bed rest, diet, propranolol, and sedation (as above) and with propylthiouracil (for 2–4 weeks). Iodide (2–10 drops daily of saturated solution of potassium iodide for 10–21 days) may be of value. Continue for 1 week after surgery.

Course & Prognosis

Medical treatment is usually effective within 2–3 years. With medical treatment alone, prolonged remissions may be expected in about one-third of cases. Hypothyroidism is likely in later life. The risk of developing leukemia or carcinoma of the thyroid after treatment with radioactive iodide has not been determined.

CARCINOMA OF THE THYROID
(See also Chapter 29.)

Carcinoma of the thyroid is uncommon. It is most likely to occur following irradiation of the neck and chest. Findings include goiter, neck discomfort, dysphagia, and voice changes or a nodule of the thyroid that fails to regress despite therapy with a large dose of thyroid hormones for a period of 1–2 months. Surgical extirpation of the entire gland, with removal of all involved nodes, is the treatment of choice. Radical neck dissection is seldom necessary. Postoperatively, the patient may be allowed to become hypothyroid and a diagnostic scan with radioactive iodide then done; metastases, if present, can be treated with ^{131}I or removed surgically, if feasible. Subsequent thyroid replacement therapy should consist of larger than maintenance doses. Patients with papillary carcinoma have a good prognosis for prolonged (> 10 years) survival.

Medullary carcinoma may be familial and associated with multiple endocrine adenomatosis, marfanoid body habitus, nodularities (mucosal neuromas) of the tongue and mucous membranes, and pheochromocytoma or visceral ganglioneuromas. The serum calcitonin level is elevated basally or after stimulation with pentagastrin.

GOITROUS CRETINISM
(See Familial Goiter, p 870.)

THYROIDITIS

Acute thyroiditis produces an acute inflammatory goiter and may be due to almost any pathogenic organism (viral or bacterial) or may be nonspecific or idiopathic. Most children are euthyroid and free of symptoms, but hypothyroidism or hyperthyroidism may be present. Specific antibiotic therapy and corticosteroids may be of value.

Subacute thyroiditis (pseudotuberculosis, de Quervain's giant cell thyroiditis) is characterized by mild and transient manifestations of hypermetabolism and an enlarged, very tender, firm thyroid gland. The T_4 concentration is elevated, and ^{131}I uptake by the gland is reduced. Aspirin (mild cases) and corticosteroids and thyroid hormone (severe disease) may be of value.

Chronic thyroiditis (lymphomatous or Hashimoto's struma, autoimmune thyroiditis) is being seen with increasing frequency, particularly in pubertal patients ("adolescent goiter"). It may be associated with other endocrine disorders (eg, Addison's disease, type I diabetes mellitus) resulting from autoimmune damage to the organ. It is characterized by firm, nontender, diffuse or nodular, "pebbly" enlargement of the thyroid with variable activity. Occasionally, there are symptoms of mild tracheal compression. Definitive diagnosis can be made only by histologic examination; thyroid function tests, antithyroid antibody tests, and scanning studies provide varying results. Needle biopsy of the gland is often diagnostic but is not generally indicated. Treatment is with thyroid hormone in full replacement dosage. Hypothyroidism is often an end result, and lifelong treatment may be required.

DISEASES OF THE PARATHYROID GLANDS

HYPOPARATHYROIDISM

Hypoparathyroidism may be idiopathic, may result from parathyroidectomy, or may be one feature of a general autoimmune disorder associated with candidiasis, Addison's disease, pernicious anemia, diabetes mellitus, thyroiditis, ovarian failure, and alopecia. Transient hypoparathyroidism may occur in the neonate as a result of parathyroid gland immaturity; the condition is more common in the offspring of diabetic and of hyperparathyroid mothers.

Clinical Findings

A. Symptoms and Signs:

1. Tetany–Symptoms and signs include numbness, cramps and twitchings of extremities, carpopedal spasm, laryngospasm, a positive Chvostek sign (tapping of the face in front of the ear produces spasm of the facial muscles), a positive peroneal sign (tapping the fibular side of the leg over the peroneal nerve produces abduction and dorsiflexion of the foot), and a positive Trousseau sign (prolonged compression of the upper arm produces carpal spasm).

2. Prolonged hypocalcemia–In addition to the findings listed above, prolonged hypocalcemia may be associated with growth retardation, blepharospasm and chronic conjunctivitis, cataracts, unexplained bizarre behavior, diarrhea, photophobia, irritability, loss of consciousness, convulsions, poor dentition, skin rashes, ectodermal dysplasias, fungal infections *(Candida)*, "idiopathic" epilepsy, symmetric punctate calcifications of basal ganglia, and steatorrhea. Candidiasis, Addison's disease, thyroiditis, and pernicious anemia may precede or follow the hypoparathyroidism in the familial "autoimmune" form.

B. Laboratory Findings: See Table 28–4. Serum parathyroid levels are inappropriately low.

Treatment

The objective of treatment is to maintain serum calcium at a low normal level.

A. Tetany: In patients with acute or severe tetany, immediate correction of hypocalcemia is indicated. Give calcium intravenously and orally. Thiazide diuretics may be used to increase urinary calcium reabsorption.

B. Prolonged Hypocalcemia: For maintenance therapy in patients with hypoparathyroidism and chronic hypocalcemia, use calciferol 1,25 dihydroxycholecalciferol or dihydrotachysterol (see Chapter 38). The diet should be high in calcium, with added calcium lactate or carbonate, and should be adequate in phosphorus.

PSEUDOHYPOPARATHYROIDISM
(Seabright Bantam Syndrome)

Pseudohypoparathyroidism consists of a group of disorders generally having a familial X-linked dominant syndrome in which there is no lack of parathyroid hormone but a failure of response in the end organs (eg, the renal tubule). The symptoms and signs

Table 28–4. Laboratory findings in rickets and disorders of calcium metabolism.[*]

Condition	Serum Concentration				Urinary Excretion	
	Ca^{2+}	P	Alk P'tase	PTH	Ca^{2+}	P
Chronic renal insufficiency	↓ (N)	↑	↑ (N)	↑	↓ (N)	↓
Hypoparathyroid states	↓	↑	N		↓	↓
Malabsorption syndrome	↓ (N)	↓ (N)	↑ (N)	↑ (N)	↓	N (↑ ↓)
Rickets						
Familial hypophosphatemic vitamin D-resistant	N (↓)	↓	N	N (↑)	N	↑
Hereditary vitamin D-refractory	↓	↓ (N)	↑	↑	↑	↑
Vitamin D-deficient	↓ (N)	↓	↑	↑	↑	↑
Transient tetany of the newborn	↓	↓ (N)	↓ (N)	↓ (N)	↓ (N)	↓ (N)

[*]Tubular reabsorption of phosphate (TRP) normally is 83–98%; the lower values are associated with higher serum levels of phosphorus. In hypoparathyroidism, TRP values vary from 40 to 70%. Low TRP values are also found in some forms of inherited renal tubular disease, eg, vitamin D-resistant rickets.

of hypocalcemia are the same as in idiopathic hypoparathyroidism. Patients with pseudohypoparathyroidism have round, full faces, stubby fingers (shortening of the first, fourth, and fifth metacarpals), mental subnormality, shortness of stature, delayed and defective dentition, and early closure of the epiphyses. X-rays may show dyschondroplastic changes in the bones of the hands, demineralization of the bones, thickening of the cortices, exostoses, and ectopic calcification of the basal ganglia and subcutaneous tissues. Corneal and lenticular opacities may be present.

Treatment is with vitamin D and supplementary oral calcium lactate or carbonate.

Pseudohypoparathyroidism type II is the result of a cellular defect in which neither cAMP nor parathyroid hormone produces a phosphaturic effect.

HYPERPARATHYROIDISM

Hyperparathyroidism may be primary (occasionally familial) or secondary. Primary hyperparathyroidism may be due to adenoma or diffuse parathyroid hyperplasia. The most common causes of the secondary form are chronic renal disease (glomerulonephritis, pyelonephritis), congenital anomalies of the genitourinary tract, pseudohypoparathyroidism, and vitamin D-refractory rickets. Rarely, it may be found in osteogenesis imperfecta, cancer with bony metastases, and vitamin D-resistant rickets.

Clinical Findings

A. Symptoms and Signs:

1. Due to hypercalcemia*–Findings include hypotonicity and weakness of muscles; nausea, vomiting, and poor tone of the gastrointestinal tract, with constipation; loss of weight; hyperextensibility of joints; bradycardia; and shortening of the QT interval.

2. Due to increased calcium and phosphorus excretion–Polyuria, hyposthenuria, polydipsia, and precipitation of calcium phosphate in the renal parenchyma or as urinary calculi (ie, sand or gravel) may occur.

3. Related to changes in the skeleton–Findings include oste-

---

*Hypercalcemia may also be secondary to immobilization, excess intake of vitamin D, sarcoidosis, milk-alkali syndrome, extensive fat necrosis of the newborn, or certain types of cancer, or it may occur as a familial disease.

itis fibrosa, absence of lamina dura around the teeth, spontaneous fractures, and a "moth-eaten" appearance of the skull.

B. Laboratory Findings: Serum calcium and parathyroid hormone, urinary phosphorus, cAMP, and hydroxyproline excretion are increased (Table 28–5).

C. Imaging: Bone changes usually do not occur in children with an adequate calcium intake. When bone changes occur, there is a generalized demineralization with a predilection for the subperiosteal cortical bone. The distal clavicle and phalanges are usually first affected. Nephrocalcinosis is an important additional x-ray finding.

Treatment

Complete removal of tumor or subtotal removal of hyperplastic parathyroid glands is indicated. Preoperatively, fluids should be forced and the intake of calcium restricted. Postoperatively, the diet should be high in calcium, phosphorus, and vitamin D.

Treatment of secondary hyperparathyroidism (viz renal disease) is directed at the underlying disease. Decrease the intake of phosphate by use of aluminum hydroxide orally and by reduction of milk consumption.

Course & Prognosis

Although the condition may recur (particularly in patients with familial forms of hyperparathyroidism), the prognosis following subtotal parathyroidectomy or removal of an adenoma is usually quite good. The prognosis in the secondary forms depends on correcting the underlying defect. Renal function may remain abnormal.

IDIOPATHIC HYPERCALCEMIA

Idiopathic hypercalcemia (Williams's syndrome) is an uncommon disorder probably related to either excessive intake or increased sensitivity to vitamin D. The disease is characterized in its severe form by peculiar facies (receding mandible, depressed bridge of nose, relatively large mouth, prominent lips, hanging jowls, large low-set ears, "elfin" appearance), failure to thrive, mental and motor retardation, irritability, purposeless movements, constipation, hypotonia, polyuria, polydipsia, hypertension, and heart disease (especially supravalvular aortic stenosis). Generalized osteosclerosis is common, and there may be premature craniosynostosis and nephrocalcinosis with evidence of urinary tract disease. Hypercholesterolemia, azotemia,

Table 28–5. Laboratory findings in hypercalcemia.

| Condition | Metabolic Features | | | | | Bone Pathology |
| | Serum Concentration | | | Urinary Excretion | | |
	Ca²⁺	P	P'tase	Ca²⁺	P	
Excessive vitamin D	↑	↑	N	↑	N (↑)	
Hyperparathyroidism	↑	↓	N (↑)	↑	↑	Generalized osteitis fibrosa
Hyperparathyroidism with impaired renal function	↑	N (↑)	↑	↑	↑	Generalized osteitis fibrosa
Hyperproteinemia	↑ (total) N (ionized)	N	N	N	N	
Idiopathic hypercalcemia	↑	N	N	↑	N	See text
Neoplasms of bone	N (↑)	N	N (↑)	↑	N (↑)	Bone destruction

882

and serum vitamin A elevations may be present. Familial benign hypercalcemia has been reported.

Clinical manifestations may not appear for several months. Severe disease may end in death. Mild disease may occur without the typical facies and other findings and has a good prognosis.

Treatment is by rigid restriction of dietary calcium and vitamin D and, in severely involved children, the administration of corticosteroids in high doses.

HYPOPHOSPHATASIA

Hypophosphatasia is an uncommon heritable condition characterized by rickets and a deficiency of alkaline phosphatase. The earlier the age at onset, the more severe the condition. Failure to thrive, premature loss of teeth, widening of the sutures, bulging fontanelles, convulsions, bony deformities, dwarfing, and renal lesions have been reported. Premature closure of cranial sutures may occur. Late features include osteoporosis, pseudofractures, and rachitic deformities. Signs and symptoms may be similar to those of idiopathic hypercalcemia. The serum calcium level is frequently high. The urinary hydroxyproline level is low during infancy. The plasma and urine contain phosphoethanolamine in excessive amounts. No specific treatment is available; corticosteroids may be of value.

DISEASES OF THE ADRENAL CORTEX

ADRENOCORTICAL HYPOFUNCTION
(Adrenal Crisis, Addison's Disease)

Adrenocortical hypofunction may be due to atrophy; autoimmune disease; destruction of the gland by a tumor, hemorrhage (Waterhouse-Friderichsen syndrome), or infection (eg, tuberculosis); congenital absence of the adrenal cortex; or congenital hyperplasia of the cortex associated with glucocorticoid insufficiency with or without androgen excess. It may occur as a consequence of inadequate secretion of corticotropin (ACTH) due to anterior pituitary or hypothalamic disease. Any acute illness, surgery, trauma, or exposure to excessive heat may precipitate an adrenal crisis. A temporary salt-losing disorder (possibly due to hypoaldosteronism) may occur during infancy.

Adrenogenital syndrome and associated adrenal insufficiency, congenital adrenocortical insufficiency, autoimmune adrenal insufficiency, and neoplasms are the most common causes of chronic adrenocortical insufficiency. Autoimmune Addison's disease may be associated with hypoparathyroidism, lymphocytic thyroiditis, candidiasis, pernicious anemia, ovarian failure, alopecia, and diabetes mellitus. Antiadrenal antibodies may be present.

Clinical Findings

A. Symptoms and Signs:

1. Acute form (adrenal crisis)–Signs and symptoms include nausea and vomiting; diarrhea; dehydration; fever, which may be followed by hypothermia; circulatory collapse; and confusion or coma.

2. Chronic form (Addison's disease)–Signs and symptoms include vomiting (which becomes forceful and sometimes projectile), diarrhea, weakness, fatigue, weight loss or failure to gain weight, increased appetite for salt, dehydration, opisthotonos (rare), increased pigmentation (both generalized and over pressure points and scars and on mucous membranes), hypotension, and small heart size.

B. Laboratory Findings:

1. Adrenal insufficiency–Findings suggestive of adrenal insufficiency include the following:

a. Serum sodium, chloride, and carbon dioxide levels are decreased.

b. Serum potassium* and blood urea nitrogen levels are increased.

c. Urinary sodium levels are increased despite low serum sodium levels.

d. Eosinophilia and moderate neutropenia occur.

e. Fasting blood glucose levels are generally normal but may be low in crisis.

f. There is inability to excrete a water load.

2. Adrenal cortex function–Results of confirmatory tests to measure the functional capacity of the adrenal cortex include the following:

a. Blood cortisol and urinary 17-hydroxycorticosteroid levels and ketogenic steroid excretion levels are decreased. ACTH levels are increased in primary adrenal insufficiency.

---

*Hyperkalemia may persist for 2 or 3 months in infants with adrenogenital syndrome despite treatment.

b. Urinary 17-ketosteroid levels are decreased except in cases due to congenital hyperplasia or tumor of the cortex.

c. Circulating eosinophil counts are elevated. If the blood eosinophil count is under $50/\mu L$, the diagnosis of primary adrenocortical insufficiency is doubtful.

d. Corticotropin and metyrapone tests.

e. In the prolonged corticotropin (ACTH) test, blood and urine levels of cortisol on the day before and on the day of ACTH infusion are compared. A rise of 50–100% or more in cortisol excludes primary adrenal insufficiency.

Treatment

A. Acute Form (Adrenal Crisis):

1. Treat infections with large doses of the appropriate antibiotics or other antimicrobial agents.

2. Treat hypovolemia with adequate fluid and electrolyte therapy. Infusion of a solution of human albumin may be necessary in severe cases.

3. In Waterhouse-Friderichsen syndrome with fulminant infections, adrenocorticosteroids and isoproterenol should be used.

4. For replacement therapy, use the following:

a. Initially, hydrocortisone sodium succinate (Solu-Cortef), 2 mg/kg diluted in 2–10 mL of water intravenously, is given over 2–5 minutes. Follow this with an infusion of normal saline and 5–10% glucose, 100 mL/kg/24 h intravenously.

b. Hydrocortisone sodium succinate, 1.5 mg/kg (12.5 mg/m^2), is given intravenously every 4–6 hours until stabilization is achieved and oral therapy tolerated.

c. Ten percent glucose in normal saline, 20 mL/kg intravenously in the first 2 hours, may be of value, particularly in infants with adrenal crisis who have congenital adrenal hyperplasia. Avoid overtreatment.

5. Fruit juices, ginger ale, milk, and soft foods should be started as soon as possible.

B. Chronic Form (Addison's Disease):
There may be variable response to different glucocorticoids in some patients. (See Table 28–6 for conversion of other corticosteroids to hydrocortisone equivalents.) Maintenance therapy following initial stabilization generally requires the use of a corticosteroid together with a liberal intake of salt and a fluorinated steroid. Children requiring prolonged adrenocorticosteroid administration should have periodic determinations of height, weight, and blood pressure (taken in the recumbent position) and assay of blood glucose, ACTH, sodium, and potassium.

Table 28–6. Corticosteroids.

Generic and Chemical Name	Potency per Milligram Compared with Hydrocortisone*	
	Glucocorticoid Effect	Mineralocorticoid Effect
Glucocorticoids		
Hydrocortisone	1	1
Betamethasone	33	
Dexamethasone	30	Minimal
Fluprednisolone	13	
Methylprednisolone	5	Minimal
Paramethasone	10–12	
Prednisolone	4	Minimal
Prednisone	4	Minimal
Triamcinolone	5	Minimal
Mineralocorticoids		
Aldosterone	30	500
Fludrocortisone		15–20

*To convert hydrocortisone dosage to equivalent dosage in any of the other preparations listed in this table, divide by the potency factors shown.

1. **Hydrocortisone**–Dosages are as follows:

a. Physiologic replacement–

(1) Intramuscularly–0.44 mg/kg or 13–20 mg/m^2 once daily.

(2) Orally*–0.66 mg/kg or 20 mg/m^2/d.

b. Therapeutic use–

(1) Intramuscularly–4.4 mg/kg or 130 mg/m^2 once daily.

(2) Orally*–6.6 mg/kg or 200 mg/m^2/d.

c. Therapeutic maintenance–

(1) Intramuscularly–1.3–2.2 mg/kg or 40–65 mg/m^2 once daily.

(2) Orally*–2–3.3 mg/kg or 60–100 mg/m^2/d.

d. Development of infection–If infection occurs while the patient is receiving a large dose of glucocorticoid, give about 2–3 times the physiologic maintenance dose for 3 or 4 days and then resume the larger dose.

e. Long-term maintenance–Except when used for replacement therapy (ie, in the treatment of Addison's disease and the adrenogenital syndrome) and in the treatment of certain malignant states, the total 2-day dose of glucocorticoid for long-term

*In 4 doses 6 hours apart (preferred) or 3 doses every 8 hours, providing approximately 50% of the total dose in the early morning.

maintenance therapy may be administered as a single dose once every 48 hours. This will not diminish the therapeutic efficacy but will diminish the side effects; there may be normal growth and decreased tendency to cushingoid appearance.

2. Fludrocortisone–Give fludrocortisone, 0.05–0.2 mg daily in 2 divided doses.

3. Sodium chloride–Give 1–3 g/d (as enteric-coated salt pills if they can be taken). Reduce the dose if edema appears.

4. Increased dosages–Additional glucocorticoids (2–3 times the maintenance dose) may be necessary with acute illness, surgery, trauma, or other stress reactions after optimal glucocorticoid stabilization has been achieved.

C. Other Recommendations:

1. If corticosteroids have been administered for more than 1 month, terminate their use gradually. Abrupt withdrawal may cause a severe "rebound" of the disease or produce symptoms of adrenal insufficiency.

2. Give corticosteroids to any child undergoing surgery, severe infection, or other significant stress who has received prolonged therapy with corticosteroids in the past.

3. If a child receiving maintenance doses of corticosteroids develops chickenpox, the dosage of glucocorticoids should be increased to pharmacologic levels (eg, 3 times maintenance). Corticosteroid withdrawal in these circumstances may have a fatal outcome.

4. Use of topical corticosteroids for the treatment of inflammatory skin conditions may result in absorption of significantly large amounts of corticosteroid.

D. Corticosteroids in Patients Requiring Surgery: In patients with current or previous adrenocortical insufficiency who undergo surgery, corticosteroids are given as follows:

1. Preoperatively–Give cortisone acetate intramuscularly in a single dose (100% of maintenance) 24 hours before surgery and in a single dose (200% of maintenance) 1 hour before surgery.

2. During operation–Give hydrocortisone sodium succinate (Solu-Cortef), 1–2 mg/kg by intravenous infusion over a 6- to 12-hour period.

3. Postoperatively–Give cortisone acetate intramuscularly, 100–200% of maintenance daily, for 1–2 days. Begin oral preparation as soon as possible, and give full maintenance doses daily. If the maintenance dose is unknown, give 1.25 mg/kg intramuscularly as follows: 100% of total dose at 8:00 AM and 50% of dose at 2:00 PM and at 10:00 PM. If significant stress occurs postoperatively, give 3–5 times the maintenance dose.

ADRENOCORTICAL HYPERFUNCTION

1. CUSHING'S SYNDROME

The principal findings in Cushing's syndrome in children result from excessive secretion of glucocorticoid and androgenic hormones, leading to varying degrees of abnormal carbohydrate, protein, and fat metabolism and virilization. There may also be lesser degrees of overproduction of mineralocorticoids.

Cushing's syndrome is more common in females; in children under 12 years of age, noniatrogenic disease is usually due to adrenal tumor. Hemihypertrophy may be present. Cushing's syndrome is a common result of therapy with corticotropin or one of the corticosteroids. Rarely, it may be associated with an apparently primary adrenocortical hyperplasia or hyperplasia secondary either to basophilic adenoma of the pituitary gland or to an ectopic ACTH-producing tumor. Spontaneous remission has been reported.

Clinical Findings

A. Symptoms and Signs:

1. Due to excessive secretion of the carbohydrate-regulating hormones–"Buffalo type" adiposity, most marked on the face, neck, and trunk, may occur; a fat pad in the interscapular area is characteristic. Other findings include easy fatigability and muscle weakness, striae, plethoric facies, easy bruisability, osteoporosis, increased appetite, growth failure, diabetes (usually latent), psychologic disturbances, and pain in the back.

2. Due to excessive secretion of androgens–Findings include hirsutism, acne, varying degrees of clitoral or penile enlargement, advanced skeletal maturation, and deepening of the voice. Menstrual irregularities occur in older girls.

3. Due to excessive production of mineralocorticoids–Sodium retention with hypertension (rarely edema) occurs.

B. Laboratory Findings:

1. Serum chloride and potassium levels may be low.

2. Serum sodium, pH, and carbon dioxide content may be elevated.

3. Plasma and urine cortisol levels are increased, and plasma diurnal variation may not occur.

4. Excretions of urinary 17-ketosteroids, 17-hydroxycorticosteroids, 17-ketogenic steroids, and free cortisol are generally increased; the test for free cortisol is the assay of choice. Increased secretion of ACTH occurs in patients with adrenal hyperplasia and with ACTH-secreting nonendocrine tumors but

not with other adrenal tumors. Suppression of blood cortisol and 17-hydroxycorticosteroids by high doses of dexamethasone occurs with adrenal hyperplasia but not with adrenal tumors.

5. Eosinophil counts are below 50/μL.

6. Glycosuria alone or with carbohydrate intolerance and hyperglycemia may be present ("diabetic" type of glucose tolerance curve).

7. Abdominal ultrasonography, CT or MRI scanning, and radioactive cholesterol uptake studies may be helpful in localizing a tumor.

Treatment

Since almost all cases of primary adrenal hyperfunction in childhood are due to tumor, surgical removal (if possible) is indicated. Corticotropin has been recommended for pre- and postoperative use to stimulate the nontumorous adrenal cortex, which is generally atrophied. Corticosteroids should be administered for 1 or 2 days before surgery and continued during and after operation. Supplemental potassium, normal saline solution, and fludrocortisone may be necessary.

Pituitary surgery, irradiation, or cyproheptadine may be of value to control Cushing's disease resulting from adrenal hyperplasia. If these measures are ineffective, bilateral adrenalectomy and hypophysectomy may be tried.

Prognosis

If the tumor is malignant, the prognosis is poor. If it is benign, cure should result following proper preparation and surgery. Following total bilateral adrenalectomy, pituitary tumors may appear in Cushing's disease.

2. ADRENOGENITAL SYNDROME

Adrenogenital syndrome is most commonly the result of tumor or congenital adrenal hyperplasia; maternal androgens from endogenous and exogenous sources and tumor may also be causative.

The congenital form of adrenogenital syndrome (due to adrenal hyperplasia) is an autosomal recessive disease due to an inborn error of metabolism with a deficiency of an adrenocortical enzyme. Various types are recognized, including the following:

(1) Deficiency of 21-hydroxylase (approximately 90% of cases), resulting in inability to convert 17-hydroxyprogesterone into 11-deoxycortisol. Mild forms result in androgenic changes

(virilization) alone, but severe cases are associated with salt loss and electrolyte imbalance.

(2) Deficiency in 11β-hydroxylation and a failure to convert 11-deoxycortisol to cortisol. This is associated with virilization and usually with hypertension.

(3) A defect in 17-hydroxylase, with the enzyme deficiency in both the adrenals and the gonads. Hypertension, virilization, amenorrhea, and eunuchoidism may be present.

(4) A partial or complete defect in 3β-hydroxysteroid dehydrogenase activity and a failure to convert Δ^5-pregnenolone to progesterone. This is associated with incomplete masculinization, hypospadias, and cryptorchidism in the male. Some degree of masculinization may occur in the female. Severe sodium loss occurs, and the infant mortality rate is high in the complete form.

(5) Cholesterol desmolase deficiency with congenital lipoid adrenal hyperplasia. Clinical features are similar to those of 3β-hydroxysteroid dehydrogenase deficiency (above).

Adrenogenital Syndrome in Females (Pseudohermaphroditism)

In congenital bilateral hyperplasia of the adrenal cortex (pseudohermaphroditism), abnormalities of the external genitalia include an enlarged clitoris with partial to complete labial fusion and a common urogenital sinus. Growth in height is excessive and "bone age" advanced, and patients may have excessive muscularity and sexual development. Pubic hair appears early; acne may be excessive; and the voice may deepen.

Pseudohermaphroditism in the female may also be produced as a result of the administration of androgens, progestins, diethylstilbestrol, and related hormones to the mother during the first trimester of pregnancy or as a result of virilizing maternal tumors. In these cases, the condition regresses after birth.

Adrenogenital Syndrome in Males (Macrogenitosomia Praecox)

In males, precocious sexual development is along isosexual lines. With congenital bilateral hyperplasia of the adrenal cortex, the infant may appear normal at birth; however, during the first few months of life, the penis enlarges, the scrotum darkens, the rugae become more prominent, and acne and pubic and axillary hair appear. The testicles generally remain small, and spermatogenesis does not occur. Other symptoms and signs are similar to those of the congenital form in females. If an adrenal or testicular tumor is the cause, the tumor may be palpable. Rarely, an adrenal tumor in either sex produces feminization, with gynecomastia resulting in males.

Laboratory Findings

1. 21-Hydroxylase deficiency–Blood and urine adrenal androgens and testosterone are elevated and the 17 OH progesterone level is elevated to diagnostic levels in cord and newborn blood. During the first 3 weeks of life, normal infants may excrete up to 2.5 mg/d. Aldosterone may be reduced, and excessive sodium loss occurs in salt-losing forms.)

2. 11β-Hydroxylase deficiency–11-Deoxycortisol (and its tetrahydro derivative), 17-hydroxycorticoid, deoxycorticosterone, 17-ketosteroid, and testosterone levels are increased.

3. 17-Hydroxylase deficiency–17-Ketosteroid and 17-hydroxycorticoid levels are decreased; aldosterone, corticosterone, and deoxycorticosterone levels are increased.

4. 3β-Hydroxysteroid dehydrogenase deficiency–With the exception of Δ^5 compounds all adrenal steroid levels in the blood and urine are low.

5. Cholesterol desmolase deficiency–All steroid excretion is markedly decreased.

6. Tumor–Excretion of dehydroepiandrosterone may be greatly elevated.

7. Other findings–Urinary excretion of gonadotropins may be elevated for age.

Dexamethasone Suppression Test. If the administration of dexamethasone, 2–4 mg/d orally in 4 doses for 7 days, reduces 17-ketosteroid levels to normal, hyperplasia rather than adenoma is the probable diagnosis.

Imaging

Genitograms using contrast material may indicate the presence of a urogenital sinus. Displacement of the kidney and calcification in the area of the adrenal may be seen on urograms or plain films of patients with tumors. "Bone age" is typically advanced with 21- and 11β-hydroxylase defects after the first year of life in the untreated child.

Treatment

A. Congenital Hyperplasia of the Adrenal Cortex:

1. Hydrocortisone–Approximately 20–25 mg/m^2/d orally will produce adrenal suppression and normal linear growth. Dosages of 10–25 mg/d for infants and 25–100 mg/d for older children initially are usually necessary. The drug should be given orally in divided doses several times a day, two-fifths of the total dose given as the first morning dose and two-fifths as the last dose at night.

2. Mineralocorticoids–For patients with salt-losing forms of adrenogenital syndrome, therapy with fludrocortisone and sodium chloride is necessary (see pp 885–887).

3. Glucocorticoids–Glucocorticoids should be increased (by 3–4 times) during acute severe stress or infection.

4. Surgical measures–Recession or partial clitoridectomy is occasionally indicated in a girl with an abnormally large or sensitive clitoris but may be delayed for 1 or 2 years until the effect of therapy is determined. Surgical correction of the labial fusion and urogenital sinus may require several operations.

B. Tumor: Because the malignant lesions cannot be distinguished clinically from the benign ones, surgical removal is indicated whenever a tumor has been diagnosed. Preoperative and postoperative treatment are as for Cushing's syndrome due to a tumor (see Cushing's Syndrome, above).

Course & Prognosis

Untreated patients with congenital adrenal hyperplasia will show precocious virilization throughout childhood. Because of excessive skeletal maturation, these individuals will be tall as children but short as adults. Adequate corticosteroid treatment permits normal growth and sexual maturation.

Female pseudohermaphrodites mistakenly raised as males for more than 3 years may have serious psychologic disturbances if their sex role is changed after that time.

When the adrenogenital syndrome is caused by a tumor, progression of signs and symptoms will cease after successful surgical removal; pubic hair, pigmentation, and deepening of the voice may regress or persist.

3. PRIMARY ALDOSTERONISM

Primary hyperaldosteronism may be caused by an adrenal tumor or by adrenal hyperplasia. It is characterized by paresthesias, tetany, weakness, periodic "paralysis," polyuria, low serum potassium levels, hypertension, alkaline urine, proteinuria, metabolic alkalosis, carbohydrate intolerance, suppressed plasma renin activity, and hyposthenuria that does not respond to vasopressin. The urinary aldosterone level is increased, but other steroid levels are variable. Adrenal tumors may be visualized with CT scanning ultrasonography or MRI. Treatment of the tumor is by surgical removal. With hyperplasia, subtotal or total adrenalectomy is recommended if pharmacologic doses of gluco-corticoid are ineffective after 2 months.

A form of secondary hyperaldosteronism, possibly due to increased prostaglandins, occurs in which both renin and aldosterone levels are elevated in the absence of hypertension (Bartter's syndrome). There is associated renovascular disease, with hyperplasia of the juxtaglomerular apparatus and renal electrolyte wasting.

DISEASES OF THE ADRENAL MEDULLA

PHEOCHROMOCYTOMA
(Chromaffinoma)

Pheochromocytoma is an uncommon tumor that may be located wherever there is any chromaffin tissue (eg, adrenal medulla, sympathetic ganglia, carotid body). The condition may be familial (eg, multiple endocrine adenomatosis type II), and in children the tumors are often multiple and bilateral.

Clinical Findings

Clinical manifestations of pheochromocytoma are due to excessive secretion of epinephrine or norepinephrine (or both). Attacks of anxiety and headaches should arouse suspicion. Other findings are palpitation, dizziness, weakness, nausea, vomiting, diarrhea, dilated pupils with blurring of vision, abdominal and precordial pain, rapid pulse, hypertension (usually persistent), and discomfort from heat. The symptoms may be sustained, producing all of the above findings plus papilledema, retinopathy, and cardiac enlargement.

Urine and serum catecholamine levels are increased. The 24-hour urine collection shows markedly increased urinary excretion of total catecholamines, metanephrine, and vanilmandelic acid. *Caution:* Attacks may be provoked by mechanical stimulation of the tumor or by histamine or tyramine. Results of the phentolamine (Regitine) test are positive, but the test is not specific for pheochromocytoma and may not be necessary for diagnosis. Displacement of the kidney may be shown by routine x-ray. The tumor may be defined by ultrasonography or by CT scanning or MRI of the abdomen.

Treatment

Surgical removal of the tumor is the treatment of choice, but a sudden paroxysm and death during surgery are not uncommon. The oral administration of propranolol and phentolamine preoperatively has been recommended to prevent the extreme fluctuations of blood pressure that sometimes occur during surgery. Medical treatment includes phenoxybenzamine to reduce hypertension and propranolol to lessen tachycardia and ventricular dysrhythmias.

Prognosis

Complete relief of symptoms, except those due to longstanding vascular or renal changes, is the rule after recovery. If no treatment is given, severe cardiac, renal, and cerebral damage may result.

DIABETES MELLITUS

Diabetes mellitus is a generalized hereditary metabolic disorder that leads to derangement of carbohydrate, protein, and fat metabolism, followed by glycosuria, dehydration, ketoacidosis, coma, and (eventually) death. The administration of insulin corrects these deficiencies but is not curative.

Diabetes in the newborn may be transient, may not require insulin, and may disappear after weeks or months. Transient hyperglycemia, acetonuria, and glycosuria have been noted in young children who have had infections or hyperglucagonemia.

Heredity is an important predisposing factor in the onset of type I (insulin-dependent) diabetes mellitus, and 40% of discordant identical twins develop diabetes after the onset in the first twin. An association with HLA types is known, and over 95% of people with type I diabetes have HLA-DR3 or HLA-DR4. Environmental factors may also be important.

Clinical Findings

A. Symptoms and Signs:

1. Early manifestations–Early manifestations in patients with chemical and overt disease (1–2 months or less) include thirst and polydipsia, polyuria and nocturia or enuresis, loss of weight or failure to gain, increase in appetite (less common in children than in adults; anorexia is often noted), lassitude and easy fatigability, cramping pains in the limbs or abdomen, dizziness, confusion, hyperventilation, and coma or stupor (due to diabetic acidosis).

2. Chronic complications–Stunting of growth and hepatomegaly occur in patients with uncontrolled diabetes of long standing (Mauriac's syndrome). Many children with diabetes develop contractures of finger joints. Serious psychologic difficulties are not infrequent. Characteristic "small vessel" changes occur. Diabetic retinopathy develops in most juvenile diabetics 10–20 years after onset of symptoms. Premature atherosclerosis and coronary vascular disease may also develop, as well as intercapillary glomerulosclerosis (Kimmelstiel-Wilson syndrome), with hypertension, edema, proteinuria, and atherosclerosis.

B. Laboratory Findings: Findings include glycosuria, fasting hyperglycemia, and hyperglycemia 2 hours after a meal. (A fasting blood glucose level of > 120 mg/dL in the absence of obesity or drugs is generally indicative of diabetes mellitus; however, a normal fasting blood glucose level does not rule out diabetes.) Other findings may include ketonuria, hyperlipidemia, hemoconcentration, and ketoacidemia. Hemoglobin A_{IC} levels may be elevated in new, long-standing, or poorly controlled patients. Insulin concentration is usually low but may be elevated, especially in obese adolescents who have maturity-onset diabetes in youth (MODY). A glucose tolerance test is abnormal, but generally not indicated.

Treatment
A. Insulin: Insulin therapy (Table 28–7) is necessary in almost all cases of childhood diabetes. Initially (7–14 days), the insulin requirements may be high, followed by a period of considerably lower needs, but requirements will soon rise again after that. The initial dose of insulin may be determined primarily by trial and error in relation to blood glucose determinations; in many cases, it will be approximately 0.5 unit/kg initially with a gradual increase to 1 unit/kg in later years. Patients with type I diabetes mellitus should usually be started on long-acting preparations with 1 part of regular to 2 or 3 parts of neutral protamine Hagedorn or isophane (NPH) insulin as soon as the initial ketoacidosis has cleared. Regular insulin should be available for emergency situations and as a supplemental dose with injections for other critical changes. Many children may achieve better control on a regimen of 2 injections daily, with two-thirds of the total dose given in the morning and one-third given before dinner. Injections should be given 20–30 minutes before meals, enabling the regular insulin to act at the time of food intake. When pure pork or human insulin is readily available, patients are now

Table 28–7. Summary of bioavailability characteristics of the insulins.

	Insulin Type	Onset	Peak Action	Duration
Short-acting	Regular, Actrapid, Velosulin	15–30 min	1–3 h	5–7 h
	Semilente, Semitard	30–60 min	4–6 h	12–16 h
Intermediate-acting	Lente, Lentard, Monotard	2–4 h	8–10 h	18–24 h
	NPH, Insulatard, Protaphane	2–4 h	8–10 h	18–24 h
Long-acting	Ultralente, Ultratard, PZI	4–5 h	8–14 h	25–36 h

usually started on one of these preparations. Both result in a lower incidence of insulin antibodies and of skin changes.

B. Oral Hypoglycemic Agents: These drugs play a minimal role in the management of type I diabetes mellitus, although they are occasionally employed in the adolescent with type II (non-insulin-dependent) diabetes mellitus.

C. Diet: The diet should be well balanced and consistent in amount from day to day, allowing approximately 1000 kcal plus an additional 100 kcal per year of age. Give 50–55% as carbohydrate, 25–30% as fat, and 20% as protein. Many believe that the patient may be allowed freedom to eat according to appetite within sensible limits but that foods high in sugar should be limited. The patient should know about the American Diabetes Association exchange diet, which uses household measurements rather than weights. With the use of long-acting or intermediate-acting insulin, one must give a bedtime feeding to prevent hypoglycemia during the night. This should include protein and fat, which last longer during the night than does carbohydrate. Consistency is very important. A small feeding in the afternoon or before exercise may also be indicated. In general, weight should be kept at normal levels. An attempt should be made to maintain normal serum lipoprotein, cholesterol, and triglyceride levels.

D. Outpatient Management: In most children and adolescents, blood should be tested 3 times each day (in the morning, before supper, and at bedtime). This can be done with diagnostic paper strips (eg, Chemstrip bG Strips), which permit visual estimation of the glucose concentration when compared to a color chart, or by use of a meter. If the blood glucose concentration is above 240 mg/dL or if the patient feels ill, urine ketone levels should also be checked. Physical examination every 3 months with particular attention to the retinas, thyroid, liver, injection sites, fingers (for blood test pricks and for contractures), and neurologic examination is recommended. The patient's understanding of the disease should be reviewed. After puberty, hemoglobin A_{IC} (glycosylated hemoglobin) levels should be determined every 3–6 months. In the young child hemoglobin A_{IC} levels may be determined only once or twice yearly.

E. Other Factors Influencing the Regulation of Diabetes:

1. Activity–Strenuous exercise tends to lower the insulin requirement. Exercise in moderation (and without significant day-to-day variations) is beneficial. However, patients should be cautioned against strenuous exercise unless they take extra carbohydrate beforehand or reduce the insulin dosage.

2. Infection–Any infection is serious in a diabetic patient; it completely upsets the equilibrium established by therapy, usually increasing the need for insulin. Infection may precipitate ketoacidosis. During severe infections, it is often necessary to add small doses of supplemental regular insulin every 2–4 hours until acetonuria clears. Supplements of approximately 10% of the total daily insulin dose are given every 3 hours as regular insulin if the patient has moderate or severe ketonuria and a blood glucose level above 150 mg/dL. When vomiting is present without ketoacidosis, it is often best to reduce the daily insulin dose by half; regular insulin may be supplemented later if high glucose and ketone levels develop. It may also be necessary to give beverages containing sugar (eg, soda pop) to keep the blood glucose level normal if vomiting is a problem.

3. Surgery–Prior to elective surgery, the patient should be given half the usual dose of long-acting insulin in the morning; following this, 5 or 10% dextrose in water should be administered slowly intravenously before, during, and after surgery to cover the insulin. Blood glucose levels should be monitored during surgery and the early postoperative period. If blood glucose levels exceed 300 mg/dL or if abnormally high levels of ketones appear, regular insulin may be administered as a continuous intravenous solution at the rate of 0.05 unit/kg/h. If the patient is unable to return to oral food intake promptly, intravenous glucose and electrolytes are continued and intravenous insulin may be continued as necessary. On the day after surgery, if the patient is able to resume eating, the usual amount of long-acting insulin should be administered. As soon as possible, feedings by mouth and the usual insulin regime should be reinstituted.

4. Control of glucose level–Hypoglycemia and posthypoglycemic hyperglycemia (Somogyi's reflex) may be due to overdosage with insulin. This should be suspected in children receiving an insulin dosage that exceeds 1.5 units/kg/d, although the relative insulin resistence of adolescence may result in insulin doses of 1.5 units/kg/d or more during the adolescent growth spurt. Poor control of blood glucose levels may also be due to an inadequate insulin dosage or to missed insulin injections.

DIABETIC ACIDOSIS
(Diabetic Coma)

Clinical Findings

A. Symptoms and Signs: Diabetic acidosis is characterized by marked thirst and polyuria, followed by nausea and vomiting, abdominal pain, and general malaise. Dehydration and acidosis (pH < 7.3) develop rapidly. Respirations then become long, deep, and labored; headache, irritability, drowsiness, stupor, and (finally) coma may develop. On physical examination, the patient is irritable, drowsy, or unconscious, and there is marked dehydration. The skin and mucous membranes are usually dry, lips cherry-red, eyeballs soft, blood pressure low, pulse usually rapid and thready, hyperventilation present, temperature low, and a sweetish ("fruity") acetone breath may be detected. The abdomen may show diffuse spasm and tenderness suggestive of an acute abdominal disorder. The signs and symptoms of the precipitating cause (infection, trauma, missed injection, emotional upset, etc) will usually be found.

A syndrome of hyperosmolar nonketotic diabetic coma in children has been described. It is characterized by the presence of severe hyperglycemia, severe dehydration, and metabolic acidosis and may occur secondary to hypernatremia. The duration of illness is short. There is little or no polydipsia and polyuria, and these children are frequently insulin-resistant. In treatment, sufficient insulin (and isotonic parenteral fluid initially) should be used to normalize glucose metabolism; insulin may not be necessary when the disorder follows hypernatremia.

B. Laboratory Findings: Findings include glycosuria, ketonemia, ketonuria, and hyperglycemia. Acidosis results, and the pH may be below 7.1 (severe ketoacidosis), between 7.1 and 7.2 (moderate ketoacidosis), or between 7.2 and 7.3 (mild ketoacidosis). Serum sodium and chloride levels and the plasma carbon dioxide content are low. Serum potassium and inorganic phosphorus levels may be increased initially, but there is a major total body depletion of these elements, and levels usually decline rapidly with correction of acidosis. Total protein, hemoglobin, and blood urea nitrogen levels may be increased. Leukocytosis and increased hematocrit are often present.

Treatment

A. Objectives: Objectives are the restoration of circulation, correction of fluid and electrolyte deficit, reestablishment of normal carbohydrate metabolism, and eradication of the cause of acidosis and the hyperosmolar state.

B. Emergency Measures:

1. Hospitalize the patient if diabetic acidosis is severe. Patients with mild acidosis can be treated without hospitalization. Keep the patient warm, but avoid excessive warmth. Do not give narcotics or barbiturates.

2. Treat shock, if present, with albumin and other antishock measures (see Chapter 6).

3. Evaluate the degree of dehydration and shock by physical examination and by close inquiry to determine if there is a history of recent weight loss.

4. Obtain urine for estimation of glucose and ketone levels, specific gravity, and evidence of infection.

5. Take venous blood for measurement of pH and determination of levels of carbon dioxide, sodium chloride, potassium, glucose, inorganic phosphorus, urea nitrogen, and ketone bodies. Measurement of the blood lactic acid level may also be of value in the acidotic nonketotic patient.

6. Insulin is given as follows:

a. Intravenous insulin should not be given until the blood glucose level is known, particularly if subcutaneous injections were given previously.

b. A constant intravenous infusion of regular insulin, 0.1–0.2 unit/kg/h, is given by use of a constant infusion pump if that method of delivery is available. One method to prepare an insulin infusion is to add regular insulin, 30 units, to 150 mL of 0.9% sodium chloride to give a dilution of 1 unit/5 mL. If 50 mL of this solution is run through the tubing prior to use, the insulin binding sites on the tubing will be saturated. A similar dose of insulin may be given intramuscularly instead of intravenously but will then need to be repeated every hour. With either route of administration, blood glucose levels should be determined hourly. Insulin may be given subcutaneously every 2–4 hours in less severely involved patients, except in markedly dehydrated patients who may have varied absorption of the drug.

7. Gastric lavage may rarely be necessary to relieve distention of the stomach and to reduce vomiting.

8. Fluids and electrolytes are given as follows:

a. First correct extracellular dehydration, shock, anoxia, and impaired renal function with normal saline solution or, if acidosis is severe (pH < 7.0), a solution containing the following: sodium, 150 meq/L; chloride, 100 meq/L; and bicarbonate, 50 meq/L. Give 20–40 mL/kg over the first 1 or 2 hours of therapy. If shock is present, the use of albumin or other volume expander is essential.

b. Then give 50% physiologic solution (usually without bicarbonate) at a rate calculated to restore deficits, supply maintenance amounts, and replace intercurrent losses.

c. When urine flow and circulatory efficiency are satisfactory, the blood pH level is above 7.1, and signs of hyperpnea have begun to subside (generally in 1–2 hours), replace intracellular electrolytes (potassium and phosphorus). Although serum potassium and phosphorus concentrations are usually normal or high early in acidosis, they may fall to low levels following correction of acidosis.

    d. Replace the remainder of the water deficit, and when the blood glucose level falls below 250 mg/dL, 5% glucose should be added to the intravenous fluids.

C. General Measures:

    1. Ascertain the precipitating cause of the acidosis, and initiate appropriate treatment.

    2. Use an indwelling catheter if spontaneous voidings are not possible (rarely necessary).

    3. Measure urinary glucose and acetone, blood glucose and carbon dioxide, venous pH, and serum electrolytes at frequent intervals.

    4. Continuous or intermittent monitoring of the ECG is helpful to follow the effect of potassium therapy.

    5. After 12–18 hours, if there is no vomiting, the remainder of the day's fluid and electrolyte requirements may be given orally in a suitable vehicle (orange juice, ginger ale, or milk). Vomiting generally subsides after ketosis has been corrected.

    6. For continued fluid and electrolyte therapy, see Chapter 5.

Prognosis

    With prompt and adequate therapy, the prognosis is good. The largest number of serious side effects and sequelae result from central nervous system complications. The risk of these may be minimized by attention to correction of fluid and electrolyte losses and avoidance of overzealous correction of the hyperglycemia, dehydration, or acidosis. Recurrent episodes of acidosis are due to failure to take the proper insulin or diet, to emotional problems, to omitting insulin altogether, or to chronic or repeated infections.

HYPOGLYCEMIA
(See also Neonatal Hypoglycemia, Chapter 11.)

    Low blood glucose levels can occur when a patient with diabetes receives excessive insulin, fails to eat, or exercises too strenuously. In children who do not have diabetes, the diagnosis of hypoglycemia *should not be made* unless the blood glucose level is below 40 mg/dL or, in a newborn, below 30 mg/dL. The diagnosis is unfortunately assigned frequently to children with behavioral or other problems who have never had a documented low blood glucose level.

The most common known cause of hypoglycemia in infants during the first year of life is inappropriate insulin secretion. During episodes of hypoglycemia, the insulin level remains above 20 μU/mL even though the blood glucose level is low. When the pancreas is examined histologically, the islet cells may be hypertrophied in some cases; in other cases, there may be excessive numbers of islet cells, which may be arising from pancreatic ductules (nesidioblastosis). A trial of diazoxide, 10–20 mg/kg, to inhibit insulin release should be attempted. Because leucine may stimulate insulin production, it is also necessary to restrict leucine intake in some infants. If this is unsuccessful, partial pancreatomy may be indicated.

The most frequent known cause of hypoglycemia in children between 1 and 5 years of age is ketotic hypoglycemia. This is hypoglycemia associated with the presence of ketones in the urine. Ketotic hypoglycemia is more common in males and in children who had birth weights below 2500 g, who were small for gestational age, or who have minor neurologic or behavioral disorders. There is often a history of vomiting or of decreased appetite or failure to eat during the previous 24 hours. Ketotic hypoglycemia is characterized by early morning seizures with the concurrent appearance of ketones in the urine. Treatment should consist of preventing excessive fasting and monitoring the urine for ketones whenever the child is ill or appears to be deviating from normal behavior patterns. If ketones are present, foods high in simple sugars should be encouraged. If the child is vomiting, parenteral glucose should be administered.

Islet cell adenoma represents an increasingly more frequent cause of primary-onset hypoglycemia in patients over 4 years of age and probably is the most frequent known cause in patients over 6 years of age. Inappropriate ratios of insulin to glucose are noted, and the tumor can sometimes be detected by means of ultrasonography or arteriography. Treatment is surgical removal.

There are some cases in which a cause for hypoglycemia cannot be found (group IV, idiopathic spontaneous hypoglycemia; Table 28–8). Sometimes a genetic metabolic disorder (group VI; Table 28–8) is suspected on the basis of the family (or other) history or the physical examination (eg, large liver). In other cases, particularly in association with poor growth, a primary endocrine deficiency (group VII; Table 28–8) or nutritional liver disease (group VIII; Table 28–8) may be the suspected cause of hypoglycemia.

Table 28–8. Hypoglycemia.

Classification	Clinical and Laboratory Findings	Treatment
I. Antenatal period disorders (1) Fetal malnutrition (placental insufficiency) (2) Sepsis Offspring of diabetic mothers Erythroblastosis fetalis (3) Neonatal cold injury (4) Hypoglycemia, cardiomegaly, and pulmonary edema	Offspring of diabetic mothers and infants with erythroblastosis fetalis may have hyperinsulinemia with rebound hypoglycemia to insulinogenic stimuli; blood ratios of insulin to glucose are elevated. The other conditions listed have in common depleted hepatic glycogen and fat stores and fasting hypoglycemia.	Infusion of 10–20% glucose by peripheral vein. Frequent oral feedings. Avoidance or cautious administration of insulinogenic agents (eg, arginine, 50% dextrose) in hyperinsulinism states.
II. Hyperinsulin states (1) Islet cell hyperplasia (2) Islet cell adenoma or adenocarcinoma (3) Islet cell nesidioblastosis (4) Leucine sensitivity (5) Beckwith-Wiedemann syndrome	As a whole, this group is prone to fasting hypoglycemia and rebound hypoglycemia to insulinogenic stimuli. Diagnosis is dependent on finding of abnormally elevated insulin or proinsulin levels during the fasting state or following insulin provocation with glucose, amino acids (ie, leucine, arginine), glucagon, or tolbutamide (1–5); or finding of clinical characteristics of the EMG triad, ie, exomphalos, macroglossia, and gigantism with abdominal organomegaly (5).	(1) Avoidance of insulinogenic stimuli. (2) Catecholamines or diazoxide (or both). (3) A diet low in simple sugars and, sometimes, low in leucine. (4) Pancreatectomy.

903

Table 26–8. (cont'd). Hypoglycemia.

Classification	Clinical and Laboratory Findings	Treatment
III. Ketotic hypoglycemia	Findings include a history of low birth weight for gestational age; onset between ages 1 and 6 yr; and triad of hypoglycemia, ketosis, and blunted glycemic response to glucagon. Patients may have abnormalities in gluconeogenesis with abnormalities in hepatic handling of alanine during a fast.	Frequent feedings with diet high in carbohydrates and protein. Avoid periods of prolonged fasting.
IV. Idiopathic spontaneous hypoglycemia	Fasting hypoglycemia occurs within the first 2 yr of life in 90% of cases. There is no determinable cause.	Frequent feedings with diet high in carbohydrates.
V. Primary neurologic disorders ("central")	Hypoglycemia is frequently observed in children with neurologic disorders of various types. No definite pattern or consistent metabolic abnormality has been demonstrated, although hyperinsulinemia has not been a feature.	Frequent feedings. Anticonvulsants when indicated.

VI. Metabolic disorders	Definitive diagnosis is dependent on enzyme determination. Blunted hyperglycemia response to glucagon (1, 2, and 5), history of hypoglycemia after fructose ingestion (3), and a characteristic odor (4) are helpful for diagnosis.	(1 and 2) Frequent feedings with diet high in carbohydrates. Hyperalimentation. Portacaval diversion in severe type 1 glycogen storage disease may be indicated.
(1) Liver glycogen storage disease		
(2) Liver glycogen synthase deficiency		
(3) Fructose intolerance		
(4) Maple syrup urine disease		(3 and 4) Rigid avoidance of offending substrate.
(5) Deficiency of liver 1,6-diphosphatase activity		
VII. Endocrine insufficiency syndromes	Definitive diagnosis is dependent on biochemical establishment of hormone deficiency. History of failure to thrive, growth retardation, and features of hypopituitarism (1 and 2), excessive tanning (3), and abnormal weight for gestational age (4) are helpful for diagnosis.	Replacement of deficient hormone or hormones.
(1) Hypopituitarism		
(2) Hypopituitarism and hyperinsulinemia		
(3) Adrenocortical insufficiency		
(4) Adrenomedullary insufficiency (Broberger–Zetterström syndrome)		
(5) Congenital hypothyroidism		
(6) Glucagon deficiency		
VIII. Severe malnutrition states	Characteristics include fasting hypoglycemia and depleted glycogen and fat stores.	Nutritional rehabilitation.
(1) Chronic diarrhea		
(2) Liver disease		

Clinical Findings

A. Symptoms and Signs: Findings include weakness, hunger, irritability, faintness, sweating, changes in mood, epigastric pain, vomiting, nervousness, hypothermia, unsteadiness of gait, semiconsciousness, tremors, and convulsions. All of these are relieved by administration of glucose. If left untreated, hypoglycemia may lead to extensive central nervous system damage. Symptomatic hypoglycemia is more commonly associated with mental deterioration, disintegration of the personality, and death, but some infants may have prolonged and severe hypoglycemia and subsequently develop normally.

B. Laboratory Findings: (See Table 28–8.)

1. Blood glucose levels are low during an attack. There is no sharp dividing line below which a level can be regarded as abnormal, but consistent or repeated levels below 40 mg/dL, except during the neonatal period, generally are considered to be significantly lowered.

2. Serum insulin levels may be inappropriately elevated in hyperinsulinemic states when compared with the simultaneous glucose level.

3. No single test of blood glucose regulation reliably confirms the diagnosis of hypoglycemia, and no combination of tests reliably establishes the mechanism of hypoglycemia in all children.

Treatment

Long-term treatment for specific types of hypoglycemia is outlined in Table 28–8. Acute treatment is usually necessary prior to definitive diagnosis and includes the following:

A. Glucose:

1. Infuse 10–20% dextrose via peripheral vein, at a constant rate, maintaining a blood glucose level that controls central nervous system symptoms (eg, 30 mg/dL in newborns and 40–50 mg/dL in children). If hyperinsulinemia is suspected or is a possibility, avoid bolus ("push") infusions of concentrated dextrose solutions. (Fifty percent dextrose solutions are seldom necessary for use during infancy and childhood.)

2. Instruct the patient's family to give glucose as follows if the patient is unconscious and a physician is not available: Place Insta-Glucose between the child's cheek and gums or under the tongue. If there is no response in 10 minutes, give an initial deep intramuscular injection of glucagon, usually 0.5 mL (0.5 mg). If there is no response, wait 10 more minutes and inject an additional 0.5 mL of glucagon.

3. If a diagnosis of hypoglycemia not due to hyperinsulinism has been established, carbohydrates can be safely administered via any route without risk of hypoglycemic rebound.

4. If a diabetic patient is unconscious and a diagnosis of coma or insulin reaction is impossible or in doubt, give 50% glucose intravenously, up to 1 mL/kg. This will definitely overcome the insulin reaction and will not harm the patient with diabetic acidosis.

B. Drugs:

1. In general, drug therapy should be employed only after a definite diagnosis (see Table 28–8) is established.

2. If the cardiorespiratory status permits, catecholamines (oral ephedrine sulfate; subcutaneous epinephrine in oil [Sus-Phrine]) may be useful and have the unique advantage in the undiagnosed case of avoiding insulin stimulation.

3. Corticosteroids, corticotropin, and glucagon may be helpful in controlling hypoglycemia, but they may stimulate insulin production, and the action of glucagon in neonates is unpredictable.

4. In severe chronic hyperinsulinism states, an oral preparation of diazoxide is useful. Diazoxide, a nondiuretic benzothiadiazine, may be of value in controlling chronic idiopathic hypoglycemia and certain cases of hyperinsulinism. The dosage has varied from 5 to 20 mg/kg/d. Side effects include hypertrichosis, advancement of epiphyseal maturation, hyperuricemia, fluid retention, neutropenia, and depression of immunoglobulin G. Failure of adequate response to therapy with diazoxide should prompt consideration of subtotal pancreatectomy.

5. Recent experience suggests that somatostatin analogs may be useful and safe in children with hyperinsulinism. Somatostatin inhibits insulin secretion.

6. Sedatives and anticonvulsant therapy may be helpful to reduce convulsions and neuromuscular irritability. (Phenytoin has the added effect of reducing insulin stimulation.)

C. Diet: In leucine-sensitive patients, a low-leucine diet is indicated. In patients with ketotic hypoglycemia, provide a liberal carbohydrate diet and place a moderate restriction on ketogenic foods.

1. Give no concentrated forms of carbohydrate; these should be avoided because they will stimulate the pancreas to secrete insulin. Rapidly utilized carbohydrates should be replaced by slow-acting ones.

2. Give small frequent feedings (6 or more meals a day). It may be necessary to feed the patient at regular intervals

throughout the 24 hours and to give small carbohydrate feedings 30–45 minutes after regular meals.

D. Surgical Measures: Surgical removal of a portion of the pancreas (or of a tumor if present) should be undertaken for any individual who cannot be controlled by the above measures.

Prognosis

Excellent results have been reported in some treated patients with the idiopathic form of the disease and following removal of a tumor. Otherwise, the results depend on the underlying condition.

GALACTOSEMIA

Galactosemia is an autosomal hereditary (recessive) disease due to congenital absence of the activity of the enzyme galactose-1-phosphate uridyl transferase, which is necessary to convert galactose-1-phosphate to glucose-1-phosphate. There is decreased activity of the enzyme in heterozygous individuals. Galactosemia is characterized by feeding difficulties, hepatomegaly with or without splenomegaly, cataracts, mental retardation (not universal), and jaundice during the neonatal period. Pseudotumor cerebri may occur. Other findings include hypoglycemia (*total* reducing substance in blood may be normal or even elevated), galactosuria, aminoaciduria, proteinuria, and increased levels of galactose-1-phosphate in erythrocytes. A screening test is available to diagnose the condition during the newborn period.

A second form of galactosemia is due to galactokinase deficiency and does not affect the liver, kidneys, or central nervous system. However, cataracts may develop in patients during the first few months of life.

Treatment consists of excluding galactose (especially milk and its derivatives) from the diet. This prevents development of the signs and symptoms of the disease or may result in improvement after they have developed. A more normal diet may be tolerated later in childhood. Administration of progesterone may minimize progression of cataract formation and mental deficiency.

The mother of a known galactosemic child should be on a restricted galactose diet during subsequent pregnancies.

GLYCOGEN STORAGE DISEASE

There are numerous types of glycogen storage diseases. The following is a partial listing:

Type I, Von Gierke's Disease: Type I, the most common glycogen storage disease, is an autosomal recessive disorder that involves the liver and kidneys. It may be associated with debranching enzyme deficiency. It starts at birth or in early infancy and is characterized by anorexia, weight loss, vomiting, convulsions, and coma. Organomegaly of the liver and kidneys, growth retardation, obesity with a "doll-like" appearance, and bleeding tendencies may be noted. Cardiac failure, intermittent cyanosis, muscular weakness, neurologic abnormalities, hepatic cirrhosis, and marked enlargement of the tongue may occur in some cases. Laboratory findings include a deficiency in glucose 6-phosphatase, flat epinephrine and glucagon tolerance curves, elevated blood lactic and pyruvic acid levels, and abnormal glycogen deposition in the liver. Findings may also include acetonuria, hypoglycemia, hyperlipemia, and impaired glucose tolerance with insulinopenia. Treatment includes frequent high-carbohydrate feedings, sometimes including nighttime intragastric tube feedings. Portacaval shunts have been shown to be helpful in some patients. The prognosis is variable.

Type II, Pompe's Disease (Generalized Glycogenosis): Findings include muscle weakness, cardiomegaly, macroglossia, hepatomegaly, normal mental development, and deficiency of the lysosomal enzyme α1,4-glucosidase.

Type III, Cori's Disease: Type III involves the liver, striated muscle, and red blood cells. The clinical features are similar to those of type I but less severe. A defect in debranching enzymes (amylo-1,6-glucosidase or oligo-1,4-glucantransferase) and hepatomegaly may be present.

Type IV, Andersen's Disease (Amylopectinosis): Findings include abnormal levels of glycogen in the liver and reticuloendothelial system, diminished response to glucagon and epinephrine, a defect in the branching enzyme (amylo-1,4 $\rightarrow$ 1,6-transglucosidase), hepatosplenomegaly, cirrhosis, ascites, and normal mental development.

Type V, McArdle's Syndrome: Type V involves the skeletal muscle. There is a defect in muscle phosphorylase.

Type VI, Hers' Disease: Type VI is clinically similar to type I but less severe. There is a deficiency in liver phosphorylase.

Type VII: Other types involve reduced activity of phospho-glucomutase, phosphofructokinase, or phosphohexoisomerase. Findings include weak muscles, partial defect of other glycolytic enzymes, and elevated levels of AST (SGOT), serum aldolase, and phosphocreatine kinase.

PHENYLKETONURIA
(Phenylpyruvic Oligophrenia)

Phenylketonuria is a hereditary (recessive) familial disease usually caused by a deficiency of phenylalanine hydroxylase.

Clinical Findings
Affected children (most often blond and blue-eyed) appear normal at birth but soon develop vomiting, irritability, a peculiar odor, patchy eczematous lesions of the skin, convulsions, schizoid personality, and abnormal findings on EEG. Mentality is retarded. (An occasional patient may have normal intelligence without treatment.) Affected children are hyperactive, with erratic behavior. Perspiration is excessive. Serum and urinary phenylalanine levels are markedly high as determined by ferric chloride test, Phenistix Reagent Strips, or Guthrie bacterial inhibition assay (of particular value in young infants). Some normal infants, particularly those with physiologic jaundice of the newborn, may have transiently elevated (> 6 mg/dL) blood levels of phenylalanine. Orthohydroxyphenylacetic acid is usually present in the urine.

Treatment
A diet low in phenylalanine (58 ± 18 mg/kg) should be instituted to keep plasma phenylalanine levels between 5 and 10 mg/dL; when started in patients during the first weeks of life, this diet prevents severe retardation. It has also been shown that it is possible to breast-feed an infant in combination with giving a milk substitute that is deficient in phenylalanine. The diet should be titrated against the nutritional status of the child and the serum phenylalanine levels to ensure that the diet is restricted enough to prevent manifestations of the disease but liberal enough to prevent hypophenylalaninemia with resultant malnutrition and cerebral damage. It is now generally recommended that weekly serum phenylalanine assays be done during the first year of life. In established cases, proper diet may arrest the condition and produce improvement in personality and in symptoms other than the mental deficiency. It may be discontinued after several years.

The blood phenylalanine levels of phenylketonuric females

should be maintained in the normal range during the childbearing years to decrease the risk of abnormalities (eg, growth and mental retardation, microcephaly) in their offspring who may be nonphenylketonuric.

Hyperphenylalaninemia may be a transient phenomenon in some newborns who have normal urinary metabolites and do not require treatment.

29 | Neoplastic Diseases

Linda C. Stork, MD

Cancer in children differs biologically from cancer in adults. (See Fig 29–1.) Neoplastic disease is the second leading cause of death in the pediatric age group in the USA. Solid tumors represent 70% of cases and acute leukemia the remaining 30%.

For solid tumors in general, the less the tumor burden and the more localized the tumor at diagnosis, the better the chance of cure. For the leukemias, various clinical and laboratory features present at diagnosis correlate with ultimate prognosis. Present-day treatment of pediatric cancers is complex, multimodal, and multidisciplinary and should be carried out under the direction of centers specializing in the care of children with neoplastic diseases.

BRAIN TUMORS
(See Table 29–1.)

Brain tumors represent the second most common type of childhood cancer, with leukemia being the most common. Over 75% of these arise in the posterior fossa. The most prominent general symptom of central nervous system (CNS) tumor of childhood is headache. The most prominent physical findings are enlargement of the head and papilledema.

In the newborn, the various forms of hydrocephalus are the most common causes of abnormal enlargement, but tumors may cause enlargement. If abnormal skull enlargement occurs in children between 2 months and 1 year of age, subdural hematoma is more likely responsible. The most common cause of abnormal increase in the size of the head after 1 year of age is tumor.

Differential Diagnosis of Intracranial Lesions

The entire symptom complex of an intracranial space-consuming lesion, including vomiting, increase in intracranial pressure, and papilledema, can be caused by lesions that are not neoplastic. The principal ones are granulomatous abscess (in-

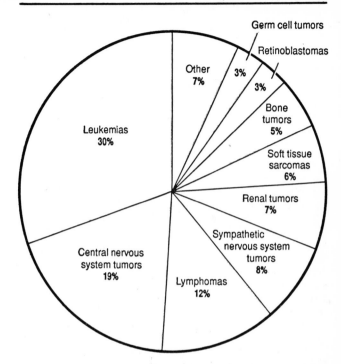

Figure 29–1. Approximate incidence of the principal cancers in children less than 15 years old (SEER program, 1973–1982).

cluding tuberculoma), pyogenic abscess, hemorrhage (subdural hematoma), CNS infections, and venous sinus thrombosis. CT scan and MRI can help differentiate among these lesions. An elevated white blood cell count and a rapid sedimentation rate, even in the absence of fever, suggest a diagnosis of pyogenic brain abscess rather than neoplasm.

TUMORS OF THE SOFT TISSUE

The most common malignant soft tissue tumor seen in children is rhabdomyosarcoma. The child usually presents with a firm mass in the region of the tumor. Rhabdomyosarcoma is one of the tumors associated with neurofibromatosis. The most common primary site of occurrence is the head and neck, followed in

Table 29–1. Brain tumors.

Part Affected	Symptoms and Signs	Radiologic Findings	Tumor Type and Characteristics	Treatment and Prognosis
Brainstem	Cranial nerve palsies (IX–X, VII, VI, V; chiefly sensory root). Pyramidal tract signs (hemiparesis). Cerebellar ataxia. Rarely, signs of increased intracranial pressure or emaciation.	CT scan of posterior fossa shows displacement of cerebral aqueduct and fourth ventricle. Calcifications may be present. MRI often better at delineating brainstem lesions than CT.	Gliomes and astrocytomas (varying grades); often rapid growth and recurrence.	Stereotactic biopsy, if possible. X-ray therapy to site; steroids to control edema from radiation. Benefit of chemotherapy unclear. Prognosis poor. Average survival 1 yr. 25% of patients survive 5 yr.
Cerebellum and fourth ventricle	Evidence of increased intracranial pressure.* Cerebellar signs.† Signs due to pressure on adjacent structures.‡ Personality and behavioral changes. Occasionally, emaciation.	CT scan of posterior fossa shows displacement or obliteration of fourth ventricle and resultant hydrocephalus. Contrast enhanced CT demonstrates the differing densities of tumors common to this region and shows their calcification.	Astrocytoma; often slow growth, frequently cystic.	Surgical removal. Follow by localized x-ray therapy and chemotherapy for high-grade tumors. Prognosis good if removal complete.
			Medulloblastoma; rapid growth; seen mostly in children age 2–6 yr; seeds along cerebrospinal fluid pathways; myelogram necessary at diagnosis to evaluate for "drop mets."	Surgical decompression of posterior fossa and x-ray therapy to site, cerebrum, and spinal canal. Chemotherapy. Shunt (ventriculopleural, etc) for relief of cerebrospinal fluid obstruction. 50% of patients survive 5 yr.

914

			Less common: ependymoma, hemangioblastoma, choroid plexus papilloma.	Surgical cure possible with hemangioblastoma and choroid plexus papilloma. Ependymomas probably best treated like medulloblastomas.
			Gliomas; astrocytomas; glioblastomas. Meningiomas rare. Leptomeningeal sarcoma.	Surgical biopsy or excision where possible. X-ray treatment. Prognosis varies with tumor type and grade. Chemotherapy for high grade tumors.
Cerebral hemispheres and lateral ventricles	Evidence of increased intracranial pressure.* Seizures (generalized, psychomotor, focal) in about 40% of cases. Neurologic deficits, including hemiparesis (40% of cases), visual field defects, ataxia, personality changes.	CT scan is highly diagnostic (nearly 100% of cases) and shows edema, ventricular deformation, shift. Increased density with contrast enhancement correlates with vascularity of lesion. Tumors as small as 0.5 cm in diameter may be detected.	Ependymoma and choroid plexus papilloma.	Surgical excision. Occasionally, hydrocephalus persists and requires shunt.

(Continued)

*Evidence of increased intracranial pressure includes headache, vomiting (often without nausea and before breakfast), diplopia, blurred vision, papilledema. Personality changes, including irritability, apathy, disturbances in sleep and eating patterns, are frequent. Sudden enlargement of the head if head circumferences have been plotted is detectable when sutures are still open or after sutures have split. Alterations of consciousness and stiff neck with tonsillar herniation may be seen.

†Cerebellar signs include ataxia, dysmetria, and nystagmus. Truncal ataxia in the absence of lateralizing signs is most common in vermis tumors.

‡Signs due to pressure on adjacent structures may include head tilting, cranial nerve signs, pyramidal tract signs, suboccipital tenderness, and stiff neck.

Table 29–1. (cont'd). Brain tumors.

Part Affected	Symptoms and Signs	Radiologic Findings	Tumor Type and Characteristics	Treatment and Prognosis
Diencephalon	Emaciation; good intake (diencephalic syndrome). Often, very active and euphoric. Few neurologic findings (occasionally, vertical nystagmus, tremor, ataxia). Frequently, eosinophilia, decreased T_4 and pituitary reserve.	CT scan shows defect in floor of third ventricle and other midline findings. MRI may delineate tumor better than CT.	Usually astrocytomas; less common, oligodendroglioma, glioma, ependymoma, glioblastoma.	Stereotactic biopsy, if possible. X-ray therapy. Shunt for relief of cerebrospinal fluid obstruction. Prognosis variable; generally poor. Possible chemotherapy.
Midbrain and third ventricle	Personality and behavioral changes, often early. Evidence of increased intracranial pressure.* Pyramidal tract signs.† Inability to rotate eyes upward. Sudden loss of consciousness. Rarely, seizures.	CT scan shows displacement or obliteration of third ventricle and resultant-hydrocephalus. Pineal is rarely calcified in children.	Astrocytomas, germinomas including pinealoma (macrogenitosomia praecox in boys), ependymoma.	Shunt (ventriculocisternal, etc) for relief of cerebrospinal fluid obstruction. Intensive x-ray therapy. Germinomas require radiotherapy to entire cerebrospinal axis. Benefit of chemotherapy unclear.
Suprasellar region	Visual disorders (visual field defects, optic atrophy). Hypothalamic disorders (including	Skull films show suprasellar calcification (about 90% of cases), deformity of sella turcica	Optic glioma (commonly associated with neurofibromatosis). Feet and hands may be large in	X-ray if optic chiasm is involved. Surgical removal if only one optic nerve is involved. Conservative

		infants and young children if the diencephalon is involved.	approach advised. Benefit of chemotherapy is unclear. Prognosis fair to good.
diabetes insipidus, adiposity). Pituitary disorders (growth arrest, hypothyroidism, delayed sexual maturation). Evidence of increased intracranial pressure.*	(frequent), and enlarged optic foramens in optic gliomas. CT scan shows deformity and obliteration of suprasellar cistern; shows hydrocephalus if foramens of Monro blocked. Optic nerves are thickened in optic glioma and may show calcification. CT scan may miss cystic craniopharyngioma, isodense with brain, in which case MRI may be helpful.	Craniopharyngioma; often dormant for years.	Complete excision of craniopharyngioma, with hormone replacement, now often feasible; or drainage of cyst and irradiation. Prognosis good if removal is complete. Repeated surgery often necessary if complete removal cannot be achieved.

*Evidence of increased intracranial pressure includes headache, vomiting (often without nausea and before breakfast), diplopia, blurred vision, papilledema. Personality changes, including irritability, apathy, disturbances in sleep and eating patterns, are frequent. Sudden enlargement of the head if head circumferences have been plotted is detectable when sutures are still open or after sutures have split. Alterations of consciousness and stiff neck with tonsillar herniation may be seen.

†Cerebellar signs include ataxia, dysmetria, and nystagmus. Truncal ataxia in the absence of lateralizing signs is most common in vermis tumors.

‡Signs due to pressure on adjacent structures may include head tilting, cranial nerve signs, pyramidal tract signs, suboccipital tenderness, and stiff neck.

decreasing frequency by genitourinary, extremity, trunk, and retroperitoneal sites. Orbital rhabdomyosarcomas often present with proptosis. Middle ear and parameningeal tumors may present with chronic otitis media, cranial nerve palsies, and headaches. After CT scan of the mass, pathologic evaluation of a biopsy specimen or of the completely removed tumor (depending on size and location) is necessary to distinguish rhabdomyosarcoma from other soft tissue sarcomas, lymphomas, and neuroblastoma.

Laboratory studies should include complete blood counts, lactate dehydrogenase, liver function studies, blood urea nitrogen, and uric acid. Evaluation for metastatic disease should include skeletal survey and bone scan, CT of the abdomen and lungs, and bone marrow aspiration and biopsy. Treatment depends on the location of the tumor, histologic type, and extent of disease. Treatment modalities include surgery, chemotherapy, and radiotherapy. The most commonly used chemotherapy includes vincristine, dactinomycin, and cytoxan (See Table 29–5). The overall disease-free survival is about 70%. Orbital tumors have the best prognosis.

Fibrosarcomas and liposarcomas are rare lesions and should be surgically excised when possible. In certain circumstances, electron beam therapy (4000–6000 rads) may be of benefit. The role of adjuvant chemotherapy is unclear.

Benign tumors are generally slow-growing and nontender. Most commonly seen are the fibromas and lipomas. These may be excised if they are symptomatic.

TUMORS OF BONE

The most frequent age groups affected by malignant bone tumors are the preadolescent, adolescent, and young adult groups. Osteosarcoma, Ewing's sarcoma, chondrosarcoma, fibrosarcoma, and synovial sarcoma may all present with a painful mass, limitation of motion, and x-ray changes in the bones involved. Osteogenic sarcoma typically arises in the metaphyses of long bones. The distal femur is the most common site, followed by the proximal tibia and proximal humerus. Ewing's sarcoma arises in long and flat bones, including the pelvis. Plain x-rays of osteogenic sarcoma typically display a "sunburst" appearance with lytic and blastic elements within the lesion. X-rays of Ewing's sarcoma typically show a moth-eaten and lytic appearance with elevation of the periosteum ("onion-skinning"). CT or MRI scan of the lesion allows assessment of extent of disease and involvement of the neurovascular bundle. Metastatic disease is not uncommon at diagnosis and should be sought prior to planning therapy.

Survival rates for patients with osteosarcoma was less than 20% with surgical amputation alone, but significant improvement has resulted from the combination of aggressive surgery (amputation or complex limb-preservation surgery) and multiple drug chemotherapy. Some chemotherapy is usually given prior to definitive surgery. Effective chemotherapeutic agents for osteogenic sarcoma include high-dose methotrexate with leucovorin rescue, doxorubicin, and cisplatin (see Table 29–5). Local high-dose radiation therapy (5000–6000 rads) has traditionally been used along with chemotherapy for Ewing's sarcoma. However, many centers now advocate full surgical resection, when possible, as for osteogenic sarcoma. Effective chemotherapy for Ewing's sarcoma includes cytoxan, adriamycin, vincristine, actinomycin, and ifosfamide (see Table 29–5). The 5-year disease-free survival for osteogenic sarcoma is about 60%, and for Ewing's sarcoma about 50%. Patients who present with metastatic disease have the worst prognosis. Ewing's sarcoma can recur many years after completion of treatment.

There are a number of fibrous, cartilaginous, and osseous benign tumors. Some have classic x-ray findings. In general, they should be biopsied or excised to rule out the possibility of a malignant tumor. Osteoid osteoma is a relatively common benign tumor of bone in adolescents and young adults. It is characterized by pain, limp (if the lower extremity is involved), atrophy of muscle, normal laboratory findings, and prompt and dramatic relief of pain in response to aspirin.

WILMS' TUMOR
(Nephroblastoma)

The most common abdominal masses encountered in early childhood are hydronephrosis, neuroblastoma, and Wilms's tumor. Wilms's tumor is believed to be embryonal in origin. It develops within renal parenchyma and enlarges with distortion and invasion of adjacent renal tissue. It occurs most commonly in children between 2 and 5 years old. Bilateral Wilms's tumors occur in up to 5% of patients. This tumor may be associated with congenital anomalies such as hemihypertrophy, aniridia, ambiguous genitalia, hypospadias, undescended testes, duplications of ureters or kidneys, horseshoe kidney, multiple nevi, and Beckwith's syndrome.

Clinical Findings

A. Symptoms and Signs: Ninety percent of patients present with an abdominal mass, but only about 30% complain of abdominal discomfort. Anemia is observed at diagnosis in about 24% of patients, hypertension in 20%, and hematuria in 15%.

B. Laboratory Findings: Results of urinalysis are usually normal, but hematuria or pyuria may be found. Blood urea nitrogen levels are usually normal; uric acid may be increased. A normochromic, normocytic anemia may be present.

C. Imaging: A soft tissue mass may be seen on a plain film of the abdomen and calcification may occur in a marginal concentric fashion. Hepatomegaly may be present if the liver has extensive metastases. Intravenous urography may show distortion and displacement of the renal pelvis and calices in any direction; hydronephrosis may also be present. Abdominal ultrasound and CT scan can define the mass, which usually appears well encapsulated. Ultrasound may demonstrate tumor thrombus in the renal vein or inferior vena cava. CT scan of chest or 4-view chest x-ray may reveal metastases.

Treatment

Surgical excision of the entire mass, without prior biopsy, is the currently recommended surgical procedure. A transabdominal approach is essential to allow adequate mobilization, prevent excess manipulation of the tumor, and allow examination of abdominal viscera, nodes, and the opposite kidney. Conservative surgery is appropriate when bilateral disease is present at diagnosis.

Treatment of Wilms' tumor depends on surgical staging and histology (Table 29–2). Improvement in survival has resulted

Table 29–2. Wilms' tumor stages.

Stage	Findings
I	Tumor *limited* to kidney; intact capsule; completely resected
II	Tumor extension *beyond capsule* into perirenal soft tissues or renal vessels but *no* residua beyond margin of resection; surgical rupture: *flank* only
III	*Residual* tumor in abdomen: 1) + lymph nodes 2) massive rupture 3) peritoneal implants 4) not fully resected secondary to local infiltration into vital structures
IV	Hematogenous metastases
V	Bilateral; each side staged as above

from cooperative clinical trials in the USA and Europe. Chemotherapy agents used to treat Wilms's tumor include dactinomycin and vincristine for the lower stages, with the addition of doxorubicin and occasionally cytoxan for the higher stages or unfavorable histology. Radiotherapy to the tumor bed is no longer recommended in stages I and II disease, but appears to be of benefit in stages III and IV disease.

Prognosis

The survival rate is best in children with localized disease and favorable histology. Survival rates have significantly improved over the past 30 years, and the overall 5-year survival rate is now about 80%.

NEUROBLASTOMA

Neuroblastoma is a tumor arising from cells in the sympathetic ganglia and adrenal medulla. It is the third most frequent pediatric neoplasm seen in children less than 5 years old. This tumor may be seen in the newborn period; the highest incidence is at 2 years of age. The tumors may regress spontaneously in infants less than 1 year old. Presentation in the abdominal area is most commonly associated with distant metastases and carries a poor prognosis.

Clinical Findings

A. Symptoms and Signs: General symptoms include failure to thrive, anorexia, fatigue, periorbital ecchymoses, chronic diarrhea, hypertension, pallor, irritability, bone pain, limp, and bluish skin nodules. Opsoclonus and myoclonus ("dancing eyes and dancing feet") have been associated with neuroblastoma.

1. Cervical tumors–Tumors commonly present with a mass in the neck and may be associated with Horner's syndrome.

2. Posterior thoracic tumors–Tumors may present with respiratory symptoms such as cough, croup, dysphagia, and fatigue, or with symptoms of spinal cord compression.

3. Abdominal tumors–Tumors may cause abdominal swelling from adrenal or paraspinal tumor. They may be very large and cross the midline or may be deep and difficult to palpate. Other findings include abdominal pain, change in bowel habits, delay in walking, paraplegia, or shock if a large tumor has ruptured.

B. Laboratory Findings: Anemia is common at diagnosis and results from chronic disease, hemorrhage into tumor, or marrow invasion. Thrombocytosis is common. Bone marrow is a common site of metastases and may reveal classic rosettes or sheets of anaplastic neuroblasts. Urine levels of catecholamines (vanillylmandelic acid [VMA] and homovanillic acid [HVA]) are elevated in nearly 90% of patients. An elevated VMA or HVA and evidence of metastatic disease in bone marrow is sufficient for the diagnosis of neuroblastoma and can obviate the need to biopsy the primary mass. Uric acid, lactate dehydrogenase, and liver and renal function should be evaluated as baseline studies. Elevated levels of serum ferritin (> 150 ng/mL), serum neuron-specific enolase (> 100 ng/mL), and amplification of the n-*myc* oncogene in the tumor itself are indicators of poor prognosis.

C. Imaging: Multiple destructive lesions of bone with a "moth-eaten" appearance may be seen in all bones. Pathologic fracture may also occur.

1. Thoracic tumors–Chest x-ray often shows soft tissue areas with clear borders and scattered calcifications close to the spine and in the upper chest. There may be erosion and separation of posterior ribs. CT scan should be obtained to define the tumor mass and its involvement with adjacent vital structures.

2. Abdominal tumors–Abdominal x-ray reveals a soft tissue mass in the region of the adrenal gland or along the spine. Many tumors show calcification. Intravenous urograms reveal downward and lateral displacement of the kidney. CT scan should be obtained to delineate the tumor and to look for hepatic metastases. Myleogram or spinal MRI may be necessary to evaluate for intercanalicular disease.

Treatment

Current therapy recommendations include surgery alone with close follow-up for patients with stage I disease. Patients with stage II disease and small or microscopic residua after surgery can also be safely treated with surgery alone and close follow-up. Improved treatments for advanced disease continue to be evaluated. Agents shown to be effective in neuroblastoma include vincristine, cytoxan, dacarbazine, etoposide, doxorubicin, cisplatin, and melphalan (see Table 29–5). Neuroblastoma is very radiosensitive. Very-high-dose chemotherapy with total body irradiation, followed by either autologous or allogeneic bone marrow transplant, is currently being evaluated in treatment of advanced disease.

Course & Prognosis

The most important variables for prediciting prognosis are age and stage. Children diagnosed at less than 1 year of age have about an 80% survival rate, while survival of children diagnosed at older than 2 years (of whom two-thirds present with metastatic disease) is about 10%. Patients with stage I disease (confined to the structure of origin and completely excised) have a survival rate of about 80%, whereas survival in stage IV disease (metastatic) treated with conventional chemotherapy is close to 10%.

RETINOBLASTOMA

Retinoblastoma is a malignant ocular tumor that occurs before the age of 5 in over 90% of cases. The tumor may arise sporadically or be inherited. Patients with inherited retinoblastoma often have bilateral disease, while those with the sporadic form have unilateral disease. The most common presenting complaint is leukocoria (white "cat's eye reflex") noted by parents. Strabismus, signs of orbital inflammation, and retinal detachment may be associated. The diagnosis is usually made by inspection of the globe under anesthesia by an ophthalmologist experienced with these tumors. The differential diagnosis includes lesions of *Toxocara canis,* toxoplasmosis, and retrolental fibroplasia. The tumor is typically confined to the globe but is extraocular in about 15% of cases. Metastatic evaluation should include CT scan (MRI) of the head and orbits, cerebrospinal fluid cytology, bone marrow aspirate, and biopsy.

Eradication of the tumor by enucleation depends on the potential for useful vision. Since the majority of unilateral tumors involve over one-half the retina by the time of diagnosis, enucleation is most commonly advised. For smaller lesions where vision may be saved, cryotherapy, photocoagulation, or radiotherapy have been successful treatments. Combination chemotherapy should be given to patients with regional or distant extraocular spread. Ophthalmologic evaluation of the uninvolved eye should be performed at regular intervals for several years in order to detect early bilateral disease.

Survival of retinoblastoma is greater than 90%. Patients with the inherited form have a high risk of second cancers throughout their lives, the most common being osteogenic sarcoma. Genetic counseling is important for families of patients with retinoblastoma. The risk of a subsequent sibling developing retinoblastoma varies from 1 to 50%, depending on the presence of other affected family members. Siblings should be carefully examined and followed by an ophthalmologist.

HODGKIN'S DISEASE

Hodgkin's disease occurs twice as frequently in men as in women, with its peak incidence in the third decade. It has been reported in children as young as 3 years of age. The cause is not known. The clinical and surgical staging system is shown in Table 29–3.

Clinical Findings

A. Symptoms and Signs: Painless lymph node enlargement, variable degrees of anorexia, weight loss, fatigue, weakness, fever, malaise, pruritus, and night sweats (see Table 29–3). The most common site of nodal involvement is the cervical region. Involved nodes are usually firm and nontender and may produce pressure symptoms depending upon their location, which may be anywhere. Hepatosplenomegaly and extranodal disease in any organ may be present. Splenomegaly does not necessarily imply splenic involvement with Hodgkin's disease, however. Other infections and inflammatory causes of lymphadenopathy are in the differential diagnosis, including infectious mononucleosis and atypical mycobacterial infections.

Table 29–3. Staging classification for Hodgkin's disease.*
(Ann Arbor classification.)

Stage†	Distinctive Features
I	Involvement of a single lymph node region (I) or a single extralymphatic organ or site (I$_E$).
II	Involvement of 2 or more lymph node regions on the same side of the diaphragm (II) or localized involvement of an extralymphatic organ or site and of one or more lymph node regions on the same side of the diaphragm (II$_E$).
III	Involvement of lymph node regions on both sides of the diaphragm (III), which may be accompanied by localized involvement of an extralymphatic organ or site (III$_E$) or of spleen (III$_S$) or both (III$_{SE}$).
IV	Diffuse or disseminated involvement of one or more extralymphatic organs with or without associated lymph node involvement. The organs involved should be identified by a symbol.

*Modified and reproduced, with permission, from Kempe CH, Silver HK, O'Brien D (editors): *Current Pediatric Diagnosis & Treatment,* 8th ed. Lange, 1984.
†Stages are also classified as IA, IB, IIA, IIB, etc. on the basis of symptoms and signs: A = asymptomatic; B = fever, night sweats, or weight loss > 10% of body weight in the 6 months prior to diagnosis.

B. Laboratory Findings: Hematologic findings may be normal or may show anemia, leukocytosis, leukopenia, thrombocytosis, thrombocytopenia, eosinophilia, or elevated sedimentation rate. Acute phase reactant proteins, including fibrinogen, ceruloplasmin, C-reactive protein, and ferritin, may be elevated in serum and can serve as sensitive markers of response to therapy and of early recurrent disease. Kidney and liver function tests or scans may reflect abnormalities if these organs are involved with disease. Cell-mediated immunity is often impaired in patients with Hodgkin's Disease. Hemolytic anemia and abnormal levels of immunoglobulins may also occur. The diagnosis of Hodgkin's disease is made by biopsy of the involved node followed by clinical staging with a number of x-ray modalities (chest x-ray, abdominal CT, gallium scan, lymphangiogram; see below) and bone marrow biopsies. Surgical staging by laparotomy, with splenectomy, liver biopsy, and lymph node sampling is still recommended in fully grown patients who may be successfully treated with radiation therapy alone. However, many pediatric oncologists prefer to treat growing children with chemotherapy and limited radiation, thus eliminating the need for laparotomy and the risk of postsplenectomy sepsis.

C. Imaging: Chest x-rays or chest CT scan may show parenchymal or mediastinal nodal disease. Skeletal survey and bone scan may show bone involvement. Lymphangiography may reveal a "foamy" enlarged node, which implies tumor filling the node. Abdominal CT scan may show enlarged periaortic nodes or spleen and liver abnormalities. Gallium scan may help identify areas of occult disease.

Treatment

Fully grown patients with surgical stages I and II disease can be successfully treated with extended field irradiation alone. Therapy for growing children with low-stage disease remains controversial, but chemotherapy with or without low-dose radiation to involved areas is becoming widely used. Chemotherapy is the primary treatment modality for stages III and IV disease. Chemotherapeutic agents commonly employed in combination are vincristine, mechlorethamine or cyclophosphamide, procarbazine, and prednisone. Other effective agents include lomustine (CCNU), vinblastine, bleomycin, doxorubicin, and dacarbazine (see Table 29–5).

Prognosis

In adequately treated patients, 5-year survival rates have improved greatly. In stages I and II disease, rates range from 85 to 90%. In stages III and IV disease, rates range from about 50% to 80%. Late side effects of treatment include infertility, impaired bony growth, hypothyroidism, and second cancers.

NON-HODGKIN'S LYMPHOMA

Classification of this diverse group of lymphomas is based on the architecture of the node, on whether the disease is nodular or diffuse, on the cytologic differentiation of lymphocytes and histiocytes, and on the surface membrane markers (T cell, B cell) of lymphocytes. Histologic classification into 2 main groups, lymphoblastic and nonlymphoblastic, is important in childhood lymphomas for determining appropriate therapy and prognosis.

Burkitt's tumor (African lymphoma) is a special type of childhood lymphoma found principally in Africa. This tumor is responsible for half of all cancer deaths in children in Uganda and Central Africa. A viral cause has been assumed and the role of Epstein-Barr virus in this disease is under scrutiny. The tumor is characterized by (1) predilection for the facial bones and mandible *or* (2) primary involvement of abdominal nodes and viscera and (3) massive proliferation of primitive lymphoreticular cells. When Burkitt's tumor is seen in patients outside of Africa, it generally presents as an abdominal tumor.

Clinical Findings

A. Symptoms and Signs: Non-Hodgkin's lymphoma of childhood tends to grow rapidly. The gastrointestinal tract in the region of the terminal ileum, cecum, appendix, ascending colon, and mesenteric nodes is the most common site of nonlymphoblastic lymphoma (aside from African Burkitt's). Acute abdominal pain, intussusception, gastrointestinal tract perforation, and hemorrhage may occur. Lymphoblastic lymphoma presents most commonly with a mediastinal mass, with or without pleural effusion. Chronic cough, dyspnea, and orthopnea are often associated. Involvement of the tonsillar region, cervical nodes, and nasopharynx may be diagnosed by the presence of a mass or compression symptoms. Other less common sites of primary disease include bone, ovaries, skin, and CNS. Spread to the bone marrow and CNS often occurs with lymphoblastic or disseminated nonlymphoblastic lymphoma.

B. Laboratory Findings: These patients should be evaluated radiographically as is done for Hodgkin's disease patients, with the exception of lymphangiogram. Staging laparotomy is not recommended in non-Hodgkin's lymphoma. Laboratory findings depend on organ, nodal, or marrow involvement. Uric acid, lactate dehydrogenase, and sedimentation rate are often elevated. Lumbar puncture with cytocentrifuge examination is necessary to evaluate for CNS disease.

Treatment

Complete surgical resection of nodal, extranodal, or gastrointestinal disease, when possible, is advocated. However, debulking of widespread abdominal disease or mediastinal mass is not advised. Multiple-drug chemotherapy should be started as soon as possible after diagnosis. Duration of therapy depends on location, type of lymphoma, and extent of disease, and currently ranges from 6 to 18 months. The drugs most commonly employed are vincristine, cyclophosphamide, doxorubicin, prednisone, methotrexate, bleomycin, and cytarabine (see Table 29–5). In patients at high risk for CNS involvement, prophylactic intrathecal therapy should be given. Irradiation to the site of the primary lesion is often part of initial therapy, but its benefit is currently in question.

Prognosis

The prognosis in children with non-Hodgkin's lymphoma depends primarily on histologic findings, extent of disease, and the receipt of appropriate therapy. Overall, at least 70% of children with non-Hodgkin's lymphoma can be cured.

GERM CELL TUMORS

Germ cell tumors are derived from primordial germ cells and can be benign or malignant, gonadal or extragonadal. Extragonadal sites are involved in about two-thirds of cases, including the sacrococcygeal area, mediastinum, retroperitoneum, and CNS. Patients with gonadal dysgenesis (as in Turner's syndrome) and those with undescended testes are at increased risk of developing germ cell tumors, particularly gonadoblastomas and germinomas. Teratomas can be benign or malignant, depending on the degree of maturity of the tissue elements involved. Since therapy is different for benign and malignant teratomas, very careful pathologic evaluation of the tumor is necessary. Malignant germ cell tumors characteristically secrete alpha-fetoprotein (AFP) or beta-subunit human chorionic gonadotropin (β-hCG), which are valuable serum markers of disease activity.

Sacrococcygeal teratomas are found more often in neonates than in older infants and children. The vast majority of these tumors have an external component, allowing for rapid diagnosis. Most of these tumors are benign at the time of diagnosis. However, since benign teratomas have the capacity to become malignant, full surgical excision is necessary. The coccyx should be removed as well since the chance of recurrence in that area is high.

Tumors of the Ovary and Testis

Tumors of the ovary are characterized by an enlarging palpable mass in the lower abdomen or pelvis. Severe abdominal pain may occur due to a twisted pedicle. The majority of ovarian tumors in children are benign teratomas; about 25% are malignant germ cell tumors. Sexual precocity, uterine bleeding, and advanced bone age as a result of excessive estrogen production occur only in patients with granulosa cell tumors (which are almost always large enough to palpate). These tumors arise from stromal rather than germ cell elements and may be malignant or benign.

Treatment of ovarian tumors is by complete surgical removal for localized disease. Postoperative chemotherapy is used to treat malignant germ cell tumors, whether completely or incompletely excised. The best treatment results so far have been obtained with cisplatin, vinblastine or etoposide, and bleomycin. Prognosis is generally very good.

Testicular tumors vary from highly malignant (embryonal carcinoma, germinoma, or malignant teratoma) to relatively benign (Leydig cell tumor or benign teratoma). They are rare in boys under 15 years of age. Paratesticular rhabdomyosarcoma may also present as a scrotal mass in the male child. Tumors are characterized by painless, solid swelling of the testicle, which does not transilluminate and appears to have a purplish discoloration. Hydrocele may be associated. Although evidence of endocrine activity usually is absent, pseudoprecocious puberty occasionally occurs. AFP or β-hCG levels may be elevated in malignant germ cell tumors and should be followed for activity of disease.

Orchiectomy with high ligation of the cord is indicated in all testicular tumors. Radiographic staging with abdominal and chest CT scan, bone scan, and skeletal survey is necessary prior to treatment of malignant tumors. Metastases may occur in lungs, mediastinum, bones, and regional and abdominal lymph nodes. For boys without radiographic evidence of lymphatic or hematologic spread, orchiectomy without chemotherapy but with close serial follow-up of serum AFP levels appears to be adequate initial treatment. The most successful chemotherapy for malignant testicular germ cell tumors is as described for ovarian primaries. The prognosis is very good.

LEUKEMIAS IN CHILDHOOD

Most leukemias (97.5%) in childhood are acute. The most common type is acute lymphoblastic leukemia (ALL), which accounts for about 80% of cases (Table 29–4). The highest incidence of leukemia occurs in patients between 2 and 5 years of age. There is an increased risk of leukemia in patients with chromosomal abnormalities or immune deficiency states.

Clinical Findings

A. Symptoms and Signs: Initial signs and symptoms, in order of decreasing frequency, include fever, pallor, petechiae and purpura, lymphadenopathy, hepatosplenomegaly, anorexia, fatigue, bone and joint pain, abdominal pain, and weight loss. Nonmalignant conditions in the differential diagnosis include juvenile rheumatoid arthritis, immune thrombocytopenic purpura, Epstein-Barr viral disease, and aplastic anemia. CNS infiltration may cause manifestations simulating meningitis, with increased intracranial pressure and cranial nerve palsies, and may be associated with findings of pleocytosis, increased protein levels, and lowered glucose levels in cerebrospinal fluid. Septicemia may occur during the course of the disease due to neutropenia.

B. Laboratory Findings:

1. Blood–Red blood cell counts and hemoglobin levels are usually low. The white blood cell count may be elevated, normal, or reduced. In some cases, large numbers of abnormal cells (blasts) are seen on smear; in others, no peripheral blasts are noted. Thrombocytopenia is very frequent.

2. Bone marrow–By definition, leukemia is present when more than 25% of cells in a bone marrow aspirate are malignant blasts. In almost all cases, 50–98% of nucleated cells are blast forms with marked reduction in the normal erythroid, myeloid, and platelet precursors. Blasts from the majority of cases of childhood ALL have an antigen present on the cell surface called the common ALL-antigen (CALLA). These blasts are derived from B-cell precursors early in their development. Less commonly, lymphoblasts are of T-cell origin or of mature B-cell origin.

Table 29-4. Acute leukemias of childhood.

Type	Approximate Frequency	Morphology	Immunophenotype (Histochemical Staining)
Lymphoblastic (ALL)	80%		
B-Cell Precursor ALL	84%*	Typically small blasts (≤ 2 RBC diameters), scant cytoplasm, indistinct nucleoli.†	Majority are CALLA (+)
T-Cell ALL	15%		E-rosette or T-cell surface antigen (+)
B-Cell ALL	1%	Blasts with deeply basophilic cytoplasm and vacuolization.	Surface immunoglobulin (+)
Nonlymphoblastic (ANLL)	20%		
Myeloblastic	45%‡	Blasts with few or many cytoplasmic granules; may have Auer rods.	Myeloperoxidase (MP) (+)
Promyelocytic	4%	Promyelocytes with numerous cytoplasmic granules.	MP (+)
Myelomonocytic	26%	Myeloblasts with cytoplasmic granules and monoblasts.	MP (+) and nonspecific esterase (NSE) (+)
Monocytic	21%	Monoblasts with smooth or irregular, folded nuclear contour.	NSE (+)
Erythroid	2%	Erythroblasts amid dyserythropoiesis.	
Megakaryocytic	2%§	Blasts look like lymphoblasts or undifferentiated myeloblasts.	Platelet peroxidase (+) endoplasmic reticulum on electron microscopy

*% of ALL.
†Some lymphoblasts are larger, with more cytoplasm and more prominent nucleoli, similar morphologically to undifferentiated myeloblasts.
‡% of ANLL.
§Frequency may be underestimated since megakaryocytic leukemia has only recently been recognized.

930

3. Chromosomes–A variety of chromosome abnormalities have been reported in the blasts of all forms of acute leukemia. Certain abnormalities, including reciprocal translocations [eg, t(4;11) and t(9;22)] or monosomy 7 are associated with a very poor prognosis.

4. Serum–Levels of uric acid and lactate dehydrogenase are usually elevated.

5. Cerebrospinal fluid–Pleocytosis (consisting of blast forms), elevated levels of protein, and decreased levels of glucose may be seen.

Treatment of Acute Leukemias

A. Acute Lymphoblastic Leukemia:

1. Remission induction–Most patients (95%) achieve complete remission following 4 weeks of treatment with vincristine, prednisone, asparaginase, and intrathecal methotrexate (Table 29–5).

2. Central nervous system leukemia–Because of the risk of CNS leukemia, patients should be treated prophylactically with intrathecal chemotherapy and sometimes CNS irradiation as well.

3. Maintenance–One commonly used maintenance therapy lasts 2–3 years, with daily oral mercaptopurine and weekly methotrexate as mainstays of treatment, along with monthly vincristine and prednisone.

4. Relapse–If the disease recurs, another remission may be induced with selected combinations of the above drugs or other antineoplastic agents. Ultimate prognosis for patients who relapse depends on when relapse occurs in relation to completion of initial therapy. Allogeneic bone marrow transplant may improve the chance of cure for patients who relapse.

B. Acute Nonlymphocytic Leukemia (ANLL): ANLL of childhood is more difficult to cure than ALL. Remission induction has been successful with a number of agents; the most commonly used are cytarabine and daunorubicin (Table 29–5). CNS prophylaxis with intrathecal cytarabine (but without cranial irradiation) is necessary. Questions that remain to be answered include the optimal length of maintenance therapy and the advantages of bone marrow transplantation over conventional chemotherapy for long-term cure in patients who achieve remission.

C. Supportive Measures: Transfusions of packed red blood cells and platelets should be given as needed. Fevers in the face of neutropenia should be treated with broad-spectrum antibiotics. Hyperuricemia due to the degradation of nucleic acids may

Table 29–5. Antineoplastic agents.*

Agent	Indications	Toxicity
Asparaginase (Elspar)	Acute lymphoblastic leukemia.	Nausea, vomiting, fever, hypersensitivity, pancreatitis, hyperglycemia thromboses.
Bleomycin (Blenoxane)	Hodgkin's disease, non-Hodgkin's lymphoma, testicular tumors.	Nausea, vomiting, stomatitis, fever, chills, pulmonary fibrosis, hyperpigmentation, alopecia.
Carmustine (BCNU)	Malignant gliomas, medulloblastoma, advanced Hodgkin's disease and other sarcomas, neuroblastoma, malignant melanoma.	Nausea, vomiting, hepatotoxicity, chemical dermatitis. Bone marrow depression (3- to 4-wk delay).
Cisplatin (Platinol, CDDP)	Germ cell tumors, osteogenic sarcoma, brain tumors, neuroblastoma.	Nausea, vomiting, anorexia, alopecia, bone marrow depression, renal failure, magnesium and calcium wasting hearing impairment.
Cyclophosphamide (Cytoxan)	Leukemia, Hodgkin's disease, neuroblastoma, sarcomas, retinoblastoma, hepatoma, rhabdomyosarcoma, Ewing's sarcoma.	Nausea, vomiting, anorexia, alopecia, bone marrow depression, hemorrhagic cystitis.
Cytarabine (cytosine arabinoside; Cytosar-U)	Acute myeloblastic and acute lymphocytic leukemia.	Nausea, vomiting, anorexia, bone marrow depression, hepatotoxicity.
Dacarbazine (DTIC)	Hodgkin's disease, neuroblastoma, sarcomas.	Bone marrow depression, flulike syndrome, rash, liver failure, pain at IV infusion site.
Dactinomycin (Cosmegan)	Wilms's tumor, sarcomas, rhabdomyosarcoma.	Nausea, vomiting, anorexia, bone marrow depression, alopecia. Chemical dermatitis if leakage at intravenous site.

Table 29–5. (cont'd). Antineoplastic agents.*

Agent	Indications	Toxicity
		Tanning of skin if used with radiation therapy.
Daunorubicin (daunomycin)	Acute myelogenous, monomyelogenous, and monoblastic leukemias.	Same as for doxorubicin (below).
Doxorubicin (Adriamycin)	Acute lymphoblastic and myelocytic leukemia, lymphoma, Hodgkin's disease, Wilms' tumor, neuroblastoma, ovarian or thyroid carcinoma, Ewing's sarcoma, osteogenic sarcoma, rhabdomyosarcoma, other soft tissue sarcomas.	Alopecia, stomatitis, esophagitis, nausea, vomiting. Severe chemical cellulitis and necrosis if extravasated. Bone marrow depression, irreversible myocardial damage (rare if cumulative dose less 350 mg/m^2).
Etoposide (VP-16)	Leukemias, germ cell tumors, neuroblastoma, brain tumors, sarcomas.	Allergic reactions, bone marrow depression, nausea and vomiting, neurotoxicity.
Fluorouracil (Adrucil)	Hepatoma, gastrointestinal carcinoma.	Nausea, vomiting, oral ulceration, bone marrow depression, gastroenteritis, alopecia, anorexia.
Ifosfamide	Sarcomas, recurrent solid tumors.	Bone marrow depression, hemorrhagic cystitis, nausea and vomiting, renal failure, alopecia, neurotoxicity.
Lomustine (CCNU; CeeNu)	Brain tumors, Hodgkin's disease.	Nausea, vomiting, alopecia, stomatitis, hepatotoxicity. Bone marrow depression (4- to 6-wk delay).
Mechlorethamine (nitrogen mustard)	Hodgkin's disease, non-Hodgkin's lymphoma.	Nausea, vomiting, bone marrow depression, strong vesicating effect on skin and veins.

Table 29–5. (cont'd). Antineoplastic agents.*

Agent	Indications	Toxicity
Mercaptopurine (Purinethol)	Acute myeloblastic and acute lymphocytic leukemia.	Nausea, vomiting, rare oral ulcerations, bone marrow depression.
Methotrexate	Acute lymphocytic leukemia, central nervous system leukemia, lymphoma, choriocarcinoma, brain tumors, Hodgkin's disease.	Oral ulcers, gastrointestinal irritation, bone marrow depression, hepatotoxicity. Do not use in presence of impaired renal function.
Prednisone	Acute myeloblastic and lymphocytic leukemia, lymphoma, Hodgkin's disease, bone pain from metastatic disease, central nervous system tumors.	Increased appetite, sodium retention, hypertension, osteoporosis, provocation of latent diabetes or tuberculosis.
Procarbazine (Matulane)	Hodgkin's disease, lymphoma.	Nausea, vomiting, anorexia. Bone marrow depression (3-wk delay). Do not give with narcotics or sedatives; has "disulfiram effect." Monitor liver and renal function.
Vinblastine	Histiocytosis, Hodgkin's disease, germ cell tumors.	Bone marrow depression, alopecia, mucositis, neurotoxicity, chemical dermatitis.
Vincristine (Oncovin)	Acute lymphocytic and myeloblastic leukemia, lymphoma, Hodgkin's disease, rhabdomyo-sarcoma, Wilms' tumor, neuroblastoma, Ewing's sarcoma, retinoblastoma, hepatoma, sarcomas, osteogenic sarcoma, brain tumors.	Alopecia, constipation, abdominal cramps, jaw pain, paresthesia, myalgia, muscle weakness, neurotoxicity, decrease in deep tendon reflexes, chemical dermatitis. Do not use in presence of severe liver impairment.

*Since the dosage of these agents varies widely depending on number of drugs used simultaneously, type of tumor being treated, bone marrow reserve, and previous toxicities and therapies (eg, irradiation), the dosages are not given in this handbook.

occur following the initiation of antileukemic therapy. Allopurinol taken orally is effective in reducing the hyperuricemia. Intravenous hydration and alkalinization (to decrease uric acid precipitation in kidneys) is also of value. Hyperphosphatemia and hypocalcemia can occur during initial treatment as well. Hyperkalemia, severe hyperphosphatemia, tetany, or oliguria may require temporary hemodialysis.

Course & Prognosis

Aggressive combination chemotherapy and supportive therapy with blood products and antibiotics have contributed to improved survival. As many as 95% of children with ALL will achieve remission within 1 month of starting therapy, and long-term "cure" rates are between 50 and 85%, depending on various prognostic features (including age and white blood cell count) present at diagnosis. In general, children diagnosed with ALL between the ages of 2 and 10 with a white blood cell count of less than 50,000/μL at diagnosis have the best chance of cure. Children with ANLL have a poorer prognosis, with long-term cure rates between 25 and 40%.

LANGERHANS CELL HISTIOCYTOSIS
(Histiocytosis X)

The diseases discussed under this heading comprise a heterogeneous group of proliferative disorders of the reticuloendothelial system. The disorders are of unknown cause, but immune system dysfunction may be involved in their pathogenesis. They differ in behavior from true neoplasms. Eosinophilic granuloma of bone, Hand-Schüller-Christian disease, and Letterer-Siwe disease constitute a complex of diseases previously grouped under the term **histiocytosis X.** Langerhans histiocytes—phagocytes normally found in skin—appear to be the proliferating cells in these disorders. Whether these cells are immature, normal, or malignant is unclear. Various immunologic abnormalities have been observed in patients with these diseases.

Certain patients present primarily with signs and symptoms of lytic lesions limited to the bones—especially the skull, ribs, clavicles, and vertebrae. These lesions are well demarcated on x-ray and occasionally are painful. Biopsy reveals eosinophilic granuloma, which may be the only lesion the patient will develop, although further bone and even visceral lesions may occur.

Another group of patients present with otitis media, seborrheic skin rash, and evidence of bone lesions, usually in the mastoid or skull area. They frequently also have visceral involvement, which may be indicated by lymphadenopathy and hepatosplenomegaly. This chronic disseminated form is usually known as Hand-Schüller-Christian disease. The classic triad of Hand-Schüller-Christian disease (bony involvement, exophthalmos, and diabetes insipidus) is rarely seen; however, diabetes insipidus is a common complication.

A third group of patients present early in life primarily with visceral involvement. They often have a petechial or macular skin rash, generalized lymphadenopathy, enlarged liver and spleen, pulmonary involvement, and hematologic abnormalities such as anemia and thrombocytopenia. Bone lesions can occur. This acute visceral form, Letterer-Siwe disease, is often fatal.

The principal diseases to be differentiated from histiocytosis X are infections with histiocyte proliferation (eg, toxoplasmosis, tularemia), bone tumors (primary or metastatic), lymphomas or leukemias, immune deficiency states, and storage diseases. The diagnosis is established by biopsy of abnormal areas of bone, skin, bone marrow, lymph node, or liver. Complete immunologic evaluation is essential to distinguish Letterer-Siwe disease from severe combined immune deficiency.

Isolated bony lesions, if progressive or symptomatic (or both), are best treated by curettage and local radiotherapy. Multiple bony involvement and visceral involvement often respond well to prednisone, vinblastine, cyclophosphamide, methotrexate, and etoposide (see Table 29–5). Combination chemotherapy does not appear to offer significant advantage over single- or double-agent chemotherapy. Immunotherapy may also play a role in the treatment of these disorders.

If diabetes insipidus occurs, treatment with vasopressin gives good control.

In patients with Langerhans histiocytosis, the prognosis is often unpredictable. Many patients with considerable bony and visceral involvement have shown apparent complete recovery. The disease can also smolder for years, causing significant morbidity without mortality. In general, the younger the patient and the more extensive the visceral involvement, the worse the prognosis.

INFECTIONS IN THE IMMUNODEFICIENT PATIENT

Immunodeficiency may be congenital but more often is due to suppression of the immune system by diseases or drugs. Deficiencies of polymorphonuclear (PMN) cells, T lymphocytes, or B lymphocytes tend to predispose the host to infection with different agents. For example, PMN deficiency predisposes to infection with gram-negative or gram-positive bacteria and fungi; B lymphocyte deficiency, infection with extracellular bacteria such as pneumococci and staphylococci; and T lymphocyte deficiency, infection with intracellular bacteria (mycobacteria, *Listeria,* etc), fungi (*Candida, Aspergillus,* etc), protozoa (*Pneumocystis,* etc), and viruses (herpes simplex, etc).

Many opportunistic organisms do not produce disease except in the immunodeficient host. Such hosts are often infected with a number of pathogens simultaneously.

Infections caused by common organisms may present uncommon clinical manifestations. Determination of the specific infecting agents is essential for effective treatment.

Immunodeficient Hosts

Immunodeficient patients fall into several groups:

(1) Children with congenital immune defects of cellular or humoral immunity or a combination of both (eg, Wiskott-Aldrich syndrome).

(2) Patients with cancer, particularly lymphomas.

(3) Patients receiving immunosuppressive therapy. These include patients with neoplastic disease and those bearing transplants who are receiving corticosteroids or other immunosuppressive drugs.

(4) Patients who have very few PMNs ($< 500/\mu$L) or those whose PMNs do not function normally with respect to phagocytosis or the intracellular killing of phagocytosed microorganisms (eg, chronic granulomatous disease). Such patients often do not manifest signs of localized infection.

(5) Splenectomized patients (surgically removed or infarcted, as in sickle cell disease) who are at increased risk of pneumococcal or *Haemophilus influenzae* bacteremia.

(6) A larger group of patients who are not classically immunodeficient but whose host defenses are seriously compromised by debilitating illness, surgical or other invasive procedures (eg, intravenous drug abuse or intravenous hyperalimentation), burns, massive antimicrobial therapy, or acquired immune deficiency syndrome (AIDS).

Infectious Agents

A. Bacteria: Any bacterium pathogenic for humans can infect the immunosuppressed host. Furthermore, noninvasive and nonpathogenic organisms (opportunists) may also cause disease in such cases. Examples include gram-negative bacteria, particularly *Pseudomonas, Serratia,* and *Aeromonas.* Many of these come from the hospital environment and may be resistant to most antimicrobial drugs.

B. Fungi: *Candida, Aspergillus, Cryptococcus, Nocardia,* and *Mucor* can all cause disease in the immunosuppressed host. Candidiasis is by far the most common and is often found in patients receiving intensive antimicrobial therapy or prednisone.

C. Viruses: Cytomegalovirus is the most common, but varicella-zoster and herpes simplex viruses are also important. Vaccinia virus may cause serious problems if inadvertently inoculated.

D. Protozoa: *Pneumocystis carinii* is an important cause of pneumonia in many immunodeficient patients. It is particularly important to make this diagnosis early, because reasonably effective therapy is available. *Toxoplasma gondii* is also important in this group of patients.

Approach to Diagnosis

A systematic approach is necessary, including the following steps:

(1) Review carefully the patient's current immune status, absolute neutrophil count, presence of indwelling central lines, previous antimicrobial therapy, and *all* previous culture reports.

(2) Obtain pertinent cultures for bacteria, fungi, and viruses.

(3) Consider which of the serologic tests for fungal, viral, and protozoal diseases are pertinent.

(4) Consider special diagnostic procedures, eg, lung biopsy or lung puncture or endobronchial brush biopsy to demonstrate *Pneumocystis.*

(5) Consider whether the infection (eg, candidiasis) is superficial or systemic. Therapeutic considerations are quite different in each case.

Approach to Treatment

Caution: It is essential to avoid aggravating the patient's underlying condition and to avoid gross alterations of the host's normal microbial flora.

Provide general therapeutic measures to improve host defenses, correct electrolyte imbalance, offer adequate caloric intake, etc. Improve the patient's immune status whenever possible. This includes a temporary decrease in the immunosuppressive drug dosage in transplant patients and modification of chemotherapy in cancer patients.

For patients with absolute neutropenia [WBC $\times$ (% bands + segs) $< 500/\mu L$] and temperature $> 38.5°C$ (oral), broad-spectrum antibiotics should be initiated immediately after blood, throat, and urine cultures are obtained. Central venous catheters may have to be removed if bacteremia persists. If disseminated varicella or herpes zoster is suspected, IV acyclovir should be started immediately, prior to culture confirmation. Fungal infection should be suspected in a patient who remains febrile after a number of days on broad-spectrum antibiotics. Granulocyte transfusions may be able to tide the patient over a period of profound PMN deficiency when appropriate antibiotics have failed to eradicate bacteremia. Injection of immune globulin at regular intervals may compensate for certain B cell deficiencies.

Once an infectious agent is identified, antimicrobial drug therapy should be specific and lethal for it. Combinations of antibiotics may be necessary, since multiple infectious agents may be involved in some cases.

30 | Allergic Diseases

David S. Pearlman, MD

Allergic reactivity, that is, the specific ability to reject foreign substances, is normal. Some forms of allergy, however, occur only in certain individuals in whom a presumably hereditary predisposition is important. These disorders—allergic rhinitis, asthma, and atopic dermatitis—are called "atopic disorders." In most instances allergic reactivity based on IgE antibody to innocuous inhaled or ingested materials is an important cause of the disorder. The most important of these materials are animal allergens, insect allergens, spores from indoor and outdoor molds, and tree, grass, and weed pollen. Inhalants generally induce symptoms in the upper and/or lower respiratory tract. Sensitivity to foods, drugs and stinging insects, and other ingested materials contribute to perennial, seasonal, or episodic problems, some of which can be life-threatening.

PRINCIPLES OF DIAGNOSIS

Diagnosis is based first on the history and physical findings. Identification of the allergic antibody that may be involved is helpful and sometimes essential for determining the nature of the reaction and the environmental culprit. **These tests are not diagnostic in themselves, and their interpretation requires knowing the child,** including his or her environmental exposures. Atopic disorders tend to occur in families, and multiple disorders often occur in the same child. A history of time and place (eg, at school or at home) where a reaction occurs is helpful in determining environmental culprits. Some reactions occur within minutes ("early reaction"), but others can develop hours after allergen exposure.

Laboratory Tests

The principal allergic antibody identified belongs to the IgE class, also called reaginic or skin sensitizing antibody. There are two basic kinds of tests for IgE antibody: skin tests and serologic tests.

A. Skin Tests: These are very sensitive "biologic" tests and measure allergic antibody as a manifestation of the local release of mediators from sensitized cells on which the allergic reaction takes place. Sensitized mediator cells are found throughout the body, including the skin, which provides an extremely convenient site for testing. Prick tests generally are done first, since they are relatively painless, a large number of allergens can be applied conveniently, and they are safer in highly sensitive children than are intradermal tests. Intradermal tests are significantly more sensitive than are prick tests but are reserved for allergens that do not elicit a positive prick test but are still considered to be likely culprits of the disorder. The end point of these tests is a wheal and erythema reaction (hive), which occurs rapidly and peaks within 15–20 minutes. Skin testing is potentially dangerous in highly sensitive individuals. Most test materials are impure and in high concentration can produce an irritant reaction easily misinterpreted as positive for antibody ("false-positive test"). Positive tests may or may not be of significant clinical relevance, hence it is important to interpret test results strictly within the context of the clinical circumstances of the patient.

B. Serologic Tests: These tests measure serum IgE antibody per se. The best known is the radioallergosorbent test (RAST), a radioimmunoassay, but various enzymatic immunoassay variations are commonly available (ELISAs). Serologic tests correlate best with skin tests when high levels of antibody are present, but are less sensitive than skin tests. Theoretically, these tests should be especially useful for testing severe drug and stinging insect hypersensitivity. However, particularly with drug sensitivity, the important drug metabolites responsible for drug sensitivity rarely are available for serologic or skin testing and the lesser sensitivity of serologic tests make these tests less valuable for determining potentially life-threatening sensitivity.

C. Immunoglobulin Levels: IgE levels are measured by radioimmunosorbent or ELISA tests. Elevated IgE levels do occur in some allergic disorders, but the frequency of this occurrence and correlation with the presence or absence of allergy is so imperfect that this is not generally a useful screening procedure. Greatly elevated IgE levels in infancy are highly predictive of an atopic diathesis but a normal or low IgE level does not rule out either an atopic disorder or specific allergic sensitization.

D. Provocative Testing: Challenging the patient with a suspected allergen and observing the response also is useful, particularly with possible food sensitivity. It should never be used when life-threatening sensitivity is suspected, however. A positive response can establish a cause-and-effect relationship but not necessarily the mechanism involved (eg, a positive challenge to milk may be due to allergy or to lactase deficiency).

Eosinophils are a component of allergic inflammation, and the presence of a large number in secretions or in blood often is seen in atopic disorders. Large numbers are suggestive but not diagnostic of an allergic reaction, and their absence does not rule out allergy. Nasal eosinophilia is especially helpful in diagnosing allergic rhinitis, but nasal eosinophilia in infants up to 3 months of age can be normal.

Controversial Techniques for Diagnosis and Treatment

Intracutaneous end-point titration (sometimes called the "Rinkel test"), sublingual and serial intracutaneous provocation titration tests, and sublingual desensitization—all used for diagnosing or treating "allergy"—are not scientifically validated. They are rarely used by trained allergists certified by the American Board of Allergy and Immunology.

GENERAL PRINCIPLES OF TREATMENT

Controlling the Environment

Avoiding the offending allergen is the most effective treatment of all allergic disorders. Although complete avoidance may be impossible, often it is feasible to reduce the degree of exposure to the point that reactions are trivial. The avoidance of nonallergic add-on irritants such as smoke also is important. The single most important area of exposure is a child's bedroom. Here the greatest effort is made to control house dust (the most allergenic ingredients of which are house dust mites or other insects and animal saliva or dander), mold, feathers, cotton linters, and kapok. Overnight exposure to pollens and molds can be diminished by keeping the bedroom window closed overnight or employing an air conditioner as a partial filter in the bedroom or centrally. Animals should not be allowed in the bedroom if there is any question of animal sensitivity and should be kept out of the house or eliminated from the environment altogether depending upon the degree of the child's sensitivity. The remainder of the house is the second most important environmental area, but exposures at babysitters', preschools or schools, or at friends' houses can be problematic and may require alternative arrangements.

Allergy Injection Therapy (Hyposensitization or Immunotherapy)

Specific hyposensitization is attempted if the allergen is not sufficiently avoidable and is considered a significant problem. Its value is documented both for upper respiratory tract inhalant allergy and for allergic asthma, and it is effective for Hymenoptera insect sting allergy. Evidence for effectiveness is greatest for pollens, house dust mites, and Hymenoptera venom. It also may be efficacious for mold sensitivity. Injection therapy to foods has not been shown to be efficacious and may be dangerous. The use of bacterial extracts is of little value.

The procedure involves injecting extremely small amounts of allergen subcutaneously in gradually increasing dosage at frequent intervals (generally once or twice a week) until a top or maintenance dose is reached. This is usually the highest tolerated dose, or the amount that induces a state of clinical hyporeactivity to the allergen as demonstrated after natural contact. The top dose is used as the maintenance dose with carefully regulated lengthening of intervals, eventually to perhaps every 4 weeks if tolerated. Injection therapy is given for a minimum of 2 years, often 3–5 years, and occasionally for longer periods.

Drug Therapy

The following are principal groups of therapeutic agents used for the treatment of allergic disorders:

A. Adrenergic Agents: Epinephrine is the single most important agent for treating acute severe allergic reactions. It is used to decrease bronchospasm in acute severe asthma, although more selective beta-2 adrenergic agents such as terbutaline by injection are available. Moreover, selective beta-2 adrenergic drugs used by inhalation are generally as effective as injectable adrenergic agents in relieving asthma and are associated with fewer side effects. Orally active beta-2 agents also can be effective. The vasoconstrictive properties of certain adrenergic agents such as phenylephrine and pseudoephedrine also are useful in decongestion of allergic and nonallergic rhinitis. They can be used topically in the nose for short (5 days or less) periods, or orally, alone or in conjunction with antihistamines.

B. Antihistamines: Antihistamines are specific antagonists of histamine and are useful therefore when histamine is an important mediator of the reaction. Since histamine is only one of the numerous mediators involved, however, antihistamines rarely are completely therapeutic. There are two major classes of antihistamines; H_1-receptor inhibitors, which are the classic antihistamines used for many years in allergic disorders, and H_2-

receptor inhibitors, marketed for inhibiting gastric acid secretion
but which also have vascular properties. H_1 antihistamines are
particularly useful for allergic rhinitis and urticaria and as a part
of the treatment of anaphylaxis. The addition of H_2 antihistamines (eg, cimetidine and ranitidine) to an H_1 antihistamine can
help control urticaria not controlled by H_1 antihistamines alone,
and the use of both classes is recommended for the treatment of
anaphylaxis. Antihistamines are *not* the drugs of first choice in
allergic emergencies—epinephrine is—but they may be administered after epinephrine has been given. Since antihistamines are
competitive antagonists, they are best used in advance of histamine liberation and of anticipated symptoms. Most antihistamines are potentially soporific and they should be used cau-
tiously during school hours. Antihistamines are most effective in
reducing symptoms of rhinorrhea, nasal itching and sneezing,
eye tearing, itching, and hives. In contrast to general warnings in
the *PDR*, antihistamines can be used when asthma is present
(and may even have some beneficial effects in asthma!).

C. Theophylline and Aminophylline: Theophylline and its
ethylene diamine derivative aminophylline are effective but
potentially toxic bronchodilators, the improper use of which has
been associated with severe reactions and in some instances
even death. Recognition of subtle CNS side effects of learning
and behavioral changes emphasizes the need for close monitoring of patients on long-term theophylline therapy. Theophylline
can be therapeutic over a wide range of blood concentrations,
but levels between 10 and 20 μg/mL have been considered "optimal" for severe asthma since *major* toxicity rarely occurs with
peak blood levels below 20 μg/mL. Since levels can vary significantly owing to viral infections, diet, the use of erythromycin and
other drugs, peak levels higher than 15 μg/mL on a long-term
basis are discouraged. In early to mid-infancy, metabolism is
markedly diminished and these drugs should be employed with
extreme caution at these ages.

D. Expectorants: Glyceryl guaiacolate (guaifenesin) is
used mainly to thin mucus in asthma and upper respiratory tract
disorders but it is not clear how effective it is. Iodides appear to
be more effective but, especially with prolonged use, goiter,
salivary gland inflammation, gastric irritation, and skin eruptions
such as acne can occur.

E. Corticosteroids: These are extremely potent antiallergic
drugs but side effects associated with prolonged therapy limit
their use mainly to those conditions that are refractory to other
measures or are life-threatening. Topically active corticosteroids
which are inactivated rapidly upon absorption have been devel-

oped, giving them a high local therapeutic potency with low systemic effects. Intranasal topical steroids, and inhalant topical steroids for chronic asthma, have been shown to be relatively safe and effective in these conditions, as have topical steroids for eczema. In the latter case, however, significant absorption of active drug occurs with extensive use over inflamed skin or with occlusive dressings, especially with the halogenated preparations. Systemic corticosteroids should be considered for short-term use for acute severe asthma not immediately responsive to nonsteroid therapy, for severe contact dermatitis, and for medical emergencies due to allergic reactions as a second- or third-line medication after adrenergic agents and antihistamines have been given. Long-term use of systemic steroids should be considered when nonsteroid agents or topical steroids cannot control symptoms sufficiently. When long-term use is necessary, alternate-day therapy with a short-acting preparation such as prednisone in the early morning should be attempted, using the least amount necessary to control symptoms.

F. Sedatives: Sedatives have little place in the treatment of allergic disorders and are contraindicated in asthma since they can depress the respiratory center. Anxiety associated with extreme asthma is more a reflection of the severity of asthma than its cause.

G. Oxygen: Oxygen is extremely important in the treatment of severe asthma since hypoxemia virtually always is present with severe obstruction.

H. Antibiotics: There are no special indications for antibiotics in allergic disorders. In most instances viral infections precipitate respiratory problems such as asthma.

I. Cromolyn Sodium (Intal, Nasalcrom, and Opticrom): Cromolyn sodium is a topically active agent useful in treatment of asthma, allergic rhinitis, and conjunctivitis. In asthma it is effective particularly as a preventive when used 15–20 minutes prior to contact with an asthmogenic agent such as an allergen or exercise. It can be used alone or in conjunction with adrenergic or other agents. If used routinely on a long-term basis, it is best given 3–4 times a day, although twice a day usage may be effective. It is a relatively safe and nonirritating drug.

PROPYHLAXIS OF ATOPIC ALLERGIC DISORDERS

There is evidence that avoidance of certain foods in the first few months of life, specifically cow products, eggs, wheat, and chicken, with or without concomitant dust and animal control, can lessen development of food sensitivity, allergic rhinitis, asthma, or eczema at least in the first year or so of life. Although some studies show no benefit from these procedures, it seems prudent to institute dietary and environmental restrictions in the first few months of life in children with a strong family history of atopy.

MEDICAL EMERGENCIES DUE TO ALLERGIC REACTIONS

Anaphylactic shock, angioedema particularly of the airway, and bronchial obstruction, alone or in combination, are the principal life-threatening manifestations of severe allergic reactions. Sweating, flushing, palpitations, lightheadedness, paresthesias, and urticaria may precede or accompany severe reactions.

Treatment

A. Immediate:

1. Epinephrine, aqueous, 1/1000, 0.2–0.4 mL should be injected intramuscularly without delay, and may be repeated at intervals of 15–20 minutes as necessary. If the reaction is due to the injection of a drug, serum, or sting on an extremity, a tourniquet should be applied proximal to the site to delay absorption and 0.1 mL of adrenaline injected into the site to delay absorption.

2. Antihistamines should be given intramuscularly, or **slowly** intravenously. An H_1 antihistamine such as diphenhydramine should be used initially; the addition of an H_2 antihistamine (eg, cimetidine) is recommended.

3. An asthmatic component should be treated with aminophylline and inhaled adrenergics, with other treatment appropriate for asthma as indicated.

4. Tracheostomy can be life-saving in cases of profound laryngeal edema.

5. Hypovolemia secondary to massive transudation of intravascular fluid can be a part of the reaction; maintenance of proper fluid volume by IV replacement may be necessary.

B. Subsequent Measures: Adrenocorticosteroids should be given only after epinephrine and antihistamines have been administered. The patient should be watched for 24 hours since a recurrence (''delayed anaphylaxis'') can occur many hours after the initial reaction and treatment.

Insect Sting Sensitivity

Life-threatening insect allergy is due mostly to the venom of stinging insects of the class Hymenoptera (bees, wasps, hornets, and fire ants). Venom immunotherapy in children is reserved mainly for those instances in which a life-threatening reaction—for example, involving the cardiovascular or respiratory tract—has occurred. A large local reaction or generalized urticaria without respiratory or cardiovascular compromise probably is not an indication for hyposensitization. Venom antigens for diagnosis and treatment are more efficacious than whole-body extracts. Treatment kits for anaphylactic reactions (ANA-KIT) or spring-loaded epinephrine injectables (Epi-Pen or Epi-Pen, Jr.) should be made available for immediate use for children with extreme insect sensitivity and should be kept in the home or taken along by a responsible person in times of travel. The single most important item in such a kit is epinephrine.

ALLERGIC RHINITIS

Major symptoms include chronic or recurrent nasal congestion generally with nasal itching and sneezing, with serous to mucoid discharge. Itching of the eyes with or without tearing also occurs, particularly in the seasonal or episodic variety. The appearance of the nasal mucosa can vary from somewhat hyperemic to very edematous with purplish pallor. Rhinitis may be perennial owing to exposure to perennially present allergens, seasonal owing to pollens or seasonal molds, episodic owing to occasional encounter with allergens such as animals, or any combination of these. The disease can occur even in infancy, but becomes more frequent and intense with age due to increased exposure to environmental allergens. "Allergic facies" can include allergic shiners, suborbital edema that takes on a bluish discoloration secondary to nasal congestion, flattened malar eminences, and a transverse crease across the nose from pushing the nose upward in an attempt to relieve nasal itching ("allergic salute"). Differential diagnosis includes chronic sinusitis and nonallergic, noninfectious (so-called "vasomotor") rhinitis. Other conditions to be considered in chronic nasal "congestion" include adenoid hypertrophy, foreign bodies (usually unilateral), choanal stenosis or atresia, nasopharyngeal neoplasms, and palatal malformations. Helpful laboratory findings include nasal eosinophilia; this is not a universal finding, however, nor does its presence establish an allergic etiology. Allergy tests reveal IgE antibody to offending allergens.

Associated Conditions

Allergic rhinitis is a risk factor for chronic or recurrent otitis media with effusion. Nasal polyps are unusual in children and even though they often contain eosinophils, generally they are not caused by allergy. They can be associated with cystic fibrosis. Sinusitis may accompany allergic rhinitis.

Treatment

Known or suspected allergens need to be avoided. When symptoms are severe or other symptomatic measures have failed, or when associated with complications, immunotherapy should be considered.

A. Drug Therapy: Table 30–1 lists various drugs useful in treating rhinitis and the symptoms and signs most relieved by each. Chronic rhinitis is more of a congestive problem, whereas acute or seasonal rhinitis tends to involve more itching, sneezing, and rhinorrhea. Antihistamines, with or without decongestants, and nasal and ocular cromolyn are first-line drugs, whereas topical corticosteroids are reserved for more resistant cases.

BRONCHIAL ASTHMA

Asthma is an obstructive disorder of the tracheal bronchial tree, in which the obstruction is variable and largely reversible. The major symptoms of asthma are cough and wheezing, a high-pitched squeaky sound from the partially obstructed large airways, shortness of breath, and chest tightness. **Wheezing is not an invariable symptom or sign;** asthma may present with chronic cough ("cough variant asthma"). Obstruction is due to mucosal edema, bronchospasm, increased and unusually viscid secretions, and chronic inflammation of mucosal walls often with sloughing of epithelium. Asthma is a chronic disorder, the symptoms of which may be only episodic. It can be mild, severe, infrequent, or constant. Because of great pulmonary reserve, obstruction can be profound without causing death, but deaths from asthma do occur. The adolescent age group is at special risk. It is a very common disorder, grossly underdiagnosed; its severity often is underestimated and generally undertreated, and it may be diagnosed as recurrent bronchitis or pneumonia. A large proportion of childhood asthma begins before age 3. Approximately twice as many males are affected as females before adolescence, after which there is not a major difference between the sexes.

Table 30–1. Drugs useful in treating rhinitis.

	Decongestant	Antihistamine	Cromolyn	Anticholinergic	Steroid
Sneezing	(x)	x	(x)		x
Itching	(x)	x	(x)		x
Rhinorrhea	(x)	(x)	(x)	x	x
Congestion	x	±			x

Most children with asthma eventually demonstrate evidence of allergy, which can play a minor to major role in asthma. Especially early in life viral respiratory infection is a frequent precipitating event; precipitants most often are multifactorial and can include irritants, exercise, some medications (aspirin infrequently), and sometimes emotional factors (mainly indirectly, through maladaptive behaviors with asthma). Asthma can occur alone or with allergic rhinitis and/or atopic dermatitis. Inhalants are most important in causing symptoms, but occasionally foods, especially early in life, may be causative. The prognosis of asthma is variable; the likelihood that asthma will be "outgrown" increases with the milder form of the disorder **but probably no more than half of even milder asthmatics outgrow the disorder.** Moderate or severe asthma generally is not outgrown. If symptoms *are* lost, the most common time is around puberty.

An important feature of at least chronic symptomatic asthma is an extraordinary generalized hyperreactivity of the tracheobronchial tree to various chemical inflammatory mediators and in turn to numerous insulting environmental agents or events. Because of this feature, asthma sometimes is called "reactive airways disorder." Reactions to allergens and irritants may be immediate, occurring within minutes of exposure, but with sufficient sensitization and strong allergen exposure, a second kind of reaction occurs 4–12 hours after allergen exposure and can be prolonged. There is a large inflammatory component to chronic asthma. Beta-2 adrenergic drugs, and cromolyn as a preventive, are most effective for immediate responses, whereas corticosteroids and cromolyn are the most effective for late inflammatory responses. Signs and symptoms of asthma are only a crude reflection of the obstructive process, and in many patients, neither the child's nor the physician's assessment of the asthma are very accurate. *The most accurate indicator of the degree of obstruction is measurement of airflow with a pulmonary function device.* A reliable simple peak flowmeter such as a Wright Peak Flow Meter, *used properly* (by patient and medical personnel), is important to the diagnosis and treatment of children with asthma.

In infancy, predominant symptoms may be dyspnea, excessive secretions, noisy and rattly breathing, cough, and intercostal or suprasternal retractions rather than the typical pronounced expiratory wheezes that occur in older children. Physical findings depend upon the degree of obstruction. Between episodes, findings can be normal. With progressive obstruction, air exchange diminishes, expiration becomes prolonged, and wheezing generally occurs and increases in intensity; with greater obstruction, wheezing will decrease due to poor air exchange, hyperinflation may be apparent, and in later stages retractions and use of accessory respiratory muscles increases. Pulsus paradoxicus may be present. There may be pallor; **cyanosis is a very late sign.** Tachycardia may occur and ultimately there can be respiratory failure. The hallmark of asthma is responsiveness to bronchodilators, both a therapeutic and diagnostic point. In the later stages of an asthmatic paroxysm or simply with severe asthma, response to bronchodilators is poor, a condition sometimes called "status asthmaticus."

Eosinophil accumulations in bronchial secretions and blood are common. The hematocrit can be elevated with dehydration or in severe chronic obstructive disease. In severe asthma, the first blood gas abnormality is hypoxemia without CO_2 retention. Since hyperpnea is usual in an attack, $Paco_2$ tends to be low with the hypoxemia so that "normal" Pco_2 in an attack should be taken as CO_2 retention. Particularly in young children, some metabolic acidosis is not unusual. Early in asthmatic paroxysms, the pH tends to be alkaline from hyperventilation. If obstruction is severe, there can be CO_2 retention with a respiratory acidosis, often with a metabolic component. X-ray may show bilateral hyperinflation, bronchial thickening, peribronchial infiltration, and areas of density that may represent patchy atelectasis (common) or associated bronchopneumonia. The former is often confused as the latter. In uncomplicated asthma, a chest x-ray is not always necessary. Lung functions reveal a decrease in flow rates, particularly FEV_1. There is hyperinflation of the chest with increased residual volume and functional residual capacity. During asymptomatic intervals, all of the above may be normal, but there frequently is residual hyperinflation on a chronic basis even in asthmatic children asymptomatic for prolonged periods. Allergy tests may reveal IgE antibodies to potentially causative allergens.

Bronchial asthma may be confused with acute bronchiolitis, laryngotracheobronchitis, bronchopneumonia, or pertussis, especially in the very young. Some children with immunodeficiency disease, particularly in the first 3 years of life, have associated cough and wheezing due to chronic lower respiratory tract infection. Nasal wheezes can be transmitted to the chest especially in infants, and other forms of upper airway obstruction such as adenoidal hypertrophy and foreign body may cause wheezing sounds. The predominant wheeze from lower airway obstruction is expiratory, although inspiratory wheezing along with expiratory wheezing can occur. Wheezing that is predominantly inspiratory more often than not is laryngeal or higher in origin. In tracheal or bronchial foreign body obstruction, dyspnea and wheezing is usually of sudden onset and often uni-lateral, although it may be bilateral. Characteristic x-ray findings are not always present. The differentiation between bronchial asthma and cystic fibrosis is made on the basis of high sweat chloride in the latter, and a history often present in cystic fibrosis of serious pulmonary infections since birth, along with a personal and family history of associated intestinal disturbances with pro-fuse, bulky stools and pancreatic enzyme deficiency. In asthma, chronic inflammatory changes generally are not seen on chest x-ray, in contrast to that seen in cystic fibrosis and other chronic infectious lower pulmonary disorders. Cystic fibrosis and asthma can and frequently do coexist. Tracheal or bronchial compres-sion by extramural forces may be due to the presence of a foreign body in the esophagus, anomalous vessels, or neoplastic of in-flammatory lymphadenopathy.

Treatment

A. General: Identify and avoid known or suspected aller-gens and irritants!

Hyposensitization should be considered for allergens that cannot be avoided and that play a substantial role in the disorder. Educate the parents and the child, if old enough, to understand asthma, the importance of avoidance or other therapy, and the proper use of medications. The major pharmacotherapeutic agents are bronchodilators of the adrenergic and methylxanthine (theophylline or aminophylline) classes, preventives (cromolyn sodium), and anti-inflammatory drugs (corticosteroids).

Adrenergic aerosols are extremely useful but must not be abused. Overreliance on these drugs can lead to delays in obtain-ing other therapy needed. Adrenergic inhalants can be as effec-tive as injected drugs in reversing acute severe asthma and is attended with fewer side effects. Cromolyn sodium is used on an around-the-clock basis 3–4 times daily for chronic symptoms, or acutely to prevent asthmatic insults from allergenic or irritant agents, or before exercise; it is used alone or in conjunction with inhaled adrenergic drugs. Encourage exercise in children with asthma, as in all children. The use of a peak flowmeter at home to assist in assessment of airflow can be useful and even lifesaving. Children with frequent overt asthma attacks (eg, 1 or 2 per week other than from exercise alone) and evidence of more-or-less constant pulmonary obstruction should be on constant pharma-cologic therapy.

Cromolyn sodium or theophylline can be considered first-line drugs for chronic symptomatic asthma. Adrenergic drugs by inhalation, with or without additional oral adrenergic agents, are adjuncts. In patients who do not require constant bronchodilator therapy, adrenergic agents by inhalation are first-line drugs. Systemic corticosteroids are used acutely (days) for the treatment of acute severe asthma not responsive to nonsteroidal bronchodilators; they also are employed chronically (weeks to months) and occasionally even longer, mainly on an alternate-day early morning dosage regimen when all other measures are not sufficient to keep the asthma under control. Inhalant corticosteroids are used in addition or in place of theophylline and cromolyn for long-term therapy, and as a substitute for long-term alternate-day systemic steroid therapy.

TREATMENT OF ACUTE SEVERE ASTHMA
(Status Asthmaticus)

This is a medical emergency and requires prompt and aggressive treatment. Injectable adrenergic agents, or if the child is sufficiently cooperative, aerosolized adrenergic drugs given by a compressed air device or preferably by oxygen are the drugs of first choice (see Table 30–2). Sensitivity to adrenergic drugs may improve after initiation of other therapy, particularly corticosteroids, and responsiveness may occur even as early as 1–2 hours after their administration.

Hospital or Emergency Room Care

(1) Give moisturized oxygen by face mask or nasal prong, at a flow rate of approximately 4 L/min.

(2) Give 5% dextrose solution with 0.2% saline IV with poor responsiveness to initial therapy, poor fluid intake, vomiting, or dehydration. *Do not overhydrate.* Particularly if corticosteroids are used, add potassium (approximately 10–20 mEq/L of intravenous fluids) after urination is established.

(3) Give aminophylline, 4–6 g/kg in intravenous tubing over a 10–20 minute period if not used in the previous 3 hours, and either repeat in 4–6 hours or give as a constant infusion using a rate of 0.6–1 mg/kg/hr. The rate should be determined, however, by measurement of theophylline blood levels, aiming for a level of $15 \pm 3\ \mu g/mL$ on a constant basis. Average total daily dosages of theophylline to achieve levels between 10–20 $\mu g/mL$ are listed below, but there is much individual variation in requirements. Also, viral infections, diet, and medications can alter metabolism (eg, erythromycin impedes metabolism).

Table 30–2. Adrenergic drugs.

Drug	Route*	Dose	Frequency
Terbutaline mg/mL (1:1000)	SC	0.01 mg/kg up to 0.30 mL	q 20 min × 2
Epinephrine aqueous 1:1000	SC	0.01 mg/kg up to 0.30 mL	q 20 min × 3
Epinephrine suspension 1:200 (Sus-Phrine)	SC	0.005 mL/kg up to 0.15 mL	single dose
Albuterol 0.5%†	NA	0.25–0.5 mL in 2 mL saline	q 30 min
Metaproterenol 5%†	NA	0.10–0.20 mL in 2 mL saline	q 30 min
Isoetharine 1%†	NA	0.25–0.50 mL in 2 mL saline	q 30 min
Terbutaline 0.1%†	NA	1 mL in 2 mL saline	q 30 min

*SC = subcutaneous; NA = nebulized aerosol.
†Each of these is also available as a metered dose inhaler and can be used, 2 inhalations per dose. For mild to moderate asthma, use every 4 hours.

Age	Average Total Daily Dose ± SD
1–8 yr	25 ± 5 mg/kg
8–16 yr	20 ± 5 mg/kg
>16 yr	12 ± 3 mg/kg

(4) Take an arterial blood sample for pH, Pco_2, and Po_2, or use oximetry for Po_2 determination (but this does *not* tell you the $Paco_2$). Repeated monitoring of gases and pH may be necessary.

(5) Correct acidosis of pH of ≤ 7.3 with sodium bicarbonate. The appropriate bicarbonate dose can be calculated with the following formula:

$$\text{mEq bicarbonate needed} = \text{negative base excess} \times 0.3 \times \text{body weight in kg}$$

(6) Give albuterol 0.5% by inhalation every 20 minutes to 1 hour until there is a response. Interval can be extended to every 4 hours as tolerated.

(7) If the patient is already receiving corticosteroids, increase the dose temporarily. Patients requiring hospitalization or who have severe asthma not responsive to other therapy within the first 2 hours should receive corticosteroids promptly. Give the equivalent of 2 mg/kg of prednisone every 4–6 hours until a therapeutic response is obtained, following which taper the dosage as rapidly as possible over a 3–7-day period.

(8) Give antibiotics if specifically indicated.

(9) Consider intravenous isoproterenol therapy in younger children with respiratory failure unresponsive to the above therapy. This is not recommended for older adolescents or adults, however, because of the increased risk of inducing cardiac arrest in these age groups. Such an infusion should be undertaken in an intensive care unit where continuous cardiac and blood pressure monitoring facilities are available. Alternatively, mechanical ventilation using a volume respirator capable of producing high expiratory pressures can be used, by personnel expert in such use. Failure to respond adequately to the previously defined measures can be considered as 2 arterial $Paco_2$ determinations above 45 mm Hg over a 15–30 minute period.

(10) Obtain a chest x-ray if there is a question of pneumothorax, massive atelectasis, or other *significant* intrathoracic complication.

Do Not's

(1) Do not use narcotics or barbiturates (they depress the respiratory center).

(2) Do not use epinephrine excessively; inhaled beta-2 adrenergic agents are preferred.

(3) Do not treat acute severe paroxysm as purely an acute problem. Follow-up therapy including eventually adequate fluid intake with shifting from IV to oral medications and the continued use of pharmacotherapy out of hospital is important until pulmonary functions reverse to essential normality. Treatment in hospital generally is not required for more than 2 or 3 days for acute severe asthmatic paroxysms but aggressive therapy on an outpatient basis must be continued for many days thereafter.

ATOPIC DERMATITIS
(Infantile Eczema)

This ordinarily begins in early infancy after age 2 months. It is a condition of itchy skin in which the threshold for itching is abnormally low, and it usually is associated with skin dryness and sometimes ichthyosis. The majority of children exhibit evidence of IgE antibody to a variety of allergens, but the role of IgE antibody in the disease process often is unclear. Food allergens by ingestion, and inhalant allergens (mites, pollens, molds, animal allergens) particularly by direct contact can play an important role in some children. Foods most often implicated are milk, egg white, peanuts, and, to a lesser extent, peas, wheat, pork, beef, and corn.

Lesions generally begin as erythematous papules, sometimes secondary to scratching, which can result in variable degrees of scaling, vesicular oozing lesions, and, in the more chronic forms, lichenification. In infants, there is predilection for the cheeks and extensor areas; in older children and adolescents, the flexural creases are most commonly affected. Pruritus is characteristic and frequently intense. Scratching plays a major role in the pathogenesis and predisposes to secondary infection. Skin dryness, sweating, and contact with rough materials and detergents all can aggravate itching. Psychologic factors also can intensify itching.

Differential Diagnosis

Seborrheic dermatitis, contact dermatitis, and scabies with a secondary eczematoid reaction may be confused with atopic dermatitis. Disorders in which skin eruptions can resemble atopic dermatitis include Wiscott-Aldrich syndrome, x-linked agammaglobulinemia, ataxia-telangiectasia, phenylketonuria, severe combined immunodeficiency, Hurler's and Hartnup syndromes, and ahistidinemia. Although this disorder may be lost by age 3, it persists into later childhood and adulthood more often than is generally appreciated. Various immune abnormalities have been identified but there are no laboratory findings that are pathognomonic. IgE antibody is found in approximately 80% of patients and IgE immunoglobulin levels are elevated in many cases as well. Secondary bacterial infections, especially with staphylococci and streptococci, occur frequently. Viral infections, mainly with herpes virus, may produce extensive viral lesions (Kaposi's varicelliform eruption).

Treatment

Good skin care, vigorous specific skin treatment, and identification and elimination of any allergens or irritants that may aggravate the disease are the mainstays of treatment. Hyposensitization is of uncertain value.

Adequate hydration is important, particularly in dry climates. There are basically two approaches, "wet" and "dry." The dry approach (Scholtz regimen) avoids bathing with water completely; instead, Cetaphil Lotion is applied liberally as a cleansing agent and wiped from the skin after foaming, leaving a thin film of lotion on the skin. In drier climates, daily baths without soap or with the occasional use of mild soaps (eg, Dove, Basis, Nutragena) are used to hydrate the skin, and the skin then is patted partly dry and covered with a bland cream or one that contains hydrocortisone if there is active inflammation. Topical corticosteroids are the mainstay of control of inflammation by both methods. A strong (eg, fluorinated) corticosteroid is used 2–3 times a day initially to control intense inflammation, but with more chronic use, the weakest corticosteroid needed is used. This generally is 1% hydrocortisone in a variety of available bases.

For acute severe dermatitis with weeping, Burow's solution (aluminum subacetate) soaks made up to $\frac{1}{20}$ solution is used for 20 minutes at a time, with gauze or cloth thoroughly moistened with solution applied 4 times a day or more for up to 3 days. Systemic antibiotics are used for secondary infections. Antihistamines can be used as antipruritic agents, but are of secondary effectiveness in controlling pruritus compared with topical corticosteroids. The use of potent topical corticosteroids frequently and extensively over inflamed skin can lead to significant systemic absorption. There is a high likelihood that a child with atopic dermatitis will develop allergic rhinitis, asthma, or both.

ADVERSE REACTIONS TO FOODS

Serious allergic reactions to foods include anaphylaxis, hives, angioedema of the upper airway, and severe asthma; however, a wide variety of signs and symptoms can be encountered. The more severe the reaction, the faster it is likely to occur; the majority of severe reactions occur within minutes to a couple of hours after ingestion of the food. Many (and probably most) reactions to foods, however, are caused by nonallergic mechanisms and include pharmacologic or metabolic, toxic, or idiosyncratic reactions. Reactions occur most frequently in infancy. Evidence of IgE antibody to a food allergen can be obtained by skin prick testing (intradermal tests are too nonspecific), serologic tests, or both. The apparent presence of IgE antibody does not in itself establish the diagnosis, nor does the apparent absence rule it out. A reaction may depend upon the amount of food ingested, rate of absorption, and other concurrent factors such as the presence of an enteric infection, which alters the intestinal permeability.

Good evidence for a reaction to a suspected food is improvement of symptoms on avoidance of the food (elimination diet), and aggravation of symptoms on adding back the food (challenge). Food challenges should never be done, however, in cases of life-threatening sensitivity.

Syndromes sometimes associated with food sensitivity include angioedema and urticaria; anaphylaxis; gastrointestinal intolerance; and allergic rhinitis, asthma, and eczema (see previous sections). In addition, "tension-fatigue syndrome"—a syndrome of symptoms ranging from irritability, disturbed behavior, sleeplessness, fatigue, lassitude, and disinterest, associated with allergic shiners, sometimes with headache and vague abdominal complaints—has been blamed on food allergy. When it occurs, however, it is not clear that allergic mechanisms are involved. There are numerous claims that various foodstuffs including sugar, food dyes, various specific foods, and natural salicylates in foods, can produce hyperactivity or other behavioral changes in children with attention deficit disorder. If these substances do contribute, it would appear to occur in an extremely small subpopulation of children. Various foods contain vasoactive material that can intensify vascular (migraine) headaches on a nonallergic basis; the most common foods implicated are chocolate, cheeses, liver, and some wines and beers. Allergic reactions to foods also may intensify vascular headaches. Eosinophilic enterocolitis, pulmonary hemosiderosis related to milk sensitivity, and villous atrophy with malabsorption also can be caused by foods. The diagnosis is based upon a suspicion that a particular food may be causing a problem, elimination of the food and then challenge to determine whether symptoms abate and then reappear. Children tend to have sensitivity only to one food at a time, occasionally two; multiple food allergies is rarely documented. A high level of IgE antibody to a food is more likely to be of clinical significance than a low level. The most common allergens implicated in young children are milk, peanut, egg, soy, and wheat. In older children, shellfish, fish, and nuts also are involved with some frequency.

Other disorders from which "food allergy" should be differentiated include those producing gastrointestinal intolerance—carbohydrate enzyme deficiency (eg, lactase), irritable bowel syndrome, gastrointestinal malformations, acute or chronic intestinal infections, celiac disease, pyloric stenosis, and cystic fibrosis.

Treatment

Treatment is based primarily on avoiding the food, although in less sensitive children, small amounts can be tolerable. *It is important to ensure nutritional adequacy when eliminating foods from the diet.* Food allergies can be outgrown—most likely to milk and soy—but when severe allergy exists, especially to peanuts, other nuts, fish, and shellfish, it is not likely. Loss of sensitivity to eggs is highly variable. In children with potential life-threatening sensitivity, an emergency medical kit with epinephrine should be available for use by the older child or a responsible adult.

DRUG SENSITIVITY

Reactions to drugs can be due to toxicity; an idiosyncratic or peculiar response to the usual action of the drug; anaphylactoid (pseudoallergic), in which the mediators associated with allergic reactants occur by nonallergic mechanisms (eg, some reactions to radio contrast dyes); or allergic, in which IgE and perhaps other immune reactions play an important role. Manifestations of drug allergy are extremely varied. Most commonly, skin eruptions occur. A prolonged syndrome of serum sickness, previously due mostly to foreign serum, can occur particularly with penicillins and sulfonamides. Some drugs given in repository forms or by mouth may linger in the body for weeks and continue to induce symptoms during this period of time. Any drug is a potential sensitizer, but the penicillins and sulfonamides are at the top of the list. Sulfonamides and tetracyclines can be photo-sensitizing.

It is often difficult to know whether a rash that develops when a drug is administered is in fact due to the agent. In many instances, the eruption is unrelated, and there is no drug sensitivity. Unfortunately, diagnostic tests for drugs are highly imperfect and particularly with antibiotics it usually is wisest to make a tentative presumption of drug sensitivity and substitute a structurally different drug. In most instances, drug reactions are due to sensitivity to by-products of the drug, and in only a few instances have these been identified. Penicillin is the best studied—reagents available for testing are useful, but tests are not foolproof.

Treatment

Treatment consists of discontinuing the drug and supportive therapy depending upon the symptoms involved (see other sections). Pretreatment with antihistamines and corticosteroids in cases in which contrast dyes that previously induced reactions must be used has been successful but *is not foolproof*. Reactions to such dyes generally are "pseudoallergic" and tests of the dye, including use of small test doses, are not accurate or advised.

URTICARIA

Urticaria, or "hives," are multiple, although occasionally single, pruritic erythematous wheals of varying sizes, consisting of localized edema and surrounding erythema. Hives can be allergic or nonallergic. Emotional tension may aggravate hives but rarely is the only cause. Angioedema, essentially urticaria of the deeper skin, results in more diffuse edema, and resolves more slowly than hives. It is a problem mainly if it affects the respiratory tract. The most common classes of allergens inducing urticaria are foods and medications. **"Physical" urticarias** include a cold-induced form in which exposure to cold air, cold water, or other cold objects induces localize urticaria or angioedema. In severe forms, death from sudden massive mediator release can occur—for example, from swimming in cold water. **"Cholinergic" urticaria** is a form relating to overheating, characterized by intense itching and small wheals with much erythema. Exercise or fever are precipitants of this form. There is a form of exercise-anaphylaxis phenomena in which urticaria and angioedema can occur with exercise, to an extent that it may be part of a more generalized anaphylactic syndrome, but generally without pulmonary involvement: it can be life-threatening. **Papular urticaria** is a term given to multiple papules induced by insect bites, found especially on the extremities. Papules secondary to infection from scratching and scabies also occurs. **Dermographism** is a familial or acquired form of "skin sensitivity" in which the threshold of the vascular response to stroking of the skin is lowered. Stroking the skin may produce erythema with or without a wheal; it is not necessarily related to allergy. **Hereditary angioedema** is a rare, nonallergic genetic disorder, characterized by periodic bouts of angioedema that are nonpruritic and can be life-threatening.

Diagnosis depends mainly upon a thorough historical review with implication of possible causative agents, and, if necessary, elimination and challenge. Allergy tests to causative agents can be useful sometimes. Inhalant or contact allergens occasionally can induce hives, the former particularly on a seasonal basis. Treatment consists of avoiding the causative factors and use of H_1 antihistamines such as diphenhydramine or hydroxyzine. With more chronic forms, the addition of an H_2 antihistamine such as cimetidine can be helpful. With severe acute urticaria and angioedema, epinephrine may be necessary. Occasionally, short courses of corticosteroids are necessary.

31 | Collagen Diseases

Elaine Van Gundy, MD

"Collagen diseases" are not limited pathologically to alterations of collagen but also involve changes in the connective tissue, and therefore, they are often called connective tissue diseases. However, although many diseases involve the connective tissue, 7 disorders with similar characteristics can accurately be called collagen diseases: rheumatic fever, rheumatoid arthritis, Lyme disease, polyarteritis (periarteritis) nodosa, systemic lupus erythematosus, scleroderma, and dermatomyositis. The similarities can be summarized as follows: (1) frequently overlapping clinical features, (2) chronicity with relapses, (3) changes in immunologic state, (4) common pathologic features (fibrinoid degeneration, granulomatous reaction with fibrosis, vasculitis with proliferation of plasma cells), and (5) improvement with use of corticosteroids (often only symptomatic).

RHEUMATIC FEVER

Rheumatic fever is the most common cause of symptomatic acquired heart disease in childhood. The incidence of rheumatic fever had been decreasing in the USA and other developed countries until the mid 1980s. Since then, there has been an increase in the incidence of rheumatic fever, with carditis being the dominant feature. It is clear that group A β-hemolytic streptococci are implicated in the etiology of rheumatic fever, but the pathogenetic mechanism remains obscure. This relation to a specific bacterial component sets rheumatic fever apart from the other collagen diseases.

A β-hemolytic streptococcal infection invariably precedes by 1–3 weeks the initial attack and subsequent relapses of rheumatic fever, although not all of these infections are clinically manifest. Since rheumatic heart disease represents a hypersensitivity reaction, it is reasonable to assume that several infections with group A β-hemolytic streptococci are necessary to trigger the first episode of rheumatic fever.

Predisposing Factors

Lower socioeconomic status (overcrowding), a familial predisposition, and reinfection with β-hemolytic streptococci place an individual at increased risk.

Clinical Findings

The diagnosis is usually certain if the child has either (a) 2 major manifestations or (b) one major and 2 minor manifestations (modified after Jones).

A. Major Manifestations:

1. Signs of active carditis.

2. Polyarthritis. Inflammation of the large joints (ankles, knees, hips, wrists, elbows, and shoulders) is usually in a migratory fashion involving one or 2 joints at a time. Occasionally, involvement is monarticular.

3. Subcutaneous nodules.

4. Erythema marginatum.

5. Chorea.

B. Minor Manifestations:

1. Fever and malaise.

2. Arthralgia.

3. Electrocardiographic changes, particularly prolonged PR intervals. Serial electrocardiographic studies may reveal useful information regarding progress. ST or T wave changes are noted if pericarditis is present. Dysrhythmias are usually minor, but occasionally second- or third-degree heart block occurs.

4. Abnormal blood test results. The sedimentation rate is greatly accelerated. The white blood cell count is raised, showing a variable polymorphonuclear leukocytosis. Levels of C-reactive protein and gamma globulin are elevated. Streptococcal antibody (antistreptolysin [ASO] or streptozyme) titers are elevated. A mild or moderate degree of anemia (normochromic or normocytic) is found.

5. Presence of β-hemolytic streptococci. Organisms are often present and can be isolated from the upper respiratory tract of the child or family contacts.

Associated manifestations include erythema multiforme; abdominal, back, or precordial pain; malaise; dyspnea on exertion; nontraumatic epistaxis; purpura; and pneumonitis with or without acute pleural effusion.

Diagnosis

There is no specific laboratory test for rheumatic fever. Combined use of clinical and laboratory findings may aid in diagnosis and subsequent evaluation of the degree of rheumatic activity. Echocardiography is helpful in diagnosis by showing that the posterior mitral valve leaflet thickens and separates from the anterior leaflet.

Treatment

A. Specific Measures:

1. Corticosteroids–Corticosteroids should be administered for management of acute-onset congestive heart failure associated with carditis. However, long-term controlled studies show no benefit from corticosteroid therapy in preventing chronic rheumatic heart disease. Thus, corticosteroids are not recommended for patients with carditis who are not in congestive heart failure.

Once initiated, corticosteroid therapy should be continued for about 6 weeks (although some recommend a much shorter course); thereafter, it should be reduced rapidly. To prevent the typical "rebound phenomenon" accompanying weaning, salicylates should be given in full dosage during the last 2 weeks of therapy.

2. Salicylates–The salicylates markedly reduce fever, alleviate joint pain, and reduce joint swelling. The rapid response of rheumatic fever to salicylates is usually quite dramatic and is a useful diagnostic test in differentiation from rheumatoid arthritis, which responds much more slowly. Salicylates should be continued as long as necessary for the relief of symptoms. If the withdrawal of salicylates results in a recurrence, they should immediately be reinstituted. The average dose of aspirin is 80–120 mg/kg/d every 4–6 hours. The highest dosage is recommended for the first 48 hours.

3. Penicillin–Penicillin in full dosage should be used in all cases for 10 days; followed by daily prophylaxis to prevent recurrences (see below). Serious and inapparent infections may occur during corticosteroid therapy but are uncommon in rheumatic fever treated as described.

B. General Measures:

Resumption of full activity should be gradual and related to the severity of the attack, particularly if a significant degree of carditis is present.

Prophylaxis

The main principle of prophylaxis is the prevention of recurrent infection with β-hemolytic streptococci.

A. Penicillin: The unequivocal treatment of choice is benzathine penicillin G, given intramuscularly every 28 days; 1.2 million units is sufficient for school-age children. In day-care settings or other extreme situations of exposure, the interval should be every 21 days. Oral penicillin G, 200,000 units twice daily, is considerably less effective and is a poor second choice. Therapeutic doses of penicillin are recommended before tooth extraction or other surgery if valvular involvement is present.

B. Erythromycin: Use of erythromycin, 125–250 mg/d orally, is of value in children who cannot tolerate penicillin.

Course & Prognosis

The course varies markedly from patient to patient. It may be fulminating, leading to death early in the course of the acute rheumatic episode, or it may be entirely asymptomatic, the diagnosis being made in retrospect on the basis of pathologic findings. Most attacks last 2–3 months. With adequate penicillin prophylaxis, recurrences are virtually eliminated. The prognosis for life largely depends on the intensity of the initial cardiac insult and the prevention of repeated rheumatic recurrences.

RHEUMATOID ARTHRITIS

Rheumatoid arthritis in childhood, commonly known as juvenile rheumatoid arthritis (JRA), is an inflammatory disease of unknown etiology. Although familial clustering of arthritis occurs, no definite genetic pattern exists. It is the most common collagen vascular disease seen in childhood. JRA is also noted to be distinctly different than rheumatoid arthritis in adults. Specifically, JRA usually has its onset in the large joints, may be associated with systemic symptoms, may be associated with iridocyclitis, and has an infrequent occurrence of rheumatoid factor (RF) and rheumatoid nodules.

There are three subgroups of JRA, distinguished by their clinical manifestations, disease course and prognosis, and serologic findings. The three types—systemic, polyarticular, and pauciarticular—are summarized in Table 31–1.

Rheumatoid arthritis should be distinguished from ankylosing spondylitis. Ankylosing spondylitis is 10 times more frequent in males. It is sometimes familial and affects the spine (particularly the sacroiliac joints). Transient and nondeforming peripheral arthritis, usually confined to a few large joints—especially in the lower extremities—occurs in about half of patients; it may occur before back complaints appear. Acute iritis and aortitis are characteristic extra-articular manifestations. Spondylitis has

Table 31–1. Types and clinical presentation of JRA.

Type	Peak age of onset	Sex	Clinical Manifestation
Systemic	no peak	F = M	Fever, rash, hepatosplenomegaly, arthritis, pericarditis, no uveitis
Polyarticular	1–3 yr & 9 yr	F > M	≥ 5 joints, symmetrical, infrequent systemic features, chronic uveitis in 5%
Pauciarticular	1–3 yr	F > M	< 5 joints, asymmetrical, no systemic features, chronic uveitis in 20%

also been associated with psoriasis, inflammatory bowel disease (eg, ulcerative colitis, regional enteritis), and Reiter's syndrome. Autoantibodies are not present, but 90% of affected individuals will carry the HLA-B27 histocompatibility antigen. Treatment with phenylbutazone and indomethacin may be of value.

Clinical Findings

All three type of JRA share the common feature of arthritis but clinically present very differently.

A. Symptoms and Signs:

1. Systemic–This onset accounts for 10% of cases of JRA. It is hallmarked by high spiking fever (usually to 39 °C or higher) once or twice a day, rapidly returning to baseline or even to a subnormal temperature. The fever may be associated with a characteristic evanescent morbilliform rash most commonly found on the trunk and proximal extremities. Arthritis may occur at any time during the course of the disease. Other features include hepatosplenomegaly, pleuritis, pericarditis, and abdominal pain. The children are characteristically quite ill-appearing while febrile but appear surprisingly well the rest of the time.

2. Polyarticular–This onset accounts for 50% of cases of JRA. This subgroup is characterized by arthritis in 5 or more joints. Joint involvement usually consists of symmetrical involvement of fingers, toes, knees, ankles, wrists, hips, and mandibular joints. Cervical spondylitis may be present. Joints are slightly swollen and tender and motion is limited. The finger joints become characteristically spindle-shaped with shiny smooth skin over them. Rheumatoid nodules are infrequent but if they occur are most common in the older female who is RF positive. Systemic features are uncommon. Uveitis occurs in a small percentage of patients (5%), although the patients that are antinuclear antibody (ANA) positive are at increased risk for eye disease.

3. Pauciarticular–This subgroup accounts for 40% of cases of JRA and its onset is characterized by involvement of 4 or fewer joints. The knees and ankles are most commonly involved, and the process is usually asymmetrical. These children do not have any systemic symptoms and appear well. Chronic uveitis is most common in this group (20%), with the majority of patients with uveitis (90%) being ANA positive.

B. Laboratory Findings: Findings include polymorphonuclear leukocytosis and accelerated sedimentation rates, especially in active disease. Moderate anemia is present. HLA-B27 antigen is frequently present in ankylosing spondylitis but is not common in juvenile rheumatoid arthritis. The rheumatoid factor is rarely positive in juvenile rheumatoid arthritis. The ANA is commonly positive in the polyarticular and pauciarticular forms of the disease. Synovial fluid may show an inflammatory reaction. Synovial biopsy demonstrates chronic inflammation, although it is not specific for rheumatoid arthritis.

C. Imaging: Findings in the early phase of disease usually include swelling of periarticular soft structures, synovial effusion, and slight widening of the joint spaces. Accelerated epiphyseal maturation, increase in size of ossification centers, and disproportionate longitudinal bone growth may occur. Later findings include obliteration of the joint space, erosions of bone, and generalized osteoporosis of all bones of the involved areas.

D. Other Findings: Electrocardiographic findings are usually normal unless cardiac involvement is present. Echocardiography often shows pericarditis.

Treatment

A. Specific Measures:

1. Nonsteroidal anti-inflammatory drugs (NSAIDs)–Aspirin is the most satisfactory anti-inflammatory agent. Its recommended anti-inflammatory dose is 80–120 mg/kg/d in divided doses. Levels of 20–30 mg/dL are therapeutic. The response of rheumatoid arthritis to salicylates occurs within 3–4 days and is usually not as dramatic as in rheumatic fever. In patients who cannot tolerate aspirin, use of tolmetin (Tolectin), 20–30 mg/kg/d, Naproxen (Naprosyn) 10–15 mg/kg/d, or other NSAIDs should be tried. Both aspirin and NSAIDs have potential deleterious effects. Some patients receiving aspirin have developed

Reye's syndrome, and renal papillary necrosis has been noted after use of NSAIDs.

2. Gold salts and penicillamine–These are being used with increasing frequency in patients who do not respond to salicylates.

3. Methotrexate–Studies of low-dose (7.5 mg once a week) methotrexate use in adults have established this immunosuppressive agent as the drug of choice in treating rheumatoid arthritis. The dose may be needed to be increased to a maximum of 15 mg/wk before clinical benefit is noted. Use in children should be restricted to those who are corticosteroid-dependent or have failed to respond to treatment with gold salts.

4. Corticosteroids–Since corticosteroids do not alter the natural remission rate, the length of the illness, or the ultimate prognosis, they are seldom indicated. However, there is a place for them (eg, prednisone, 1–2 mg/kg/d) in cases of myocarditis and in any case where the disease appears to be life-threatening. They are used topically for the treatment of uveitis and systemically in low doses (5–10 mg/d) if the uveitis is unresponsive to topical therapy. Low-dose therapy is also used in patients with severe debilitating morning stiffness, and those beginning on slow-acting anti-inflammatory drugs. Intra-articular corticosteroids have a place in the management of JRA when there is a monarticular involvement or when one or 2 joints appear to retard rehabilitation.

B. General Measures:

1. Physical therapy–The overall goal is to prevent deformities and maintain muscle strength and function. The type of therapy prescribed depends on the disease activity. Acutely inflamed joints should not be subjected to weight-bearing exercise, but range-of-motion exercises should be prescribed. Later, stretching and strengthening should be added. Heat and hydrotherapy may be a useful adjunct to a well-planned exercise program.

2. Orthopedic care–The wearing of splints during the night will ensure proper alignment of joints. Cylinder casts are to be avoided.

3. Ophthalmic care–Periodic slit lamp examination is the only means for early diagnosis of iridocyclitis, which may otherwise continue undiagnosed until vision fails.

4. Rest–As fatigue is a frequent symptom, periods of rest should be alternated with periods of activity. However, complete bed rest should be discouraged, since it can lead to osteoporosis, renal calculi, muscle atrophy, or joint deformities.

5. Psychologic care–In view of the long duration of this disease, the family should understand the necessity of fulfilling the patient's social, educational, and psychologic needs.

6. Diet–There is no special diet. Ferrous sulfate should be given if iron deficiency is present.

Course & Prognosis

Rheumatoid arthritis is a chronic disease with waxing and waning of inflammatory activity. The systemic features (fever, rash, pericarditis, etc) remit more often than the joint manifestations. It has been reported that reactivation of the disease is occasionally associated with group A β-hemolytic streptococcal or viral infection.

With good medical management, one can expect that more than 70% of patients will have complete functional recovery and less than 10% will be severely disabled. Deaths are reported in the pediatric age group, but they are rare.

LYME DISEASE
(Lyme Arthritis)

Lyme disease is a form of arthritis that is often chronic. The first case was reported in Connecticut in 1975, and is known to be due to a spirochete transmitted by a tick (*Ixodes dammini*).

The onset is usually in summer and is commonly characterized by influenzalike symptoms (fever, malaise, headache, stiff neck). A target-shaped skin rash (erythema chronicum migrans) develops and may be confused with ringworm. Progressive disease often involves the heart (myocarditis, AV block), the nervous system (aseptic meningitis, neuropathies), and the joints (arthritis). All these symptoms can recur, and the arthritis can be chronic.

The treatment is by use of either penicillin or tetracycline, and early treatment may avoid later complications.

POLYARTERITIS NODOSA

Polyarteritis (periarteritis) nodosa is a rare systemic disease characterized by inflammatory damage to blood vessels, with resulting injury to involved organs. Pathologically, there is segmental inflammation of small- and medium-sized arteries, with fibrinoid changes and (more rarely) necrosis in the vessel wall. Mucocutaneous lymph node syndrome (Kawasaki disease) and infantile polyarteritis nodosa bear many pathologic similarities to polyarteritis nodosa.

Clinical Findings

Clinical manifestations vary, depending on the location of the involved arterioles.

A. Symptoms: Symptoms are generally those of a rapidly progressive, wasting disease: fever, lassitude, weight loss, and generalized pains in the extremities or abdomen (or both).

B. Signs: Skin eruptions of the urticarial, purpuric, or macular type occur. Subcutaneous nodules are frequently present along the course of the blood vessels. Involvement of the kidneys, gastrointestinal tract, heart, and nervous system often occur. Features include hypertension, myocardial infarction, seizures, and peripheral neuropathy.

C. Laboratory Findings: Abnormalities reflect the organ involved. These include anemia, with moderate leukocytosis and eosinophilia; accelerated sedimentation rate; proteinuria; intermittent microscopic hematuria and showers of casts; elevated levels of nonprotein nitrogen; sterile blood cultures; and cardiomegaly on x-ray. Muscle, skin, or testicular biopsy may show vasculitis and aid in diagnosis. Hepatitis B surface antigen (HBsAg) has been identified in a small percentage of patients, but its role in disease expression remains unknown.

Treatment

Treatment with corticosteroids usually produces symptomatic improvement and suppressive doses may prolong life, but the response is unpredictable and quite variable.

Prognosis

Prognosis is poor for patients with renal, cardiac, or central nervous system involvement, although spontaneous and corticosteroid-induced remissions are seen.

SYSTEMIC LUPUS ERYTHEMATOSUS

Systemic lupus erythematosus (SLE) is a multisystem progressive disease whose protean symptomatology and relentless course present a diagnostic and therapeutic challenge. Pathologically, immune complex vasculitis, extensive fibrinoid degeneration, and necrosis are found. The disease is 9 times more common in females than in males. In the pediatric population, the disease onset peaks during the adolescent years. The cause is unknown. It is believed that multiple factors (viral, immunologic, and genetic) play a role. A lupuslike syndrome (including positive findings in LE cell preparations and ANA tests) may occur during procainamide or anticonvulsant therapy.

Table 31–2. Clinical manifestations of SLE.

System	Presentation
Cutaneous	Butterfly rash, mucocutaneous ulcers, alopecia, photosensitivity, digital ulcerations, Raynaud's phenomenon.
Cardiac	Pericarditis (most common), endocarditis and myocarditis (less common).
Pulmonary	Pleuritis, basilar pneumonitis.
Gastrointestinal	Abdominal pain, diarrhea, esophageal dysmotility.
Renal	Nephritis, hypertension, uremia, nephrotic syndrome.
Musculoskeletal	Arthralgia, arthritis, myalgia.
Nervous system	Seizures, organic brain syndrome.
Lymphoreticular	Splenomegaly, hepatomegaly, lymphadenopathy.

Clinical Findings

A. Symptoms and Signs: Children often present with fever, rash, arthralgia, and arthritis. Myalgia, fatigue, weakness, and weight loss frequently occur. Table 31–2 summaries typical clinical presentations.

B. Laboratory Findings: Antinuclear antibodies are present in 100% of active cases; the antinuclear antibody test has replaced the LE cell preparation as the most sensitive diagnostic test. Table 31–3 summarizes common laboratory findings.

Diagnosis & Treatment

The diagnosis of SLE is based on clinical findings and presentation, although specific laboratory abnormalities aid in the diagnosis. Consistent features include the episodic nature of the disease, multisystem involvement, and positive ANA.

Nonsteroidal anti-inflammatory drugs should be given for joint symptoms. Prednisone, given in doses of at least 60 mg/

Table 31–3. Laboratory findings in SLE.

Autoantibodies
Anemia
Thrombocytopenia
Hypocomplementemia
Leukopenia
Hematuria, proteinuria
Elevated ESR
Positive Coombs'
False (+) VDRL

m²/d, not only suppresses the acute inflammatory manifestations but, in many cases, also modifies or halts progressive glomerular involvement. Antibiotics should be used at the first sign of an infection. Chloroquine may be of value for skin and joint symptoms.

The idea that lupus is the classic autoimmune disorder has led to trials with immunosuppressive agents. Both azathioprine (Imuran) and cyclophosphamide (Cytoxan) are effective in controlling renal and systemic manifestations of the disease in some children who are resistant to corticosteroids alone. Recent evidence suggests that long-term survival in cases of lupus nephritis has improved when cytoxan and prednisone are used together.

Intravenous pulse therapy with methylprednisolone sodium succinate (Solu-Medrol) should be tried in critically ill patients.

Because of their well-known photosensitivity, patients should use sunscreens when exposed to the sun.

Course & Prognosis

Renal complications and central nervous system involvement are the most frequent causes of death. With good medical management, the 5-year survival rate increased from 51% at 5 years in 1954 to 71% at 10 years in 1979, and later data are even more encouraging. If at the time of diagnosis the serum creatinine concentration is greater than 3 mg/dL and there is severe proteinuria and severe anemia, survival considerably below the average can be anticipated.

SCLERODERMA

Scleroderma is a collagen disease chiefly involving the skin, but any organ may be involved. In local benign scleroderma (morphea), there is a linear distribution of lesions that first show erythema and edema and subsequently scarring and shrinking. In the progressive generalized form (sclerodactyly), there is more extensive thickening and induration of the skin, followed by contractures. Interstitial and perivascular fibrosis may occur in the viscera.

Trophic ulcers, calcific deposits, and Raynaud's phenomenon are common. Disturbances in esophageal motility lead to dysphagia, and small bowel involvement leads to malabsorption.

There is no specific therapy. Physiotherapy given early may minimize contractures. Corticosteroids are of little value. Phenoxybenzamine (Dibenzyline) has been used to relieve peripheral vasospasm. Bethanechol, cimetidine, and antacids have been used for dysphagia. Colchicine and D-penicillamine therapy have produced inconsistent results.

The prognosis is excellent for patients with local scleroderma but only fair for those with the severe generalized form, in which death may occur within a year. Some deformity may occur with the former and is the rule with the latter. Renal or cardiac involvement implies a poor prognosis.

DERMATOMYOSITIS

Juvenile dermatomyositis is a multisystem inflammatory disease of unknown cause, involving primarily the muscles, skin, and subcutaneous tissues. It may be an autoimmune disorder. The pathologic process can and sometimes does involve the gastrointestinal tract and the central nervous system. Theoretically, since dermatomyositis in childhood appears to be a vascular process leading to arteritis and phlebitis, any organ could be involved. Muscles show segmental or focal necrosis, inflammation, fibrinoid changes in capillaries of blood vessels, and, finally, atrophy.

Clinical Findings

The diagnosis is suggested by the presence of muscle weakness and induration accompanied by dermatitis, but a biopsy of the area most intensely involved may be required to establish the diagnosis conclusively.

A. Symptoms: Symptoms include symmetrical proximal muscle weakness; fever; muscle tenderness and pain; malaise and weight loss; arthralgia and arthritis; dyspnea; and dysphagia.

B. Signs: The pathognomonic rash of this disease is a violaceous (heliotrope) discoloration of the eyelids, an erythematous malar rash, accompanied by edema. Skin lesions can occur elsewhere as well and include urticaria. Erythematous nodules—areas of dark pigmentations and telangiectasia—are frequently seen over the extensor surfaces of the joints. Calcinosis can occur along tendons or ligaments and near the joints. Muscles may be firm and atrophic, with contractures.

C. Laboratory Findings: Elevation of muscle enzymes (SGOT, CPK, aldolase) is a useful laboratory tool. Anemia, increased sedimentation rate, and increased levels of serum globulin may be present. Myopathy on electromyogram, and inflammation on muscle biopsy will aid in the diagnosis.

Treatment

Corticosteroid therapy is indicated in all patients with acute or active disease. Prednisone (1–2 mg/kg/d in divided doses) during the first month after diagnosis is usually required. The nonspecific suppressive effect of corticosteroids on systemic and local inflammatory phenomena is best achieved early in the course of the disease. Treatment should be vigorous and be modulated to produce normal muscle enzymes. The immunosuppressive drugs methotrexate and azathioprine may be of value in life-threatening disease and in children whose disease is not adequately controlled with corticosteroid therapy alone.

Physiotherapy is a very important part of the treatment; the principles outlined in the section on rheumatoid arthritis should be followed.

Course & Prognosis

The clinical course of juvenile dermatomyositis varies considerably. The prognosis is favorable in most cases with early treatment. A small percentage of children will experience a relapsing course. The majority of patients can be returned to functional normality. Calcinosis, contractures, and atrophy produce long-term residua. Intractable muscle weakness, sepsis, and gastrointestinal vasculitis can be responsible for death in a small number of patients. Unlike adults, the juvenile form of this disease is not associated with cancer.

Pediatric Procedures | 32

Nancy Carlson, MD, &
Dale William Steele, BA, MD

RESTRAINT & POSITIONING

The optimal care of children logically includes an understanding of specific procedures often required in diagnosis and management. In most cases of failure to complete a procedure successfully, the fault lies in undue haste in preparing a struggling or crying patient. The physician should therefore become acquainted with various methods of restraining pediatric patients. Before starting any procedure, all items of equipment that may be needed should be set out for immediate use as required.

If drapes cover the child, adequate monitoring of cardiorespiratory function is mandatory. In using total body restraint, be certain that cardiorespiratory function is not impaired. Adequate analgesia and sedation should be considered when appropriate.

Many of the following procedures require the use of an iodine solution; the solution must be carefully washed off to prevent severe burns in neonates.

VENIPUNCTURE

The antecubital and external jugular veins are the safest and most frequently used large vessels for venipuncture and withdrawal of blood. (The femoral vein should be employed only in emergencies.) Smaller vessels in the dorsa of the hands and feet and scalp veins may also be used for withdrawing blood samples. Applying negative pressure with a syringe attached to the needle may cause collapse of these vessels because of their small size. Therefore, for these vessels, a different technique should be employed to obtain blood (see below).

The skin should be cleansed thoroughly with alcohol or an iodine solution. The use of a "butterfly" (21- or 23-gauge) needle will facilitate entry into the vein and subsequent withdrawal of blood.

Antecubital Vein Puncture

After placing a proximal turniquet, palpation of the antecubital vein is often possible even if it is not visible.

External Jugular Vein Puncture

A. Preparation: Wrap the child firmly so that the arms and legs are adequately restrained. The wraps should not extend higher than the shoulder girdle. Place the child on a flat, firm table so that both shoulders are touching the table; the head is rotated fully to one side and extended partly over the end of the table so as to align the vein (Fig 32–1). Adequate immobilization is essential.

B. Technique: Use a 21- or 23-gauge pediatric scalp vein infusion set ("butterfly"; ie, a needle attached to plastic wings and tubing) for withdrawing blood. The child should be crying and the vein distended when entered. Thrust the needle under the skin and apply gentle, constant negative pressure with the syringe as the vein is entered. This will prevent air embolism resulting from air being drawn into the vein when the child inspires. After removing the needle, exert firm pressure over the vein for 3–5 minutes while the child is in a sitting position.

Femoral Vein Puncture

Caution: This is a hazardous procedure, particularly in the neonate, and should be employed only in emergencies. Septic

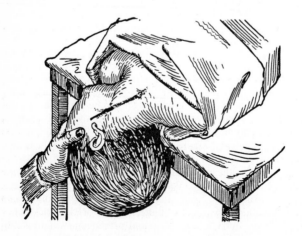

Figure 32–1. External jugular vein puncture.

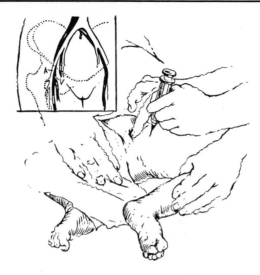

Figure 32–2. Femoral vein puncture.

arthritis of the hip may complicate femoral vein puncture as a result of accidental penetration of the joint capsule. Arteriospasm with serious vascular compromise of the lower extremity may result from hematoma formation. Great care should be exercised in cleansing the skin prior to venipuncture so as to decrease the risk of infection.

A. Preparation: Place the child on a flat, firm table. Abduct the leg so as to expose the inguinal region. Use strict sterile precautions.

B. Technique: Locate the femoral artery by its pulsation. The left femoral vein is preferable because it lies medial to the artery throughout its course (Fig 32–2). Be certain of the position of the femoral pulse at the time of puncture. Insert a short-beveled needle into the vein (perpendicularly to the skin) about 3 cm below the inguinal ligament; use the artery as a guide (see Fig 32–2). If blood does not enter the syringe immediately, withdraw the needle slowly, drawing gently on the barrel of the syringe; the needle sometimes passes through both walls of the vein, and blood is obtained only when the needle is being withdrawn. After removing the needle, exert firm, steady pressure over the vein for 3–5 minutes. If the artery has been entered, check the limb periodically during the next hour. If blanching of the extremity occurs, the application of heat may be of value.

Small Vein Puncture

After cleansing the skin, securely grasp the child's hand or foot in a manner that allows milking of the extremity. Using a 21- or 23-gauge straight needle with a clear hub, pierce the skin and advance the needle until blood flows into the hub. Gently milk the extremity and allow blood to drip into the collection vial. This technique allows sampling from small vessels that would collapse with negative pressure from a syringe.

COLLECTION OF MULTIPLE SPECIMENS OF BLOOD

When a number of blood samples must be obtained over a short period of time (eg, when glucose and electrolyte determinations are needed for a diabetic patient with ketoacidosis), multiple venipunctures may be avoided by employing an indwelling 22-gauge or larger Teflon intravenous catheter. The catheter and stylet are inserted in an arm or hand vein in the usual manner (see below). When the stylet is removed, the catheter hub is attached by means of a male Luer adapter to a heparin lock filled with heparinized saline (2 units/mL). Blood may be withdrawn at intervals by applying a tourniquet to the extremity, inserting a needle attached to a syringe through the sterilely prepared rubber port, and drawing off and discarding a minimum of 3–5 mL. A second needle and syringe are then used to collect the blood specimen. The tourniquet is removed, and the buffalo cap and catheter are subsequently cleared by injecting heparinized saline through the rubber port.

INTRAVENOUS THERAPY

Venous Access

A. Sites: For small infants, a scalp, wrist, hand, foot, or arm vein will usually be most convenient. Any accessible vein may be used in an older child. In an emergency if the vein cannot be entered, fluids may be administered by intraosseous infusion. In children with poor peripheral perfusion, attempts should focus on the antecubital, saphenous, and external jugular veins. The saphenous vein has a predictable course, and cannulation by location alone is often successful.

B. Equipment: For scalp infusions use a 25-gauge butterfly. For peripheral veins in infants use a 24- or 22-gauge Teflon catheter. It is helpful to have a T-connector set-up with a 3-mL syringe of saline available. If an IV is being placed in an extremity, it is best to secure the extremity to a padded board prior to beginning the procedure.

C. Technique:

1. Insertion of the butterfly–First flush the tubing with an isotonic solution. Insert the needle under the skin, and disconnect the syringe from the tubing so that blood return can occur when the needle tip enters the vein. Advance the needle until blood return is noted in the tubing. Holding the needle stationary, remove the tourniquet, reattach the syringe to the tubing, and attempt to flush solution into the vein. Watch carefully for evidence of fluid extravasation. Secure the needle and wings of the butterfly in place. Bolster the wings of the butterfly as needed with cotton to hold the needle at a proper angle. Coil the butterfly tubing and tape away from the needle entry site. Attach intravenous tubing.

2. Insertion of the catheter–The catheter/stylet apparatus consists of an intravenous catheter with removable stylet. Insert the apparatus under the skin, and advance it until blood appears in the catheter hub. Flushing the catheter gently after the initial blood return may facilitate cannulation, especially in infants. Holding the stylet stationary, advance the catheter over the stylet into the vessel. Withdraw the stylet and attach intravenous tubing to the catheter hub. Secure the catheter in place carefully.

D. Precautions: The rate of flow should be checked frequently. An accurate record must be kept of the amount and type of fluid added. For small infants (particularly if premature), a pump system is preferable for careful control of the volume of intravenous fluid infused. Phlebitis usually develops after a few days. Dextrose concentrations greater than 12.5 gm% should not be infused peripherally. Inspect the limb at regular intervals for evidence of undue pressure circulatory embarrassment, or extravasation.

Intraosseous Infusion

Venous access in children is often a challenge. It may be excessively delayed or impossible in children with cardiac arrest or shock. Prolonged attempts to obtain venous access may delay life-saving therapy. However, fluids and drugs that are infused into the medullary space of long bones quickly enter the venous circulation.

A. Sites: The flat medial surface of the proximal tibia is usable up to 5 or 6 years (see technique below). The medial surface of the distal tibia, proximal to the medial malleous, may be used in older children and adults.

B. Equipment: Any large-bore needle may be used. However, a needle with a stylet is preferred to prevent plugging the lumen with bone fragments. Spinal needles are commonly available, but are long and subject to dislodgement. The Kormed/Jamshidi Illinois sternal/iliac needle is somewhat easier to use, and more readily stabilized. Several commercially produced intraosseous needles are similarly useful. In children less than 18 months of age use an 18- to 20-gauge needle. In older children a 13- to 16-gauge needle may be used.

C. Technique: Palpate the tibial tuberosity with the index finger. Grasp the medial aspect of the tibia with the thumb. Insert the needle halfway between these two points 1 to 2 cm distal to the tibial tuberosity. Local anesthetic should be injected into the skin and periosteum before needle placement in the conscious patient. Advance the needle with a twisting motion until a slight decrease in resistance is met. The needle should be inserted pointing slightly away from the joint space in a caudal direction. It should remain firmly in place without support. Avoid advancing the needle through the opposite side of the bone by placing a finger on the needle approximately one cm from the bevel, or by using a preset depth indicator. It may not always be possible to aspirate blood and marrow with a syringe. If so, the needle may be flushed with saline. Minimal resistance to infusion with no evidence of extravasation indicates appropriate placement. Only a single attempt per tibia is possible, as fluid will exit from previous holes in the cortex of the bone. For volume resuscitation, fluid should be injected under pressure by syringe. Gravity may be used to infuse fluid once the patient is hemodynamically stable.

D. Complications: Extravasation occurs commonly around the puncture site, especially with pressure infusion and prolonged placement. Other potential complications are fracture, damage to the epiphyseal plate, and pulmonary fat embolus. Osteomyelitis is rare.

E. Clinical Uses: Intraosseous infusion is used for fluid resuscitation with saline, glucose, and blood. Infusion of various drugs including sodium bicarbonate, atropine, dopamine, isoproterenol, epinephrine, diazepam, antibiotics, phenytoin, pancuronium, and succinylcholine have been reported. The injection of 10 mL of saline solution following drug injection may improve transport of drugs from the marrow cavity. While this route is rapid and relatively safe, continued efforts to obtain venous access should always be made.

Venous Cutdown

Venous cutdown is indicated for small infants and for situations in which a seriously ill older child is in urgent need of fluids and difficulty is encountered in entering a vein. In these cases, expose a vein surgically and, under direct visualization, insert a Teflon catheter with an inner needle stylet.

A. Sites: The saphenous vein running anterior to the medial malleolus of the tibia will be found the most satisfactory. It can be entered at any point along its course. Hence, by starting at the ankle, the same vein can be used 2 or 3 times if necessary.

B. Equipment: A Teflon catheter with inner stylet is easiest to use. A pediatric cutdown tray containing scalpel, hemostats, forceps, and curved clamps should be available.

C. Preparation: Apply a tourniquet. Cleanse the skin and drape the leg as for a surgical procedure, using sterile precautions. The foot can be securely taped to a board splint (Fig 32–3). Make a large wheal with 1 or 2% lidocaine solution (without epinephrine) in the skin over the vein.

D. Technique:

1. Incision–With a scalpel, make an incision just through the skin. The incision should be about 1 cm long and at a right angle to the direction of the vein. Using a fine curved clamp, spread the incision widely, dissecting through the subcutaneous fat in a direction parallel to the vein.

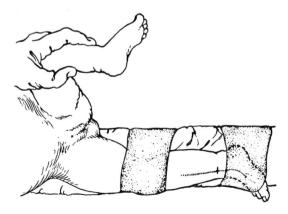

Figure 32–3. Position and taping of leg for venous cutdown.

2. Identification of the vein–Usually, the vein is seen lying on the fascia. Some dissection of subcutaneous fat may be necessary. Insert a curved clamp to the periosteum and bring the vein to the surface (Fig 32–4). Be certain it is a vein, not a nerve or tendon, by noting the flow of blood. Pass 2 silk ties (No. 00) under the isolated vein. Using a hemostat, dissect the vein free for a length of 1–2 cm. Apply gentle traction on proximal and distal ties to maximally expose the vessel. In small infants, the vein is small and fragile; great care must be taken in handling it.

3. Insertion of the catheter–Introduce the catheter with the stylet needle bevel-up. When the needle is in the vessel lumen, hold the stylet stationary and gently advance the catheter. Withdraw the stylet and release tension on the proximal tie so that the catheter may be threaded and blood return ascertained. If there is no blood flow, remove the tourniquet and attempt to inject a small amount of intravenous solution into the vein. Watch for a wheal or extravasation of fluid, indicating that the catheter is not in the vessel. If the catheter flushes easily, remove the proximal and distal ligatures and suture the plastic wings of the catheter hub to the skin. This can most easily be accomplished by placing a skin closure suture on either side of the catheter hub. Tie the suture, and then pass the free ends through holes provided in the wings of the plastic hub. Tie the suture again. This should hold

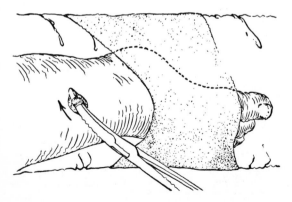

Figure 32–4. Isolation of vein for venous cutdown.

the catheter securely in the vessel. Apply tape across the hub and tubing for further security.

Arterial Access

In a pediatric intensive care unit, intra-arterial access is often necessary to monitor blood pressure and permit frequent arterial blood sampling. Access through a "line" must be carefully monitored by experienced personnel to prevent hemorrhage from the access site. Arterial lines should not be used to administer large amounts of fluid or to give any medications. Patency of the line should be maintained by use of a solution of normal saline to which heparin, 2 units/mL, has been added. The saline solution may be given at a rate of 2–4 mL/h by mechanical pump to ensure continuous infusion.

A. Sites: The radial artery and posterior tibial artery are the most appropriate vessels for cannulation because of the presence of collateral circulation. Use of more proximal arteries is dangerous because of the possibility of vessel thrombosis resulting in distal ischemia. The location of the vessel should be determined by palpating the pulse. The radial artery usually lies just medial to the radial head. The posterior tibial artery can be palpated posterior to the medial malleolus. Use of a transilluminator or doppler device may aid in locating the artery.

B. Equipment: In addition to the equipment used for venous cutdown (see above), a transducer is needed for continuous monitoring of systolic, diastolic, and mean blood pressures.

C. Preparation: Secure the child's limb on a board splint to expose the desired vessel. When using the radial artery, position the wrist in a slightly dorsiflexed position. Cleanse the skin and drape as for a surgical procedure. Make a wheal with 1% lidocaine (without epineprine) in the skin over the artery. (For cannulation under direct visualization, proceed as for venous cutdown.)

D. Technique: Insert a 22-gauge Teflon catheter with the stylet needle bevel-up (no syringe attached) at a 45-degree angle to the skin surface. Advance the stylet until the arterial blood flow is obtained. If blood flow is not obtained pull the catheter back slowly, as it is not uncommon to pierce both walls of the artery. Adjust the position of the needle until blood return is maximal. Holding the stylet stationary, lower the catheter and stylet until they are flush with the skin and then advance the catheter. Remove the stylet and attach intravenous tubing to the hub of the catheter by use of a T-connector. Secure the catheter in place as for venous cutdown.

URINE COLLECTION

Voided Urine

A pediatric urine collector (a plastic bag with a round opening surrounded by an adhesive surface that binds to the skin) may be used.

If a specimen is to be used for culture, catheterization or percutaneous bladder aspiration is advised; these are the most reliable methods that decrease the chances of contamination of the specimen. Voided midstream collections are difficult to obtain from children and are subject to contamination.

Catheterization

A. Equipment: If the procedure is being performed to obtain a single specimen for culture, use an appropriately sized plastic feeding tube (No. 5 French feeding tube for infants). If the catheter is to remain in place for continuous monitoring of urine output, use a Foley catheter with balloon and a closed sterile collection system. Have ready gloves and drapes, iodine solution, urine cup for specimen collection, normal saline solution to inflate the Foley balloon, and lubricant for the catheter; these should all be sterile.

B. Technique: Have adequate personnel available to restrain the patient during the procedure.

1. Female patients–Place the female patient in the frog-leg position to expose the urinary meatus. Separate the labia majora, and prepare and drape the patient as for a surgical procedure. Using sterile gloves, apply lubricant to the end of the catheter and pass the catheter through the urethral opening. Continue to thread the catheter gently until urine flow is obtained. Allow the first aliquot of urine to drain out of the catheter. Collect subsequent urine for culture. If a Foley catheter is used, inflate the balloon with the appropriate volume of normal saline solution (the volume is written on the catheter); inflation is through a one-way valve in the sidearm tubing. Pull back on the catheter to test that the balloon is in the bladder and that the catheter is secured. Tape the tubing to the thigh and attach the sterile collection unit and tubing.

2. Male patients–Hold the male patient's legs in extension. Prepare the glans as for a surgical procedure, retracting the foreskin if present. Proceed as above, taking special care to advance the catheter gently while applying gentle traction on the penis, with the meatus pointed cephalad. If resistance is encountered, retract the catheter slightly, change the angle of entry, and attempt to pass the catheter again.

C. Follow-Up Measures: To prevent phimosis in male patients, remember to return the foreskin to its normal position after catheter insertion.

Suprapubic Percutaneous Bladder Aspiration

Suprapubic percutaneous bladder aspiration is preferable to catheterization when a sterile urine specimen is required for culture and bacterial count.

A. Preparation: The diaper should be dry for at least 45 to 60 minutes. This procedure should not be attempted in patients with abdominal distention, bleeding diathesis, or previous abdominal surgery. Place the patient in a supine position, with the lower extremities held in the frog-leg position. Prepare the skin carefully as for a surgical procedure.

B. Technique: Introduce a 22-gauge, 1.5-in straight needle (attached to a syringe) 1 cm above the pubis, with the needle perpendicular to the skin. With a quick, firm motion, advance the needle while applying gentle traction on the syringe. Stop when urine is aspirated. After urine has been obtained, withdraw the needle with a single, swift motion. If a second attempt is unsuccessful, further attempts are usually futile.

OBTAINING SPINAL FLUID BY LUMBAR PUNCTURE

Lumbar Puncture in Children & Older Infants

The procedure should be deferred in unstable patients, or in those in whom increased intracranial pressure is suspected.

A. Preparation: Have a helper restrain the patient in the flexed lateral position on a firm, flat table. Sterile gloves should be worn. Draw an imaginary line between the 2 iliac crests and use the intervertebral space immediately above or below this line (L3–4 interspace). Prepare the skin surrounding this area as for a surgical procedure, with iodine and alcohol. Drape the area with sterile towels. Infiltrate the skin and subcutaneous tissues with 1–2% lidocaine (not necessary in infants).

B. Technique: Use a short 23-gauge spinal needle for infants; use a long 21-gauge needle for older children. Insert the lumbar puncture needle, with the stylet bevel-up, just below the vertebral spine in the midline (Fig 32–5). Keep the needle perpendicular to both planes of the back or pointing slightly cephalad. A distinct "give" is usually felt when the dura is pierced; if in doubt, remove the stylet to watch for fluid. When fluid is obtained, a 3-way stopcock and manometer may be attached to measure opening pressure (at the beginning of collec-

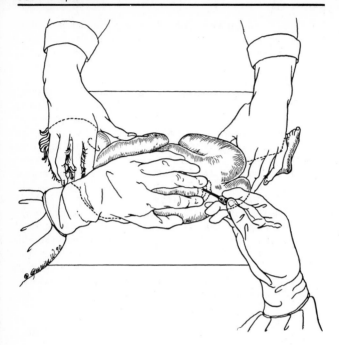

Figure 32-5. Lumbar puncture with assistance of nurse.

tion) and closing pressure (at the end of collection). Cardio-respiratory function should be monitored throughout the procedure.

Lumbar Puncture in Small Infants

For small infants, lumbar puncture may be performed at the level of the superior iliac crests, with the patient in a sitting position and leaning forward. The stylet may be removed after the needle is firmly lodged in the subcutaneous tissues. The needle should then be advanced very slowly while watching the needle hub for cerebrospinal fluid. Cerebrospinal fluid may flow very slowly, and the "give" may not be felt in small infants. Gentle aspiration with a small syringe may be necessary.

BODY CAVITY PUNCTURES

Thoracentesis

Thoracentesis is used to remove pleural fluid or air for diagnosis or treatment.

Caution: Risks include introduction of a new infection; pneumothorax or hemothorax (or both) as a result of tearing of the lung; hemoptysis; syncope (pleuropulmonary reflex or air embolus); and pulmonary edema as a result of too rapid removal of large amounts of fluid. None of these are common if reasonable care is taken.

A. Sites: Locate the fluid or air by physical examination and by x-ray. Ultrasound examination prior to thoracentesis may aid in location of fluid and selection of an optimal site. If entering at the base, locate the bottom of the opposite uninvolved lung as a guide so the puncture will not be below the pleural cavity. Enter the dependent pleural cavity to remove fluid, or enter the superior chest (usually through the second interspace anteriorly, 1–2 cm lateral to the sternum on the right side, or just left of the midclavicular line on the left side when the patient is in a supine position) to relieve pneumothorax.

B. Equipment: For evacuation of a pneumothorax, use a 19- or 21-gauge needle (butterfly) with a 20–60 mL syringe attached to the tubing via a 3-way stopcock. For removal of pleural fluid, use an 18- to 19-gauge Teflon catheter (with inner removable stylet) attached to a 20-mL syringe via a 3-way stopcock. If a large amount of fluid is to be removed, it can be pumped through a rubber tube attached to the sidearm of the stopcock, thereby avoiding leakage of air into the pleural space.

C. Preparation: The patient should sit up, if possible, and lean forward with support. If too ill or too young to sit up, the patient should be held with the involved side (ie, lung with the effusion) in the most dependent position. Prepare skin as for a surgical procedure. Use 1–2% lidocaine to infiltrate the skin and down to the pleura.

D. Technique: Insert the stylet and catheter in an interspace, passing just above the edge of the rib. The intercostal vessels lie immediately below each rib. Usually, it is not difficult to know when the pleura is pierced, but suction on the needle at any stage will show whether or not fluid has been reached. Remove the inner stylet, and quickly attach the stopcock and syringe to the hub of the catheter, thereby avoiding creation of a pneumothorax. In cases of long-standing infection, the pleura may be thick and the fluid loculated, necessitating more than one puncture site. If a large amount of fluid is present, it should be removed slowly at intervals, 100–500 mL each time, depending on the size of the patient. Pleural fluid is apt to coagulate unless it is frankly purulent; thus, to facilitate examination, an anticoagulant should be added to the fluid after it is removed.

BONE MARROW PUNCTURE

Bone marrow puncture is indicated for diagnosis of blood dyscrasias, neuroblastoma, and storage diseases. It is also used to obtain specimens for culture. The procedure should be done with great caution when a defect of the clotting mechanism is suspected.

A. Sites: In children, the posterior iliac crest is the preferred site. When the child is restrained in a prone position, the iliac crest can be located and a spot can be marked approximately 1 cm below the crest. Puncture of the sternal marrow is rarely indicated in children. The site between the tibial tubercle and the medial condyle over the anteromedial aspect is recommended by some for bone marrow puncture in infants.

B. Preparation: Prepare the skin surrounding the area as for a surgical procedure. Scrub and wear sterile gloves. Use 1% lidocaine solution to infiltrate the skin and tissues down to the periosteum.

C. Technique: Use a 21-gauge lumbar puncture needle for infants; use an 18- or 19-gauge special marrow needle with a short bevel for older children. Insert the needle with stylet in place, perpendicular to the skin, through the skin and tissues, down to the periosteum. Push the needle through the cortex, using a screwing motion with firm, steady, and well-controlled pressure. Generally some "give" is felt as the needle enters the marrow; the needle will then be firmly in place. Immediately fit a dry syringe (20- to 50-mL) onto the needle and apply strong suction for a few seconds. A small amount of marrow will enter the syringe; this should be smeared on glass coverslips or slides for subsequent staining and counting. Remove the needle after withdrawing marrow, and exert local pressure for 3–5 minutes or until all evidence of bleeding has ceased. Apply a dry dressing.

UMBILICAL VESSEL CATHETERIZATION

Umbilical Artery Catheterization

Umbilical artery catheterization is indicated for those infants who require frequent sampling of blood. Complications of umbilical artery catheterization include thrombosis, embolism, vasospasm, and perforation of the vessel. There is no consensus regarding the ideal placement of the catheter.

A. Catheter Placement: Umbilical artery catheters can be placed in one of two positions: above the diaphragm in the thoracic aorta (T6–T9; high), or just below the aortic bifurcation (L3–L4; low). The graph in Figure 32–6 may be used to estimate the appropriate length of catheter to be inserted. As a general rule, it is best to overestimate, as the catheter can always be pulled back after confirming placement by x-ray.

To use the graph, measure the distance (in cm) from the shoulder down to a line perpendicular to the umbilicus, then add the length of the umbilical stump to the appropriate catheter length determined from the graph.

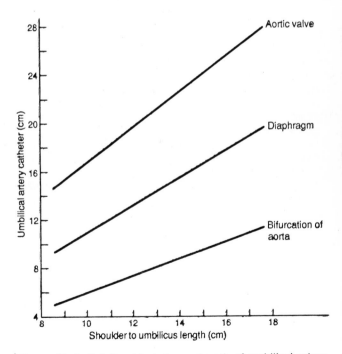

Figure 32–6. Relationship between length of umbilical artery catheter placed and shoulder–umbilicus length in an infant. (Adapted from Dunn P: *Arch Dis Child.* 1966;**41**:73.)

B. Equipment: For term infants use a 5.0 French umbilical artery catheter; use a 3.5 French for infants less than 32–34 weeks' gestation. Attach a 3-way stopcock to the catheter and flush the system with heparinized saline. Other equipment needed include a scalpel with a straight blade, umbilical tape, and 2 fine, curved, nontoothed forceps.

C. Preparation: The umbilicus and surrounding skin should be prepped and draped. As always, the infant should be monitored and placed under a radiant warmer. A snug tie of umbilical tape should be placed around the base of the cord and easily tightened if bleeding should occur.

D. Technique: The cord is cut with one slicing motion about one cm above the base preferably in a moist part of the cord. Identify the 2 (occasionally there is only one) arteries, which should be narrow, white, and thick-walled compared with the dilated, thin-walled vein. Using a fine, curved, toothless forceps, probe the artery gently; first using one tip and then inserting both tips and allowing the forceps to gently open within the vessel. This will allow adequate dilation of the vessel so that the catheter tip will easily pass into the lumen. Gentle retraction of the vessel wall will facilitate passage of the catheter. Insert the catheter to the desired distance. If resistance is met, try loosening the umbilical tape or changing the angle of the umbilical stump while applying gentle steady pressure. DO NOT FORCE THE CATHETER. If these attempts are unsuccessful, try the second artery.

Once the catheter is in place, attach a syringe to the stopcock; blood should be easily aspirated. The catheter can be sewn in place using a purse-string stitch in the Wharton's jelly and/or constructing a tape bridge. An x-ray should be taken to confirm the placement of the catheter tip.

Umbilical Vein Catheterization

An umbilical venous catheter is most commonly used for emergency intravenous access in the delivery room for the administration of fluids, glucose, and medications. Other uses include exchange transfusions and long-term intravenous access in the very-low-birth-weight infant. Complications of umbilical vein catheterization include thrombosis, embolism, vasospasm, and perforation of the vessel. Portal vein thrombosis with subsequent development of presinusoidal portal hypertension has been associated with umbilical vein catheterization.

A. Catheter Placement: The catheter tip should be placed in a low position for use in emergencies, and exchange transfusions and in a high position for long-term use. For low position,

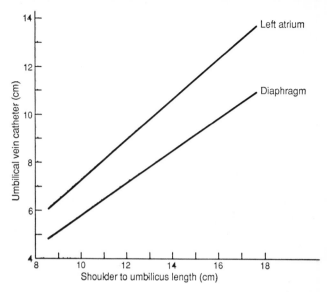

Figure 32–7. Relationship between length of umbilical venous catheter placed and shoulder–umbilicus length in an infant (Adapted from Dunn P: *Arch Dis Child*. 1966;**41**:71.)

insert the catheter only as far as is required to get good blood flow with aspiration. For a high position, the catheter tip should be placed in the inferior vena cava just above the level of the diaphragm and, therefore, above the ductus venosus, portal vein, and the hepatic veins. The graph in Figure 32–7 can be used to estimate the length of catheter needed. Measure the distance (in cm) from the shoulder to a line perpendicular to the umbilicus and add the length of the umbilical stump to the appropriate catheter length determined from the graph.

B. Equipment: Same as for umbilical artery catheterization.

C. Preparation: Same as for umbilical artery catheterization.

D. Technique: Identify the thin-walled, dilated vessel and remove any clots with a forceps. Insert the catheter to the desired length. When in place, blood should be easily aspirated. Unless it is an emergency, check catheter tip placement with an x-ray and secure with a suture and/or a tape bridge.

Appendix

NORMAL BLOOD CHEMISTRY VALUES & OTHER HEMATOLOGIC VALUES*
(Values may vary with the procedure employed.)

The following is a compilation of normal values for some laboratory tests. Where values differ with age, tables have been provided. Some laboratory values that are often ordered together are arranged in tables.

Determinations for:
(S) = Serum
(B) = Whole blood

(P) = Plasma
(RBC) = Red blood cells

Acid-Base Measurements (B)
pH: 7.38–7.42 from 14 minutes of age and older.
Pao$_2$: 65–76 mm Hg (8.66–10.13 kPa).
Paco$_2$: 36–38 mm Hg (4.8–5.07 kPa).
Base excess: −2 to +2 meq/L, except in newborns (range, −4 to −0).

Acid Phosphatase (S, P)
Values using *p*-nitrophenyl phosphate buffered with citrate (end-point determination).
Newborns: 7.4–19.4 IU/L at 37°C
2–13 years: 6.4–15.2 IU/L at 37°C
Adult males: 0.5–11 IU/L at 37°C
Adult females: 0.2–9.5 IU/L at 37°C

Alanine Aminotransferase (ALT, SGPT) (S)
Newborns (1–3 days): 1–25 IU/L at 37°C
Adult males: 7–46 IU/L at 37°C.
Adult females: 4–35 IU/L at 37°C.

Albumin
Birth–3 months: 3.2–4.8 g/dL.
Over 1 year: 3.7–5.7 g/dL.

Aldolase (S)
Newborns: 17.5–47.8 IU/L at 37°C.
Children: 8.8–23.9 IU/L at 37°C.
Adults: 4.4–12 IU/L at 37°C.

Aldosterone (P)
First year: 25–140 ng/dL.
Second year: 9–25 ng/dL.

Alkaline Phosphate (S)
(See Table, below.)

Alkaline phosphatase in serum.

Values at 37°C using *p*-nitrophenyl phosphate buffered with AMP (kinetic).

Group	Males (IU/L)	Females (IU/L)
Newborns (1–3 days)	95–368	95–368
2–24 months	115–460	115–460
2–5 years	115–391	115–391
6–7 years	115–460	115–460
8–9 years	115–345	115–345
10–11 years	115–336	115–437
12–13 years	127–403	92–336
14–15 years	79–446	78–212
16–18 years	58–331	35–124
Adults	41–137	39–118

*Adapted from Meites S (editor): *Pediatric Clinical Chemistry*, 2nd ed. American Association for Clinical Chemistry, 1982, and many other sources.

Ammonia (P)
Newborns: 90–150 μg/dL (53–88 μmol/L; higher in premature and jaundiced infants.
Thereafter: 0–60 μg/dL (0–35 μmol/L).

Amylase (S)
Neonates: Undetectable.
2–12 months: Levels increase slowly to adult levels.
Adults: 28–108 IU/L at 37°C.

α$_1$-Antitrypsin (S)
1–3 months: 127–404 mg/dL.
3–12 months: 145–362 mg/dL.
1–2 years: 160–382 mg/dL.
2–15 years: 148–394 mg/dL.

Ascorbic Acid:
See Vitamin C.

Aspartate Aminotransferase (AST, SGOT) (S)
Newborns (1–3 days): 16–74 IU/L at 37°C.
Adult males: 8–46 IU/L at 37°C.
Adult females: 7–34 IU/L at 37°C.

Base Excess:
See Acid-Base Measurements.

Bicarbonate, Actual (P)
Calculated from pH and Paco$_2$.
Newborns: 17.2–23.6 mmol/L.
2 months–2 years: 19–24 mmol/L.
Children: 18–25 mmol/L.
Adult males: 20.1–28.9 mmol/L.
Adult females: 18.4–28.8 mmol/L.

Bilirubin (S)
Levels after 1 month are as follows:
Conjugated: 0–0.3 mg/dL (0–5 μmol/L).
Unconjugated: 0.1–0.7 mg/dL (2–12 μmol/L).
For peak newborn levels, see Figure (below).

Bleeding Time
See Coagulation Factor Table.

BUN:
See Urea Nitrogen.

C Peptide (S)
5–15 years (8:00 AM fasting): 1–4 ng/mL.

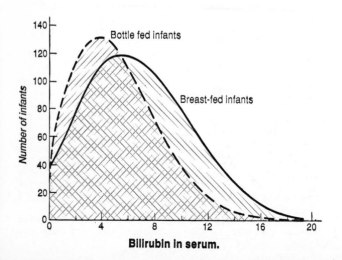

Bilirubin in serum.

Adults (8:00 AM fasting): < 4
  ng/mL.
Adults (nonfasting): < 8 ng/mL.

Calcium (S)
Premature infants (first week):
  3.5–4.5 meq/L. (1.7–2.3
  mmol/L).
Full-term infants (first week): 4–5
  meq/L (2–2.5 mmol/L).
Thereafter: 4.4–5.3 meq/L (2.2–
  2.7 mmol/L).

Calcium (Ionized)
At pH 7.4: 3.9–4.5 mg/dL (0.9–
  1.12 mmol/L).

Carotene (S, P)
0–6 months: 0–40 µg/dL (0–0.75
  µmol/L).
Children: 50–100 µg/dL (0.93–1.9
  µmol/L).
Adults: 100–150 µg/dL (1.9–2.8
  µmol/L).

Cation-Anion Gap (S,P)
5–15 mmol/L.

**Ceruloplasmin (Copper Oxidase)
(S, P)**
21–43 mg/dL (1.3–2.7 µmol/L).

Chloride (S, P)
Premature infants: 95–110 mmol/L.
Full-term infants: 96–116 mmol/L.

Children: 98–105 mmol/L.
Adults: 98–108 mmol/L.

Cholesterol (S, P)
See Lipid Profile Table.

Complement (S)
C3: 96–195 mg/dL.
C4: 15–20 mg/dL.

Copper (S)
Cord blood: 26–32 µg/dL (4.1–5.2
  µmol/L).
Newborns: 26–32 µg/dL (4.1–5.2
  µmol/L).
1 month: 73–93 µg/dL (11.5–14.6
  µmol/L).
2 months: 59–69 µg/dL (9.3–10.9
  µmol/L).
6 months–5 years: 27–153 µg/dL
  (4.2–24.1 µmol/L).
5–17 years: 94–234 µg/dL (14.8–
  36.8 µmol/L).
Adults: 70–118 µg/dL (11–18.6
  µmol/L).

Creatine (S, P)
0.2–0.8 mg/dL (15.2–61 µmol/L).

Creatine Kinase (S, P)
Newborns (1–3 days): 40–474 IU/L
  at 37°C
Adult males: 30–210 IU/L at 37°C.
Adult females: 20–128 IU/L at 37°C.

Creatinine (S, P)
(See Table, next page.)

Coagulation factors and tests.*

Factor	Level
II (Prothrombin)	81–123 U/dL
V (Proaccelerin)	61–127 U/dL
VII (Proconvertin)	6–14 U/dL
VIII (Antihemophilic globulin)	82–157 U/dL
IX (Christmas factor)	78–122 U/dL
Fibrinogen	200–500 mg/dL
Bleeding time	1–3 min
Partial Thromboplastin Time (PTT)	42–54 sec
Prothrombin Time (PT)	11–15 sec
Thrombin Time (TT)	12–16 sec

*All values are for children.

Creatinine in serum and plasma.

Group	Males mg/dL (μmol/L)	Females mg/dL (μmol/L)
Newborns (1–3 days)*	0.2–1.0 (17.7–88.4)	0.2–1.0 (17.7–88.4)
1 year	0.2–0.6 (17.7–53.0)	0.2–0.5 (17.7–44.2)
2–3 years	0.2–0.7 (17.7–61.9)	0.3–0.6 (26.5–53.0)
4–7 years	0.2–0.8 (17.7–70.7)	0.2–0.7 (17.7–61.9)
8–10 years	0.3–0.9 (26.5–79.6)	0.3–0.8 (26.5–70.7)
11–12 years	0.3–1.0 (26.5–88.4)	0.3–0.9 (26.5–79.6)
13–17 years	0.3–1.2 (26.5–106.1)	0.3–1.1 (26.5–97.2)
18–20 years	0.5–1.3 (44.2–115.0)	0.3–1.1 (26.5–97.2)

*Values may be higher in premature newborns.

Creatinine Clearance

Values show great variability and depend on specificity of analytical methods used.

Newborns (1 day): 5–50 mL/min/ 1.73 m^2 (mean, 18 mL/min/ 1.73 m^2).

Newborns (6 days): 15–90 mL/min/ 1.73 m^2 (mean, 36 mL/min/ 1.73 m^2).

Adult males: 85–125 mL/min/ 1.73 m^2.

Ferritin (S)

Newborns: 20–200 ng/mL (mean, 117 ng/mL).

1 month: 60–550 ng/mL (mean, 350 ng/mL).

1–15 years: 7–140 ng/mL (mean, 31 ng/mL).

Adult males: 50–225 ng/mL (mean, 140 ng/mL).

Adult females: 10–150 ng/mL (mean, 40 ng/mL).

Fibrinogen (P)

See Coagulation Factor Table.

Folate (S)

Prepubertal children: Mean folic acid values are reported to be slightly higher than mean adult values but remain within the normal range.

Adults: 3–21 ng/mL.

Galactose (S, P)

1.1–2.1 mg/dL (0.06–0.12 mmol/L).

Glucose (S, P)

Premature infants: 40–80 mg/dL (2.22–4.44 mmol/L).

Full-term infants: 40–100 mg/dL (2.22–5.56 mmol/L).

Children and adults (fasting): 60–105 mg/dL (3.33–5.88 mmol/ L).

γ-Glutamyl Transpeptidase (S)

0–1 month: 12–271 IU/L 37°C (kinetic).

1–2 months: 9–159 IU/L at 37°C (kinetic).

2–4 months: 7–98 IU/L at 37°C (kinetic).

4–7 months: 5–45 IU/L at 37°C (kinetic).

7–12 months: 4–27 IU/L at 37°C (kinetic).

1–15 years: 3–30 IU/L at 37°C (kinetic).

Adult males: .9–69 IU/L at 37°C (kinetic).

Adult females: 3–33 IU/L at 37°C (kinetic).

Glycohemoglobin (Hemoglobin A$_{1c}$) (B)

Normal: 6.3–8.2% of total hemoglobin. Diabetic patients in good control of their condition ordinarily have levels < 10%.

Hematologic values.

	Hct (%)	MCV (fL)	HgB (g/dL)
Birth	44–64	85–125	14–24
2 weeks–3 months	35–49	94–102	11–17
6 months–1 year	30–40	78	11–15
4 years–10 years	31–43	80–82	12.5–15

Values tend to be lower during pregnancy.

Immunoglobins (S)
(See Table, below.)

Iron (S, P)
Newborns: 20–157 µg/dL (3.6–28.1 µmol/L).

6 weeks–3 years: 20–115 µg/dL (3.6–20.6 µmol/L).

3–9 years: 20–141 µg/dL (3.6–25.2 µmol/L).

9–14 years: 21–151 µg/dL (3.8–27 µmol/L).

14–16 years: 20–181 µg/dL (3.6–32.4 µmol/L).

Adults: 40–175 µg/dL (7.2–31.3 µmol/L).

Iron-Binding Capacity (S, P)
Newborns: 59–175 µg/dL (10.6–31.3 µmol/L).

Children and adults: 250–400 µg/dL (45–75 µmol/L).

Lactate (B)
Venous blood: 5–18 mg/dL (0.5–2 mmol/L).

Arterial blood: 3–7 mg/dL (0.3–0.8 mmol/L).

Lactate Dehydrogenase (LDH) (S, P)
Values using lactate substrate (kinetic).

Newborns (1–3 days): 30–348 IU/L at 37°C.

1 month–5 years: 150–360 IU/L at 37°C.

5–8 years: 150–300 IU/L at 37°C.

8–12 years: 130–300 IU/L at 37°C.

12–14 years: 130–280 IU/L at 37°C.

14–16 years: 130–230 IU/L at 37°C.

Adult males: 70–178 IU/L at 37°C.

Adult females: 42–166 IU/L at 37°C.

Immunoglobulins in serum.

Group	IgG (mg/dL)	IgA (mg/dL)	IgM (mg/dL)
Cord blood	766–1693	0.04–9	4–26
2 weeks–3 months	299–852	3–66	15–149
3–6 months	142–988	4–90	18–118
6–12 months	418–1142	14–95	43–223
1–2 years	356–1204	13–118	37–239
2–3 years	492–1269	23–137	49–204
3–6 years	564–1381	35–209	51–214
6–9 years	658–1535	29–384	50–228
9–12 years	625–1598	60–294	64–278
12–16 years	660–1548	81–252	45–256

Lipid profile.

	Triglycerides (mg/dL)*	Cholesterol (mg/dL)	HDL (mg/dL)	LDL (mg/dL)	VLDL (mg/dL)
Term	*	45–167	‡	‡	‡
< 1 year	*	69–174	‡	‡	‡
2–20 years	10–130	120–205	37–73	66–145	6–15
20–29 years		120–240	37–73	66–145	6–15

*= 12–14 hr fast
‡Values not determined in age range.

Lead (B)
< 30 μg/dL (< 1.4 μmol/L).

LH:
See Luteinizing Hormone.

Lipase (S, P)
20–136 IU/L based on 4-hour incubation.

Magnesium (S, P)
Newborns: 1.5–2.3 meq/L (0.75–1.15 mmol/L).
Adults: 1.4–2 meq/L (0.7–1 mmol/L).

Manganese (S)
Newborns: 2.4–9.6 μg/dL (0.44–1.75 μmol/L).
2–18 years: 0.8–2.1 μg/dL (0.15–0.38 μmol/L).

Methemoglobin (B)
0–0.3 g/dL (0–186) μmol/L).

Osmolality (S, P)
270–290 mosm/kg.

Oxygen Capacity (B)
1.34 mL/g of hemoglobin.

Partial Thromboplastin Time (P)
See Coagulation Factor Table.

Phenylalanine (S, P)
0.7–3.5 mg/dL (0.04–0.21 mmol/L).

Phosphorus, Inorganic (S, P)
Premature infants:
At birth: 5.6–8 mg/dL (1.18–2.58 mmol/L).
6–10 days: 6.1–11.7 mg/dL (1.97–3.78 mmol/L).
20–25 days: 6.6–9.4 mg/dL (2.13–3.04 mmol/L).
Full-term infants:
At birth: 5–7.8 mg/dL (1.61–2.52 mmol/L).
3 days: 5.8–9 mg/dL (1.87–2.91 mmol/L).
6–12 days: 4.9–8.9 mg/dL (1.58–2.87 mmol/L).
Children:
1 year: 3.8–6.2 mg/dL (1.23–2 mmol//L).
10 years: 3.6–5.6 mg/dL (1.16–1.81 mmol/L).
Adults: 3.1–5.1 mg/dL (1–1.65 mmol/L.)
(See also Glucose Tolerance Test.)

Potassium (S, P)
Premature infants: 4.5–7.2 mmol/L.
Full-term infants: 3.7–5.2 mmol/L.
Children: 3.5–5.8 mmol/L.
Adults: 3.5–5.5 mmol/L.

Proteins (S)
(See Table, next page.)

Prothrombin (Factor II) (P)
See Coagulation Factor Table.

Prothrombin Time (P)
See Coagulation Factor Table.

Proteins in serum.

Values are for cellulose acetate electrophoresis and are in g/dL. SI conversion factor: g/dL × 10 = g/L.

Group	Total Protein	Albumin	α_1-Globulin	α_2-Globulin	β-Globulin	γ-Globulin
At birth	4.6–7.0	3.2–4.8	0.1–0.3	0.2–0.3	0.3–0.6	0.6–1.2
3 months	4.5–6.5	3.2–4.8	0.1–0.3	0.3–0.7	0.3–0.7	0.2–0.7
1 year	5.4–7.5	3.7–5.7	0.1–0.3	0.5–1.1	0.4–1.0	0.2–0.9
> 4 years	5.9–8.0	3.8–5.4	0.1–0.3	0.4–0.8	0.5–1.0	0.4–1.3

Protoporphyrin, "Free" (FET, ZPP) (B)
Values for free erythrocyte protoporphyrin (FEP) and zinc protoporphyrin (ZPP) are 1.2–2.7 μg/g of hemoglobin.

Pseudocholinesterase (S)
2.5–5 μmol/mL/min.

Pyruvate (B)
Resting adult males (arterial blood): 50.5–60.1 μmol/L.
Adults (venous blood): 34–102 μmol/L.

Pyruvate Kinase (RBC)
7.4–15.7 units/g of hemoglobin.

Sedimentation Rate (Micro) (B)
< 2 years: 1–5 mm/h.
> 2 years: 1–8 mm/h.

SGOT:
See Aspartate Aminotransferase.

SGPT:
See Alanine Aminotransferase.

Sodium (S, P)
Children and adults: 135–148 mmol/L.

Thrombin Time (P)
See Coagulation Factor Table.

Thyroid-Stimulating Hormone (TSH) (S)
See Thyroid Function Table.

Thyroxine (T_4) (S)
See Thyroid Function Table.

Thyroxine, "Free" (Free T_4) (S)
See Thyroid Function Table.

α-Tocopherol:
See Vitamin E.

Transaminase:
See Alanine Aminotransferase and Aspartate Aminotransferase.

Thyroid Function Tests

T4 (mg/dL)		T3 (ng/dL)	TSH (μL/mL)
1–2 days:	11.4–25.5	89–405	30–40
3–4 days:	9.8–25.2	91–300	1.6–10.9
1–6 years:	5–15.2	119–218	
11–13 years:	4–13	55–170	
> 18 years:	4.7–11	55–170	
Free T4 (ng/dL)	1.0–2.3		

Triglycerides (S, P)
See Lipid Profile Table.

Triiodothyronine (T₃) (S)
See Throid Function Table.

Trypsinogen, Immunoreactive (S, P)
Newborns: 5–97 ng/mL.
99.5th percentile: 136 ng/mL.
99.8th percentile: 162 ng/mL.

Tyrosine (S,P)
Premature infants: 3–30.2 mg/dL
(0.17–1.67 mmol/L).
Full-term infants: 1.7–4.7 mg/dL
(0.09–0.26 mmol/L).
1–12 years: 1.4–3.4 mg/dL (0.08–
0.19 mmol/L).
Adults: 0.6–1.6 mg/dL (0.03–
0.09 mmol/L).

Urea Nitrogen (S, P)
1–2 years: 5–15 mg/dL (1.8–
5.4 mmol/L).
Thereafter: 10–20 mg/dL (3.5–
7.1 mmol/L).

Uric Acid (S, P)
Males: 0–14 years: 2–7 mg/dL (119–
416 μmol/L).
> 14 years: 3–8 mg/dL (178–
476 μmol/L).
Females: 0–14 years: 2–7 mg/dL
(119–416 μmol/L).
> 14 years: 2–7 mg/dL (119–
416 μmol/L).

Vitamin A (S, P)
Values of < 20 μg/dL (0.7 μmol/L)
should be considered abnormally low.

Vitamin B₁₂ (S, P)
330–1025 pg/mL (243–756 pmol/L).

Vitamin C (Ascorbic Acid) (S, P)
0.2–2 mg/dL (11–114 μmol/L).

Vitamin D (S)
1.25-Dihydroxycholecalciferol:25–
49 pg/mL.
25-Hydroxycholecalciferol: 26–31
ng/mL.

Vitamin E (α-Tocopherol) (S, P)
Premature infants: 0.05–0.35 mg/
dL (1.2–8.4 μmol/L).
Full-term infants: 0.10–0.35 mg/dL
(2.4–8.4 μmol/L).
2–5 months: 0.2–0.6 mg/dL (4.8–
14.4 μmol/L).
6–24 months: 0.35–0.8 mg/dL (8.4–
19.2 μmol/L).
2–12 years: 0.55–0.9 mg/dL (13.2–
21.6 μmol/L).
Breast-fed infants: 0.6–1.1 mg/dL
(14.4–26.4 μmol/L).

Zinc (S)
Males: 83–88 μg/dL (12.7–13.5
μmol/L).
Females: 85–91 μg/dL (13–13.9
μmol/L).
Females taking oral contraceptives: 86–93 μg/dL (13.2–14.2
μmol/L).
At 16 weeks of gestation: 66–
70 μg/dL (10.1–10.7 μmol/L).
At 38 weeks of gestation: 54–
58 μg/dL (8.3–8.9 μmol/L).

NORMAL VALUES: URINE, SWEAT, & CSF*

URINE

Calcium
4–12 years: 4–8 meq/L (2–4 mmol/L).

Catecholamines (Norepinephrine, Epinephrine)
(See Table, next page.)

Chloride
Infants: 1.7–8.5 mmol/24 h.
Children: 17–34 mmol/24 h.
Adults: 140–240 mmol/24 h.

Coproporphyrin:
See Porphyrins.

Epinephrine:
See Catecholamines.

Metanephrine & Normetanephrine
< 2 years: < 4.6 μg/mg of creatinine (23.3 nmol).
2–10 years: < 3μg/mg of creatinine (15.2 nmol).
10–15 years: <2μg/mg of creatinine (10.3 nmol).
> 15 years: < 1μg/mg of creatinine (5.1 nmol).

Norepinephrine:
See Catecholamines.

Normetanephrine:
See Metanephrine & Normetanephrine.

Osmolality
Infants: 50–600 mosm/kg.
Older children: 50–1400 mosm/kg.

Porphobilinogen:
See Porphyrins.

Porphyrins
δ-Aminolevulinic acid: 0–7 mg/24 h (0–53.4 μmol/24 h).
Porphobilinogen: 0–2 mg/24 h (0–8.8 μmol/24 h).
Coproporphyrin: 0–160 μg/24 h (0–244 nmol/24 h).
Uroporphyrin: 0–26 μg/24 h (0–31 nmol/24 h).

Potassium
26–123 mmol/L.

Catecholamines in urine.

Group	Total Catecholamines μg/24 h	Norepinephrine μg/24 h (nmol/24 h)		Epinephrine μg/24 h (nmol/24 h)	
< 1 year	20	5.4–15.9	(32–94)	0.1–4.3	(0.5–23.5)
1–5 years	40	8.1–30.8	(48–182)	0.8–9.1	(4.4–49.7)
6–15 years	80	19.0–71.1	(112–421)	1.3–10.5	(7.1–57.3)
> 15 years	100	34.4–87.0	(203–514)	3.5–13.2	(19.1–72.1)

*Adapted from Meites S (editor): *Pediatric Clinical Chemistry*, 2nd ed. American Association for Clinical Chemistry, 1982, and many other sources.

Sodium
Infants: 0.3–3.5 nmol/24 h (6–10 mmol/m²).
Children and adults: 5.6–17 mmol/24 h.

Uroporphyrin:
See Porphyrins.

Vanilmandelic Acid (VMA)
Because of the difficulty in obtaining an accurately timed 24-hour collection, values based on microgram per milligram of creatinine are the most reliable indications of VMA excretion in young children.
1–12 months: 1–35 μg/mg of creatinine (31–135 μg/kg/24 h).
1–2 years: 1–30 μg/mg of creatinine.
2–5 years: 1–15 μg/mg of creatinine.
5–10 years: 1–14 μg/mg of creatinine.
10–15 years: 1–10 μg/mg of creatinine.
Adults: 1–7 μg/mg of creatinine (1–7 mg/24 h; 5–35 μmol/24 h).

SWEAT

Electrolytes
Values for sodium or chloride or both. Elevated values in the presence of a family history or clinical findings of cystic fibrosis are diagnostic of cystic fibrosis.
Normal: < 55 mmol/L.
Borderline: 55–70 mmol/L.
Elevated: > 70 mmol/L.

CSF VALUES

Appearance
clear, colorless

Cells
White blood cells
Birth: 0–30
> 3 months: 0–5
Red blood cells
Birth: 2–50
> 3 months: 0

Glucose (mg/dL):
50–80 (two-thirds of blood glucose)

Protein (mg/dL)
Birth: 40–150
1–6 months: 20–65
> 6 months: 15–35

BEDSIDE LABORATORY TESTS

1. **Apt test**–used to distinguish maternal from fetal blood. Mix specimen (vomitus, stool) with an equal amount of tap water; centrifuge. Proceed only if supernatant is pink. To 5 parts supernatant add 1 part 0.25 N (1%) NaOH. If the pink color persists > 2 minutes it means fetal Hgb is present. If the pink turns yellow it means adult Hgb is present (denatured by NaOH).

2. **Clinitest**–used to detect reducing substances in stool; reflects carbohydrate malabsorption.
Mix 1 part stool with 2 parts water (use 1N HCI if testing for sucrose). Add 15 drops of this mixture to one Clinitest tablet. Compare color of suspension with chart for percentage of reducing substances. Abnormal if ≥ ½%.

3. **Cold agglutinins**–present in *Mycoplasma* disease. Collect 4–5 drops of blood in small purple-top tube (0.2 mL EDTA). Place

tube in ice water for 30–60 seconds. Rotate tube and look for clumping. Agglutination that occurs when cold and resolves with warming is interpreted as a cold agglutinin titer > 1:64.

4. **Fecal leukocytes**–present in inflammatory enterocolitis. Place stool mucus on microscope slide. Add 2 drops 0.5% methylene blue. Wait 2–3 minutes. Examine under microscope.

5. Ferric chloride urine test of aminoaciduria*–

SPECIMEN: Random urine; an early morning specimen is preferred to reduce variations due to diet. If not analyzed immediately, the urine should be acidified to a pH less than 4; if necessary, freeze at −20°C for no longer than one week.
REFERENCE RANGE: Negative; that is, no color change.
METHOD: Add 10% $FeCl_3$ by drops to 1–2mL of urine.
INTERPRETATION: The ferric chloride test is *nonspecific* and gives color reactions with *metabolities from amino acid disorders,* other metabolites and *drugs* as shown in the table:

Ferric Chloride Test in Urine	
Disorder and Urinary Product	*Color Change*
Phenylketonuria (PKU)	
Phenylpyruvic acid	Blue or blue-green, fades to yellow
Tyrosinosis (emia)	
p-Hydroxyphenylpyruvic acid	Green, fades in seconds
Alkaptonuria	
Homogentisic acid	Blue or green, fades quickly
Maple Syrup Urine Disease	
Alpha-Ketoisovaleric acid	Blue
Alpha-Ketoiscaproic acid	Blue
Alpha-keto-beta-methyl valeric acid	Blue
Histidinemia	
Imidazole pyruvic acid	Green or blue-green
Diabetics, Alcoholics, Starvation	
Acetoacetic acid	Red or red brown
Other Products:	
Bilirubin	Blue-green
Ortho-hydroxphenyl acetic acid	Mauve
Ortho-hydroxphenyl pyruvic acid	Red
Alpha-ketobutyric acid	Purple; fades to red-brown
Pyruvic acid	Deep gold-yellow or green
Xanthurenic acid	Deep green, later brown
Drugs:	
Salicylates	Stable purple
Aminosalicylic acid	Red-brown
Phenothiazine derivatives	Purple-pink
Antipyrines and acetophenetidines	Red
Phenol derivatives	Violet
Cyanates	Red

*From Bakeman S: *ABC's of Interpretive Laboratory Data,* 2nd ed. Interpretive Lab Data, Inc., 1984.

Table 1. Normal peripheral blood values at various age levels.

Value	1st d	2nd d	6th d	2 wk	1 mo	2 mo
Red blood cells* (million/µL)	5.9 (4.1–7.5)	6 (4.0–7.3)	5.4 (3.9–6.8)	5 (4.5–5.5)	4.7 (4.2–5.2)	4.1 (3.6–4.6)
Hemoglobin (g/dL)	19 (14–24)	19 (15–23)	18 (13–23)	16.5 (15–20)	14 (11–17)	12 (11–14)
White blood cells* (per µL)	17,000 (8–38)		13,500 (6–17)	12,000	11,500	11,000
PMNs (%)	57	55	50	34	34	33
Eosinophils* (total) (per µL)	20–1,000				150–1,150	
Lymphocytes (%)	20	20	37	55	56	56
Monocytes (%)	10	15	9	8	7	7
Immature white blood cells (%)	10	5	0–1	0	0	0
Platelets (per µL)	350,000		325,000	300,000		
Nucleated red blood cells/100 white blood cells*	0–10		0.0–0.3	0	0	0
Reticulocytes (%)	3 (2–8)	3 (2–10)	1 (0.5–5.0)	0.4 (0.0–2.0)	0.2 (0.0–0.5)	0.5 (0.2–2.0)
Mean diameter of red blood cells (µm)	8.6				8.1	
MCV† (fl)	85–125		89–101	94–102	90	
MCHC† (%)	36		35	34		
MCH† (pg)	35–40		36	31	30	
Hematocrit (%)	54 ± 10		51	50	35–50	

*Total nucleated red blood cells: first day, < 1000/µL.
†MCV = mean corpuscular volume. MCHC = mean corpuscular hemoglobin concentration. MCH = mean corpuscular hemoglobin.

Table 1 (cont'd). Normal peripheral blood values at various age levels.

Value	3 mo	6 mo	1 yr	2 yr	5 yr	8-12 yr	Adults Males	Adults Females
Red blood cells* (million/μL)	4 (3.5-4.5)	4.5 (4-5)	4.6 (4.1-5.1)	4.7 (4.2-5.2)	4.7 (4.2-5.2)	5 (4.5-5.4)	5.4 (4.6-6.2)	4.8 (4.2-5.4)
Hemoglobin (g/dL)	11 (10-13)	11.5 (10.5-14.5)	12 (11-15)	13 (12-15)	13.5 (12.5-15.0)	14 (13.0-15.5)	16 (13-18)	14 (11-16)
White blood cells* (per μL)	10,500	10,500	10,000	9,500	8,000	8,000	7,000 (5-10)	
PMNs (%)	33	36	39	42	55	60	57-68	
Eosinophils* (total) (per μL)	70-550	70-550					100-400	
Lymphocytes (%)	57	55	53	49	36	31	25-33	
Monocytes (%)	7	6	6	7	7	7	3-7	
Immature white blood cells (%)	0	0	0	0	0	0	0	
Platelets (per μL)	260,000			260,000		260,000	260,000	
Nucleated red blood cells/100 white blood cells*	0	0	0	0	0	0	0	
Reticulocytes (%)	2 (0.5-4.0)	0.8 (0.2-1.5)	1 (0.4-1.8)	1 (0.4-1.8)	1 (0.4-1.8)	1 (0.4-1.8)	1 (0.5-2.0)	
Mean diameter of red blood cells (μm)	7.7		7.4		7.4	7.5	7.5	
MCV† (fl)	80	78	78	80	80	82	82-92	
MCHC† (%)		33		32	34	34	34	
MCH† (pg)	27	26	25	26	27	28	27-31	
Hematocrit (%)	35	30-40	36	37	31-43	40	40-54	37-47

*Total nucleated red blood cells: first day, <1000/μL.
†MCV = mean corpuscular volume. MCHC = mean corpuscular hemoglobin concentration. MCH = mean corpuscular hemoglobin.

APPENDIX

TABLE A-1. BODY SURFACE AREA: ADULTS

Height	Body surface	Mass
cm 200 — 79 in	2.80 m²	kg 150 — 330 lb
195 — 78, 77	2.70	145 — 320
— 76	2.60	140 — 310
190 — 75, 74	2.50	135 — 300
185 — 73, 72	2.40	130 — 290, 280
180 — 71, 70	2.30	125 — 270
175 — 69, 68	2.20	120 — 260
170 — 67, 66	2.10	115 — 250
165 — 65, 64	2.00	110 — 240
160 — 63, 62	1.95, 1.90	105 — 230
155 — 61, 60	1.85, 1.80	100 — 220
150 — 59, 58	1.75, 1.70	95 — 210
145 — 57, 56	1.65, 1.60	90 — 200
140 — 55, 54	1.55, 1.50	85 — 190
135 — 53, 52	1.45, 1.40	80 — 180
130 — 51, 50	1.35, 1.30	75 — 170
125 — 49, 48	1.25, 1.20	70 — 160
120 — 47, 46	1.15, 1.10	65 — 150
115 — 45, 44	1.05	60 — 140, 130
110 — 43, 42	1.00	55 — 120
105 — 41, 40	0.95	50 — 110, 105
cm 100 — 39 in	0.90, 0.86 m²	45 — 100, 95
		40 — 90, 85
		35 — 80, 75
		kg 30 — 70, 66 lb

To determine the body surface area in an adult, use a straight edge to connect the height and mass.
The point of intersection on the body surface line gives the area in m².
From Lentner C (ed): Geigy Scientific Tables, ed 8. Basle, CIBA-GEIGY, 1981, vol 1, p 226

Index